Interpersonal Relationships

PROFESSIONAL
COMMUNICATION SKILLS
FOR NURSES

GHAM

SIXTH EDITION

Elizabeth C. Arnold, PhD, RN, PMHCNS-BC
Associate Professor, Retired
University of Maryland
Baltimore, Maryland

Family Nurse Psychotherapist
Montgomery Village, Maryland

Kathleen Underman Boggs, PhD, FNP-CS
Family Nurse Practitioner

Associate Professor Emeritus
College of Health and Human Services
University of North Carolina Charlotte
Charlotte, North Carolina

ELSEVIER
SAUNDERS

ELSEVIER
SAUNDERS

3251 Riverport Lane
St. Louis, Missouri 63043

INTERPERSONAL RELATIONSHIPS: PROFESSIONAL
COMMUNICATION SKILLS FOR NURSES, SIXTH EDITION

ISBN: 978-1-4377-0944-5

Notices

Knowledge and best practice in this field are constantly changing. As new research and experience broaden
our understanding, changes in research methods, professional practices, or medical treatment may become
necessary.

Practitioners and researchers must always rely on their own experience and knowledge in evaluating and
using any information, methods, compounds, or experiments described herein. In using such information or
methods they should be mindful of their own safety and the safety of others, including parties for whom they
have a professional responsibility.

With respect to any drug or pharmaceutical products identified, readers are advised to check the most
current information provided (i) on procedures featured or (ii) by the manufacturer of each product to be
administered, to verify the recommended dose or formula, the method and duration of administration, and
contraindications. It is the responsibility of practitioners, relying on their own experience and knowledge of
their patients, to make diagnoses, to determine dosages and the best treatment for each individual patient,
and to take all appropriate safety precautions.

To the fullest extent of the law, neither the Publisher nor the authors, contributors, or editors, assume any
liability for any injury and/or damage to persons or property as a matter of products liability, negligence or
otherwise, or from any use or operation of any methods, products, instructions, or ideas contained in the
material herein.

International Standard Book Number: 978-1-4377-0944-5   2599476X

Managing Editors: Jean Fornango and Michele D. Hayden
Developmental Editors: Maria Broeker and Heather D. Bays
Publishing Services Manager: Deborah Vogel
Design Direction: Kim Denando

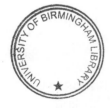

Printed in the United States of America

Last digit is the print number: 9 8 7 6 5 4 3 2

To Jacob D. Goering, PhD
His influence on my life as an educator and clinician
was life changing and long lasting.

Elizabeth C. Arnold

In Memoriam,
Richard Daniel Underman, beloved brother.

Kathleen Underman Boggs

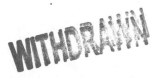

ACKNOWLEDGMENTS

This sixth edition of *Interpersonal Relationships: Professional Communication Skills for Nurses* continues to reflect the ideas and commitment of our students, valued colleagues, clients, and the editorial staff at Elsevier. As noted in earlier editions, the origin of the text began in conjunction with the development of an interpersonal relationship seminar at the University of Maryland School of Nursing. This seminar was designed by faculty to facilitate understanding of therapeutic communication across clinical settings through experiential simulations. Developing effective communication was important then, and it remains central to effective clinical practice in contemporary health care. The vitality of its contents reflects the commitment of faculty and students from many nursing programs and clinical nurses who have deepened the understanding of the materials presented in this text through their positive support, ideas, and constructive feedback. Their voices still find consistent expression in each chapter of this revision.

We acknowledge important past and present faculty and student contributors to the development of *Interpersonal Relationships: Professional Communication Skills for Nurses,* in particular, Verna Benner Carson, PhD, RN, PCNS (Chapter 8); Judith W. Ryan, PhD, RN, CRNP (Chapter 19); Michelle Michael, PhD, APRN, PNP; Barbara Harrison, RN, PMH-NP; Ann O'Mara, PhD, RN, AOCN, FAAN; Barbara Dobish, MS, RN; Anne Marie Spellbring, PhD, RN, FAAN; Kristin Bussell, MS, RN, CS-P; Patricia Harris, MS, APRN, NP; and Jacqueline Conrad, BS, RN, from the University of Maryland, and Ann Mabe Newman, DSN, RN, CS (Chapter 4); and David R. Langford, RN, DSNc, from the University of North Carolina Charlotte.

This book is the result of the unique team effort of several talented developmental editors who worked hard to make the process of revision as seamless as possible. We are most grateful for their expertise and commitment to the completion of this book. Each went out of her way to make the revision a positive, quality experience. Tiffany Trautwein worked with us during the first part of the preparation for this edition. Maria Broeker stepped in during the next phase of the text, and Heather D. Bays worked with us to finish the book in the final phase of the project. Maria Broeker deserves special acknowledgment for her dedication to the preparation of this book. Her support and encouragement have been invaluable. We also express our appreciation to Jeff Somers from Graphic World Publishing Services, who coordinated the final production of this book for publication, and to Jeanne Robertson for the revised artwork in this edition.

Finally, we acknowledge the loving support of our families and Michael J. Boggs for their unflagging support and encouragement.

Elizabeth C. Arnold
Kathleen Underman Boggs

Recognition of the importance of therapeutic communication and professional relationships with clients and families as a primary means of achieving treatment goals in health care continues to be the underlying theme in *Interpersonal Relationships: Professional Communication Skills for Nurses*. This sixth edition has been thoroughly revised, rewritten, and updated to meet the challenge of continuing to serve as a primary communication resource for nursing students and professional nurses. Although the content, exercises, and case examples continue to be written in terms of nurse-client relationships, they are applicable to clinical practice relationships conducted by other health care providers. This edition, like previous editions can be used as individual teaching modules, as a primary text, or as a communication resource integrated across the curriculum. Two new chapters related to communication strategies for client safety, and contemporary realities in continuity of care reflect the latest applications of communication in contemporary health care delivery.

The text is divided into five parts, using a similar format to that of previous editions. Part I, Conceptual Foundations of Nurse-Client Relationships, provides a theory-based approach to therapeutic relationships and communication in nursing practice, and identifies professional, legal, and ethical standards guiding professional actions. Chapters on the relevance of critical thinking and understanding of self-concept aid the students' comprehension of the many variables involved in communication. Part II, The Nurse-Client Relationship, discusses the fundamental structure and characteristics of effective nurse-client relationships and alliances, taking into account the context of short-term realities found in contemporary health care systems. Chapter 7, Role Relationship Patterns, establishes a framework for considering the issues surrounding new models of nursing education and explores role relationships as a nursing diagnosis. This section ends with a comprehensive discussion about palliative care and communication strategies in end-of-life care. Part III, Therapeutic Communication, explores basic concepts of therapeutic communication and applications of strategies nurses can use with different population groups: culturally diverse, family, and group communication. Applying therapeutic communication strategies in conflict situations and special attention to health promotion community strategies and health teaching complete this section. Part IV, Responding to Special Needs, focuses on the special communication needs of children, older adults, clients with communication deficits, and those experiencing stress or crisis. Part V, Professional Communication, describes communication issues with other health professionals and nursing applications in the use of electronic health records with accompanying taxonomies. Two new chapters address issues in contemporary health care related to the role of communication in promoting safety in the health care environment and principles related to supporting continuity of care within and across care settings. Major changes in managing health care data and transmitting vital health information including the place of the Internet for continual transmission of information in real time are addressed. The role of electronic communication as an increasingly important form of communication is highlighted at point of care and across clinical settings.

Each chapter is designed to illuminate the connection between theory and practice by presenting basic concepts, followed by clinical applications, using updated references and instructive case examples. *Developing an Evidence-Based Practice* boxes offer a summary of a research article related to each chapter subject and are intended to stimulate awareness of the need to link research with practice. The *Ethical Dilemmas* presented at the end of each chapter offer the student an opportunity to reflect on common ethical situations, which occur on a regular basis in health care relationships. The art program for the sixth edition has been enhanced with photos and drawings, which provide contemporary visual representations of chapter concepts.

Experiential exercises provide students with the opportunity to practice, observe, and critically evaluate their professional communication skills in a safe learning environment. The learning exercises are planned to encourage self-reflection about how one's personal practice fits with the larger picture of contemporary nursing, health practice models, and interdisciplinary communication. Through active experiential involvement with relationship-based communication principles, students can develop confidence and skill with using patient-centered communication in real-life clinical settings. The comments and reflections of other students provide a unique, enriching perspective on the wider implications of communication in clinical practice.

The text gives voice to the centrality of communication as the basis for helping clients, families, and communities make sense of relevant health issues and develop effective ways of coping with them. Our hope is that the sixth edition will continue to serve as a primary reference source for nurses seeking to improve their communication and relationship skills across traditional and nontraditional community-based health care settings. As the most consistent health care provider in many clients' lives, the nurse bears an awesome responsibility to provide communication that is professional, honest, empathetic, and knowledgeable in a person-to-person relationship that is without equal in health care. As nurses, we are answerable to our clients, our profession, and ourselves to communicate with clients in a therapeutic manner and to advocate for their health care and well-being in the larger sociopolitical community. We invite you as students, practicing nurses, and faculty to interact with the material in this text, learning from the content and experiential exercises but also seeking your own truth and understanding as professional health care providers.

Instructor Resources are available on the textbook's Evolve Web site. Additional experiential exercises can be found in the *Instructor's Manual,* together with strategies for teaching and learning, and brief chapter summaries with teaching tips. A revised Test Bank reflecting the updated content in the text is also included. Instructors are encouraged to contact their Elsevier sales representative to gain access to these valuable teaching tools.

Elizabeth C. Arnold
Kathleen Underman Boggs

CHAPTER 1

Theoretical Perspectives and Contemporary Dynamics

Elizabeth C. Arnold

OBJECTIVES

At the end of the chapter, the reader will be able to:

1. Describe the role of nursing theory in clinical practice, education, and research.
2. Discuss the historical development of nursing theory.
3. Describe the different types and levels of nursing theory.
4. Identify relevant nursing theory frameworks used in the nurse-client relationship.
5. Identify applications of psychodynamic, developmental, and behavior concepts in nurse-client relationships.
6. Describe the use of communication theory in nursing practice.
7. Discuss contemporary social perspectives and dynamics that influence nurse-client relationships in clinical practice.

Every nurse, regardless of specialty, uses the nurse-client relationship as a fundamental means for providing safe, effective, patient-centered nursing care. The nurse-client relationship is based on an integration of scientific evidence-based practice (EBP) guidelines and values-based application of nursing principles in health care.

This chapter introduces selected theory frameworks and contemporary perspectives related to communication and the nurse-client relationship. Included in this chapter are concepts related to nursing, developmental, psychological, and communication theories. A brief introduction to changes in the health care system and contemporary issues influencing nursing practice and the nurse-client relationship is included.

BASIC CONCEPTS

THE DISCIPLINE OF NURSING

Monti and Tingen (2006) define **discipline** as "a community of interest that is organized around the accumulated knowledge of an academic or professional group" (p. 28). Nurses globally represent the largest group of health care providers and are in a unique position to have a major impact on present and future nursing practice. They can be expected to take a key role in mapping a quality health care system in which nurses will increasingly support individuals and communities in self-managing their own health. As part of a collaborative team of health care professionals, nurses are able to seamlessly and appropriately link clients with health

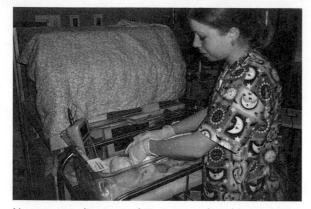

Nurses see clients at their most vulnerable in health situations.

services and health professionals at the right time, across health care settings. Electronic records and communication technologies provide nurses with capabilities and clinical supports that were not possible even a decade ago, to assist clients at entry points to an increasingly complex health care system. According to Donaldson and Crowley (1978), the discipline of nursing is concerned with the following factors:

- "Principles and laws that govern the life processes, well-being, and optimum functioning of human beings, sick or well;
- Patterning of human behavior in interaction with the environment in critical life situations; and
- Processes by which positive changes in health status are affected." (p. 113)

NURSING THEORY

The fundamental knowledge base required of nurses includes human growth and development, pathophysiology, pharmacology, epidemiology, genetics, immunology, microbiology, health assessment and chronic disease management, psychology, and sociology. The theoretical foundations of nursing are drawn from philosophy, theory, research, and the practice wisdom of the profession (Smith & Liehr, 2008).

A **theory** represents a theorist's thoughtful examination of a phenomenon, defined as a concrete situation, event, circumstance, or condition of interest. Theory defines the relationships among its concepts, assumptions, and propositions in a formal, systematic manner, and provides a conceptual foundation for nursing research studies (Polit & Beck, 2007).

TYPES OF THEORY

Four types of theory are used in nursing practice, education, and research:

- *Descriptive theory* describes the properties and components of nursing as a professional discipline and explains what is important about the phenomenon.
- *Explanatory theory* identifies the functions of nursing and describes how the properties and components relate to each other.
- *Predictive theory* forecasts the relationships between the components of the model, how they occur, and what happens if an intervention is applied.
- *Prescriptive theory* identifies the conditions under which relationships occur and focuses on nursing therapeutics (Polit & Beck, 2007).

HISTORICAL DEVELOPMENT

Theory development is essential to maintaining the truth of any discipline (Reed & Shearer, 2007). The first nursing theorist was Florence Nightingale. She wrote the first published work on nursing theory, in which she differentiated the practice of nursing from other disciplines. She linked health with the environmental factors and offered guidelines for influencing the client's environment to help clients heal. In her classic work *Notes on Nursing,* Nightingale demonstrated through medical statistics that environmental cleanliness and hand washing were major factors in preventing infection in clinical situations. An early advocate for high-quality care, Nightingale's use of statistical data marks her as one of the first nurse researchers (Dossey et al., 2005; Kudzma, 2006).

Nursing theory development was relatively dormant until the middle of the 20th century, when nursing leaders in major universities began to describe a theoretical body of knowledge unique to professional nursing. Their graduate students provided ideas, struggled to understand the language and meaning of concepts, critiqued ideas, and developed important research studies to test the validity of nursing concepts (Fawcett, 2005).

Because nursing practice is embedded in a sociocultural context, nursing theory as a framework for practice has evolved as new information developed. Early nursing theorists, such as Virginia Henderson (1966) and Dorothy Johnson, supported the medical model, which focused primarily on identifying and modifying illness and disability. Modern nursing theorists, such as Rosemarie Parse and Betty Newman, incorporate a stronger emphasis on health promotion, client strengths, and preventive nursing strategies to facilitate health and well-being in line with today's conceptualization of health and well-being.

NURSING'S METAPARADIGM

Nursing's metaparadigm, or worldview, distinguishes the nursing profession from other disciplines and emphasizes its unique functional characteristics. Four key concepts—person, environment, health, and nursing—form the foundation for all nursing theories. Although each theorist's theoretical interpretation differs, person, environment, health, and nursing are reflected as central constructs in all nursing theories (Marrs & Lowry, 2006). Despite major transformational changes in the health care system from a medical model to a public health model, the conceptual strength of person, environment, health, and nursing as the cornerstone of nursing theory persists.

Concept of Person

Person, defined as the recipient of nursing care, is considered from a holistic perspective as having unique biopsychosocial and spiritual dimensions. The term *person* is applied to individuals, family units, the community, and target populations such as the elderly or mentally ill. Personal factors "comprise features of the individual that are not part of a health condition or health states" (World Health Organization [WHO], 2001, p. 17). For example, gender, lifestyle, coping styles, habits, among others, are a part of person, to be considered in conjunction with health and environment factors. The complexity of "person" as a key concept in nursing is evidenced in the increasingly robust explanations provided by current nursing theorists (Greene, 2009). Knowledge of the client as a person—his or her preferences, perceptions, beliefs, and values—is combined with the nurse's self-awareness as a basic understanding needed in all professional nursing relationships. This knowledge is an essential characteristic of "patient-centered care" currently identified as a central goal for the nation's health care system (Institute of Medicine [IOM], 2001; Shaller, 2007). Preserving and protecting a client's basic integrity and health rights as a unique individual is a unique ethical responsibility of nurse to client, whether the person is a contributing member of society, a critically ill newborn, a comatose client, or a seriously mentally ill individual. The concept of "person"

supersedes health diagnosis, apart from and before a specific health care problem is considered (American Holistic Nurses Association, 2004).

Concept of Environment

Environment refers to the internal and external context of the client, as it shapes and is affected by a client's health care situation. The WHO (2001) states, "Contextual Factors include both personal and environmental factors" (p. 8). Person and environment are so intertwined that to consider person as an isolated variable in a health care situation is impracticable. The concept of environment includes the cultural, developmental, and biopsychosocial conditions that influence a client's perceptions or behavior. For example, poverty, education, religious or spiritual beliefs, type of community (rural or urban), family strengths and challenges, and access to resources are part of a client's environmental context. Even climate, space, pollution, and food choices are important dimensions of environment that nurses may need to consider in choosing the most appropriate nursing interventions. Hegyvary (2007) urges nurses to "take the lead in health ecology" (p. 103). The concept of environment and health ecology becomes increasingly important as health care becomes a global enterprise and nursing responsibility.

Concept of Health

Nursing actions emphasize health and well-being. The word *health* derives from the word *whole*. Weil (2004) defines **health** as "a dynamic and harmonious equilibrium of all elements and forces making up and surrounding a human being" (p. 51). The concept of health exists on a continuum, and encompasses the entire life span, beginning with birth, and including palliative care and a peaceful death. Health involves individuals, families, and communities as a multidimensional concept having physical, psychological, sociocultural, developmental, and spiritual elements. Health includes disease prevention and promoting healthy lifestyle behaviors, regardless of clinical diagnosis (Morgan & Marsh, 1998).

Healthy People 2010, the health agenda for the United States for the next decade, considers quality of life as a desired outcome of health and health promotion activities. **Quality of life** is defined as a personal experience of subjective well-being and general satisfaction with life that includes, but is not limited to, physical health. *Health is a social concern*, particularly for people

---

EXERCISE 1-1 | **Understanding the Meaning of Health as a Nursing Concept**

Purpose: To help students understand the dimensions of health as a nursing concept.

Procedure:
1. Write a one-page description about the characteristics of a healthy person that you know.
2. In small groups of three or four, read your stories to each other. As you listen to other students' stories, write down themes that you note.
3. Compare themes, paying attention to similarities and differences, and developing a group definition of health derived from the stories.

4. In a larger group, share your definitions of health and defining characteristics of a healthy person.

Discussion:
1. Were you surprised by any of your thoughts about being healthy?
2. Did your peers define health in similar ways?
3. Based on the themes that emerged, how is health determined?
4. Is illness the opposite of being healthy?
5. In what ways can a nurse support the health of a client?

---

who do not have personal control over their health or the necessary resources to enhance their health status (Meleis, 1990). Exercise 1-1 provides an opportunity to explore the multidimensional meaning of health. Health is a cultural concern because people explain health, wellness, pathology, and treatment from the perspective of their cultural beliefs. For example, depression is explained as sadness in the Asian culture. Nurses play a major role in assessing health behaviors, and in recommending and working with individuals and families to achieve and maintain a healthy lifestyle.

Concept of Nursing

In 1956, Margaret Mead noted that nurses are invariably found wherever there is human pain and suffering. This statement has been expanded in modern times to include health promotion and disease prevention strategies designed to offset the occurrence of pain and suffering, and to minimize its effects once it has occurred. The International Council of Nursing (ICN) defines **nursing** as "encompassing autonomous and collaborative care of individuals of all ages, families,

groups and communities, sick or well and in all settings" (ICN, 2006).

The overarching goal of all nursing activities is to empower clients by providing them with the support they need to achieve optimal health and well-being. Nursing services are designed to build on and strengthen the natural capacities of individuals, families, and communities through a continuum of services ranging from health promotion and health education, to direct care, rehabilitation, and research evaluation.

Contemporary roles associated with nursing include advanced practice, community advocacy in shaping public health policies, and leadership in nursing management and education. Health behavior changes are strongly influenced by person-centered interventions promoted through normal nurse-client relationships. Exercise 1-2 looks at professional nursing.

LEVELS OF NURSING THEORY

The levels of nursing theory are categorized according to their level of abstraction: grand theory, mid-range theory, and practice theory (Marrs & Lowry, 2006).

EXERCISE 1-2 | **What Is Professional Nursing?**

Purpose: To help students develop an understanding of professional nursing.

Procedure:
1. Interview a professional nurse. Ask for descriptions of what he or she considers professional nursing to be today, in what ways he or she thinks nurses make a difference, and how the nurse feels the role might evolve within the next 10 years.

2. In small groups of three to five students, discuss findings and develop a group definition of professional nursing.

Discussion:
1. What does nursing mean to you?
2. Is your understanding of nursing different from those of the nurse(s) you interviewed?
3. As a new nurse, how would you want to present yourself?

- **Grand theories** address the key concepts and principles of the discipline as a whole. Examples include Martha Rogers's theory of unitary beings, Margaret Neuman's theory of expanding consciousness, Parse's theory of human becoming, and Dorothea Orem's self-care deficit theory of nursing.
- **Mid-range theories** cover more discrete aspects of a phenomenon specific to professional nursing, exploring them in depth rather than exploring the full phenomena of nursing (Marrs & Lowry, 2006). To be classified as a mid-range theory, the concepts must be applicable to many nursing situations, easily recognized, operationalized in nursing practice, and capable of being tested (Whall, 2004). A mid-range theory can derive from a grand theory, or from inductive research methodologies such as concept analysis or grounded theory (Meleis, 2006). Examples include Peplau's theory of interpersonal relationships and Pender's theory of health promotion.
- **Practice theories** are the most limited form of nursing theory. Walker and Avant (2005) believe that practice theories should receive greater attention in guiding the direction of modern nursing. The value of practice theory lies in the development of situation-producing guidelines for EBP, based on the day-to-day experiences of professional nurses. Marrs and Lowry (2006) note that "practice theories may be as simple as a single concept that is operationalized, and may be linked to a special population or situation" (p. 47). Exercise 1-3 provides an opportunity to critique an article using nursing theory in clinical practice.

THEORY AS A GUIDE TO PRACTICE

Donaldson and Crowley (1978) characterize a discipline as having "a unique perspective, a distinct way of viewing all phenomena, which ultimately defines and limits the nature of its inquiry" (p. 113). Nursing theory informs nursing practice by furnishing a distinct body of nursing knowledge that nurses universally recognize as being unique to their discipline. They offer a systematic, organized way to view and interpret nursing care. In addition, concepts, drawn from multiple interdisciplinary perspectives and sources, serve as a guide for curriculum development and clinical practice.

Nursing theories provide a basis for research and a framework for understanding study results. Theoretical frameworks guide nursing research by generating hypotheses that can be supported or refuted from a theoretical perspective. When the researcher completes a study, the discussion will contain an interpretation of the findings in relation to the identified theoretical framework.

THE ART OF NURSING

Theoretical understandings do not describe variations in a client's individual needs, perceptual or educational skills, or socioeconomic and cultural differences that require accommodations in therapeutic approach. This comes from the art of nursing, which includes caring and presence in combination with scientific applications to define nursing from a different, yet integrated perspective (Fingeld-Connett, 2008).

Integration occurs as a seamless interactive process in which nurses combine knowledge, skills, and scientific medical understandings with an individualized

---

| EXERCISE 1-3 | Critiquing a Nursing Theory Article |

Purpose: To provide students with an opportunity to understand the connection of nursing theory to research and clinical practice.

Procedure:
1. Select an article from a professional journal that describes the use of nursing theory or nursing concepts. Suggestions for journals include *Nursing Science Quarterly, Journal of Advanced Nursing, Journal of Professional Nursing,* and *Advances in Nursing Science.*

2. Read the article carefully and critique the article to include the following: (a) how the author applied the theory or concept; (b) relevance of the concept or theory for nursing practice; (c) how you could use the concept in your own clinical practice; and (d) what you learned from reading the article.

Discussion:
In your class group, share some of the insights you obtained from the article and engage in a general discussion about the relevance of nursing theory for professional nursing practice.

knowledge of the humanity of each client as a unique individual with physical, cognitive, emotional, and spiritual needs. Gramling (2004) describes the **art of nursing** as the "nurse's mode of being knowing, and responding" and suggests that it represents "an attunement rather than an activity" (p. 394). It is the element of care that nurses and clients tend to remember best.

Patterns of Knowing

In her classic work, Carper (1978) describes four patterns of knowing embedded in nursing practice: empirical, personal, aesthetic, and ethical. Although the patterns of knowing are described as individual prototypes, in practice, they inform care as an integrated focus of knowledge. Together they lay the epistemological and ontological foundation of nursing practice (Zander, 2007). Holtslander (2008) notes that "this integrated, inclusive, and eclectic approach is reflective of the goals of nursing, which are to provide effective, efficient, and compassionate care while considering individuality, context, and complexity" (p. 25). The four patterns of knowing include:

- **Empirical** ways of knowing, which are grounded in the science of nursing. Nurses incorporate empirical ways of knowing as the basis for scientific rationales when choosing appropriate nursing interventions.

- **Personal** ways of knowing, which help nurses connect with and acknowledge the humanness of another. Personal knowing occurs when a nurse is able to intuitively understand and treat individual clients as unique human beings because of the nurse's own personal experience and awareness of his or her own humanness.

- Carper equates esthetics with the art of nursing. **Aesthetic** ways of knowing are intangible, but they allow for creative applications in the relationship through meaningful connections with the larger environment and life experience. Esthetic ways of knowing link the art of nursing with its scientific application. An example of aesthetic ways of knowing is found in storytelling, in which the nurse seeks to understand the experience of the client's journey through illness (Leight, 2002). Nurses can use stories to clarify or enhance a variety of themes and supplement instructions.

- **Ethical** ways of knowing refer to the moral aspects of nursing. Ethical ways of knowing encompass knowledge of what is right and wrong, attention to standards and codes in making moral choices, responsibility for one's actions, and protection of the client's autonomy and rights (Altmann, 2007). Exercise 1-4 provides an application of patterns of knowing in clinical practice.

EXERCISE 1-4	Relevance of Patterns of Knowing for Clinical Practice

Purpose: To help students understand how patterns of knowing can be used effectively in clinical practice.

Procedure:
1. Break into smaller groups of three to four students. Identify a scribe for each student group.
2. Using the following case study, decide how you would use empirical, personal, ethical, and aesthetic patterns of knowing to see that Mrs. Jackson's holistic needs were addressed in the next 48 hours.

Case Study:
Mrs. Jackson, an 86-year-old widow, was admitted to the hospital with a hip fracture. She has very poor eyesight because of macular degeneration and takes eye drops for the condition. Her husband died 5 years ago, and she subsequently moved into an assisted housing development. She had to give up driving because of her eyesight and sold her car to another

resident 5 months ago. Although her daughter lives in the area, Mrs. Jackson has little contact with her. This distresses her greatly, as she describes being very close with her until 8 years ago. She feels safe in her new environment but complains that she is very lonely and is not interested in joining activities. She has a male friend in the complex, but recently he has been showing less interest. Her surgery is scheduled for tomorrow, but she has not yet signed her consent form. She does not have advance directives.

Discussion:
1. In a large group, have each student share their findings.
2. For each pattern of knowing, write the suggestions on the board.
3. Compare and contrast the findings of the different groups.
4. Discuss how the patterns of knowing add to an understanding of the client in this case study.

Developing an Evidence-Based Practice

Awa M, Yamashita M: Persons' experience of HIV/AIDS in Japan: application of Margaret Newman's theory, *International Nursing Review* 55:454–461, 2008.

This qualitative study was designed to describe the lived experience of clients diagnosed with HIV/AIDS using Margaret Newman's theory of health as expanding consciousness. The findings are based on the narratives of five men who had participated in a self-help group for men afflicted with HIV/AIDS. Each was interviewed twice, and study informants were asked to confirm, clarify, or revise the pattern inherent in his story. Expanding consciousness was noted as informants recognized the importance of significant personal relationships with family and significant others.

Study Findings: Although their experiences were different, the five men experienced a unified sense of expanding consciousness described as an evolving five-stage pattern of the illness trajectory. The trajectory consisted of "a pattern of self consciousness of (their) own sexual orientation, chaos, stagnation, turning point and regaining a new identity" (p. 456). The process, enhanced by participation in a support group, allowed the men to accept their illness as a part of their identity and improved their ability to take responsibility for their actions. Acceptance of self and their chronic illness as part of the whole allowed for deeper, more enriching relationships with others. Peer support was acknowledged as an important facilitator of expanding consciousness.

Application to Your Clinical Practice: As a profession, nurses need to develop theory-based research evidence to support effective practice. How do you see the role of self-help and support groups helping to improve the health and well-being of clients with chronic illness through expanded consciousness? What steps would you need to take as an individual nurse to encourage expanded consciousness as a part of your routine nursing care?

APPLICATIONS

USING NURSING THEORY FRAMEWORKS IN CLINICAL PRACTICE

Nursing theory and practice represent reciprocal interactive processes. Theory frameworks are used to guide critical thinking and actions in nursing practice; practice informs nursing theory. Different theories and nursing models provide a variety of lenses from which to approach the nursing process.

This section addresses a short list of selected nursing theories with particular relevance for use with nurse-client relationships. Alligood (2010) notes a shift in the 21st century from theory development to a new era of theory applicability and utilization. Contemporary nurses will play an important role in this process.

NURSING THEORY AND THE THERAPEUTIC RELATIONSHIP

Hildegard Peplau's (1952; 1997) mid-range theory of interpersonal relationships is considered an essential nursing theory framework for the study of interpersonal relationships. The model describes how the nurse-client relationship can facilitate the identification and accomplishment of therapeutic goals to enhance client and family well-being (see Chapter 5). In today's health care environment, nurse-client relationships are of short duration, and nursing interventions have to be brief, concise, and effective. Despite the brevity of the relationship, Peplau's basic principles of building rapport, developing a working partnership, and terminating a relationship remain relevant. Originally conceptualized as a central phenomenon in psychiatric nursing, Peplau's framework for interpersonal relationships is applicable to all areas of nursing (McCarthy and Aquino-Russell (2009).

Holistic nursing theories focus on the meaning of a health experience and are used as guides in nurse-client relationships to help clients create a productive way of understanding and responding to difficult health situations. Exemplars include Rosemarie Parse's (1998) theory of human becoming and Margaret Newman's (1986) theory of expanding consciousness. Parse's theory, which focuses on valuing a person's health situation and quality of life from the client's perspective, is an important consideration in developing patient-centered approaches. Newman patterned her theory of health based on Martha Rogers's earlier theory of unitary human beings and interconnectedness with the environment. Her theory emphasizes mutual interaction between nurse and client unique to each client situation. Each therapeutic interaction is designed to move the human system toward making health choices that transcend physical limitations. Her theory is useful in helping clients with chronic illness find meaning in their situation through expanding consciousness about new possibilities for living with illness and maximizing patterns needed for health and well-being.

Caring

Caring is recognized as a hallmark of quality nursing practice and an essential concept in effective nurse-client relationships. Crowe (2000) suggests, "Caring does not involve specific tasks, instead it involves the creation of a sustained relationship with the other" (p. 966). Characteristics of professional caring, as identified by graduate nurses, include: (a) giving of self, (b) involved presence, (c) intuitive knowing and empathy, (d) supporting the patient's integrity, and (e) professional competence (Arnold, 1997). Caring is a relationship attitude and a commitment to the well-being of clients and families, demonstrated through actions for and on behalf of them.

Caring is a primary construct in nursing theories developed by Jean Watson (1988), and Madeleine Leininger (1985; 2002). Both theorists believe caring is central to the practice of nursing. Watson's theory promotes caring as a primary transpersonal value, and moral imperative concerned with protecting and preserving the dignity and humanity of the client. Her model describes the empathetic features of caring (Jasmine, 2009). Watson identified 10 carative factors, which are applicable to nurse client relationships (Box 1-1). These factors have, over time, evolved into a broader concept of "clinical caritas" and "caritas processes," terms that Watson considers to be a more fluid and mature framework for nursing in the 21st century. This expanded version is identified on Jean

---

| BOX 1-1 | Watson's Carative Factors |

1. The formation of a humanistic-altruistic system of values.
2. The instillation of faith-hope.
3. The cultivation of sensitivity to one's self and to others.
4. The development of a helping-trust relationship.
5. The promotion and acceptance of the expression of positive and negative feelings.
6. The systematic use of the scientific problem-solving method for decision making.
7. The promotion of interpersonal teaching-learning.
8. The provision for a supportive, protective, and (or) corrective mental, physical, sociocultural, and spiritual environment.
9. Assistance with the gratification of human needs.
10. The allowance for existential-phenomenological forces.

From Watson J: *Nursing: human science and human care: a theory of nursing* (pp. 9–10), New York, 1988, National League for Nursing.

Watson's website: http://www.nursing.ucdenver.edu/faculty/jw_evolution.htm.

Leininger's theory of cultural care expands on the concept of caring within a broader cultural context. Transcultural nursing theory incorporates cultural perspectives in applying relationship and nursing process concepts to culturally diverse clients. Leininger's sunrise diagram outlines the dimensions of cultural assessment).

THEORETICAL PERSPECTIVES FROM OTHER DISCIPLINES

Professional nursing includes concepts and theoretical perspectives from other disciplines as a foundation for practice, related to the nurse-client relationship (Villarruel, Bishop, Simpson, Jemmott, & Fawcett, 2001). Exemplar concepts from models are identified in this chapter and reintroduced in later chapters. They are not meant to be inclusive but were selected because of their relevance in implementing nurse-client relationships.

PSYCHODYNAMIC MODELS

Sigmund Freud (1937), acknowledged as the Father of Psychiatry, recognized the therapeutic value of talking about stressful life experiences as a way of reducing their impact, and problem-solving difficult life problems. Freud's ideas about **transference**, defined as projecting irrational attitudes and feelings from the past onto people in the present, are useful in understanding the origin of difficult behaviors in nurse-client relationships. For example, the client who says to the young nurse, "Get me a real nurse! You're young enough to be my daughter, and I don't want to talk with you about my personal life," may be having a transference reaction having little to do with the nurse's competence. Recognizing this statement as a transference reaction helps the nurse depersonalize the client's comment, allowing for a more appropriate response.

Transference feelings can also occur within the nurse. Unless these feelings are recognized and resolved, they can compromise the effectiveness of the therapeutic relationship. Referred to as **countertransference**, these feelings represent unconscious attitudes or exaggerated feelings a nurse may develop toward a client. Not all transference feelings are negative. Positive countertransferences of strong attraction, oversolicitousness, or special treatment can represent transference feelings that lead to boundary crossings or violations.

Freud was the first clinician to identify age-related sequential stages of personality development. His theory of linear psychosexual development focused on children from birth through adolescence. Failure to resolve stages of development result in immature behavioral response patterns such that the person remains "fixated" at an earlier stage of development. For example, a person experiencing little parental support in early childhood may find it difficult to trust that health providers will help.

Freud believed that people protect themselves against anxiety through the use of unconscious **ego defense mechanisms** (see Chapter 20). Defensive behaviors that compromise the development of a therapeutic relationship can reflect a person's use of ego defense mechanisms.

Carl Jung

Carl Jung's (1971) theoretical perspectives provide nurses with a basis for examining the complex dimensions of gender roles and our universal heritage as human beings. He referred to a person's universal heritage as the collective unconscious and suggested that forces from the past continue to influence behaviors in the present. Jung characterized the first half of life as a search for self, and the second half as a search for soul. Jung's personality theory for mid-life and beyond is relevant in helping nurses to understand and support the older adult's shifting needs to find new inner meaning and direction in the second half of life.

Interpersonal Relationship Approaches

Harry Stack Sullivan

Harry Stack Sullivan (1953) introduced the idea of the therapeutic relationship as a human connection that heals. Hildegard Peplau (1997) credits Sullivan's model of therapeutic relationship as a foundation for her mid range theory of interpersonal relationships in nursing practice. A corrective interpersonal experience with a helping professional can help individuals discover their strength and value through relationship.

Sullivan introduced the concept that people cannot always relate easily to a helping person and may need ongoing, compassionate, supportive encouragement to make use of the therapeutic relationship even when the helper is extremely empathetic. This is especially true for individuals experiencing shock, panic, serious mental illness, or brain damage. Further explanation of Sullivan's theory as it relates to therapeutic relationships is presented in Chapter 5.

PSYCHOSOCIAL DEVELOPMENT THEORIES

Two developmental theories, adapted from psychology, guide the study of interpersonal relationships in health care. Nurses use Erik Erikson's (1950) theory of psychosocial development to assess developmental client needs, and to design *developmentally* age-appropriate nursing interventions (see Chapter 4). Erikson modified Freud's age-related developmental stages to focus on progressive stages of psychosocial, rather than psychosexual, maturation. Erikson believed that people continue to mature throughout life. Exercise 1-5 offers an opportunity to review a person's perception of different developmental life stages.

Different life experiences and culture—for example, the death or divorce of a parent, frequent moves, family abuse, and ethnic norms—can affect the actual timetable and expression of psychosocial development of individuals. When life crises coincide with normal developmental crises, the developmental crisis can be

EXERCISE 1-5	Completing the Life Cycle

Purpose: To help students understand the integration of psychosocial development through the life cycle.

Procedure:
1. Interview an adult who has reached at least the sixth decade of life.
2. Identify Erikson's psychosocial tasks, and ask the person to identify what factors in his or her life contributed to or interfered with mastery of the task for each stage.

3. Describe in short summary the factors that you believe contributed or interfered with each stage of the person's adult life.

Discussion:
1. In a larger group, share your examples.
2. For each stage, compile on the board a list of the factors identified.
3. Discuss the impact certain factors may have on the outcome of development through the life span.

| TABLE 1-1 | Distinguishing Freud's Psychosexual and Erikson's Psychosocial Stages of Personality Development | | | | |

FREUD'S PSYCHOSEXUAL STAGES OF PERSONALITY DEVELOPMENT			**ERIKSON'S PSYCHOSOCIAL STAGES OF PERSONALITY DEVELOPMENT**		
Stage	Characteristics	Age (years) Range	Stage	Strengths	Tasks
Oral	*Physical:* Mouth *Psychological:* Dependency	0–2	Trust vs. mistrust	Hope	To receive, to give
Anal	*Physical:* Elimination *Psychological:* Self control/obedience	2–4	Autonomy vs. shame/doubt	Willpower	To control, let go
Phallic (Oedipal)	*Physical:* Penis *Psychological:* sexual identity	4–6	Initiative vs. guilt	Purpose	To make, play-act
Latency	Calm period, little psychosexual activity	6–puberty	Industry vs. inferiority	Competence	To make things, put things together
Genital	*Physical:* Sexuality *Psychological:* Intimacy, mature Adult	⇐Post puberty 13-19⇒	Identity vs. identity diffusion	Fidelity	To be oneself: develop self-identity
Freud does not identify progressive adult stages of psychosexual development		Young adult, 20s	Intimacy vs. isolation	Love	To share one's self with another
N/A		Middle adult, 30s–50s	Generativity vs. self-absorbtion	Caring	To take care of, to make be
N/A		Older adult, over 50	Integrity vs. despair	Wisdom	To be, to face death

Data Source: Erikson E: Childhood and society, New York, 1950, WW Norton.
Sigelma C, Rider E. Life-Span Human Development, 6th edition. Belvont CA: 2009, Wadsorth Cengage Learning.

more difficult to resolve, for example, a diagnosis of breast cancer occurring at menopause. Table 1-1 presents the key stage development theories. Exercise 1-6 provides an opportunity to look at the influence of life circumstances on psychosocial development.

Abraham Maslow

Nurses use Abraham Maslow's needs theory (1970) as a framework to *prioritize* client needs and develop related nursing approaches. Maslow's hierarchy of needs theory proposes that people are motivated to

EXERCISE 1-6	Time Line

Purpose: To give students experience with understanding psychosocial development through the life span.

Procedure:
1. Draw a time line of your life to date. Include all significant events and the age at which they occurred.
2. Insert Erikson's stages as markers in your time line.

Discussion:
1. In what ways did Erikson's stages provide information about expected tasks in your life?
2. In what ways did they deviate?
3. To what would you attribute the differences?
4. How could you use this exercise in your nursing care of clients?

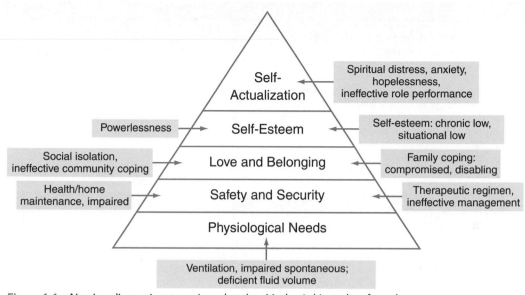

Figure 1-1 Nursing diagnosis categories related to Maslow's hierarchy of needs.

meet their needs in an ascending order beginning with meeting basic survival needs, moving into psychological and social spheres as essential needs are satisfied, and ending with self-actualization. Figure 1-1 illustrates Maslow's model with associated nursing diagnoses.

Physiologic needs required for survival are the most fundamental. Maslow referred to basic needs as "deficiency" needs, meaning that if they cannot be met, the person is at risk for survival. Basic needs include satisfying hunger, thirst, and sexual appetites, and sensory stimulation. Maslow's second level, safety and security needs, includes physical safety and emotional security, for example, housing and freedom from abuse. Once a person meets safety and security needs, love and belonging needs, related to being a part of a family or community, become the focus. Basic need satisfaction allows for the attention to growth needs for self-esteem and self-actualization. A sense of dignity, respect, and approval by others for the self within is the hallmark of successfully meeting self-esteem needs.

Maslow's highest level of need satisfaction, self-actualization, represents humanity at its best. Self-actualized individuals are not superhuman; they are subject to the same feelings of insecurity that all individuals experience, but they recognize and accept their vulnerability as part of the human condition. Box 1-2

BOX 1-2	Characteristics of Self-Actualization

- Quality of genuineness
- Passion for living
- Ability to get along well with others
- Strong sense of personal worth
- View of life situations as opportunities, not threats
- Ability to experience each moment fully
- Moments of intense emotional meaning, "peak experience"
- Full acceptance of self and others
- Identification with fellow human beings
- High sense of responsibility with a strong desire to serve humanity
- Integrity of purposes

presents characteristics of self-actualization. Not everyone reaches Maslow's self-actualization stage.

Although nurses routinely use Maslow's theory to prioritize nursing interventions, how the client and/or family prioritize health care needs is an important assessment. This consideration will enhance client cooperation, and family support will affect compliance. Exercises 1-7 and 1-8 provide practice with using Maslow's model in clinical practice.

EXERCISE 1-7	Maslow's Hierarchy of Needs

Purpose: To help students understand the usefulness of Maslow's theory in clinical practice.

Procedure:
1. Divide the class into small groups, with each group assigned to a step of Maslow's hierarchy. Each group will then brainstorm examples of that need as it might present in clinical practice.
2. Identify potential responses from the nurse that might address each need.

3. Share examples with the larger group and discuss the concept of prioritization of needs using Maslow's hierarchy.

Discussion:
1. In what ways is Maslow's hierarchy helpful to the nurse in prioritizing client needs?
2. What limitations do you see with the theory?

EXERCISE 1-8	Case Application of Maslow's Theory

Purpose: To examine the use of Maslow's theory in a specific case.

Procedure:
In groups of three or four students, consider the following case study and apply Maslow's hierarchy of needs theory to Mr. Rodgers's case, from the time of admission to the coronary care unit until his discharge and follow-up care. Include any considerations for changing priorities because of fluctuations in his condition.

Case Study:
Mr. Rodgers was admitted to the cardiac intensive care unit with an acute myocardial infarction. He is an internationally known, middle-aged businessman, a corporate vice president of a major company, and very

well liked by his employees. His blood pressure for the past two years has never fallen below a diastolic reading of 95, and he is being treated with a mild diuretic. Before this hospitalization, he had never been admitted to a hospital. Mr. Rodgers is anxious and perspiring profusely. He has many of the predisposing factors for heart problems present in his history, family, and lifestyle.

Discussion:
1. At what stage of Maslow's hierarchy is this client?
2. With what needs is the client likely to require nursing intervention during his hospitalization and after discharge?
3. In a large group, share your conclusions and recommendations for prioritizing Mr. Rodgers's care with a rationale.

PERSON-CENTERED MODELS
Carl Rogers

Carl Rogers's person-centered model forms a solid theoretical foundation for examining the current concepts of "client-centered care" as a key dimension of quality nurse-client relationships, as described in later chapters. Rogers emphasized an equal partnership between client and health care provider. He pointed to the primacy of client as the agent of healing. According to Rogers (1961), "If I can provide a certain type of relationship, the other person will discover within himself the capacity to use that relationship for growth and change, and personal development will occur" (p. 33).

Rogers identified three "helper" characteristics essential to the development of client-centered relationships: unconditional positive regard, empathetic understanding, and genuineness. He later added a fourth characteristic: a spiritual or transcendental presence as an intuitive way of being with a client (Anderson, 2001).

Rogers's concepts of a person-centered relationship also are applicable for nurse-client health teaching formats (see Chapter 16). They have found merit as a foundation for the patient-centered health care approaches advocated by the IOM.

Aaron Beck. Concepts from Aaron Beck's (1991) cognitive behavioral therapy (CBT) model uses a person-centered approach aimed at helping individuals troubled by faulty thinking reframe the meaning of difficult situations. Beck believed that there is a relationship between a person's thoughts, feelings, and behaviors. By helping people become aware of and modify negative or dysfunctional thoughts, beliefs, and perceptions (cognitive distortions), it is possible for individuals to change behavior patterns, resulting in a more constructive approach to a problem situation. The focus of treatment is not on the behavior itself, but rather on the internal perceptions and thoughts that create and perpetuate self-defeating

TABLE 1-2	Irrational Beliefs and Common Triggers	
Orientation	**Example**	**Common Triggers**
Self	"I must do everything perfectly, and put 110% into everything I do. Otherwise, I will never be a good nurse."	Failing a test, being criticized by a client or instructor
Others	"Everyone must like and respect me. No one should be angry with me. I should always be able to get what I want, when I want it. Otherwise, I am not worth much."	Having someone cut in front of me, reject or challenge my opinions, waiting in line for services
World	"The world and everything in it should be predictable, and things should happen as I believe they should. Otherwise, there is no point to my doing anything."	Elections, allocation and availability of resources, taxes, lack of equal opportunities, prejudice

behaviors. Table 1-2 identifies irrational beliefs and common triggers.

Faulty or negative thinking causes a person to interpret neutral situations in an unrealistic, exaggerated, or negative way. These automatic negative thoughts are classified as **cognitive distortions**. Examples include magnifying or minimizing the impact of a single behavior as being a commentary on the whole person, selective attention, mind reading, rigid rules about what a person "should" do, and so forth. Related to the concept of distortions is the concept of *schema or schemata*. This a term used to describe a person's learned rules and understandings of the stimulus world, and his/her relationship to it. A core schema becomes a template for understanding the meaning of incoming information and appraising its value to the self. It is more pervasive

and harder to dislodge. Although distortions seem to be legitimate assessments, they are not valid. Cognitive distortions and schemata are related to behaviors of self, others, and the world (Hale-Evans, 2006).

Nurses can teach people to challenge distortions through Socratic questioning. By gathering and weighing evidence to support a position, people are able to distinguish between a distorted perception and a realistic appraisal of its validity. Ridding oneself of unrealistic expectations and negative self-thoughts allows cognitive space for thinking about possible options and broader choices. Once a problem is appropriately categorized, the solutions become more apparent.

COMMUNICATION THEORIES

Communication theories are concerned with the transmission of information. Communication is an essential characteristic of human functioning. Through communication, we construct meaning and share it with others. Most of us take communication for granted until it is no longer a part of our lives. Communication can take place intrapersonally (within the self) or interpersonally (with others).

Intrapersonal communication takes place within the self in the form of inner thoughts and beliefs that are colored by feelings and influence behavior. **Interpersonal communication** is defined as a cyclic, reciprocal, interactive, and dynamic process, with value, cultural, and cognitive variables that influence its transmission and reception. Interpersonal communication has a content and a relationship dimension. The content dimension (verbal component) refers to the data. The relationship dimension (nonverbal metacommunication) helps the receiver interpret the message. People tend to pay more attention to nonverbal communication than to words when they are noncongruent with each other.

Human communication is unique. Only human beings have large vocabularies and are capable of learning new languages as a means of sharing their ideas and feelings. Communication includes language, gestures, and symbols to convey intended meaning, exchange ideas and feelings, and share significant life experiences. Basic assumptions serving as the foundation for the concept of communication are presented in Box 1-3.

BOX 1-3	Basic Assumptions of Communication Theory

- It is impossible not to communicate (Bateson, 1979).
- Every communication has a content and a relationship (metacommunication) aspect.
- We only know about ourselves and others through communication.
- Faulty communication results in flawed feeling and acting.
- Feedback is the only way we know that our perceptions about meanings are valid.
- Silence is a form of communication.
- All parts of a communication system are interrelated and affect one another.
- People communicate through words (digital communication) and through nonverbal behaviors and analog-verbal modalities, which are equally necessary to interpret a message appropriately.
- Interpersonal communication processes are either symmetric or complementary, and can reflect differences in the equality of the relationship (Waltzlawick, Beavin-Bevalas & Jackson, 1967).

LINEAR MODEL

Linear models consist of three components:
- The **sender** is the source or initiator of the message. The sender encodes the message (i.e., puts the message into verbal or nonverbal symbols that the receiver can understand). Encoding a message appropriately requires a clear understanding of the receiver's mental frame of reference (e.g., feelings, personal agendas, past experiences) and knowledge of its purpose or intent.
- The **message** consists of the transmitted verbal or nonverbal expression of thoughts and feelings. Effective messages are relevant, authentic, and expressed in understandable language.
- The **receiver** is the recipient of the message. Once received, the receiver decodes it (i.e., translates the message into word symbols and internally interprets its meaning to make sense of the message). An open listening attitude and suspension of judgment strengthens the possibility of accurately decoding the sender's message. The **channels** of communication through which a person receives messages are the five senses: sight, hearing, taste, touch, and smell.

CIRCULAR TRANSACTIONAL MODELS

A circular model is a transactional model that expands linear models to include the context of the communication, feedback loops, and validation (Figure 1-2). With this model, the sender and receiver construct a mental picture of the other, which influences the message and includes perceptions of the other person's attitude and potential reaction to the message. In this sense, transactional models reflect system theory with

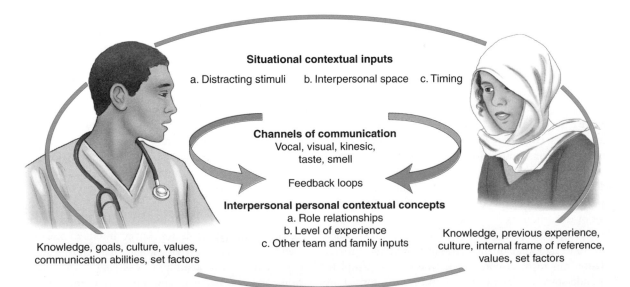

Figure 1-2   Circular transactional model of communication.

feedback and context added to the linear model. Communication is conceptualized as a continuous, interactive activity in which sender and receiver continuously influence each other as they converse. The human system (client) receives information from the environment (input), internally processes the information and reacts to it based on its own internal functions (throughput), and produces new information or behavior (output) as a result of the process. Feedback (from the receiver or the environment) allows the system to correct or maintain its original information.

Circular models take into account the role relationships between communicators. People take either symmetric or complementary roles in communicating. Symmetric role relationships are equal, whereas complementary role relationships typically operate with one person holding a higher position than the other in the communication process. Nurses assume a complementary role of clinical expert when helping the client to achieve mutually determined health goals, and a symmetric role in working with the client as partner on developing mutually defined goals and the means to achieve them. Exercise 1-9 provides an opportunity to contrast linear versus circular models of communication.

THERAPEUTIC COMMUNICATION

Therapeutic communication is a term originally coined by Ruesch (1961) to describe a goal-directed form of communication used in health care to achieve goals that promote client health and well-being. Doheny et al. (2007) observed that "when certain skills are used to facilitate communication between nurse and client in a goal directed manner, the therapeutic communication process occurs" (p. 5). Nurses use therapeutic communication skills to provide new information, correct misinformation, promote understanding of client responses to health problems, explore options for care, assist in decision making, and facilitate client well-being.

CONTEMPORARY SOCIAL ISSUES AND DYNAMICS

Theoretical frameworks sensitize nurses to perceive, think about, and act on relevant client information in a systematic way. In today's practice environment, theory is insufficient as a guide to practice. Recognition that nursing practice is deeply embedded in the political factors, and the cultural context in which nursing is practiced is critical. Engebretson (2003) notes that cultural constructions of health and illness determine the nature of helpful provider-client interactions and influence the ways in which people make decisions and use health care services. Many factors (e.g., economics, unprecedented changes in demographics, multidisciplinary approaches to health care delivery, and advances in technology) are changing nursing's professional landscape (Booth et al., 1997). Nurses must be knowledgeable about the contemporary societal issues and political dynamics that currently influence the conduct of the nurse-client relationship in fundamental ways. The clinical skill sets for nurses in the past need to be replaced with expanded competencies that reflect the changing health care delivery system.

CHANGES IN HEALTH CARE DELIVERY

A key change is a shift from health care delivery provided mainly in hospitals to care delivered in primary care settings in the community. Figure 1-3 displays fundamental characteristics of contemporary

---

EXERCISE 1-9	Differences Between Linear and Circular Models of Communication

Purpose: To help students see the difference between linear and circular models of communication.

Procedure:
1. Role-play a scenario in which one person provides a scene that might occur in the clinical area using a linear model: sender, message, and receiver.
2. Role-play the same scenario using a circular model, framing questions that recognize the context of the message and its potential impact on the receiver, and provide feedback.

Discussion:
1. Was there a difference in your level of comfort? If so, in what ways?
2. Was there any difference in the amount of information you had as a result of the communication? If so, in what ways?
3. What implications does this exercise have for your future nursing practice?

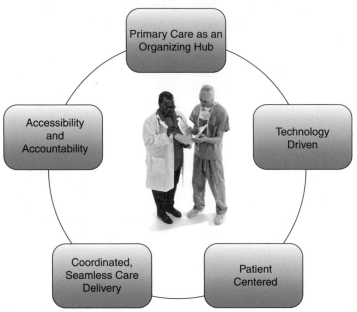

Figure 1-3   Characteristics of Contemporary Health Care Systems of Delivery.

health care delivery systems. Science and technology are keeping people living longer with a better quality of life than could have been imagined even a few decades ago. Clients are discharged quicker and sicker than in previous decades, partly because of capitated management of health care. Most will require additional education and support to self-manage chronic health conditions. The emphasis in health care has changed from a focus solely on service delivery to an expanded population focus on health promotion for health and well-being. People are expected to take responsibility for their own health and well-being. These changes provide the impetus for exploring nursing practice from a broader perspective.

As a result of these changes, the scope of practice and nature of work for contemporary nurses is multidimensional, multirelational, and highly complex. Managed care, the emergence of integrated interdisciplinary professional roles as the preferred model of provider service delivery, public reporting of clinical outcomes, and inclusion of client quality of life and satisfaction with care as expected clinical outcomes have revolutionized previous thinking about what needs to be included in nurse-client relationships. The length of the relationship is brief, with a focus on the client as the central person on the health care team.

Nurses practice across a wider range of clinical settings. They are expected to be multiskilled and able to function competently in a variety of health care environments. Health care relationships between clients and providers, and among interdisciplinary professional colleagues are collaborative and complementary.

Health care consumers expect more. They are better informed about their health conditions and are expected to take an active role in self-management of chronic diseases. The level of knowledge about health information on the Internet, medications, drug interactions, and health promotion/disease prevention strategies has increased exponentially.

New Professional and Consumer Roles

Nurses need to appreciate the larger number of stakeholders, including clients and families involved in health care relationships. Incorporating multiple perspectives in health care management across a continuum of care that extends into the community is the norm. Nurses are expected to have knowledge about and apply a variety of paradigms to real-life situations in clinical practice. Client roles have evolved from being passive recipients of health care into active autonomous partners, with providers involving shared authority over decision making in their treatment.

The context of the nurse-client relationship includes a broader connection with other clinicians, health care decision makers, and even occasionally policy makers. New interprofessional relationships are influencing the need for and provision of nursing services. Nurses have professional accountability, not only as a member of their profession but as members of a professional team. Instruction about interdisciplinary roles is evolving as a national curriculum thread in medical, nursing, social work, and pharmacy with combined student courses (see Chapter 7).

DEMOGRAPHIC CHANGES AND HEALTH DISPARITIES

Health care in the United States is not equally accessible. There are glaring gaps in access to care, with many segments of a growing minority population receiving inadequate or no health care. Regulation and surveillance of quality in health care with reliance on performance measures to describe the nation's progress has made the quality of health care more transparent and has highlighted the plight of major segments of the nation's population (Institute of Medicine (IOM, 2003)).

Health disparities disproportionately impact the elderly, children, and minority populations. Demographic changes with a marked increase in the percentage of older adults and ethnically diverse consumers needing ongoing health care raise important ethical and medical issues.

Healthy People 2010 (U.S. Department of Health and Human Services, 2000) identifies "reducing health disparities" as a primary goal for health care. Appreciation for the rapidly increasing diversity of our society is compelling in health care, not only because of differences in health-related characteristics, but because of language, economic, and social barriers to seeking health care.

On March 23, 2010, President Obama signed an historic health care reform bill, passed by Congress. The Patient Protection and Affordable Care Act is designed to provide better health care insurance coverage for consumers of health care services. Included in the bill is health insurance for children with preexisting conditions, and access to affordable insurance for previously uninsured adults. Funding to increase the number of nurses, physicians, and other health professionals is included. Like all sweeping changes imposed by law, health care reform will take time to implement and will undergo modification as it is put into practice.

Health care reform is necessary to provide access to care and the level of health care services needed to reduce health disparities. Nurses can and should be in the forefront of helping the nation provide affordable, culturally congruent health care as an essential means of reducing health disparities.

EVIDENCE-BASED PRACTICE

The IOM (2001) calls for an innovative health care system that is evidence based, patient centered, and systems oriented. Porter-O'Grady (2010) suggests that EBP represents an integration of client concerns and individual clinical applications with external evidence from clinical data and research, and best practices. The strength of the connection requires the blending of extensive clinical experience with sound clinical research and professional judgment in real-time situations with clients.

Quality nursing practice, implemented through the nurse-client relationship, is theory guided and evidence based. EBP is dynamically related to nursing theory through empirical ways of knowing. Nursing theory provides a reference framework for understanding the complex features of human responses in health care. This is a necessary, but insufficient condition for excellence. Since the late 1990s, EBP has emerged as a primary means to advance professional standards in nursing practice and to enhance the quality of care for clients (Van Achterberg, Holleman, & Van de Ven, 2006).

Sackett, Rosenberg, and Gray (1996) define EBP as "the conscientious explicit and judicious use of current best evidence in making decisions about the care of individual patients" (p. 71). Systematic review of all randomized, controlled, clinical trials and EBP guidelines based on findings and opinions of expert committees provide the strongest evidence. EBP consists of four elements:

- Best practices, derived from consensus statements developed by expert clinicians and researchers
- Evidence from scientific findings in research-based studies found in published journals
- Clinical nursing expertise of professional nurses, including knowledge of pathophysiology, pharmacology, and psychology
- Preferences and values of clients and family members (Sigma Theta Tau International, 2003)

All health care disciplines are being called on to deliver quality health care according to standardized, evidence-based guidelines that in the future will be used "to define best practices rather than to support existing practices" (Youngblut & Brooten, 2001, p. 468).

PERSON-CENTERED CARE

Scientific guidelines need to be balanced by values-based nursing knowledge. Person-centered care is mandated as an essential characteristic of contemporary health care. Ironically, it is a value that nursing has always championed. Gottlieb and Gottlieb (1998) identify nursing values important to health care in the 21st century as caring, holism, health promotion, continuity of care, family-based care, and working in partnership with individual and community agendas (see Chapters 15 and 24).

Patterns of knowing help nurses individualize care tailored to the particular needs of each client (Mead, 2000; Fawcett, Watson, & Neuman, 2001). Issues related to making "the health care system patient centered and performance focused" include:

- "Continuous healing relationships,
- Customization as the source of control

- Shared knowledge and the free flow of information
- Safety as a system priority,
- Anticipation of patient needs rather than reacting to events" (Harris, 2001, p. 86)

In contemporary clinical practice, the client is recognized as a central person on the health care team. There is a clear assumption that clients and family will assume greater responsibility for maintaining health and well-being, as well as for primary self-management of chronic illness. Access to care, client safety, and continuity of care, health promotion, and maintenance of health represent an evolving emphasis in health care delivery. A person centered nursing framework developed by McCormack and McCance (2006) identifies environmental characteristics, pre-requisites and person centered outcomes associated with providing patient centered care.

Frist (2005) asserts that the focus of the 21st century health care system must be on the "patient, such that health care system will ensure that patients have access to the safest and highest-quality care, regardless of how much they earn, where they live, how sick they are, or the color of their skin" (p. 468). The concept of mutuality in treatment planning has been strengthened to include active involvement in shared decision making about treatment (Mead and Bower, 2000).

BOX 1-4	Pew Commission's Recommendations to Nursing Programs: 21 Nursing Competencies Needed for the 21st Century

1. Embrace a personal ethic of social responsibility and service.
2. Exhibit ethical behavior in all professional activities.
3. Provide evidence-based, clinically competent care.
4. Incorporate the multiple determinants of health in clinical care.
5. Apply knowledge of the new sciences.
6. Demonstrate critical thinking, reflection, and problem-solving skills.
7. Understand the role of primary care.
8. Rigorously practice preventive health care.
9. Integrate population-based care and services into practice.
10. Improve access to health care for those with unmet health needs.
11. Practice relationship-centered care with individuals and families.
12. Provide culturally sensitive care to a diverse society.
13. Partner with communities in health care decisions.
14. Use communication and information technology effectively and appropriately.
15. Work in interdisciplinary teams.
16. Ensure care that balances individual, professional, system, and societal needs.
17. Practice leadership.
18. Take responsibility for quality of care and health outcomes at all levels.
19. Contribute to continuous improvement of the health care system.
20. Advocate for public policy that promotes and protects the health of the public.
21. Continue to learn and help others learn.

From Bellack J, O'Neil E: Recreating nursing practice for a new century: recommendations and implications of the Pew Health Professions Commission's final report, *Nursing and Health Care Perspectives* 21(1):20, 2000.

New models of client-centered care can include shift reports in client rooms, reviewing care plans for the day early in the shift with clients, asking about their priorities, and working closely with other health team members to deliver quality care (Jasovsky, Morrow, Clementi, & Hindle, 2010).

SYSTEM ORIENTED CONTINUITY OF CARE

Continuity of care delivered through a networked health care delivery system rather than an individualized clinical approach to health care is quickly becoming the norm in service delivery (see Chapter 24). The Pew Commission (Bellack & O'Neil, 2000) set forth 21 competencies that nurses will need to incorporate into their nursing care to be successful practitioners in the 21st century (Box 1-4). Communication skills and the development of team-based professional interpersonal relationships with clients, other professionals, and families will be key to achieving and integrating these competencies in health care delivery.

ADVANCES IN TECHNOLOGY

Advances in technology have revolutionized health care delivery, documentation, and availability of medical information. With technology, communication is possible to any location at any time. Malloch (2010) notes, "What has not changed is the need for effective personal relationships in the evaluation and selection of new technologies; human to human sensitivity, acknowledgment, and respect for the patient care experience" (p. 1).

Nurses increasingly face the challenge of being present in relationships to clients and other health professionals in a digital age dominated by technology. Technologic advances such as the electronic house call, Internet support groups, and the virtual health examination are still in their infancy but may well take the place of office visits and become a major health care resource in the future, particularly in remote areas (Kinsella, 2003). Telehealth is fast becoming an integral part of the health care system, used both as a live interactive mechanism (particularly in remote areas, where there is a scarcity of health care providers) and as a way to track clinical data. Two important outcomes are reduction of health costs and access to care (Peck, 2005).

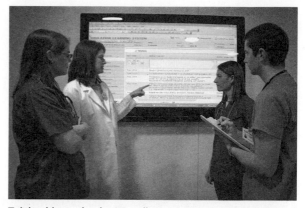

Telehealth technologies allow nurses a new level of interaction with clients and other health providers.

The Internet serves as a vital source of health information for consumers and health care providers, instantly linking them with current scientific and medical breakthroughs in diagnosis and treatment. Sophisticated technology allows health experts in geographically distant areas throughout the world to share information and to draw important conclusions about health care issues in real time. New technologies have the capacity to bring highly trained specialists into the home through the Internet and teleconferencing. Clark (2000) describes a "virtual" application of technology from the perspective of a Canadian nurse caring for a client in a remote area as it might occur in the year 2020.

Case Example

The computer gently hums to life as community health nurse Rachel Muhammat logs into Nursenet. She asks a research partner, a cyberware specialist in London, England, for the results from a trial on neurologic side effects of ocular biochips. Rachel, as part of a 61-member team in 23 countries, is studying 6 clients with the chips. Then it's down to local business. Rachel e-mails information on air contaminant syndrome to a client down the street whose son is susceptible to the condition and tells her about a support group in Philadelphia. She contacts a qigong specialist to see if he can teach the boy breathing exercises and schedules an appointment with an environmental nurse specialist. Moments before her 9:45 appointment, Rachel gets into her El-van and programs it to an address 2 kilometers away. Her patient, Mr. Chan, lost both legs in a subway accident and needs to be prepared for a bionic double-leg transplant. Together, they assess his needs and put together a team of health workers, including a surgeon, physiotherapist, acupuncturist, and home care

Continued

Case Example—cont'd

helpers. She talks to him about the transplant, and they hook up to his virtual reality computer to see and talk to another client who underwent the same procedure. Before leaving, Mr. Chan grasps her hand and thanks her for helping him. Rachel hugs him and urges him to e-mail her if he has any more questions (Sibbald, 1995, p. 3 [quoted in Clark, 2000]).

Positioning Nurses as Key Players

Nursing has had a long and honorable commitment to providing care for poor, marginalized, and vulnerable populations, consistent with the goal of reducing health disparities. Table 1-3 identifies seven conditions and their evolutionary correlates needed to secure a key player role for nurses in the new health care delivery system.

TABLE 1-3	Criteria for Survival of the Nursing Profession Based on Evolutionary Principles
Criteria or Condition	**Evolutionary Principle**
Nursing needs to be relevant.	In nature, an organism will survive only if it occupies a niche, that is, performs a specific role that is needed in its environment.
Nursing must be accountable.	In every environment there is a limited amount of resources. Organisms that are more efficient and use the available resources more effectively are much more likely to be selected by the environment.
Nursing needs to retain its uniqueness while functioning in a multidisciplinary setting.	In nature, an organism will survive only if it is unique. If it ceases to be so, it is in danger of losing its niche or role in the environment. In other words, it might lose out if the new species is slightly better adapted to the role, or if physically similar enough, it might even breed with that species and thus completely lose its identity. Successful organisms must also learn to coexist with many different species so that their role complements that of the other organisms.
Nursing needs to be visible.	In nature, organisms often are required to defend their niche and their territory usually by an outward display that allows other similar species to be aware of their presence. By being "visible," similar species can avoid direct conflict. In addition, visibility is also important for recognition by members of their own species, to allow for the formation of family and social units, based on cooperation and respect.
Nursing needs to have a global impact.	In nature, if a species is to survive, it must make its presence felt not just to its immediate neighbors but to all the members of its environment. Often, this results in a species adapting a unique presence, whether it is a color pattern, smell, or sound.
Nurses need to be innovators.	In evolution, the organisms that survive are, more often than not, innovators that have the flexibility to come up with new and different solutions to rapid changes in environmental conditions.
Nurses need to be both exceptionally competent and strive for excellence.	During evolution, when new niches open up, it is never possible for more than one species to occupy one niche. Only the best adapted and most competent among the competing organisms will survive; all others, even if only slightly less competent, will die.

From Bell (1997) as cited in Gottlieb L, Gottlieb B: Evolutionary principles can guide nursing's future development, *Journal of Advanced Nursing* 28(5):1099, 1998.

SUMMARY

This chapter presents theoretical concepts important to the understanding of the nurse-client relationship. These models bring order to nursing practice, and provide a cognitive structure for developing a body of knowledge for professional nursing and a theoretical basis for nursing research. Four theoretical concepts found in all nursing theories are person, health, nursing, and environment. The art of nursing helps nurses integrate scientific understandings with a personalized approach to individual clients.

Hildegard Peplau's theory of interpersonal relationships form the theoretical basis for understanding the nurse's role in the nurse-client relationship. Concepts from other developmental and psychological theories broaden the nurse's perspective and understanding of client behaviors. Nurses use Erikson's model of psychosocial development to provide nursing care in line with developmental needs of their clients and Maslow's need theory to prioritize care activities. Carl Rogers offered basic concepts concerning the characteristics the nurse needs for developing effective interpersonal relationships with clients. Therapeutic communication is used in the nurse-client relationship as a primary means of achieving treatment goals.

Changes in the health care delivery system require nurses to embrace new skill sets consistent with contemporary health care changes. What nurses bring to the table, the essential values of professional nursing practice—caring relationships with clients, a holistic view of persons, a wide range of scientific and value-based knowledge combined with critical thinking and clinical reasoning skills—remain unchanged. Nurses have an unprecedented opportunity to make a difference and shape the future of nursing practice through communication at every level in health care delivery.

ETHICAL DILEMMA

Note: Refer to Chapter 3, Clinical Judgment: Applying Critical Thinking and Ethical Decision Making, and values clarification as you consider the ethical dilemma.

Countertransference refers to strong feelings that nurses hold about clients that act as a major barrier in therapeutic relationships. These feelings interfere with fully understanding and appreciating the humanness of clients in professional relationships. In the following example, identify what you see as the countertransference issues involved in caring authentically and compassionately for this client. What would you do to resolve the countertransference issues?

Craig Montegue is a difficult client to care for. As his nurse, you find his constant arguments, poor hygiene, and the way he treats his family very upsetting. It is difficult for you to provide him with even the most basic care, and you just want to leave his room as quickly as possible. What are the ethical elements in this situation, and how would you address them in implementing care for Craig?

REFERENCES

Alligood M: *Nursing Theory: Utilization and Application*, ed 4, Maryland Heights, MO, 2010, Mosby Elsevier.

Altmann T: An evaluation of the seminal work of Patricia Benner: theory or philosophy? *Contemp Nurs* 25:114–123, 2007.

American Holistic Nurses Association: *What is holistic nursing?* 2004. Available online: http://www.ahna.org/about/whatis.html.

Anderson H: Postmodern collaborative and person-centered therapies: what would Carl Rogers say? *Journal of Family Therapy* 23:339–360, 2001.

Arnold E: Caring from the graduate student perspective, *International Journal of Human Caring* 1(3):32–42, 1997.

Awa M, Yamashita M: Persons' experience of HIV/AIDS in Japan: application of Margaret Newman's theory, *Int Nurs Rev* 55:454–461, 2008.

Bateson G: *Mind and nature*, New York, 1979, Dutton.

Beck AT: *Cognitive therapy and the emotional disorders*, London, 1991, Penguin Books.

Bell G: *Selection: The Mechanism of Evolution*, New York, 1997, Chapman & Hall.

Bellack J, O'Neil E: Recreating nursing practice for a new century: recommendations and implications of the Pew Health Professions Commission's final report, *Nurs Health Care Perspect* 21(1):14–21, 2000.

Booth K, Kenrick M, Woods S: Nursing knowledge, theory and method revisited, *J Adv Nurs* 26(4):804–811, 1997.

Carper B: Fundamental patterns of knowing in nursing, *ANS Adv Nurs Sci* 1:13–23, 1978.

Clark DJ: Old wine in new bottles: delivering nursing in the 21st century, *J Nurs Scholarsh* 32(1):11–15, 2000.

Crowe M: The nurse-patient relationship: a consideration of its discursive content, *J Adv Nurs* 31(4):962–967, 2000.

Doheny M, Cook C, Stopper M: *The discipline of nursing*, Stamford, CT, 2007, Appleton & Lange.

Donaldson SK, Crowley DM: The discipline of nursing, *Nurs Outlook* 26:113–120, 1978.

Dossey B, Selander L, Beck D, et al: *Florence Nightingale today: healing, leadership, global action*, Silver Spring, MD, 2005, American Nurses Association.

Engebretson J: Cultural constructions of health and illness: recent cultural changes toward a holistic approach, *J Holist Nurs* 21(3):203–227, 2003.

Erikson E: *Childhood and society*, New York, 1950, WW Norton.

Fawcett J: *Contemporary nursing knowledge: Analysis and evaluation of nursing models and theories*, ed 2, Philadelphia, 2005, Davis.

Fawcett J, Watson J, Neuman B, et al: On nursing theory and evidence, *J Nurs Scholarsh* 33(2):115–119, 2001.

Fingeld-Connett D: Qualitative convergence of three nursing concepts: art of nursing, presence and caring, *J Adv Nurs* 63(5):527–534, 2008.

Freud S: *The basic writings of Sigmund Freud* (Brill AA, translator), New York, 1937, Modern Library.

Frist W: Health care in the 21st century, *N Engl J Med* 352:267–272, 2005.

Gottlieb L, Gottlieb B: Evolutionary principles can guide nursing's future development, *J Adv Nurs* 28(5):1099–1105, 1998.

Gramling K: A narrative study of nursing art in critical care, *J Holist Nurs* 22(4):379–398, 2004.

Greene C: A comprehensive theory of the human person from philosophy and nursing, *Nurs Philos* 10(4):263–274, 2009.

Hale-Evans R: *Mind performance hacks*, Seastopol, CA, 2006, O'Reilly Media, Inc.

Harris J: Shaping the system and culture of health care, *Dermatol Nurs* 13(2):86, 2001.

Hegyvary S: An agenda for nursing as a means to improve health, *J Nurs Scholarsh* 39(2):103–104, 2007.

Henderson V: *The nature of nursing*, New York, 1966, Macmillan.

Holtslander L: Patterns of knowing hope: Carper's fundamental patterns as a guide for hope research with bereaved palliative care givers, *Nurs Outlook* 56(4):25–30, 2008.

Institute of Medicine (IOM): *Unequal treatment: confronting racial and ethnic disparities in health care*, Washington, D.C., 2003, National Academies Press.

Institute of Medicine (IOM): *Crossing the quality chasm: a new health system for the 21st century*, Washington, D.C., 2001, National Academies Press.

International Council of Nurses: *The ICN definition of nursing*, [International Council of Nurses website]. 2006. Available online: http://www.icn.ch/definition.htm.

Jasmine T: Art, science or both? Keeping the care in nursing, *Nurs Clin North Am* 44(4):415–421, 2009.

Jasovsky D, Morrow M, Clementi P, et al: Theories in action and how nursing practice changed, *Nurs Sci Q* 23(1):29–38, 2010.

Jung CG: The stages of life. In Campbell J, editor: *The portable Jung*, New York, 1971, Viking.

Kinsella A: Telemedicine connection, *Advance for Providers of Post-Acute Care* (May-June):24–26, 2003.

Kudzma E: Florence Nightingale and health care reform, *Nurs Sci Q* 19(1):61–64, 2006.

Leininger M: *Transcultural care diversity and university: a theory of nursing*, Thorofare, NJ, 1985, Charles B. Slack.

Leininger M: *Transcultural Nursing: Concepts, Theories, Research, and Practice*, ed 3, New York, 2002, McGraw Hill.

Leight S: Starry night: using story to inform aesthetic knowing in women's health nursing, *J Adv Nurs* 37(1):108–114, 2002.

Malloch K: Innovation leadership: new perspectives for new work, *Nurs Clin North Am* 45(1):1–9, 2010.

Marrs J, Lowry L: Nursing theory and practice: connecting the dots, *Nurs Sci Q* 19(1):44–50, 2006.

Maslow A: *Motivation and personality*, ed 2, New York, 1970, Harper & Row.

McCarthy C, Aquino-Russell C: A comparison of two nursing theories in practice: Peplau and Parse, *Nurs Sci Q* 22(1):34–40, 2009.

McCormack B, McCance T: Development of a framework for person centred nursing, *J Adv Nurs* 56(5):472–479, 2006.

Mead N, Bower P: Patient centredness: a conceptual framework and review of the empirical literature, *Soc Sci Med* 51:1087–1110, 2000.

Mead P: Clinical guidelines: Promoting clinical effectiveness or a professional minefield? *J Adv Nurs* 31(1):110–116, 2000.

Meleis A: Being and becoming healthy: the core of nursing knowledge, *Nurs Sci Q* 3(3):107–114, 1990.

Meleis A: *Theoretical nursing: development and progress*, ed 4, Philadelphia, 2006, Lippincott.

Monti E, Tingen M: Multiple paradigms of nursing science. In Cody W, editor: *Philosophical and theoretical perspectives for advanced practice nursing*, ed 4, Sudbury, MA, 2006, Jones and Bartlett Publishers.

Morgan I, Marsh G: Historic and future health promotion contexts for nursing, *Image J Nurs Sch* 30(4):379–383, 1998.

Newman M: *Health as expanding consciousness*, St. Louis MO, 1986, Mosby.

Parse RR: *The human becoming school of thought*, Thousand Oaks, CA, 1998, Sage Publications.

Peck A: Changing the face of standard nursing practice through telehealth and telenursing, *Nurs Adm Q* 29(4):339–343, 2005.

Peplau H: *Interpersonal relations in nursing*, New York, 1952, Putnam.

Peplau H: Peplau's theory of interpersonal relations, *Nurs Sci Q* 10(4):162–167, 1997.

Polit D, Beck C: *Nursing research: generating and assessing evidence for nursing practice*, ed 8, Philadelphia, 2007, Lippincott Williams & Wilkins.

Porter-O'Grady T: A new age for practice: creating the framework for evidence. In Malloch K, Porter-O'Grady T, editors: *Introduction to evidence-based practice in nursing and health care*, ed 2, Sudbury, MA, 2010, Jones and Bartlett Publishers, pp 1–29.

Reed P, Shearer N: *Perspectives on nursing theory*, Philadelphia, 2007, Lippincott.

Rogers C: *On becoming a person*, Boston, 1961, Houghton Mifflin.

Ruesch J: *Therapeutic communication*, New York, 1961, Norton.

Sackett D, Rosenberg W, Gray J, et al: Evidence based medicine: what it is and what it isn't, *Br Med J* 312(7023):71–72, 1996.

Shaller D: *Patient-centered care: what does it take?* October 2007, The Commonwealth Fund. Available online: http://www. commonwealthfund.org/Content/Publications/Fund-Reports/2007/ Oct/Patient-Centered-Care–What-Does-It-Take.aspx. Accessed December 18, 2009.

Sibbald B: 2020 vision, *Can Nurse* 91(3):3, 1995.

Sigelma C, Rider E. Life-Span Human Development, 6th edition. Belvont CA: 2009, Wadsorth Cengage Learning.

Sigma Theta Tau International: *Sigma Theta Tau International's position statement on evidence-based nursing*, [Sigma Theta Tau International's website]. 2003. Available online: http://www.nursingsociety.org.

Smith MJ, Liehr P: Theory-guided translation: emphasizing human connection, *Arch Psychiatr Nurs* 22(3):175–176, 2008.

Sullivan HS: *The interpersonal theory of psychiatry*, New York, 1953, Norton.

United States Department of Health and Human Services: *Healthy people 2010*, McLean, VA, 2000, International Medical Publishing.

Van Achterberg T, Holleman G, Van de Ven M, et al: Promoting evidence-based practice: the roles and activities of professional nurses' associations, *J Adv Nurs* 53(5):605–612, 2006.

Villarruel AM, Bishop TL, Simpson EM, et al: Borrowed theories, shared theories, and the advancement of nursing knowledge, *Nurs Sci Q* 14(2):158–163, 2001.

Walker L, Avant K: *Strategies for theory construction in nursing*, ed 4, Upper Saddle River, NJ, 2005, Pearson Prentice Hall.

Watzlawick P, Beavin-Bavelas J, Jackson D: Some tentative axioms of communication. In *Pragmatics of Human Communication—A Study of Interactional Patterns, Pathologies and Paradoxes*, New York, W. W. Norton, 1967.

Watson J: *Nursing: human science and human care: a theory of nursing,* New York, 1988, National League for Nursing.

Weil A: *Health and healing,* New York, 2004, Houghton Mifflin.

Whall A: The structure of nursing knowledge: analysis and evaluation of practice, middle-range and grand theory. In Fitzpatrick J, Whall A, editors: *Conceptual models of nursing: analysis and application,* ed 4, Stamford, CT, 2004, Appleton & Lange.

World Health Organization (WHO): *International classification of functioning, disability and health,* Geneva, 2001, WHO.

Youngblut J, Brooten D: Evidence-based nursing practice: why is it important? *AACN Clin Issues* 12(4):468–476, 2001.

Zander P: Ways of knowing in nursing: the historical evolution of a concept, *Journal of Theory Construction & Testing* 11(1):7–11, 2007.

CHAPTER 2

Professional Guides to Action in Interpersonal Relationships

Elizabeth Arnold

OBJECTIVES

At the end of the chapter, the reader will be able to:

1. Describe the use of professional standards of care and professional performance standards in nurse-client relationships.
2. Identify regulatory bodies and state laws guiding the conduct of professional nursing practice.
3. Discuss legal standards used in nursing practice.
4. Discuss ethical standards and issues of professional nursing practice.
5. Apply the nursing process and SBAR format to structure professional nursing care.
6. Discuss client privacy, Health Insurance Portability and Accountability Act of 1996 (HIPAA) regulations, confidentiality, and informed consent as guides to action in nurse-client relationships.

This chapter introduces the student to the professional, legal, and ethical standards of practice that provide essential parameters for professional therapeutic activities occurring within the nurse-client relationship. Included in this chapter is an overview of the nursing process, which is used to sequence nursing actions in the nurse-client relationship and as a guide to chart client progress.

BASIC CONCEPTS

STANDARDS AS GUIDES TO ACTION IN CLINICAL NURSING PRACTICE

All legitimate professions have standards of conduct. Nursing's professional, legal, and ethical standards identify principles of professional nursing practice and govern its actions. Professional nurses, regardless of setting, are expected to follow these standards in

their clinical practice, research, and education. The Code of Ethics for Nurses (ANA, 2001) establishes principled guidelines designed to protect the integrity of clients related to their care, health, safety, and rights. Nurses are held to federal and state regulatory laws for hospital and other health care facilities, and to the nursing standards, policies, and procedures of the health care facility in which they are employed (Guido, 2009). Professional nursing practice is legally regulated through state licensure, with additional education and national certification required for advanced practice. The American Nurses Credentialing Center (ANCC) certifies nurses for advanced practice in a nursing specialty once the applicant completes all requirements for national certification. Each state sets forth professional nursing standards and interpretive guidelines through its Nurse Practice Act. Professional, ethical, and legal standards are complementary but distinct guides to action in nurse-client relationships. They each reflect societal values.

PROFESSIONAL STANDARDS OF CARE AND NURSING PERFORMANCE STANDARDS

The national professional organization for registered nurses (ANA), publishes standards of care and nursing performance that help ensure professional nursing competence and safe ethical clinical practice. Professional standards of practice serve the dual purpose of providing a standardized benchmark for evaluating the quality of their nursing care and offering the consumer a common means of understanding nursing as a professional service relationship. They inform the public what they can expect from professional nurses.

Specified competencies identified in nursing standards represent a uniform legal yardstick against which care can be measured. In legal situations, professional standards of practice would be used as a first-line defense, in conjunction with what a "reasonable and prudent nurse" would do in a similar nursing situation, to determine nursing accountability. Failure to adhere to established nursing practice and professional performance standards could result in a negative civil judgment against a professional nurse.

The Joint Commission (TJC, 2007) mandates that written nursing policies with specific standards of care be available on all nursing units. Professional standards of practice provide definitions of the minimum competencies needed for quality professional nursing practice Presented as principled statements, they designate the knowledge and clinical skills required of nurses to practice competently and safely.

Professional performance standards describe a competent level of professional role behaviors related to quality of care, practice evaluation, continuing education, collegiality, collaboration, ethics, research, resource utilization, and leadership. Nurses are expected to competently perform professional role behaviors consistent with published standards and appropriate to their education, position, and the practice setting. They are expected to refrain from performing any nursing activities for which they are not trained.

Professional nurses are accountable for adhering to professional standards regardless of their particular nursing role or the acuity of individual nursing circumstances. Additional specialty practice guidelines provide a customized set of standards for care of specific populations (e.g., children, the elderly, and psychiatric patients) and specialty areas of clinical practice (e.g., acute care or perioperative nursing).

Nursing's Social Policy Statement

Nursing's Social Policy Statement spells out the discipline's covenant with society and contractual obligations for care (LaSala, 2009). Nursing is conceptualized as a dynamic profession, operating within a social context, and being responsive to the ever-changing nature of societal health care needs. The American Nurses Association Social Policy Statement (American Nurses Association, 2003) describes the social values and assumptions inherent in professional nursing practice and identifies nursing's stewardship commitment to society. The ANA recently published a revised edition of Nursing's Social Policy Statement: The Essence of the Profession in 2010 (American Nurses Association, 2010).

REGULATORY BODIES: STATE BOARDS OF NURSING

Each state has its own Board of Nursing. The National Council of State Boards of Nursing states, *"Boards of Nursing* are state governmental agencies that are responsible for the regulation of nursing practice in each respective state. Boards of Nursing are authorized to enforce the Nurse Practice Act, develop administrative rules/regulations and other responsibilities per the Nurse Practice Act" (National Council of State Boards of Nursing, 2008).

In addition to issuing professional licenses to practice nursing, the state Board of Nursing is responsible for establishing and maintaining standards for safe nursing care in that state, and monitoring nurses' compliance with state laws governing their practice. Each state Board of Nursing has the authority to take disciplinary action against the licenses of those nurses who have exhibited unsafe nursing practice.

Nurse Practice Acts

Nurse Practice Acts are the most important statutory laws governing the provision of professional nursing care through the nurse-client relationship. *Nurse Practice Acts* are legal documents that communicate professional nursing's scope of practice, and outline nurses' rights, responsibilities, and licensing requirements in providing care to individual clients, families, and communities. Nurses appointed by the governor to serve on a state Board of Nursing develop the statutes' governing nursing practice in each state.

Each state's Board of Nursing develops and executes its own Nurse Practice Act. If a nurse practices in one state and then moves to another, the nurse has to follow the Nurse Practice Act guidelines in his or her new state of residence. Because all Nurse Practice Acts reflect standards of nursing care developed by the ANA, they do not usually differ significantly, but nurses are advised to have a working knowledge of the Nurse Practice Act in each state of planned employment.

Nurse Practice Acts authorize state boards of nursing to interpret the legal boundaries of safe nursing practice and give them the authority to punish violations, with suspension or loss of professional licensure.

Scope of Practice

Scope of practice is a broad term referring to the legal and ethical boundaries of practice for professional nurses The ANA (2010) recently published its latest revised edition of *Nursing: Scope and Standards of Nursing*. In addition to national standards, each state's Board of Nursing establishes the scope of nursing practice within its state. Scope of practice is defined in written state statutes. Scope of practice in most states reflects different levels of nursing practice, based on the nurse's education, special skill training, supervised experience, state and national professional credentials, and appropriate professional experience.

Scope of practice includes a broad range of nursing activities such as providing direct care, effectively managing emergency and crisis situations, administering medications, monitoring changes in client conditions, teaching and coaching clients and their families, prioritizing and coordinating care, delegating of nursing tasks, and supervision of unlicensed personnel.

Professional Licensure

The registered nurse's professional license ensures that each individual nurse has successfully completed an accredited nursing program and can demonstrate the knowledge, skills, and competencies to function as a health provider of safe, effective nursing care. All graduates must pass a national licensure examination (National Council Licensure Examination [NCLEX]) that tests core nursing knowledge before being granted a professional RN license to practice nursing. Practicing nursing without a license can result in legal prosecution.

Nursing licensure helps maintain standards for nursing. Although the NCLEX is a national examination, each nurse must apply for RN state licensure through the state Board of Nursing in his or her state of residence to practice as a registered nurse.

Compact State Recognition Model

In 2000, the National Council of State Boards of Nursing (NCSBN) developed a mutual recognition model of nurse licensure, permitting registered nurses licensed and residing in a compact state to practice in other compact states without obtaining a second license. The multistate license is issued by the compact state in which the nurse resides. The registered nurse is held to the state's nursing practice laws and regulations in which he or she is actually practicing at the time. The multistate license is valid only between compact states. Over the past few years, more than half the nation's state boards of nursing have enacted the RN and LPN/VN nurse licensure compact legislation. This legislation is particularly helpful for nurses working in states with large rural populations and few nurses.

LEGAL STANDARDS

Professional nurses are held legally accountable for all aspects of the nursing care they provide to clients and families, including documentation and referral. As the registered nurse's professional responsibilities have increased in depth and complexity, requiring greater levels of clinical judgment, so has the potential for legal liability (Aiken, 2004). Of special relevance to the nurse-client relationship are issues of professional liability, informed consent, and confidentiality.

Classifications of Laws in Health Care

Nurses need to take into consideration two types of law related to the care they provide for clients and families. *Statutory laws* are legislated laws, drafted and enacted at federal or state levels. Medicare and Medicaid amendments to the Social Security Act are examples of federal statutory laws. Nurse practice acts are examples of statutory laws enacted at the state level (Aiken, 2004).

Civil laws are developed through court decisions, which are created through precedents, rather than written statutes. Most infractions for malpractice and negligence are covered by civil law and are referred to as *torts*. A tort is defined as a private civil action that causes personal injuries to a private party. Deliberate intent is not present. Four elements are necessary to qualify for a claim of malpractice or negligence.

- The professional duty was owed to client (professional relationship)
- A breach of duty occurred in which the nurse failed to conform to an accepted standard of care
- Causality in which a failure to act by professional was a proximate cause of the resulting injury
- Actual damage or injuries resulted from breach of duty (Dimond, 2008).

Definitions of negligent actions and related examples are found in Table 2-1.

TABLE 2-1	Definition and Examples of Negligent Actions
Definition of Negligent Action	**Example**
Performing a nursing action that a prudent nurse would not perform	Carrying out a physician's order that would have been questioned by other reasonably prudent nurses in similar circumstances
Failing to perform a nursing action that a reasonably prudent nurse would perform	Failing to report suspected physical or sexual child abuse
Failure to provide routine or customary care	Failing to check vital signs before and after surgery; failing to perform postpartum checks on a client
Exhibiting conduct that a reasonably prudent nurse would recognize as posing an unreasonable risk to a client	Failing to give accurate information in a manner that the client can understand regarding choice of treatment and known adverse effects; sharing confidential information with a client's family or workplace without the client's permission
Failing to protect a client from unnecessary harm	Not putting up the guardrails on a bed with a newly diagnosed client suffering from a stroke; allowing unlicensed personnel to do a nursing procedure without appropriate experience or supervision

The nurse is bound legally by the principles of civil tort law to provide reasonable standard of care, defined as a level of care that a reasonably prudent nurse would provide in a similar situation (Catalano, 2008). If taken to court, this standard would be the benchmark against which the nurse's actions would be judged.

Criminal law is reserved for cases in which there was intentional misconduct, and/or the action taken by the health care provider represents a serious violation of professional standards of care (Scott, 2006). The most common violation of nurses related to criminal law is failure to renew a professional nursing license, which, in effect, means that a nurse is practicing nursing without a license (Calalano, 2008).

Legal Liability in Nurse-Client Relationships

In the nurse-client relationship, the nurse is responsible for maintaining the professional conduct of the relationship. Examples of unprofessional conduct in the nurse-client relationship include:

- Breaching client confidentiality
- Verbally or physically abusing a client
- Assuming nursing responsibility for actions without having sufficient preparation
- Delegating care to unlicensed personnel, which could result in client injury
- Following a doctor's order that would result in client harm
- Failing to assess, report, or document changes in client health status
- Falsifying records
- Failing to obtain informed consent
- Failure to question a physician's orders, if they are not clear
- Failure to provide required health teaching
- Failure to provide for client safety (e.g., not putting the side rails up on a client with a stroke)

Scott (2006) claims that effective and frequent communication with clients and other providers is one of the best ways to avoid and/or minimize the possibility of claims of malpractice or negligence. In-depth communication provided in simple layperson's language about what the nurse is doing, the status of the client's health care, the meaning of diagnostic tests for client care, and so forth allows clients to make more informed choices and leads to greater satisfaction.

ETHICAL STANDARDS AND ISSUES

Nurses have an ethical accountability to the clients they serve that extends beyond their legal responsibility in everyday nursing situations. Ethical issues of particular relevance to the nurse-client relationship relate to caring for clients in ambulatory managed care settings, the rights of clients participating in research, caring for mature minors, client education, right to die issues, transfer to long-term care of elderly clients, and telehealth nursing (Guido, 2009).

American Nurses Association Code of Ethics

The revised ANA Code of Ethics for Nurses (ANA, 2001) with interpretive statements provides ethical guidelines for nurses designed to protect client rights, provide a mechanism for professional accountability, and educate professionals about sound ethical conduct. The new provisions of the Code of Ethics for Nurses are identified in Box 2-1. Similar codes of ethics for nurses exist in other nations. For example, in Canada, nursing practice is guided by the Canadian Nurses Association Code of Ethics for Registered Nurses (1997).

The ANA Code of Ethics for Nurses provides a broad conceptual framework outlining the principled behaviors and value beliefs expected of professional nurses in delivering health care to individuals, families, and communities. Ethical standards of behavior require a clear understanding of the multidimensional aspects of an ethical dilemma, including intangible human factors that make each situation unique (e.g., personal and cultural values or resources).

When an ethical dilemma cannot be resolved through interpersonal negotiation, an ethics committee composed of biomedical experts reviews the case and makes recommendations (Otto, 2000). Of particular importance to the nurse-client relationship are ethical directives related to the nurse's primary commitment to

- The client's welfare
- Respect for client autonomy
- Recognition of each individual as unique and worthy of respect, advocacy
- Truth telling

Exercise 2-1 provides an opportunity to consider the many elements in an ethical nursing dilemma.

Advance Directives

In 1991, the U.S. Congress passed the Patient Self-Determination Act. This legislation requires health care institutions to inform their clients, on admission, of their right to choose whether to have life-prolonging treatment should they become mentally or physically unable to make this decision (Westley & Briggs, 2004). An *advance directive* is a legal document, executed by a competent client or legal proxy, specifically

---

BOX 2-1   American Nurses Association Code of Ethics for Nurses

1. The nurse, in all professional relationships, practices with compassion and respect for the inherent dignity, worth and uniqueness of every individual, unrestricted by considerations of social or economic status, personal attributes, or the nature of health problems.
2. The nurse's primary commitment is to the patient, whether an individual, family, group, or community.
3. The nurse promotes, advocates for, and strives to protect the health, safety, and rights of the patient.
4. The nurse is responsible and accountable for individual nursing practice and determines the appropriate delegation of tasks consistent with the nurse's obligation to provide optimum patient care.
5. The nurse owes the same duties to self as to others, including the responsibility to preserve integrity and safety, to maintain competence, and to continue personal and professional growth.
6. The nurse participates in establishing, maintaining, and improving health care environments and conditions of employment conducive to the provision of quality health care and consistent with the values of the profession through individual and collective action.
7. The nurse participates in the advancement of the profession through contributions to practice, education, administration, and knowledge development.
8. The nurse collaborates with other health professionals and the public in promoting community, national, and international efforts to meet health needs.
9. The profession of nursing, as represented by associations and their members, is responsible for articulating nursing values, for maintaining the integrity of the profession and its practice, and for shaping social policy.

Reprinted from ANA (2001), by permission.

EXERCISE 2-1	Applying the Code of Ethics for Nurses to Professional and Clinical Situations

Purpose: To help students identify applications of the Code of Ethics for Nurses.

Procedure:
Break into small groups of four or five students. Consider the following clinical scenarios:*

1. Mrs. Jones has consented to participate in a phase I clinical trial for her cancer. She tells you that she feels very lucky to have met the criteria because now she has a good chance of "beating the cancer."
2. Barbara Kohn is a 75-year-old woman who lives with her son and daughter-in-law. She reveals to you that her daughter-in-law keeps her locked in her room when she has to go out because she does not want her to get in trouble. She asks you not to say anything as that will only get her into trouble.
3. The nursing supervisor asks you to "float" to another unit that will require some types of skills that you believe you do not have the knowledge or skills to perform. When you explain your problem, she tells you that she understands, but the unit is short staffed and she really needs you to do this.

4. Bill Jackson is an elderly client who suffered a stroke and is uncommunicative. He is not expected to live. The health care team is considering placement of a feeding tube based on his wife's wishes. His wife agrees that he probably won't survive, but wants the feeding tube just in case the doctors are wrong.
5. Dr. Holle criticizes a nurse in front of a client and the client's family.
   Share each ethical dilemma with the group and collaboratively come up with a resolution that the group agrees on, using the nurse's code of ethics to work through the situation.

Discussion:
1. What types of difficulty did your group encounter in resolving different scenarios?
2. What type of situation offers the most challenge ethically?
3. Were there any problems in which the code of ethics was not helpful?
4. How can you use what you learned in this exercise in your nursing practice?

*An alternative would be to use an actual ethical dilemma you have experienced either as a student nurse, as a patient, or with a family member in a clinical situation.

identifying individual preferences for the level of care at end of life, related to treatment, medications, hydration, and nutrition (Basanta, 2002). Advance directives allow individuals to specify what actions should be taken on their behalf should they be unable to make health-related decisions. Types of advance directives are identified in Table 2-2. Because life-threatening medical emergencies can occur at any time, all adults—even the healthiest—can benefit from having advance directives in place concerning preferred end-of-life care. Advance

TABLE 2-2	Types of Advance Directives
Living will	Documents the client's preferences for medical treatment, artificial life support, nutrition, use of antibiotics, pain medication) should the client be unable or incompetent to state them (Legal status of living wills varies from state to state.)
Medical power of attorney for health care decisions	Legal document with designation of a proxy who is authorized to make health care decisions for a person should the individual be unable to express his or her wishes
Durable power of attorney	Legal document with designation of a proxy authorized to make financial decisions and to represent the client's interests should the client be unable to do so; durable power of attorney can be revoked in writing at any time, as long as the client is competent
Do-not-resuscitate (DNR) orders	Written directions about not resuscitating the client if the client's breathing or heartbeat stops
Durable mental health power of attorney	Legal document with designation of a proxy who is authorized to make mental health care decisions for a person should the individual be unable to do so because of mental symptoms

EXERCISE 2-2	Role Playing with Advance Directives

Purpose: To help students understand advance directives and their use in health care.

Procedure:

1. Obtain a copy of an advance directive from your hospital, or from the web.
2. Review the advance directive, and then in groups of 3 students, role play introducing the advance directive with one person taking the role of the client, another of the client's spouse or sibling, and the third taking the role of the nurse.

Case Study:

1. Greg Atkins has been diagnosed with stage IV colon cancer. He has metastasis to the liver and lung, and has been growing gradually weaker. This is his first admission to the hospital. He has been advised to get his affairs in order, as he is not expected to live too much longer. He is discouraged by his latest report as he is not ready to die.

Discussion:

1. How difficult was it to introduce the topic of the advance directive to the client and family?
2. What made it harder or easier to discuss the advance directive?
3. How could you use this experience in your clinical practice?

directives can be revoked or revised at any time by its author. Exercise 2-2 provides an opportunity to understand the use of advance directives in clinical practice.

Psychiatric advance directives are legal, written documents used by people with mental illness to indicate their preference for treatment in the event that they are unable to make decisions about treatment because of mental symptoms (Vuckovich, 2003). A psychiatric advance directive specifies the person who the client wants to accept legal responsibility for making clinical decisions if the client is unable to do so. The document can identify the client's preferences for medication, treatment, and treatment setting. Having an advance directive in place helps decrease family anxiety and provides direction for health care, endorsed by the client.

APPLICATIONS

The most common configuration for collecting, organizing, and analyzing data, and for sharing information with other professionals is the nursing process. The nursing process is an interpersonal, client-centered process. Assessment data, nursing diagnosis, and goals for treatment are systematically documented on treatment plans that can be easily shared with nurses and other health professionals.

USING THE NURSING PROCESS IN NURSE-CLIENT RELATIONSHIPS

The nursing process is the primary framework used to structure and organize nursing care. Nurses use the nursing process to apply problem-solving strategies to complex health problems and to develop individualized care plans. The Joint Commission has identified six interrelated elements required of the nursing care plan; these are presented in Box 2-2.

The nursing process consists of five progressive phases: assessment, problem identification and diagnosis, outcome identification and planning, implementation, and evaluation. As a dynamic, systematic clinical

---

Developing an Evidence-Based Practice

Shapiro S: Evaluating clinical decision rules, *Western Journal of Nursing Research* 271(5):655–664, 2005.

This study examines the role of decision support tools needed to combine different clinical evidence into bedside tools for practice.

Results: Clinical decision-making tools are similar to clinical pathways and treatment algorithms used to guide treatment and nursing care. To be effective, clinical decision rules (CDRs) must follow strict protocols and be research based, valid, and reflective of multiple sources of data. The impact of CDRs on client outcomes and costs of care is measured through implementation trials and cost-effectiveness analysis.

Application to Your Clinical Practice: In today's health care arena, nurses find themselves increasingly dependent on methodologies developed to standardized practice protocols based on the best research evidence currently available. What do you see as the role of CDRs for clinical practice? What would be important to consider in protecting the integrity of the rules as an evidence-based rationale for improving client outcomes?

BOX 2-2	Joint Commission on Accreditation of Health Care Organizations Requirements for Nursing Care Plans

1. Initial assessment, modified as needed
2. Nursing diagnosis of patient care needs
3. Specified nursing interventions that address client health care needs
4. Provision of appropriate nursing interventions
5. Documentation of the client's response and achievement of treatment outcomes
6. Discharge plan providing direction to client and others involved in care to manage continuing health care needs after discharge

From TJC (1991).

management tool, it functions as a primary means of directing the sequence, planning, implementation, and evaluation of nursing care to achieve specific health goals. Communication plays an important role in all aspects of the nursing process by

- Helping clients to promote, maintain, or restore health, or to achieve a peaceful death
- Facilitating client management of difficult health care issues through communication
- Providing quality nursing care in a safe and efficient manner

The nursing process is closely aligned with meeting professional nursing standards in the total care of the client. Table 2-3 illustrates the relationship.

TABLE 2-3	Relationship of the Nursing Process to Professional Nursing Standards in the Nurse-Client Relationship
Assessment	**Related Nursing Standard**
Collects data	The nurse collects data throughout the nursing process related to client strengths, limitations, available resources, and changes in the client's condition.
Analyzes data	The nurse organizes cluster behaviors and makes inferences based on subjective and objective client data, combined with personal and scientific nursing knowledge.
Verifies data	The nurse verifies data and inferences with the client to ensure validity.
Diagnosis	
Identifies health care needs/problems and formulates biopsychosocial statements	The nurse develops a comprehensive biopsychosocial statement that captures the essence of the client's health care needs/problems and validates the accuracy of the statement with the client and family; this statement becomes the basis for the nursing diagnoses.
Establishes nursing diagnosis	The nurse develops relevant nursing diagnoses and prioritizes them based on the client's most immediate needs in the current health care situation.
Outcome Identification and Planning	
Identifies expected outcomes	The nurse and client mutually and realistically develop expected outcomes based on client needs, strengths, and resources.
Specifies short-term goals	The nurse and client mutually develop realistic short-term goals and choose actions to support achievement of expected outcomes.
Implementation	
Takes agreed-on action	The nurse encourages, supports, and validates the client in taking agreed-on action to achieve goals and expected outcomes through integrated, therapeutic nursing interventions and communication strategies.
Evaluation	
Evaluates goal achievement	The nurse and client mutually evaluate attainment of expected outcomes and survey each step of the nursing process for appropriateness, effectiveness, adequacy, and time efficiency, modifying the plan as indicated by evaluation.

The nursing process begins with the nurse's first encounter with a client and family, and ends with discharge, referral, or both. There is an ordered sequence of nursing activities, with each activity linked to the trustworthiness of the activity that preceded it. Although the sequence of activities follows a distinctive order, each phase is flexible, flowing into and overlapping with other phases of the nursing process. For example, in providing a designated nursing intervention, the nurse might discover a more complex need than what was originally assessed. This could require a modification in the nursing diagnosis, identified outcome, intervention, or the need for a referral.

The nursing process is not complete until treatment outcomes and client responses are documented on the client's chart using correct spelling and terminology. Nurses are expected to report all relevant data to appropriate health care personnel at regular intervals and when there is a change in the client's condition.

ASSESSMENT

A client-centered approach to assessment uses a systematic, dynamic process to gather data about the client seeking service. The assessment process begins when when you first meet the client and family. Introducing yourself and explaining the purpose of the assessment interview helps put the client at ease and sets the stage for the information that needs to be gathered. The next step is to ask the client to tell his or her story as it relates to the current request for nursing services. A simple statement, such as "Can you tell me what prompted you to seek treatment at this time?" usually is sufficient to start the conversation. Clients sometimes seek treatment for reasons that one would not ordinarily expect, so this type of open-ended question provides valuable information that otherwise might not emerge so quickly.

The intake assessment, usually completed on admission to the health care agency, serves as baseline data. Using open-ended and focused questions, you should collect data about

- The current problem for which the client seeks treatment
- The client's perception of his or her health patterns
- Presence of other health risk and protective factors
- Relevant social, occupational, and family history
- The client's medical and psychiatric history (e.g., previous hospitalizations, family history, medical and psychiatric treatment, and medications)

- The client's coping patterns
- Level and availability of the client's support system

Assessment of client needs should take the client's entire experience of an illness or injury into account, rather than simply focusing on clinical data related to the diagnosis. This is what is meant by "patient-centered" care. The behavior, attitude, and appearance of the client also are important sources of information. For example, does the client appear anxious, angry, apathetic, lethargic, cooperative, or uncooperative?

Assessment data should reflect behavioral observation and information from as many sources as is needed for complete accuracy. Sources of data include interview, history, physical assessment, review of records, family interviews, and in some instances, contact with previous health care providers, schools, or other referral sources. As new information becomes available, nurses are expected to refine and update the original assessment.

Two types of data are collected during an assessment interview. **Subjective data** refers to the client's perception of data and what the client or family says about the data (e.g., "I have a severe pain in my chest"). Client data about alternative forms of treatment, medications, and previously used care systems are relevant pieces of information. **Objective data** refers to data that are directly observable or verifiable through physical examination or tests (e.g., an abnormal electrocardiogram). Combined, these data will present a complete picture of the client's health problem.

Observations of the client's appearance and nonverbal behaviors can help nurses make inferences. An inference is an educated guess about the meaning of an observed behavior or statement. To be sure that the inference represents a correct interpretation of an observation or statement, you must validate the data with the client. For example, if a client is withdrawn and distractible, the nurse may infer that the client is struggling with an internal emotional issue. To validate this inference, you might comment, "You seem withdrawn, as though something is troubling you. Is that true for you right now?"

You also can use *data cues,* defined as small pieces of data that would not reveal much when taken by themselves but, when considered within the total assessment picture, can lead the nurse to ask further questions (Avant, 1991). For example, hesitancy about a certain topic, complaints of hunger or thirst, dry skin, or agitation is a data cue that can help nurses to seek a fuller explanation.

The assessment should consider more than client problems. Appraisal of client strengths is an important dimension of the assessment process as it provides a built-in resource asset for resolving health problems. Identifying client strengths is particularly important in today's health care environment, when clients have to assume much more responsibility for their health care than previously. Analysis of the client's support systems including level of utilization, availability, and social role is relevant data, as is the client's spiritual or philosophical beliefs and values. Environmental, economic, and legal factors also should be included when related to the client's health and well-being.

Throughout the assessment phase, you will need to validate the information you receive from the client and significant others to make sure that the data are complete and accurate. Ask the client for confirmation that your perceptions and problem analysis are correct periodically throughout the assessment interview, and summarize your impressions at the end. An assessment summary should highlight important elements in ways that are easily understood and retrievable by everyone involved in the client's care. After the summary, you should thank the client or health informant for giving you the information, with a brief explanation of what will happen with this information. Respectful, regular communication represents an important intersection between the nurse-client relationship and the nursing process.

Once the assessment is complete, the next step is to analyze the information and identify gaps in the data collection or content. One way to do this is to compare individual client data with normal health standards, behavior patterns, and developmental norms. Gordon's 11 Functional Health Patterns (Box 2-3) provide a useful structure for clustering assessment data and help direct the choice of nursing diagnoses. The determination of whether a pattern is functional or dysfunctional is based on established norms for age and sociocultural standards (Gordon, 2007).

In each clinical situation, you should take individual differences and preferences into consideration. For example, maintaining a sufficient intake of food needs to be assessed in terms of what is adequate intake for an individual on the basis of age, activity, height-to-weight ratio, and current health status. Nutritional needs for an active teenager are greater than those for an older, sedentary adult. The nurse

BOX 2-3	Gordon's Functional Health Patterns

1. Health perception-health management pattern
2. Nutritional-metabolic pattern
3. Elimination pattern
4. Activity-exercise pattern
5. Sleep-rest pattern
6. Cognitive-perceptual pattern
7. Self-perception-self-concept pattern
8. Role-relationship pattern
9. Sexuality-reproductive pattern
10. Coping-stress tolerance pattern
11. Value-belief pattern

would ask different specific questions of a client with diabetes, anorexia, or obesity regarding nutritional intake and food choices than of those for whom potential deviations would not appear to be an issue.

Environmental factors such as socioeconomic status and culture can influence the nature of a client's health care needs. For example, diet choices and lack of prenatal care can represent financial constraints, rather than preference. Lack of knowledge about health care options, access, and experience are additional issues that nurses need to consider.

Documentation of relevant problems, observations, and assessments form the basis for planning care. A direct relationship among assessment data, nursing diagnosis, treatment goals, and intervention strategies should exist. Health care concerns judged potentially responsive to nursing intervention form the basis for the selection of nursing diagnoses.

PLANNING
Nursing Diagnosis

The planning phase begins with the development and prioritization of relevant nursing diagnoses related to identified nursing problems. Nursing diagnoses is the term used to describe the client's human responses to medical diagnoses (Carpenito-Moyet, 2008). They should complement, not compete, with the actual medical diagnosis of a health problem.

The nursing diagnosis consists of three parts: problem, cause, and evidence (North American Nursing Diagnosis Association [NANDA], 2005).

- *Problem:* A statement identifying a health problem or alteration in a client's health status, requiring nursing intervention. Using a list of the most recent NANDA diagnoses, you would pick a

NANDA diagnosis that best represents the identified problem or potential problem.

- *Cause:* A statement specifying the probable causative or risk factors contributing to the existence or maintenance of the health care problem. The cause of a problem can be psychosocial, physiologic, situational, cultural, or environmental in nature. The phrase "related to" (R/T) serves to connect the problem and causative statements. Example: "Impaired communication related to a cerebrovascular accident."
- *Evidence:* A statement identifying the clinical evidence (behaviors, signs, symptoms) that support the diagnosis. An example of a nursing diagnosis statement would be "Impaired verbal communication related to a cerebrovascular accident, as manifested by incomplete sentences and slurred words."

The nursing diagnosis should be written in such clear, precise language that any member of the interdisciplinary health care team can look at the statement and be able to identify relevant client issues.

Nurses use Maslow's Hierarchy of Needs (see Chapter 1) to prioritize goals and objectives. Examples of nursing problems associated with each level of Maslow's hierarchy are included in Table 2-4. Priority attention should be given to the most immediate, life-threatening problems. You also should consider what the client sees as his or her priorities, and incorporate this information in your prioritization. Otherwise, you and your client may be working at cross-purposes.

Nurses may be able to address more than one nursing diagnosis at a time, because attention to several interconnected nursing diagnoses can often serve the same outcome. In addition to identifying and prioritizing nursing diagnoses, nurses are expected to monitor progress and look for potential complications accompanying nursing diagnoses. Examples of monitoring include vital signs, hydration, potential fluid imbalances, electrolytes, intravenous (IV) infusions associated with health issues requiring nursing diagnosis for resolution. Clearly written nursing diagnoses helps to ensure continuity and an ordered approach to meeting the individualized needs of the client (Carpenito-Moyet, 2008). Exercise 2-3 provides practice in considering cultural, age, and gender-related themes when using the nursing process with different types of clients.

Outcome Identification

Shaughnessy (1997) defines a health care outcome as "the change in health status between a baseline time point and a final time point" (p. 1225). The outcome refers to the result or end product of an identified nursing action. Some outcomes are unexpected. When this circumstance occurs, either the assessment failed to reveal a critical piece of data, the diagnosis or other issue was not validated with the client or family, the associated risks or plans for continuity of care were not factored into the treatment goals, or the treatment plan was not executed as collaboratively developed by the stakeholders in the process. Sometimes factors beyond the control of the client and health care provider interfere, for example, a change in the client's physical or mental status. At any point in the process, ongoing assessment data can be used to revise the diagnosis, the plan itself, or implementation to meet the emerging needs in the clinical situation.

Clients should be involved in a shared decision-making process with health care providers in choosing relevant goals and outcomes (Kerr, 2009). Evidence of shared decision making can be documented with a simple statement, such as "Client states that she is satisfied that she made the right decision to decline surgery at this time."

Outcome criteria need to take into account the client's culture and life situation, present mental status, strengths and limitations, and available resources. Important client values and preferences should be factored into the development of relevant outcome criteria. Time limits need to be realistic so that the client can be successful.

Outcomes should be client-centered (e.g., "The client will...") and described in specific, measurable

TABLE 2-4	Identifying Nursing Problems Associated with Maslow's Hierarchy of Needs
Physiologic survival needs	Circulation, food, intake/output, physical comfort, rest
Safety/Security needs	Domestic abuse, fear, anxiety, environmental hazards, housing
Love and belonging	Lack of social support, loss of significant person or pet, grief
Self-esteem needs	Loss of a job, inability to perform normal activities, change in position or expectations
Self-actualization	Inability to achieve personal goals

EXERCISE 2-3   Using the Nursing Process as a Framework in Clinical Situations

Purpose: To help students develop skills in considering cultural, age, and gender role issues in assessing each client's situation and developing relevant nursing diagnoses.

Procedure:

1. In small groups of three to four students, discuss how you might assess and incorporate differences in client/family values, knowledge, beliefs, and cultural background in delivery of care for each of the following clients. Indicate what other types of information you would need to make a complete assessment.
2. Identify and prioritize nursing diagnoses for each client to ensure client-centered care.
   a. Michael Sterns was in a skiing accident. He is suffering from multiple internal injuries, including head injury. His parents have been notified and are flying in to be with him.
   b. Lo Sun Chen is a young Chinese woman admitted for abdominal surgery. She has been in this country for only 8 weeks and speaks very little English.
   c. Maris LaFonte is a 17-year-old unmarried woman admitted for the delivery of her first child. She has had no prenatal care.
   d. Stella Watkins is an 85-year-old woman admitted to a nursing home after suffering a broken hip.

Discussion:

1. In what ways might the needs of each client be different based on age, gender role, or cultural background? How would you account for the differences?
2. Were there any common themes in the types of information each group decided it needed to make a complete assessment?
3. How could you use what you learned from this exercise in your clinical practice?

---

terms. An appropriate treatment outcome for a client after surgery might be: "The client will show no signs of infection as evidenced by the incision being well-approximated and free of redness and swelling, normal temperature, and white blood cell count within normal limits by 9/21/09." Nursing outcomes should be

- Based on diagnoses
- Documented in measurable terms
- Developed collaboratively with the client and other health providers
- Realistic and achievable

Each treatment outcome specifies the action or behavior that the client will demonstrate once the health problem is resolved. Outcome criteria are stated as long- and short-term treatment goals. Using measurable action verbs to describe what the client will be doing to achieve a short-term goal is key to effective identification of treatment outcomes; for example, "The client will take his medicine, as prescribed" is measurable: He either takes his medicine or he does not. Other measurable verbs include "perform," "identify," "discuss," and "demonstrate." Broad-spectrum verbs such as "understand," "know," and "learn" are not easily measurable and should not be used. Note the conditions or circumstances for outcome achievement "as prescribed" is specifically identified. Documentation of clinical outcomes should include client response.

Planning

The care plan serves as the structural framework for providing safe quality care. Each care plan should be individualized to reflect client values, clinical needs, and preferences. The care plan provides for continuity of care and supplies a concrete basis for supportive documentation of client response. The care plan is dynamic, meaning that it needs to be continuously updated as the client's condition and health needs change.

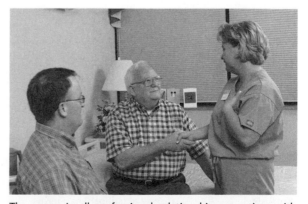

The nurse, in all professional relationships, practices with compassion and respect for the inherent dignity, worth, and uniqueness of every individual.

Implementation

During the implementation phase, the client and nurse manage the care plan through specified nursing interventions and corresponding client actions. McCloskey and Bulechek (2000) define **nursing intervention** as "any treatment, based upon clinical judgment and knowledge, that a nurse performs to enhance patient/client outcomes. Nursing interventions include both direct and indirect care, nurse-initiated, physician-initiated, and other provider-initiated treatments" (p. xix). Interventions appropriate to the purposes of the nurse-client relationship include giving direct physical, psychological, social, and spiritual support; health teaching; collaborating with other health professionals on behalf of the client; continuing to make ongoing assessments; documenting client responses; and updating or revising the care plan as needed.

Nursing interventions can be classified as independent, dependent, or collaborative (Snyder, Egan, & Nojima, 1996). Independent interventions are those that nurses can provide without a physician's order or direction from another health professional. Independent nursing interventions are permitted under Nurse Practice Acts and are protected through professional licensure and law. Many forms of direct care assistance, health education, health promotion strategies, and counseling fall into this category, and nurses are particularly well equipped to provide these functions. Dependent interventions require an oral or a written order from a physician to implement. For example, in most states, staff nurses cannot administer a medication without having a physician order it. The nurse is accountable for using appropriate knowledge, judgment, and competence in administering the medication at physician orders—and for questioning a physician about a problematic medical order. Thus, a nurse would not automatically carry out a physician's order without considering first the appropriateness of the medication or without knowing appropriate dosage, mode of action, side effects, and potential adverse reactions. Collaborative interventions are those performed by the nurse and other health care team members with the mutual goal of providing the most appropriate and effective care to clients (McCloskey & Bulechek, 2000). Box 2-4 identifies factors the nurse should consider in developing nursing interventions.

BOX 2-4	Factors for Consideration When Choosing a Nursing Intervention

- Desired client outcomes
- Characteristics of the nursing diagnosis
- Research base for the intervention
- Feasibility of doing the intervention
- Acceptability to the client
- Capability of the nurse

Evaluation

In the evaluation phase, the nurse and client mutually examine the client's progress or lack of progress toward achievement of treatment outcomes, mutually determined during the planning phase. When treatment goals are not achieved, or there is a lack of progress, the nurse needs to ask the following questions:

- Were the assessment data collected appropriate and complete?
- Was the nursing diagnosis appropriate?
- Were the treatment outcomes realistic and achievable in the time frame allotted?
- Were the nursing interventions chosen appropriate to the needs of the situation and the capabilities of the client?
- Was there any variable within the client, situation, or family that was overlooked and should have been addressed?

Issues and circumstances that can influence the achievement of treatment outcomes include the effectiveness, time efficiency, appropriateness, and adequacy of the nursing actions selected for implementation, economic barriers or assets, the motivation of the client, family obstruction or support, and obstacles in the setting, which could not have been anticipated. The nurse and client review progress, determine necessary modifications or need for referral, and terminate the relationship. Exercise 2-4 provides an opportunity to practice developing a care plan.

Documentation

Nurses are responsible for careful, accurate, and timely documentation of nursing assessments, the care given, and the behavioral responses of the client. This documentation represents a permanent record of the client's health care experience. In the eyes of the law, failure to document in written form any of these elements means the actions were not taken.

EXERCISE 2-4	Developing a Care Plan

Purpose: To provide students with experience developing care plans based on client-centered assessment data.

Procedure:

1. For a client you have been assigned to work with, develop an assessment summary from data obtained from the client, the client's chart, and other key informants.
2. Analyze and categorize specific assessment data.

  a. Indicate relationships between nursing and medical diagnoses.
3. Develop relevant, individualized nursing diagnoses.
4. Specify client goals, outcomes, and nursing interventions for the top 2 nursing diagnoses.

Discussion:

In small groups of three to five students, discuss your findings and compare rationales for the plan you developed.

This exercise can also be done with a selected case study provided by your faculty.

Two common models for documenting nursing care are the Nursing Outcomes Classification (NOC) and Nursing Interventions Classification (NIC) systems, which complement the function of the other. The NOC model is linked to the problem (nursing diagnosis), whereas the NIC intervention classification is linked to the related or contributing factors (Marrs & Lowery, 2006). These classification systems help standardize the language used to describe the nursing process. Frisch (2001) observed, "Nurses documenting practice using these systems are accomplishing three important things: appropriate documentation of care, identification of work as within the scope of professional nursing, and building a body of knowledge for nurses on the use of specific interventions" (pp. 11–12).

Clients need to trust that their health care provider is accurately and appropriately representing their voice and experience in medical care records. The medical record of care and treatment is also used to direct and improve client-centered care. Although nursing documentation usually covers documentation of biophysical issues, important aspects of nursing care related to the client's perspective, spiritual state, and learning needs are not always adequately noted (Laitinen, Kaunonen & Astedt-Kurki, 2010). Statements related to accommodations made for cultural, religious, and spiritual practices and preferences should be included in the record of care.

Verbal Reporting: Using the SBAR as a Communication Tool

Nurses need to verbally communicate assessment data and changes in health status to physicians, nurse colleagues, and others involved in the client's care on a regular basis. The SBAR format is a standardized assessment reporting format that helps nurses communicate a clear, succinct overview of critical information in an organized, thoughtful way. This can be especially important when communicating with physicians by phone (Rodgers, 2007). When communicating by phone, it is useful to have the client's chart in front of you.

SBAR is an acronym used to describe the

Situation (What is going on with the patient?)

Background (What is the key clinical background or context?)

Assessment (What do I think the problem is?)

Recommendation (What do I recommend or what do I want you to do?) (Guise & Lowe, 2006, p. 313)

Table 2-5 provides a sample of how nurses can use this structured format in communicating assessment data and changes in health status effectively.

The Joint Commission, the Institute for Health Care Improvement, and the AACN all support the use of SBAR as a desirable structured communication format. Given these approvals, Pope et al. (2008) suggest that the SBAR should be considered a "best practice" communication tool. In addition to using SBAR when there is a change in a client's health status, this communication format is used between shifts between nurse colleagues, between nurses and physicians during rounds, transfer and handoffs from one care setting or unit to another, and presurgery handoffs (Dunsford, 2009).

A distinct advantage of using SBAR as a primary communication tool between physicians and nurses is that it cuts down on professional differences in communication styles (Haig, Sutton, & Whittington, 2006). In addition to communication with professional colleagues at regular intervals or when a client's

TABLE 2-5	SBAR Example	
Step	**Components**	**Sample of Urgent Communication**
Situation	• Identify yourself, client, and client location. • Briefly describe problem and concerns. • Give highlights in 1–2 sentences.	"This is Judy Mayer on 3G. I'm calling about Mrs. Jones in room 312. She has spiked a temperature, and is experiencing pain of 7 on a scale of 0 to 10, which is not relieved by Percocet. She had her last Percocet about an hour ago."
Background	• Provide pertinent history, client diagnosis, and medical status. • Give clinical context.	"Mrs. Jones is a 62-year-old woman who was operated on for total hip replacement 2 days ago. Her surgery was successful, and her progress uneventful until a few hours ago."
Assessment	• Provide specific information regarding vital signs, mental status, and condition. • Offer a provisional clinical impression.	"Temperature 101, pulse rate 92, 1+ pedal pulse, edema in her right ankle, and local tenderness in her right calf. She is quite anxious. She is in a lot of discomfort, and feels 'crappy.' I'm concerned that she may have a DVT or an infection."
Recommendation	• Explain what you need to happen, including time frame. • Be clear about what is needed immediately to correct the problem.	"I need you to come now and evaluate the change in her condition. Would you want to order a Doppler ultrasound exam or blood work?"

Developed in consultation with Barbara Dobish, RN, MS, Assistant Professor, University of Maryland, March 10, 2010.

condition changes, nurses are accountable for orally informing ancillary clinical staff about the meaning of changes in the client's condition. They are responsible for appropriately supervising their care of the client, and for questioning unclear or controversial orders made by a physician. (See Chapter 22 and 24 for more information and related exercises).

PROTECTING THE CLIENT'S PRIVACY

Jones (1998) states: "*Privacy* refers to a client's right to have control over personal information whereas confidentiality refers to the obligation not to divulge anything said in a nurse-client relationship" (p. 5). As data is increasingly stored and transmitted through electronic record keeping, issues related to maintaining client privacy are under greater scrutiny. Institutional policies and federal law provide specific guidelines that all health care providers are required to follow. Kerr (2009) refers to the nurse's obligation to protect a client's privacy as a "sacred trust" (p. 315). The client's right to have personal control over personal information is upheld through federal HIPAA regulations. The ANA Code of Ethics (2003) specifically addresses the nurse's responsibility to safeguard the client's right to privacy.

HIPAA Regulatory Compliance

In the United States, the first federal legislation dealing with privacy of medical records was part of P.L. 104-191, the Health Insurance Portability and Accountability Act of 1996 (U.S. Department of Health and Human Services [DHHS], 2003). HIPAA regulations protect the privacy of the client's medical record and the client's right to have control over his or her identifiable information in health care records. Health care providers must provide clients with a written notice of their privacy practices and procedures. Key elements of the HIPAA privacy regulations are presented in Box 2-5.

HIPAA privacy rules govern the use and disbursement of individually identifiable health information, and give individuals the right to determine and restrict access to their health information. Clients have the right to access medical records, request copies, and/or request amendments to health information contained in the record. The Fair Health Information Practices Act of 1997 stipulates civil and criminal penalties for not allowing clients to review their medical records (Milton, 2009).

HIPAA regulations protect the confidentiality, accuracy, and availability of all electronic protected

BOX 2-5	Overview of Federal HIPAA Guidelines Protecting Client Confidentiality

- All medical records and other individually identifiable health information used or disclosed in any form, whether electronically, on paper, or orally, are covered by HIPAA regulations.
- Providers and health plans are required to give clients a clear written explanation of how their health information may be used and disclosed.
- Clients are able to see and get copies of their records and request amendments.
- Health care providers are required to obtain client consent before sharing their information for treatment, payment, and health care operations.
  - Clients have the right to request restrictions on the uses and disclosures of their information.
- People have the right to file a formal complaint with a covered provider or health plan, or with the U.S. Department of Health and Human Services (HHS), about violations of HIPAA regulations.
- Health information may not be used for purposes not related to health care (e.g., disclosures to employers to make personnel decisions) without explicit authorization.
- Disclosure of information is limited to the minimum necessary for the purpose of the disclosure.
- Written privacy procedures must be in place to cover anyone who has access to protected information related to how information will be used and disclosed.
- Training must be provided to employees about the use of HIPAA privacy procedures
- Health plans, providers, and clearinghouses that violate these standards will be subject to civil liability, and if knowingly violating client privacy for personal advantage, can be subject to criminal liability.

Adapted from HIPAA Guidelines: www.hhs.gov/ocr/hipaa.

information, whether created, received, or transmitted. Strict maintenance of written records in a protected, private environment is required. Other potential issues of concern about privacy involve cell phones, picture taking, use of hand held devices, use of fax machines, internet user ID and passwords, and use of RFID technologies or electronic monitoring devices (Kerr, 2009).

Health care providers must get written authorization from clients before disclosing or sharing any personal medical information. Client authorization is not required in situations concerning the public's health, criminal and legal matters, quality assurance, and aggregate record reviews for accreditation. In addition, "information can and must be shared between healthcare providers who have a legitimate need to know in order to provide safe and appropriate care" (Brooke, 2009, p. 11). This provision typically refers to emergency situations such as in the case of a client who is unable because of a psychotic state to give accurate information, or to sign a release of information form in the emergency department. HIPAA provisions allow nurses to gather information about the client's medical condition or drug history in an emergency for the purpose of providing immediate treatment, without having the client's written permission. When this occurs, it is important to document in the client's chart the immediacy of the need to obtain the required information.

The Office of Civil Rights enforces HIPAA regulations. Agencies and providers face severe penalties for violations, with improper disclosure of medical information punishable by fines or imprisonment. Study your agency's policies to determine to whom and under what conditions personal health information can be released. More information can be obtained through their web site (www.hhs.gov/ocr).

Protecting Client Privacy in Clinical Situations

In addition to informational privacy, which is a legal mandate, informal protection of the client's right to control the access of others to one's person in clinical situations is an ethical responsibility. The client and family usually view protecting the client's privacy in the clinical setting as a measure of respect. Simple strategies that nurses can use to protect the client's right to privacy in clinical situations include:

- Providing privacy for the client and family when disturbing matters are to be discussed
- Explaining procedures to clients before implementing them
- Entering another person's personal space with warning (e.g., knocking or calling the client's name) and, preferably, waiting for permission to enter
- Providing an identified space for the client's personal belongings

- Encouraging the inclusion of personal and familiar objects on the client's nightstand
- Decreasing direct eye contact during hands-on care
- Minimizing body exposure to what is absolutely necessary for care
- Using only the necessary number of people during any procedure
- Using touch appropriately

Confidentiality

Protecting the privacy of client information and confidentiality are related, but separate concepts. **Confidentiality** is defined as providing *only* the information needed to provide care for the client to other health professionals who are directly involved in the care of the client. Kerr (2009) notes that "a violation occurs when information deemed private, and divulged in confidence, is shared with others" (p. 315). The need to share information with other health professionals directly involved in care on a "need to know" basis should be made clear to the client as they enter the clinical setting. Other than these individuals, the nurse must have the client's written permission to share his or her private communication, unless the withholding of information would result in harm to the client or someone else, or in cases where abuse is suspected. Confidential information about the client cannot be shared with the family or other interested parties without the client or designated legal surrogate's written permission. Shared confidential information, unrelated to identified health care needs, should not be communicated or charted in the client's medical record.

Confidentiality within the nurse-client relationship involves the nurse's legal responsibility to guard against invasion of the client's privacy related to the following:

- Releasing information about the client to unauthorized parties
- Unwanted visitations in the hospital
- Discussing client problems in public places or with people not directly involved in the client's care
- Taking pictures of the client without consent or using the photographs without the client's permission
- Performing procedures such as testing for HIV without the client's permission
- Publishing data about a client in any way that makes the client identifiable without the client's permission (Cournoyer, 2001)

Professional Sharing of Confidential Information. Nursing reports and interdisciplinary team case conferences are acceptable forums for the discussion of health related communications shared by clients or families. Other venues include change-of-shift reports, one-on-one conversations with other health professionals about specific client care issues, and client-approved consultations with client families. Discussion of client care should take place in a private room with the door closed. Only relevant information specifically related to client assessment or treatment should be shared. Discussing private information casually with other health professionals without the client's permission is an abuse of confidentiality. The ethical responsibility to maintain client confidentiality continues even after the client is discharged from care.

Mandatory Reporting. Mandatory reporting of personal health information related to certain communicable or sexually transmitted diseases, child and elder abuse, and the potential for serious harm to another individual are considered exceptions to sharing of confidential information. Required mandatory disclosures may differ slightly from state to state. In general, nurses are required to report all notifiable infectious diseases and abuse to appropriate state and local reporting agencies. This duty to report supersedes the client's right to confidentiality or privileged communication with a health provider. Relevant client data should be released only to the appropriate local, state, or federal agency and as confidential information. The information provided must be the minimum amount needed to accomplish the purposes of disclosure, and the client needs to be informed about what information will be disclosed, to whom, and for what reason(s).

Informed Consent

Informed consent is more than a signature on a form indicating a client's willingness to undergo a treatment or procedure (Neary, Cahill, Kirwan, Kiely, & Redmond, 2008). **Informed consent** is defined as a focused communication process in which the professional nurse or physician discloses all relevant information related to a procedure or treatment, with full opportunity for dialogue, questions, and expressions of concern, before asking the client or health care agent for the client to sign a legal consent form. Unless there is a life-threatening emergency, all clients have the right to give informed consent. For legal consent to be valid, it must contain three elements (Northrop & Kelly, 1987):

- Consent must be voluntary.
- The client must have full disclosure about the risks, benefits, cost, potential side effects or adverse reactions of the proposed treatment or procedure, and should be provided with information about other treatment alternatives, if available.
- The client must have the capacity and competency to understand the information and to make an informed choice.

Before initiating an informed consent process, nurses need to assess the adequacy of a client's "hearing, sight, mental status, literacy level, and ability to understand the process or procedure" (Plawecki & Plawecki, 2009, p. 3). Essential disclosures needed to help ensure informed consent include:

- The nature and purpose of the proposed treatment or procedure
- The risks and benefits of not receiving or undergoing a treatment or procedure
- The client has the right to refuse treatment or discontinue it without penalty, unless it is an emergency situation

Clients should be given ample opportunity to ask questions and to express concerns. They should never feel coerced or pressured into consenting to treatment, as allowing a client to sign a consent form without fully understanding the meaning of what he or she is signing will invalidate the consent (Brooke, 2009). Ending the conversation leading to the actual signing of the consent form should always include the question, "Is there anything else that you think might be helpful in making your decision?" This type of dialogue gives the client permission to ask a question or address a concern that the nurse may not have given thought to in the informed consent discussion.

Guidelines Governing Legal Consent. Only legally competent adults can give legal consent; adults who are mentally retarded, developmentally disabled, or cognitively impaired cannot give legal consent (White, 2000). Evaluation of competency is made on an individual basis (e.g., in the case of emancipated adolescents no longer under their parent's control, brain-injured clients, or clients with early dementia) to determine the extent to which they understand what they are signing.

Legislation exists in all states, such that a legal guardian or personal health care agent can provide consent for the medical treatment of adults who lack the capacity to consent on their own behalf. In most cases, legal guardians or parents must give legal consent for minor children, defined as those younger than 18, unless the youth is legally considered an emancipated minor. Minors can also give consent in cases of immediate emergencies.

Emancipated minors are mentally competent adolescents younger than 18 who petition the courts for adult status. To be considered, adolescents must be financially responsible for themselves, and no longer living with their parents. Other criteria include being married, having a child, and/or being in military service.

SUMMARY

This chapter addresses the professional, legal, and ethical standards nurses use to guide their actions in the nurse-client relationship. Standards of professional practice provide a measurement benchmark, used to assess nursing competence in clinical situations regardless of specialty. Nurses are bound legally by the principles of tort law to provide a reasonable standard of care. This means that the nurse is obligated to provide a level of care that a reasonably prudent nurse with similar education and experience would provide in a similar situation. The ANA Code of Ethics for Nurses provides a conceptual framework for identifying the moral dimensions of nursing practice; it is an important guide to choice of actions in nurse-client relationships. Each state's Nurse Practice Acts defines the scope of nursing practice for nurses practicing in that state. Multistate licensure in a compact state allows registered nurses licensed and residing in a compact state to practice in other compact states without obtaining a second license.

The nursing process serves as a clinical management framework. It consists of sequential, overlapping phases: assessment, planning (including diagnosis and development of outcome criteria), implementation, and evaluation. The client is an active participant and decision maker in all phases. Nurses use the SBAR format to communicate essential information to other health professionals involved in the client's care.

Nurses are legally and ethically responsible for protecting the client's privacy. Privacy and confidentiality are related but separate concepts nurses use to protect a client's freedom of choice about sharing personal information with others. Privacy refers to a client's right to have control over personal information; confidentiality refers to the obligation not to divulge private information from a nurse-client relationship. HIPAA regulations, mandated by federal law govern the use and disbursement of personally identifiable health information, and give individuals the right to determine and restrict access to their health information.

ETHICAL DILEMMA   What Would You Do?

As a student nurse, you observe a fellow nursing student making a medication error. She is a good friend of yours and is visibly upset by her error. She also is afraid that if she tells the instructor, she could get a poor grade for clinical, and she needs to have a good average to keep her scholarship. The client was not actually harmed by the medication error, and your friend seems sufficiently upset by the incident to convince you that she would not make a similar error again. What would you do?

REFERENCES

Aiken TD: *Legal, ethical, and political issues in nursing*, Philadelphia, 2004, FA Davis Company.

American Nurses Association: *Code of ethics for nurses with interpretive statements* (approved revised), Washington, DC, 2001, Author.

American Nurses Association: *Nursing's Social Policy Statement.* 2nd ed, Washington, DC, 2003, Author.

American Nurses Association: *Nursing's Social Policy Statement: The Essence of the Profession*, Washington, DC, 2010, Author.

American Nurses Association: *Nursing: scope and standards of practice*, Washington, DC, 2010, Author.

Avant K: Paths to concept development in nursing diagnosis, *Nurs Diagn* 2(3):105–110, 1991.

Basanta WE: Advance directives and life sustaining treatment: a legal primer, *Hematol Oncol Clin North Am* 16(6):1381–1396, 2002.

Brooke P: Legal questions, *Nursing* 39(4):10–11, 2009.

Canadian Nurses Association: *The code of ethics for registered nurses*, Alberta, Canada, 1997, Author. Available online: http://www.cna-nurses.ca/CNA/practice/ethics/code/default_e.aspx.

Carpenito-Moyet LJ: *Handbook of nursing diagnoses*, ed 12, Philadelphia, 2008, Lippincott Williams & Wilkins.

Catalano J: *Nursing now: today's issues, tomorrow's trends*, ed 5, Philadelphia, 2008, FA Davis.

Cournoyer C: Legal relationships in nursing practice. In Creasia J, Parker B, editors: *Conceptual foundations: the bridge to professional nursing practice*, St. Louis, 2001, Mosby.

Dimond B: *Legal aspects of nursing*, ed 5, Essex, United Kingdom, 2008, Pearson Education Limited.

Dunsford J: Structured communication: improving patient safety with SBAR, *Nurs Womens Health* 13(5):384–390, 2009.

Frisch N: Nursing as a context for alternative/complementary modalities, *Online J Issues Nurs* [serial online] Available online: 6(2):2, 2001. http://www.nursingworld.org/ojin/topic15/ tpc15_2.htm.

Gordon M: *Manual of nursing diagnoses*, ed 11, Sudbury, MA, 2007, Jones and Bartlett Publishers.

Guido G: *Legal and ethical issues in nursing*, ed 5, Saddle River, NJ, 2009, Prentice Hall.

Guise JM, Lowe N: Do you speak SBAR? *J Obstet Gynecol Neonatal Nurs* 25(3):313–314, 2006.

Haig K, Sutton S, Whittington J: SBAR: a shared mental model for improving communication between clinicians, *J Qual Patient Saf* 32(3):167–175, 2006.

Joint Commission on Accreditation of Health Care Organizations: *Accreditation manual for hospitals*, Chicago, 1991, Author.

Joint Commission on Accreditation of Health Care Organizations: *Hospital accreditation standards*, Oakbrook Terrace, IL, 2007, Joint Commission Resources.

Jones D: *Adjunctive therapies: issues and interventions in psychiatric nursing practice*, ed 4, New Westminster, British Columbia, Canada, 1998, Douglas College.

Kerr P: Protecting patient education in an electronic age: A sacred trust, *Urol Nurs* 29(5):315–319, 2009.

Laitinen H, Kaunonen M, Astedt-Kurki P: Patient-focused documentation expressed by nurses, *J Clin Nurs* 19(1):489–497, 2010.

LaSala C: Moral accountability and integrity in nursing practice, *Nurs Clin North Am* 44:423–434, 2009.

Marrs J, Lowry L: Nursing theory and practice: connecting the dots, *Nurs Sci Q* 19:44–50, 2006.

McCloskey JC, Bulechek GM, editors: *Nursing interventions classification (NIC)*, ed 3, St Louis, 2000, Mosby.

Milton C: Information sharing: transparency, nursing ethics, and practice implications with electronic medical records, *Nurs Sci Q* 22(3):214–219, 2009.

NANDA: *Nursing diagnoses: definitions & classification*, Philadelphia, 2005, NANDA International.

National Council of State Boards of Nursing (NCSBN): Available online: https://www.ncsbn.org/boards.htm. Accessed September 5, 2008.

Neary P, Cahill R, Kirwan W, et al: What a signature adds to the consent process, *Surg Endosc* 22(12):2698–2704, 2008.

Northrop C, Kelly M: *Legal issues in nursing*, St Louis, 1987, Mosby.

Otto S: A nurse's lifeline: a nursing ethics committee offers the chance to review and learn from ethical dilemmas, *Am J Nurs* 100(12):57–59, 2000.

Plawecki L, Plawecki H: Simply stated: informed consent can be a very complex task, *J Gerontol Nurs* 35(2):3–4, 2009.

Pope B, Rodzen L, Spross G: Raising the SBAR: how better communication improves patient outcomes, *Nursing* 38(3):41–43, 2008.

Rodgers KL: Using the SBAR communication technique to improve nurse-physician phone communication, *AAACN Viewpoint* March/April 7–9, 2007.

Scott R: *Legal aspects of documenting patient care for rehabilitation professionals*, ed 3, Sudbury, MA, 2006, Jones & Bartlett.

Shapiro S: Evaluating clinical decision rules, *Western J Nurs Res* 271(5): 655–664, 2005.

Shaughnessy P: Outcomes across the care continuum: home health care, *Med Care* 35(12):1225–1226, 1997.

Snyder M, Egan EC, Nojima Y: Defining nursing interventions, *Image J Nurs Sch* 28(2):137–141, 1996.

U.S. Department of Health and Human Services (DHHS): *Summary of the HIPAA privacy rule*, 2003. Retrieved July 1, 2010, from http://www.hhs. gov/ ocr/ privacy/ hipaa/ understanding/summary/ index.Html.

Vuckovich P: Psychiatric advance directives, *J Am Psychiatr Nurses Assoc* 9(2):55–59, 2003.

Westley C, Briggs L: Stages of change model to improve communication about advance care planning, *Nurs Forum* 39(3):5–12, 2004.

White G: Informed consent, *Am J Nurs* 100(9):83, 2000.

CHAPTER 3

Clinical Judgment: Applying Critical Thinking and Ethical Decision Making

Kathleen Underman Boggs

OBJECTIVES

At the end of the chapter, the reader will be able to:

1. Define terms related to thinking, ethical reasoning, and critical thinking.
2. Identify and discuss the three principles of ethics underlying bioethical reasoning.
3. Describe the 10 steps of critical thinking.
4. Identify criteria necessary for acquisition of a value.
5. Discuss the application of ethics in nurse-client relationships.
6. Analyze the critical thinking process used in clinical judgments with clients.
7. Apply the critical thinking process to decision making in clinical nursing situations.
8. Demonstrate ability to analyze, synthesize, and evaluate a complex simulated case situation to make a clinical judgment.
9. Discuss application of findings from a research study to clinical practice.

This chapter examines the principles of ethical decision making and the process for critical thinking. Both are essential foundational knowledge for you to make effective nursing clinical judgments. These competencies, together with expert communication skills, are an integral part of nursing practice (Fero, Witsberger, Wesmiller, Zullo, & Hoffman, 2009). Ethical discussions in this book focus on the current literature in bioethics as held in Western society. In addition to basic content knowledge, throughout this book are included ethical dilemmas to help you begin applying your knowledge.

Critical thinking is a learned skill that teaches you how to "think about your thinking." In the past, expert nurses accumulated this skill with on-the-job experience, through trial and error. But this is an essential nursing skill that can be learned with practice while in school. The Applications section of this chapter specifically walks you through the reasoning process in applying the 10 steps of critical thinking.

BASIC CONCEPTS

TYPES OF THINKING

There are many ways of thinking (Figure 3-1). Students often attempt to use total recall by simply memorizing a bunch of facts (e.g., memorizing the cranial nerves by using a mnemonic such as "On Old Olympus' Towering Tops..."). At other times, we rely on developing habits by repetition, such as practicing cardiopulmonary resuscitation (CPR) techniques. More structured methods of thinking, such as inquiry, have been developed in disciplines related to nursing. For example, you are probably familiar with the scientific method. As used in research, this is a logical, linear method of systematically gaining new information, often by setting up an experiment to test an idea. The nursing process uses a method of systematic steps: assessment before planning, planning before intervention, and evaluation.

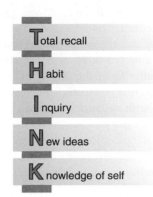

Total recall

Habit

Inquiry

New ideas

Knowledge of self

Figure 3-1 Mnemonics can be useful tools.

Knowing about your individual thinking style is vital not only for your own learning but also because your values affect the quality of relationships you are able to establish with clients. This chapter focuses on the most important concepts to help you develop your clinical judgment abilities. Completing the exercises will help you develop your skills.

ETHICAL REASONING

In clinical situations, nurses often face ethical dilemmas. Most nurses report facing ethical dilemmas in their work on a weekly basis. Examples include issues involving client choice, quality of life, and end-of-life decisions. A nurse frequently has to act in value-laden situations. For example, you may have clients who request abortions or who want "do not resuscitate" (DNR; "no code") orders. Your decisions affect the client's rights and the client's quality of life. A willingness to comply with ethical and professional standards is a hallmark of a professional.

Yet, members of many professions have difficulty applying ethical principles to clinical care situations. When various professionals answered questions about ethical dilemmas presented to them, physician responses were correctly ethically based 49.2% of the time, nurse responses 46.3%, and adult citizens 40% (Johnson, 2005). Is being ethically correct less than half the time acceptable? Student practice in applying ethical principles is important. Although it is true that most agencies have ethics committees that often are the primary party involved with the client or family in resolving difficult ethical dilemmas, on many other occasions, you, the nurse, will be called on to make ethical decisions.

As nurses, we need to have a clear understanding of the ethics of the nursing profession. Nursing organizations have formally published ethical codes, such as those from American Nurses Association (ANA) or the Federation of European Countries (Sasso, 2008). Academic programs now include application to clinical practice in the curriculum.

Case Example

During an influenza pandemic, Michaela May, RN, is reassigned to work on an unfamiliar pulmonary intensive care unit. Clients there have a severe form of infectious flu with respiratory complications and are receiving mechanical ventilation. She worries that if she refuses to care for these assigned clients, she could lose her job or even her license. But she also fears carrying this infection home to her two preschool children.

This case highlights conflicting duties: employer/client versus self/family. According to the ANA, nurses are obligated to care for all clients but there are limits to the personal risk of harm a nurse can be expected to accept. It is her *moral duty* if clients are at significant risk for harm that her care can prevent. This situation becomes a *moral option* only if there are alternative sources of care (i.e., other nurses available). For a full discussion, read Stokowski (2009).

ETHICAL THEORIES AND DECISION-MAKING MODELS

Ethical theories provide the bedrock from which we derive the principles that guide our decision making. There is no one "right" answer to an ethical dilemma: The decision may vary depending on which theory the involved people subscribe to. The following section briefly describes the most common models currently used in bioethics. They are, for the most part, representative of a Western European and Judeo-Christian viewpoint. As we become a more culturally diverse society, other equally viable viewpoints may become acculturated. This discussion focuses on three decision-making models: utilitarian/goal-based, duty-based, and rights-based models.

The **utilitarian/goal-based model** says that the "rightness" or "wrongness" of an action is always a function of its consequences. Rightness is the extent to which performing or omitting an action will contribute to the overall good of the client.

Good is defined as maximum welfare or happiness. The rights of clients and the duties of a nurse are determined by what will achieve maximum welfare. When a conflict in outcome occurs, the correct action is the one that will result in the greatest good for the majority. An example of a decision made according to the goal-based model is forced mandatory institutionalization of a client with tuberculosis who refuses to take medicine to protect other members of the community. The client's hospitalization produces the greatest balance of good over harm for the majority. Thus, "goodness" of an action is determined solely by its outcome.

The **deontologic** or **duty-based model** is person centered. It incorporates Immanuel Kant's deontologic philosophy, which holds that the "rightness" of an action is determined by other factors in addition to its outcome. Respect for every person's inherent dignity is a consideration. For example, a straightforward implication would be that a physician (or nurse) may never lie to a client. Do you agree? Decisions based on this duty-based model have a religious-social foundation. Rightness is determined by moral worth, regardless of the circumstances or the individual involved. In making decisions or implementing actions, the nurse cannot violate the basic duties and rights of individuals. Decisions about what is in the best interests of the client require consensus among all parties involved. Examples are the medical code "do no harm" and the nursing duty to "help save lives."

The **human rights–based model** is based on the belief that each client has basic rights. Our duties as health care providers arise from these basic rights. For example, a client has the right to refuse care. Conflict occurs when the provider's duty is not in the best interests of the client. The client has the right to life and the nurse has the duty to save lives, but what if the quality of life is intolerable and there is no hope for a positive outcome? Such a case might occur when a neonatal nurse cares for an infant with anencephaly (born without brain tissue in the cerebrum) in whom even the least invasive treatment would be extremely painful and would never provide any quality of life.

Ethical dilemmas arise when an actual or potential conflict occurs regarding principles, duties, or rights. Of course, many ethical or moral concepts held by Western society have been codified into law. Laws may vary from state to state, but a moral principle should be universally applied. Moral principles are shared by most members of a group, such as physicians or nurses, and represent the professional values of the group. Conflict arises when a nurse's professional values differ from the law in her state of residence. Conflict may also arise when you have not come to terms with situations in which your personal values differ from the profession's values. One example is doctor-assisted suicide (euthanasia). *Legally,* at the turn of the twenty-first century, such an act was legal in Oregon but illegal in Michigan. *Professionally,* the ANA Code of Ethics guides you to do no harm. *Personally,* your belief about whether euthanasia is right or wrong may be at variance with either of the above.

Bioethical Principles

To practice nursing in an ethical manner, you must be able to recognize the existence of a moral problem. Once you recognize a situation that puts your client in jeopardy, you must be able to take action. Three essential, guiding ethical principles have been developed from the theories cited earlier. The three principles that can assist us in decision making are autonomy, beneficence (nonmaleficence), and justice (Figure 3-2).

Autonomy versus Medical Paternalism. Autonomy is the client's right to self-determination. In the medical context, respect for a client's autonomy is a fundamental ethical principle. It is the basis for the concept of informed consent, which means your client makes a rational, informed decision without coercion (Ebbesen & Pedersen, 2008). The medical profession went from having a paternalistic relationship with clients to letting them decide. In the past, nurses and physicians often made decisions for clients based on what they thought was best for the client. This *paternalism* sometimes discounted the wishes of

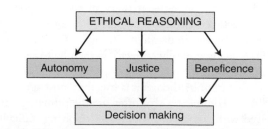

Figure 3-2 Guiding ethical principles that assist in decision making.

clients and their families. The ethical concept of client autonomy has so strongly emerged as a client right in Western countries that aspects involved in an individual's right to participate in medical decisions about his own care have become law.

This moral principle of autonomy means that each client has the right to decide about his or her health care. Clients who are empowered to make such decisions are more likely to comply with your treatment plan. Internal factors such as pain may interfere with a client's ability to choose. External factors such as coercion by a care provider may also interfere. As a nurse, you and your employer must legally obtain the client's permission for all treatment procedures. In the United States, under the Patient Self-Determination Act of 1991, all clients of agencies receiving Medicaid funds must receive written information about their rights to make decisions about their medical care. Nurses, as well as physicians, must provide clients with all the relevant and accurate information they need to make an "informed" decision whether they agree to treatments. The ANA states that it is the nurse's responsibility to assist clients to make these decisions, as discussed in Chapter 2 (see Informed Consent section).

Many of the nursing theories incorporate concepts about autonomy and empowering the client to be responsible for self-care, so you may find this easy to accept as part of your nursing role. However, what happens if the client's right to autonomy puts others at risk? Whose rights take precedence?

Case Example

A child is admitted to the emergency department with life-threatening blood loss after an automobile accident. The father refuses transfusion on religious grounds. The hospital obtains a court order, and the physician gives the transfusion.

The concept of autonomy has also been applied to the way we practice nursing, but our professional autonomy has some limitations. For example, the American Medical Association's Principles of Medical Ethics says a physician can choose whom to serve, except in an emergency; however, the picture is a little different in nursing practice. According to the ANA Committee on Ethics, nurses are ethically obligated to treat clients seeking their care. For example, you could not refuse to care for a client with AIDS who is assigned to you.

A nurse has autonomy in caring for a client, but this is somewhat limited because legally she must also follow physician orders and be subject to physician authority. Before the nurse or physician can override a client's right to autonomy, he or she must be able to present a strong case for their point of view based on either or both of the following principles: beneficence and justice.

Case Example

Dorothy Kneut, 72, refuses physician-assisted suicide after being diagnosed with Alzheimer's disease. She also refuses entry into a long-term care facility, deciding instead to rely on her aged, disabled spouse to provide her total care as she deteriorates physically and mentally. As her home health nurse, you find he is unable to provide needed care, and ask her physician to transfer her to an extended care facility.

Beneficence and Nonmaleficence

Beneficence implies that a decision results in the greatest good or produces the least harm to the client. This is based on the Hippocratic Oath and its concept of "do no harm." Avoiding actions that bring harm to another person is known as *nonmaleficence*. An example is the Christian belief of "do not kill," which has been codified into law but has many exceptions (e.g., soldiers sent to war are expected to kill the enemy).

In health care, beneficence gives care providers the moral obligation to act at all times for the benefit of their clients. Again, nursing theorists have incorporated this into the nursing role, so you may find this easy to accept. Helping others may be why you chose to become a nurse. In nursing, you not only have the obligation to avoid harming your clients, but you also are expected to advocate for your clients' best interests.

Case Example

Mr. Harper, 62, is admitted with end-organ failure. You are expected to assess for pain that he has and treat it. Do you seek a palliative order even though his liver cannot process drugs? It is estimated that more than 50% of conscious clients spend their last week of life in moderate to severe pain. Who is advocating for them?

Beneficence is challenged in many clinical situations (e.g., requests for abortion or euthanasia). Currently, some of the most difficult ethical dilemmas involve situations where decisions may be made to withhold treatment. For example, decisions are made to justify such violations of beneficence in the guise of permitting merciful death. Is there a moral difference between actively causing death and withholding treatment, when the outcome for the client is the same death? There are clear legal differences. In most states, a health care worker who intentionally acts to cause a client's death is legally liable.

Other challenges to beneficence occur when the involved parties hold different viewpoints about what is best for the client. Consider a case in which the family of an elderly, poststroke, comatose, ventilator-dependent client wants all forms of treatment continued, but the health care team doesn't believe it will benefit the client. The initial step toward resolution may be holding a family conference and really listening to the viewpoints of family members, asking them whether the client ever expressed wishes verbally or in writing in the form of an advance directive. Maintaining a trusting, open, mutually respectful communication may help avoid an adversarial situation.

Justice

Justice is actually a legal term; however, in ethics, it refers to being fair or impartial. A related concept is equality (e.g., the just distribution of goods or resources, sometimes called *social justice* or *distributive justice*). Within the health care arena, this distributive justice concept might be applied to scarce treatment resources. As new and more expensive technologies that can prolong life become available, who has a right to them? Who should pay for them? If resources are scarce, how do we decide who gets them? Should a limited resource be spread out equally to everyone? Or should it be allocated based on who has the greatest need?

Unnecessary Treatment. Decisions made based on the principle of justice may also involve the concept of unnecessary treatment. Are all operations that are performed truly necessary? Why do some clients receive antibiotics for viral infections, when we know they do not kill viruses? Are unnecessary diagnostic tests ever ordered solely to document that a client does not have Condition X, just in case there is a malpractice lawsuit?

Social Worth. Another justice concept to consider in making decisions is that of social worth. Are all people equal? Are some more deserving than others? If a client Dan is 7 years old instead of 77 years old, and the expensive medicine would cure his condition,

should these factors affect the decision to give him the medicine? If there is only one liver available for transplant today, and there are two equally viable potential recipients—Larry, age 54, whose alcoholism destroyed his own liver; or Kay, age 32, whose liver was destroyed by hepatitis she got while on a life-saving mission abroad—who should get the liver?

Veracity. Truthfulness is the bedrock of trust. And trust is an essential component of the professional nurse-client relationship. Not only is there a moral injunction against lying, but it is also destructive to any professional relationship. Generally, nurses would agree that a nurse should never lie to a client. However, there is controversy about withholding information from a client. We need clarity about truth telling. There will be times when we need to exercise some judgment about to whom to disclose information. We have an obligation to protect potentially vulnerable clients from information that would cause emotional distress. Although it is never acceptable to lie, nurses have evaded answering questions by saying, "You need to ask your physician about that." Can you suggest another response?

STEPS IN ETHICAL DECISION MAKING

The process of moral reasoning and making ethical decisions has been broken down into steps. These steps are only a part of the larger model for critical thinking. Table 3-1 summarizes a model useful for nurses that was adapted from Lincourt's model. This model covers the most essential parts of an ethical reasoning process. If you are the moral agent making this decision, you must be skillful enough to implement the actions in a morally correct way. Consider the following case.

Case Example

You are assigned to four critical clients on your unit. Mrs. Rae, 83, is unconscious, dying, and needs suctioning every 10 minutes. Mr. Jones, 47, has been admitted for observation for severe bloody stools. Mr. Hernandez, 52, has newly diagnosed diabetes and is receiving intravenous (IV) drip insulin; he requires monitoring of vital signs every 15 minutes. Mr. Martin, 35, is suicidal and has been told today he has inoperable cancer.

In deciding how to spend your limited time with these clients, do you base your decision entirely on how much good you can do for each client? Under distributive justice, what should happen when the

TABLE 3-1	Moral Decision-Making Guide	
Moral Component	**Data**	**Evaluation**
Claim	Clear statement of the claim or dilemma; issues and values are clearly identified	Are values of all parties represented? Who has a stake in the outcome? Are there any ethical conflicts between two or more values?
Evidence	Clarify the facts; list the grounds, statistics, and so on	Are they true? Relevant? Sufficient?
Warrant	Agency policy, professional standards of care, written protocols, legal precedents	Are they general? Are they appropriate?
Basis	Identify the moral basis for each individual's claim; list backing, such as ethical principle of autonomy, beneficence, or justice	Is the backing recognizable? Impressively strong?
Rebuttal	List the benefit and the burdens; weigh them for each alternative in terms of possible consequences for each of the parties involved*	How strong and compelling is the rebuttal argument? Is the decision in accord with or in conflict with the law?

*Benefits might include profit for one of the parties. Burden might include causing physical or emotional pain to one of the parties or imposing financial burden on them.

needs of these four conflict? You could base your decision on the principle of beneficence and do the greatest good for the most clients, but this is a very subjective judgment. Would one of these clients benefit more from nursing care than the others?

In using ethical decision-making processes, nurses must be able to tolerate ambiguity and uncertainty. One of the most difficult aspects for the novice nurse to accept is that there often is no one "right" answer; rather, usually several options may be selected, depending on the person or situation.

CRITICAL THINKING

Critical thinking is an analytical process in which you purposefully use specific thinking skills to make complex clinical decisions. You are able to reflect on your own thinking process. We can paraphrase the American Philosophical Association definition, which considers critical thinking as a purposeful, self-regulating process of interpretation, analysis, evaluation, and inference for the purpose of making judgments (Worell & Profetto-McGrath, 2007).

Although no consensus has been reached on a critical thinking definition in the nursing arena, current definitions are similar (Ravert, 2008). Generally, we define critical thinking as the purposeful use of a cognitive framework to identify and analyze assumptions and evidence to recognize emergent client situations, make clear, objective clinical decisions, and intervene appropriately (Mangena & Chabeli, 2005; Wilgis & McConnell, 2008). It encompasses the steps of the nursing process, but possibly in a more circular loop than we usually envision the nursing process. Critical thinking allows the nurse to modify the care plan based on the client's responses to her nursing interventions (Fero et al., 2009).

Critical thinking is more than just a *cognitive process* of following steps. It also has an *affective component*—the willingness to engage in self-reflective inquiry. As you learn to be a critical thinker, you improve and clarify your thinking process skills, so that you are more accurately able to solve problems based on available evidence. Although the cognitive skills can be taught, the affective willingness to use critical thinking process is an ingrained trait that may be difficult to change. Changing from a lecture method of nurse education to a learner-centered approach would have faculty "model" the critical thinking process for students.

CHARACTERISTICS OF A CRITICAL THINKER

Critical thinkers are skilled at using inquiry methods. They approach problem solutions in a systematic, organized, and goal-directed way when making clinical decisions. They continually use past knowledge, communication skills, new information, and observations to make these clinical judgments. Table 3-2 summarizes the characteristics of a critical thinker.

TABLE 3-2	Characteristics of a Critical Thinker
Attitude	• Develops an analytical thinking ability • Maintains an inquisitive mind set, systematically seeking solutions • Displays open-minded and flexible thinking process
Thought Processes	• Is reflective • Combines existing knowledge and standards with new information (transformation) • Thinks in an orderly way, especially in complex situations (logical reasoning) • Incorporates creative thinking • Diligently perseveres in seeking relevant information • Discards irrelevant information (discrimination) • Considers alternative solutions
Actions	• Recognizes when information is missing and seeks new input • Revises actions based on new input • Evaluates solutions and outcomes

Based on information from Facione PA: *Critical thinking: what is it and why it counts*, Milbrae, CA, 2006, California Academic Press; Scheffer BK, Rubenfeld MG: A consensus statement on critical thinking in nursing, *J Nurs Educ* 39(8):352–359, 2000; and Worrell JA, Profetto-McGrath J: Critical thinking as an outcome of context-based learning among post RN students: a literature review, *Nurse Educ Today* 27:420–426, 2007.

Expert nurses recognize that priorities change continually, requiring constant assessment and alternative interventions. When the authors analyzed the decision-making process of expert nurses, they all used the critical thinking steps described in this chapter when they made their clinical judgments, even though they were not always able to verbally state the components of their thinking processes. Expert nurses organized each input of client information and quickly distinguished relevant from irrelevant information. They seemed to categorize each new fact into a problem format, obtaining supplementary data and arriving at a decision about diagnosis and intervention. Often, they commented about comparing this new information with prior knowledge, sometimes from academic sources but usually from information gained from preceptors. They constantly scan for new information, and constantly reassess their client's situation. This is not linear. New input is always being added. This contrasts with novice nurses who tend to think in a linear way, collect lots of facts but not logically organize them, and fail to make as many connections with past knowledge. Novice nurses' assessments are more generalized and less focused, and they tend to jump too quickly to a diagnosis without recognizing the need to obtain more facts.

Because nurses are responsible for a significant proportion of decisions that affect client care, and are key gatekeepers in preventing harm, employing agencies periodically retest staff nurses for competencies. This procedure was initially done just to retest or recertify technical skills, such as CPR. Now many agencies have added other competency testing, including evaluation of critical thinking/clinical judgment skills (Rush, 2008).

BARRIERS TO THINKING CRITICALLY AND REASONING ETHICALLY
Attitudes and Habits

Barriers that decrease a nurse's ability to think critically, including attitudes such as "my way is better," interfere with our ability to empower clients to make their own decisions. Our thinking habits can also impede communication with clients or families making complex bioethical choices. Examples include becoming accustomed to acknowledging "only one right answer" or selecting only one option. Behaviors that act as barriers include automatically responding defensively when challenged, resisting changes, and desiring to conform to expectations. Cognitive barriers, such as thinking in stereotypes, also interfere with our ability to treat a client as an individual.

Cognitive Dissonance

Cognitive dissonance refers to the mental discomfort you feel when there is a discrepancy between what you already believe and some new information that does not go along with your view. In this book, we use the term to refer to the holding of two or more conflicting values at the same time.

Personal Values versus Professional Values

We all have a *personal value system* developed over a lifetime that has been extensively shaped by our family, our religious beliefs, and our years of life experiences. Our values change as we mature in our ability to think critically, logically, and morally. Strongly held values become a part of self-concept. Our education as

BOX 3-1	Five Core Values of Professional Nursing

Five *core values of professional nursing* have been identified by the American Association of Colleges of Nursing (AACN):
- Human dignity
- Integrity
- Autonomy
- Altruism
- Social justice

nurses helps us acquire a *professional value system.* In nursing school, as you advance through your clinical experiences, you begin to take on some of the values of the nursing profession (Box 3-1). You are acquiring these values as you learn the nursing role. The process of this role socialization is discussed in Chapter 7. For example, maintaining client confidentiality is a professional value, with both a legal and a moral requirement. We must take care that we do not allow our personal values to obstruct care for a client who holds differing values.

VALUES CLARIFICATION AND THE NURSING PROCESS

The nursing process offers many opportunities to incorporate *values clarification* into your care. During the assessment phase, you can obtain an assessment of the *client's values* with regard to the health system. For example, you interview a client for the first time and learn that he has obstructive pulmonary disease and is having difficulty breathing, but he insists on smoking. Is it appropriate to intervene? In this example, you know that smoking is detrimental to a person's health and you, as a nurse, find the value of health in conflict with the client's value of smoking. It is important to understand your client's values. When your values differ, you attempt to care for this client within his reality. He has the right to make decisions that are not always congruent with those of his health care providers (Bromley & Braslow, 2008).

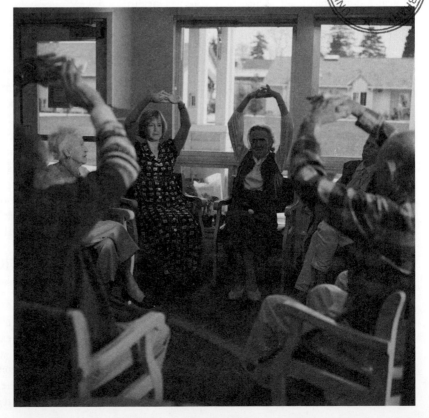

The values people hold often are observed in their interest in, involvement with, and commitment to people, places, and things.

When identifying specific nursing diagnoses, it is important that your diagnoses are not biased. Examples of value conflicts might be spiritual distress related to a conflict between spiritual beliefs and prescribed health treatments, or ineffective family coping related to restricted visiting hours for a family in which full family participation is a cultural value. In the planning phase, it is important to identify and understand the client's value system as the foundation for developing the most appropriate interventions. Plans of care that support rather than discount the client's health care beliefs are more likely to be received favorably. Your interventions include values clarification as a guideline for care. You help clients examine alternatives. During the evaluation phase, examine how well the nursing and client goals were met while keeping within the guidelines of the client's value system.

To summarize, in case of conflict (with own personal ethical convictions), nurses must put aside their own moral convictions to provide necessary assistance in a case of emergency when there is imminent risk to a patient's life (Sasso, 2008). Ethical reasoning and critical thinking skills are essential competencies for making clinical judgments, in an increasingly complex health care system (Carter & Ruckholm, 2008). To apply critical thinking to a clinical decision, we need to base our intervention on *the best evidence* available. These skills can be learned by participating in simulated patient case situations. These skills will enable you to provide higher quality nursing care (Fero et al., 2009; Ravert, 2008).

Developing an Evidence-Based Practice

Fero LJ, Witsberger CM, Wesmiller SW, Zullo TG, Hoffman LA: Critical thinking ability of new graduate and experienced nurses, *Journal of Advanced Nursing*, 65(1):139–148, 2009.

A nonrandom consecutive sample of 2,144 newly hired nurses completed a valid and reliable instrument, the Performance Based Development System Assessment (PBDS), which consists of 10 video vignettes depicting change in client status. Written answers for each nurse's response to each video were scored as meeting or not meeting expectations. The purpose of this research project was not explicitly stated, but seems to be determining which staff nurses were using critical thinking skills, and which specific skills could be identified.

Results: Expectations for critical thinking process were met by 74.9% of nurse participants. Controlling for years of experience, new graduates were less likely to meet critical thinking expectations compared with nurses having 10 or more years' experience

($P = 0.046$). Among nurses not meeting expectations, areas needing improvement included: not identifying problem correctly (57.1%), not prioritizing urgency (67%), not reporting essential data (65.4%), unable to provide rationale to support decisions (62.6%), and not anticipating relevant medical orders (62.8%). Analysis of written responses for those not meeting expectations also showed that 97.2% did not initiate appropriate nursing interventions. ADN students (associate's degree) and BSN (bachelor's degree) students were more likely to meet expectations as years of experience accrued, a trend not seen in diploma nurses.

Application to Your Clinical Practice: The PBDS tool was able to identify specific areas of learning needs in working nurses, as opposed to prior studies using student nurses. It is crucial for a client's safety that his or her nurse is able to recognize a significant change in his or her condition and make appropriate interventions. Identifying nurses unable to do so allows hospital inservice departments to initiate a learning program tailored to each individual's area of weakness to help them develop needed critical thinking abilities and to improve client care. As a student, would you be willing to use the PBDS to identify areas you need to work on?

APPLICATIONS

Accrediting agencies for nursing curriculums require inclusion of critical thinking curriculum. Accepted teaching-learning methods for assessing critical thinking include case studies, questioning, reflective journalism, client simulations, portfolios, concept maps, and problem-based learning (Sorensen & Yankech, 2008; Wilgis & McConnell, 2008). As a nurse, you are faced with processing copious amounts of information to be considered before making a decision about your client's situation. Often, you must consider more than one possibility but make your decision quickly. To provide safe care, you must be able to apply critical thinking skills to clinical situations (Fero et al., 2009; Rogal & Young, 2008).

PARTICIPATION IN CLINICAL RESEARCH

You or your clients may be called on at some time to participate in clinical research trials. The focus of this book is to examine ethical dilemmas faced in nursing practice, and this does not encompass the ethical aspect of conducting or participating in research studies. To examine what makes clinical research ethical, consult a nursing research book.

SOLVING ETHICAL DILEMMAS IN NURSING

Nurses indicate a need for more information about dealing with the ethical dilemmas they encounter, yet most say they receive little education in doing so. Exercises 3-1 (autonomy), 3-2 (beneficence), and 3-3 (justice) give you this opportunity.

The ethical issues that nurses commonly face today can be placed in three general categories: moral uncertainty, moral or ethical dilemmas, and moral distress. *Moral uncertainty* occurs when a nurse is uncertain as

to which moral rules (i.e., values, beliefs, or ethical principles) apply to a given situation. For example, should a terminally ill client who is in and out of a coma and chooses not to eat or drink anything be required to have IV therapy for hydration purposes? Does giving IV therapy constitute giving the client extraordinary measures to prolong life? Is it more comfortable or less comfortable for the dying client to maintain a high hydration level? When there is no clear definition of the problem, moral uncertainty develops, because the nurse is unable to identify the situation as a moral problem or to define specific moral rules that

---

EXERCISE 3-1   Autonomy

Purpose: To stimulate class discussion about the moral principle of autonomy.

Procedure:
In small groups, read the three case examples on page 47 and discuss whether the client has the autonomous

right to refuse treatment if it affects the life of another person.

Discussion:
Prepare your argument for an in-class discussion.

EXERCISE 3-2   Beneficence

Purpose: To stimulate discussion about the moral principle of beneficence.

Procedure:
Read the following case example and prepare for discussion:

    Dawn, a staff nurse, answers the telephone and receives a verbal order from Dr. Smith. Ms. Patton was admitted this morning with ventricular arrhythmia. Dr. Smith orders Dawn to administer a potent diuretic, Lasix 80 mg, IV, STAT. This is such a large dose that she has to order it up from pharmacy.

    As described in the text, you are legally obliged to carry out a doctor's orders unless they threaten the welfare of your client. How often do nurses question orders? What would happen to a nurse who questioned orders too often? In a research study using this case simulation, nearly 95% of the time the nurses participating in the study attempted to implement this potentially lethal medication order before being stopped by the researcher!

Discussion:
1. What principles are involved?
2. What would you do if you were this staff nurse?

EXERCISE 3-3   Justice

Purpose: To encourage discussion about the concept of justice.

Procedure:
Consider that in Oregon several years ago, attempts were made to legislate some restrictions on what Medicaid would pay for. A young boy needed a standard treatment of bone marrow transplant for his childhood leukemia. He died when the state refused to pay for his treatment.

    Read the following case example and answer the discussion questions:

    Mr. Diaz, age 74, has led an active life and continues to be the sole support for his wife and disabled daughter. He pays for health care with Medicare government insurance. The doctors think his cancer may respond to a very expensive new drug, which is not paid for under his coverage.

Discussion:
1. Does everyone have a basic right to health care, as well as to life and liberty?
2. Does an insurance company have a right to restrict access to care?

apply. Strategies that might be useful in dealing with moral uncertainty include using the values clarification process, developing a specific philosophy of nursing, and acquiring knowledge about ethical principles.

Ethical or moral dilemmas arise when two or more moral issues are in conflict. An ethical dilemma is a problem in which there are two or more conflicting but equally right answers. Organ harvesting of a severely brain-damaged infant is an example of an ethical dilemma. Removal of organs from one infant may save the lives of several other infants. However, even though the brain-damaged child is definitely going to die, is it right to remove organs before the child's death? It is important for the nurse to understand that, in many ethical dilemmas, there is often no single "right" solution. Some decisions may be "more right" than others, but often what one nurse decides is best differs significantly from what another nurse would decide.

The third common kind of ethical problem seen in nursing today is *moral distress.* Moral distress results when the nurse knows what is "right" but is bound to do otherwise because of legal or institutional constraints. When such a situation arises (e.g., a terminally ill client who does not have a "do not resuscitate" medical order and for whom, therefore, resuscitation attempts must be made), the nurse may experience inner turmoil.

Nurses in the National Rural Bioethics Project reported that three of their most commonly encountered ethics problems had to do with resuscitation decisions for dying clients with unclear, confusing, or no code orders; patients and families who wanted more aggressive treatment; and colleagues who discussed clients inappropriately.

Because values underlie all ethical decision making, nurses must understand their own values thoroughly before making an ethical decision. Instead of responding in an emotional manner on the spur of the moment (as people often do when faced with an ethical dilemma), the nurse who uses the values clarification process can respond rationally. It is not an easy task to have sufficient knowledge of oneself, of the situation, and of legal and moral constraints to be able to implement ethical decision making quickly. Expert nurses still struggle. Taking time to examine situations can help you develop skill in dealing with ethical dilemmas in nursing, and the exercises in this book will give you a chance to practice. Each chapter in this book has also included at least one ethical dilemma, so you can discuss what you would do.

Finally, in thinking about your own ethical practice, reflect on how important it is for your client to be able to always count on you. Consider the following client journal entry (Milton, 2002):

> I ask for information, share my needs, to no avail. You come and go...
>
> "Could you find out for me?" "Sure I'll check on it."
>
> [But] check on it never comes...
>
> Who can I trust? I thought you'd be here for me...
>
> You weren't. What can I do?
>
> Betrayal permeates...

PROFESSIONAL VALUES ACQUISITION

Professional values or ethics consist of the values held in common by the members of a profession. Professional values are formally stated in professional codes. One example is the ANA Code of Ethics for Nurses. Often, professional values are transmitted by tradition in nursing classes and clinical experiences. They are modeled by expert nurses and assimilated as part of the role socialization process during your years as a student and new graduate. Professional values acquisition should perhaps be the result of conscious choice by a nursing student. This is the first step in values acquisition. Can you apply it to your own life? It may also help you understand the value system of your clients. Refer to Box 3-2 for the seven criteria for aquisition of a value.

BOX 3-2	Seven Criteria for Acquisition of a Value

The value must be
1. Freely chosen.
2. Chosen from alternatives.
3. Chosen after careful consideration of each alternative.

There must be
4. Pride in and happiness with the choice.
5. Willingness to make the values known to others.

It must be acted on
6. In response to the choice.
7. In a pattern of behavior consistent with the choice (value is incorporated into the individual's lifestyle).

Values are a strong determinant in making selections between competing alternatives. Consider whether the nursing profession holds values regarding the following situation: What if you observed a nurse charting that a medicine was given to a client when you know it was not? What professional value should guide your response? Exercise 3-4 will give you an opportunity to practice explaining which of your choices are based on the profession's values.

APPLYING CRITICAL THINKING TO THE CLINICAL DECISION-MAKING PROCESS

This section discusses a procedure for developing critical thinking skills as applied to solving clinical problems. Different examples illustrate the reasoning process developed by several disciplines. Unfortunately, each discipline has its own vocabulary. Table 3-3 shows

---

EXERCISE 3-4	Professional Nurses' Values

Purpose: To begin to focus thinking on professional role values.

Procedure:
Read the following statements. Think about each situation carefully. How would you want to respond if you were the primary nurse in the situation?
1. An 8-year-old girl is admitted to the emergency department, immaculately dressed, with many bruises and welts on her arms and legs. Her mother states she was hurt on the playground.
2. You note that your student partner has alcohol on her breath when she picks up her assignments. This has happened on more than one occasion.

3. A client has been told his bone scan shows metastatic lesions. He tells you not to tell his wife because she will just worry.
4. You have an order to administer a narcotic to a client who clearly is not in pain.

Discussion:
Share the responses to this exercise in a class discussion.
1. How did your answers compare with those of your peers?
2. In what ways did your values enter into your choices?

TABLE 3-3	Reasoning Process

Generic Reasoning Process	Diagnostic Reasoning in the Nursing Process	Ethical Reasoning	Critical Thinking Skill
Collect and interpret information	Gordon's functional patterns of health assessment	Parties, claim, basis	1. Clarify concepts 2. Identify own values and differentiate
Identify problem	Statement of nursing diagnosis	Statement of ethical dilemma	3. Integrate data and identify missing data 4. Collect new data 5. Identify problem 6. Apply criteria 7. Look at alternatives 8. Examine skeptically 9. Check for change in context 10. Make decision
Plan for problem solving	Prioritization of problems/ interventions	Prioritized claims and action plan	
Implement plan	Nursing action	Moral action	
Evaluate	Outcome evaluation	Moral evaluation	Reflect/evaluate

that we are talking about concepts with which you are already familiar. It also contrasts terms used in education, nursing, and philosophy to specify 10 steps to help you develop your critical thinking skills. For example, the nurse performs a "client assessment," which in education is referred to as "collecting information" or in philosophy may be called "identifying claims."

The process of critical thinking is systematic, organized, and goal directed. As critical thinkers, nurses are able to explore all aspects of a complex clinical situation (Worrell & Profetto-McGrath, 2007). This is a learned process. Among many teaching-learning techniques helping you develop critical thinking skills, most are included in this book: reflective journaling, concept maps, role-playing, guided small group discussion, and case study discussion. An extensive case application follows. During your learning phase, the critical thinking skills are divided into 10 specific steps. Each step includes a discussion of application to the clinical case example provided.

To help you understand how to apply critical thinking steps, read the following case and then see how each of the steps can be used in making clinical decisions. Components of this case are applied to illustrate the steps and stimulate discussion in the critical thinking process; many more points may be raised. From the outset, understand that, although these are listed as steps, they do not occur in a rigid, linear way in real life. The model is best thought of as a circular model. New data are constantly being sought and added to the process.

Case Example

Day 1—Mrs. Vlios, a 72-year-old widowed teacher, has been admitted to your unit. Her daughter, Sara, lives 2 hours away from her mother, but she arrives soon after admission. According to Sara, her mother lived an active life before admission, taking care of herself in an apartment in a senior citizens' housing development. Sara noticed that for about 3 weeks now, telephone conversations with her mother did not make sense or she seemed to have a hard time concentrating, although her pronunciation was clear. The admitting diagnosis is dehydration and dementia, rule out Alzheimer's disease, organic brain syndrome, and depression. An IV of 1,000 ml dextrose/0.45 normal saline is ordered at 50 drops/hour. Mrs. Vlios's history is unremarkable except for a recent 10-pound weight loss. She has no allergies and is known to take acetaminophen regularly for minor pain.

Day 2—When Sara visits her mom's apartment to bring grooming items to the hospital, she finds the refrigerator and food pantry empty. A neighbor tells her that Mrs. Vlios was seen roaming the halls aimlessly 2 days ago and could not remember whether she had eaten. As Mrs. Vlios's nurse, you notice that she is oriented today (to time and person). A soft diet is ordered, and her urinary output is now normal.

Day 5—In morning report, the night nurse states that Mrs. Vlios was hallucinating and restraints were applied. A nasogastric tube was ordered to suction out stomach contents because of repeated vomiting. Dr. Green tells Sara and her brother, Todos, that their mother's prognosis is guarded; she has acquired a serious systemic infection, is semicomatose, is not taking nourishment, and needs antibiotics and hyperalimentation. Sara reminds the doctor that her mother signed a living will in which she stated she refuses all treatment except IVs to keep her alive. Todos is upset, yelling at Sara that he wants the doctor to do everything possible to keep their mother alive.

STEP 1: CLARIFY CONCEPTS

The first step in making a clinical judgment is to identify whether a problem actually exists. Poor decision makers often skip this step. To figure out whether there is a problem, you need to think about what to observe and what basic information to gather. If it is an ethical dilemma, you not only need to identify the existence of the moral problem, but you need to also identify all the interested parties who have a stake in the decision. Figuring out exactly what the problem or issue is may not be as easy as it sounds.

Look for Clues

Are there hidden meanings to the words being spoken? Are there nonverbal clues?

Identify Assumptions

What assumptions are being made?

Case Discussion

This case is designed to present both physiologic and ethical dilemmas. In clarifying the problem, address both domains.

- Physiological concerns: Based on the diagnosis, the initial treatment goal was to restore homeostasis. By Day 5, is it clear whether Mrs. Vlios's condition is reversible?

- Ethical concerns: When is a decision made to initiate treatment or to abide by the advance directive and respect the client's wishes regarding no treatment?
- What are the wishes of the family? What happens when there is no consensus?
- Assumptions: Is the diagnosis correct? Does the client have dementia? Or was her confusion a result of dehydration and a strange hospital environment?

STEP 2: IDENTIFY YOUR OWN VALUES

Values clarification helps you identify and prioritize your values. It also serves as a base for helping clients identify the values they hold as important. Unless you are able to identify your client's values and can appreciate the validity of those values, you run the risk for imposing your own values. It is not necessary for your values and your client's values to coincide; this is an unrealistic expectation. However, whenever possible, the client's values should be taken into consideration during every aspect of nursing care. Discussion of the case of Mrs. Vlios presented in this section may help you with the clarification process.

Having just completed the exercises given earlier should help your understanding of your own personal values and the professional values of nursing. Now apply this information to this case.

Case Discussion

Identify the values of each person involved:

- Family: Mrs. Vlios signed an advance directive. Sara wants it adhered to; Todos wants it ignored. Why? (Missing information: Are there religious beliefs? Is there unclear communication? Is there guilt about previous troubles in the relationship?)
- Personal values: What are yours?
- Professional values: The ANA says nurses are advocates for their clients; beneficence implies nonmaleficence ("do no harm"), but autonomy means the client has the right to refuse treatment. What is the agency's policy? What are the legal considerations? Practice refining your professional values acquisition by completing the values exercises in this chapter.

In summary, you need to identify which values are involved in a situation or which moral principles can be cited to support each of the positions advocated by the involved individuals.

STEP 3: INTEGRATE DATA AND IDENTIFY MISSING DATA

Think about knowledge gained in prior courses and during clinical experiences. Try to make connections between different subject areas and clinical nursing practice.

- Identify what data are needed. Obtain all possible information and gather facts or evidence (evaluate whether data are true, relevant, and sufficient). Situations are often complicated. It is important to figure out what information is significant to this situation. Synthesize prior information you already have with similarities in the current situation. Conflicting data may indicate a need to search for more information.
- Compare existing information with past knowledge. Has this client complained of difficulty thinking before? Does she have a history of dementia?
- Look for gaps in the information. Actively work to recognize whether there is missing information. Was Mrs. Vlios previously taking medications to prevent depression? For a nurse, this is an important part of critical thinking.
- Collect information systematically. Use an organized framework to obtain information. Nurses often obtain a client's history by asking questions about each body system. They could just as systematically ask about basic needs.
- Organize your information. Clustering information into relevant categories is helpful. For example, gathering all the facts about a client's breathing may help focus your attention on whether the client is having a respiratory problem. In your assessment, you note rate and character of respirations, color of nails and lips, use of accessory muscles, and grunting noises. At the same time, you exclude information about bowel sounds or deep tendon reflexes as not being immediately relevant to his respiratory status. Categorizing information also helps you notice whether there are missing data. A second strategy that will help you organize information is to look for patterns. It has been indicated that experienced nurses intuitively note recurrent meaningful aspects of a clinical situation.

Case Discussion

Rely on prior didactic knowledge or clinical experience. Cluster the data. What was Mrs. Vlios's status immediately before hospitalization? What was her status at the time of hospitalization? What information is missing? What additional data do you need?

- Physiology: Consider pathophysiologic knowledge about the effects of hypovolemia and electrolyte imbalances on the systems such as the brain, kidneys, and vascular system. What is her temperature? What are her laboratory values? What is her 24-hour intake and output? Is she still dehydrated?
- Psychological/cognitive: How does hospitalization affect older adults? How do restraints affect them?
- Social/economic: Was weight loss a result of dehydration? Why was she without food? Could it be due to economic factors or mental problems?
- Legal: What constitutes a binding advance directive in the state in which Mrs. Vlios lives? Is a living will valid in her state, or does the law require a health power of attorney? Are these documents on file at the hospital?

STEP 4: OBTAIN NEW DATA

Critical thinking is not a linear process. Expert nurses often modify interventions based on the response to the event, or change in the client's physical condition (Fero et al., 2008). Constantly consider whether you need more information. Establish an attitude of inquiry and obtain more information as needed. Ask questions; search for evidence; and check reference books, journals, the ethics sources on the Internet, or written professional or agency protocols.

Evaluate conflicting information. There may be time constraints. If a client has suspected "respiratory problems," you may need to set priorities. Obtain data that are most useful or are easily available. It would be useful to know oxygenation levels, but you may not have time to order laboratory tests. But perhaps there is a device on the unit or in the room that can measure oxygen saturation.

Sometimes you may need to change your approach to improve your chances of obtaining information. For example, when the charge nurse caring for Mrs. Vlios used an authoritarian tone to try to get the sister and brother to provide more information about possible drug overdose, they did not respond. However, when the charge nurse changed his approach, exhibiting empathy, the daughter volunteered that on several occasions her mother had forgotten what pills she had taken.

Case Discussion

List sources from which you can obtain missing information. Physiologic data such as temperature or laboratory test results can be obtained quickly; some of the ethical information, however, may take longer to consider.

STEP 5: IDENTIFY THE SIGNIFICANT PROBLEM

- Analyze existing information: Examine all the information you have. Identify all the possible positions.
- Make inferences: What might be going on? What are the possible diagnoses? Develop a working diagnosis.
- Prioritize: Which client problem is most urgently in need of your intervention? What are the appropriate interventions?

Case Discussion

A significant physiologic concern is sepsis, regardless of whether it is an iatrogenic (hospital-acquired) infection or one resulting from immobility and debilitation. A significant ethical concern is the conflict among family members and client (as expressed through her living will). At what point do spiritual concerns take priority over a worsening physical concern?

STEP 6: EXAMINE SKEPTICALLY

Thinking about a situation may involve weighing positive and negative factors, and differentiating facts that are credible from opinions that are biased or not grounded in true facts.

- Keep an open mind.
- Challenge your own assumptions.
- Consider whether any of your assumptions are unwarranted. Does the available evidence really support your assumption?
- Discriminate between facts and inferences. Your inferences need to be logical and plausible, based on the available facts.
- Are there any problems that you have not considered?

In trying to evaluate a situation, consciously raising questions becomes an important part of thinking critically. At times there will be alternative explanations or different lines of reasoning that are equally valid. The challenge is to examine your own and others' perspectives for important ideas, complicating factors, other plausible interpretations, and new insights. Some nurses believe that examining information skeptically is part of each step in the critical thinking process rather than a step by itself.

Case Discussion

Challenge assumptions about the cause of Mrs. Vlios's condition. For example, did you eliminate the possibility that she had a head injury caused by a fall? Could she have liver failure as a result of acetaminophen overdosing? Have all the possibilities been explored? Challenge your assumptions about outcome: Are they influenced by expected probable versus possible outcomes for this client? If she, indeed, has irreversible dementia, what will the quality of her life be if she recovers from her physical problems?

STEP 7: APPLY CRITERIA

In evaluating a situation, think about appropriate responses.

- Laws: There may be a law that can be applied to guide your actions and decisions. For example, by law, certain diseases must be reported to the state. If you suspect physical abuse, there is a state statute that requires professionals to report abuse to the Department of Social Services.
- Legal precedents: There may have been similar cases or situations that were dealt with in a court of law. Legal decisions do guide health care practices. In end-of-life decisions, when there is no legally binding health care power of attorney, the most frequent hierarchy is the spouse, then the adult children, then the parents.
- Protocols: There may be standard protocols for managing certain situations. Your agency may have standing orders for caring for Mrs. Vlios if she develops respiratory distress, such as administering oxygen per face mask at 5 L/min.

Case Discussion

Many criteria could be used to examine this case, including the Nurse Practice Act in the area of jurisdiction, the professional organization code of ethics or general ethical principles of beneficence and autonomy, the hospital's written protocols and policies,

state laws regarding living wills, and prior court decisions about living wills. Remember that advance directives are designed to take effect only when clients become unable to make their own wishes known.

STEP 8: GENERATE OPTIONS AND LOOK AT ALTERNATIVES

- Evaluate the major alternative points of view.
- Involve experienced peers as soon as you can to assist you in making your decision.
- Use clues from others to help you "put the picture together."
- Can you identify all the arguments—pro and con—to explain this situation? Almost all situations will have strong counterarguments or competing hypotheses.

Case Discussion

The important concept is that neither the physician nor the nurse should handle this alone; rather, others should be involved (e.g., the hospital bioethics committee, the ombudsman client representative, the family's spiritual counselor, and other medical experts such as a gerontologist, psychologist, and nursing clinical specialist).

STEP 9: CONSIDER WHETHER FACTORS CHANGE IF THE CONTEXT CHANGES

Consider whether your decision would be different if there were a change in circumstances. For example, a change in the age of the client, in the site of the situation, or in the client's culture may affect your decision. A competent nurse prioritizes which aspects of the situation are most relevant and can modify her actions based on the client's response (Fero et al., 2009).

Case Discussion

If you knew the outcome from the beginning, would your decisions be the same? What if you knew Mrs. Vlios had a terminal cancer? What if Mrs. Vlios had remained in her senior housing project and you were the home health nurse? What if Mrs. Vlios had remained alert during her hospitalization and refused IVs, hyperalimentation, nasogastric tubes, and so on? What if the family and Mrs. Vlios were in agreement about no treatment? Would you make more assertive interventions to save her life if she were 7 years old, or a 35-year-old mother of five young children?

STEP 10: MAKE THE FINAL DECISION

After analyzing available information in this systematic way, you need to make a judgment or decision. An important part of your decision is your ability to communicate it coherently to others and to reflect on the outcome of your decision for your client.

- Justify your conclusion.
- Evaluate outcomes.
- Test out your decision or conclusion by implementing appropriate actions.

The critical thinker needs to be able to accept that there may be multiple solutions that can be equally acceptable. In other situations, you may need to make a decision even when there is incomplete knowledge. Be able to cite your rationale or present your arguments to others for your decision choice and interventions.

After you implement your interventions, examine the client outcomes. Was your assessment correct? Did you obtain enough information? Did the benefits to the client and family outweigh the harm that may have occurred? In retrospect, do you know you made the correct decision? Did you anticipate possibilities and complications correctly? This kind of self-examination can foster self-correction. It is this process of reflecting on one's own thinking that is the hallmark of a critical thinker.

Case Discussion

The most important concept is to forget the idea that there is one right answer to the dilemmas raised by discussion of this case. Accept that there may be several equally correct solutions depending on each individual's point of view.

SUMMARIZING THE CRITICAL THINKING LEARNING PROCESS

The most effective method of learning these steps in critical thinking results from repeatedly applying them to clinical situations. This can occur in your own clinical care. A new graduate nurse must, at a minimum, be able to identify essential clinical data, know when to initiate interventions, know why a particular intervention is relevant, and differentiate between problems that need immediate intervention versus problems that can wait for action. Repeated practice in applying critical thinking can help a new graduate fit into the expectations of employers.

Students have demonstrated that critical thinking can be learned in the classroom, as well as through clinical experience. Effective learning can occur when opportunities are structured that allow for repeated in-class applications to client case situations. This includes using real-life case interviews with experienced nurses, which allow you to analyze their decision-making process. The interview and analysis of an expert nurse's critical thinking described in Exercise 3-5 explains how this is done using a 10-minute recording.

You may also help increase your critical thinking and clinical problem-solving skills by discussing the following additional case example. Remember that most clinical situations requiring decision making will not involve the types of ethical dilemmas discussed earlier in this chapter.

EXERCISE 3-5	Your Analysis of an Expert's Critical Thinking: Interview of Expert Nurse's Case

Purpose: To develop awareness of critical thinking in the clinical judgment process.

Procedure:
Find an experienced nurse in your community and record him or her describing a real client case. You can use a computer or cell phone with recording capability, videotape, or audiotape to record an interview that takes less than 10 minutes. During the interview, have the expert describe an actual client case in which there was a significant change in the client's health status. Have the expert describe the interventions and thinking process that took place during this situation.

Ask what nursing knowledge, laboratory data, or experience helped the nurse make his or her decision. You can work with a partner. Remember to protect confidentiality by omitting names and other identifiers.

Discussion:
Analyze the tape using an outline of the 10 steps in critical thinking. Discussion should first include citation examples of each step noted during their review of the taped interview, followed by application to the broad principles. Discussion of steps missed by the interviewed expert can be enlightening, as long as care is taken to avoid any criticism of the guest "expert."

Case Example

Mr. Gonzales has terminal cancer. His family defers to the attending physician who prescribes aggressive rescue treatment. The hospice nurse is an expert in the expressed and unexpressed needs of terminal clients. She advocates for a conservative and supportive plan of care. A logical case could be built for each position.

SUMMARY

Critical thinking is the ability to think about your thinking. It is not a linear process. Analysis of the thinking processes of expert nurses reveals that they continually scan new data and simultaneously apply these steps in clinical decision making. They monitor the effectiveness of their interventions in achieving desired outcomes for their client. A nurse's values and critical thinking abilities often have a profound effect on the quality of care given to a client, even affecting client mortality outcomes. Functioning as a competent nurse requires that you have knowledge of medical and nursing content, an accumulation of clinical experiences, and an ability to think critically. Almost daily, we confront ethical dilemmas and complicated clinical situations that require expertise as a decision maker. We can follow the 10 steps of the critical thinking process described in this chapter to help us respond to such situations. Developing skill as a critical thinker is a learned process, one requiring repeated opportunities for application to clinical situations. Reflecting on one's own thinking about case example situations provided in this chapter can assist such learning.

ETHICAL DILEMMA   What Would You Do?

Rosa Smith, RN, is a newly graduated nurse employed on a medical unit in a county hospital system. She is a single mother and sole support for her toddler daughter. Nine clients are admitted with a new virulent pandemic flu that has killed citizens internationally in a manner similar to the SARS virus in the 1990s or the H1N1 virus of 2009. You know that both of these pandemics caused deaths in health care workers.

1. Identify Rosa's conflicting obligations.
2. Should Rosa continue to work, caring for such clients, putting herself and child at risk?
3. By virtue of her choosing to become a nurse, did she assume an ethical obligation/moral duty to treat clients during this disease outbreak?
4. What if Rosa's daughter were an adult?
5. What would you do if you worked on this unit?
6. When, if ever, is it okay to say "no"?

Developed based on information in Stokowski's (2009) article, "Ethical dilemmas for healthcare professionals: can we avoid influenza?"

REFERENCES

Bromley E, Braslow JY: Teaching critical thinking in psychiatric training: a role for the social sciences, *Am J Psychiatry* 165(11): 1396–1401, 2008.

Carter LM, Rukholm E: A study of critical thinking, teacher-student interaction, and discipline-specific writing in an online educational setting for registered nurses, *J Contin Educ Nurs* 39(3):133–138, 2008.

Ebbesen M, Pedersen BD: The principle of respect for autonomy—concordant with the experience of oncology physicians and molecular biologists in their daily work? *BMC Med Ethics* 9:5, 2008.

Facione PA: *Critical thinking: what is it and why it counts*, Milbrae, CA, 2006, California Academic Press.

Fero LJ, Witsberger CM, Wesmiller SW, et al: Critical thinking ability of new graduate and experienced nurses, *J Adv Nurs* 65(1):139–148, 2009.

Johnson P: US journalists fare well on test of ethics, study finds, *USA Today* 5D, February 2, 2005.

Mangena A, Chabeli MM: Strategies to overcome obstacles in the facilitation of critical thinking in nursing education, *Nursing Education Today* 25:291–298, 2005.

Milton C: Ethical implications for acting faithfully in nurse-person relationships, *Nurs Sci Q* 15:21–24, 2002.

Ravert P: Patient simulator sessions and critical thinking, *J Nurs Educ* 47(12):557–562, 2008.

Rogal SM, Young J: Exploring critical thinking in critical care nursing education: a pilot study, *J Contin Educ Nurs* 39(1):28–33, 2008.

Rush KL, Dyches CE, Waldrop S, et al: Critical thinking among RN-to-BSN distance students participating in human patient simulation, *J Nurs Educ* 47(11):501–507, 2008.

Sasso L: *Federazione Europea delle Professioni Infermieristiche Action Plan 2007*, 2008..

Sasso L, Stievano A, Jurado MG, et al: Code of ethics and conduct for European nursing, *Nurs Ethics* 15(6):821–836, 2008.

Sorensen HA, Yankech LR: Precepting in the fast lane: improving critical thinking in new graduate nurses, *J Contin Educ Nurs* 39(5): 208–216, 2008.

Stokowski LA: Ethical dilemmas for healthcare professionals: can we avoid influenza? *Medscape Infectious Diseases* 1–7, 2009.

Wilgis M, McConnell J: Concept mapping: an educational strategy to improve graduate nurses' critical thinking skills during a hospital orientation program, *J Contin Educ Nurs* 39(3):119–126, 2008.

Worrell JA, Profetto-McGrath J: Critical thinking as an outcome of context-based learning among post RN students: a literature review, *Nurse Educ Today* 27:420–426, 2007.

Self-Concept in the Nurse-Client Relationship

Elizabeth C. Arnold

OBJECTIVES

At the end of the chapter, the reader will be able to:
1. Define self-concept.
2. Describe the features of and functions of self-concept.
3. Identify theoretical models of the self and self-concept.
4. Discuss Erikson's theory of psychosocial ego development.
5. Identify functional health patterns and nursing diagnosis related to self-concept pattern disturbances.
6. Apply the nursing process to the nursing diagnosis of body image disturbance.
7. Apply the nursing process to the nursing diagnosis of personal identity disturbance.
8. Apply the nursing process to the nursing diagnosis of self-esteem disturbance.
9. Apply the nursing process to the nursing diagnosis of spiritual distress.

This chapter explores self-concept as a key informant of behavior in human interaction and nurse-client relationships. The chapter describes theoretical frameworks for how self-concept develops. The Applications section discusses body image, personal identity, spirituality, and self-esteem as important clinical components of self-concept and applies the nursing process to self-concept disturbances. The key role of self-concept in nurse-client relationships is explored.

BASIC CONCEPTS

Self-concept is an integral component of nurse-client relationships. It is a difficult idea to conceptualize due to its many facets and abstract nature. Figure 4-1 identifies aspects that are relevant to an appreciation of the self-concept's role in communication. The nursing diagnosis Association (NANDA International, 2009)

recognizes self-concept pattern disturbances as approved nursing diagnoses. A healthy self-concept reflects attitudes, emotions and values that are realistically consistent with meaningful purposes in life and satisfying to the individual. A well-differentiated sense of personal identity permits the self-as-knower to experience a feeling of distinctness from others and a sense of sameness through time (Konig, 2009).

DEFINITION

Self-concept refers to an acquired set of thoughts, feelings, attitudes, and beliefs that individuals have about the nature and organization of their personality. Cunha and Goncalves (2009) refer to the self as an open system, which is fluid and dynamic. Like fingerprints, no two self-concepts are exactly alike. Self-concepts help people experience who they are and what they are capable of becoming physically, emotionally, intellectually,

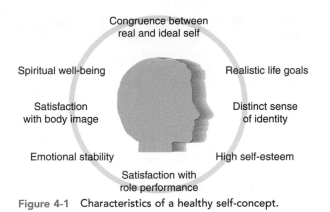

Congruence between
real and ideal self

Spiritual well-being

Realistic life goals

Satisfaction
with body image

Distinct sense
of identity

Emotional stability

High self-esteem

Satisfaction with
role performance

Figure 4-1 Characteristics of a healthy self-concept.

socially, and spiritually in relationship or community with others. McCormick & Hardy (2008) state, "identity, the definition of one's self, is the heart of one's life" (p. 405). Consciousness of one's personal identity allows a person to make authentic choices and maintain well-developed personal boundaries in relationships with others.

Self-concepts create and reflect our personal reality and worldview. The four aspects of self-concept—physical, cognitive, emotional, and spiritual—represent the holistic self, and are important determinants of behavior. Different aspects of self become more prominent, depending on the particular situation in which people find themselves (Prescott, 2006). From a patient-centered health care perspective, relevant self-concept patterns include body image (physical), personal identity (cognitive and perceptual awareness), self-esteem (emotional valuing), and spirituality (connectivity with a higher purpose or God).

FEATURES AND FUNCTIONS OF SELF-CONCEPT

Self-concept is an active, rather than static source of information about the self. Hunter (2008) suggests, "As one ages, the 'self' develops and becomes a more and more unique entity formed by personal experiences and personally developed values and beliefs" (p. 318). Self-concept is not necessarily a unified concept. It consists of multiple self-images, some of which may not match with each other or be supportive of the whole. For example, a star athlete can be a marginal student. Which is the true self-image, or are both valid? One can think of self-concept basically as the response to the question, "Who am I?" (Exercise 4-1).

Self-concepts provide important bridges to meaning. They help individuals make personal sense of their past, as it relates to the present and as it might be in the future (Lee & Oyserman, 2009). Personal decisions congruent with self-concept affirm the sense of self-identity, whereas those that are not consistent with important self-concepts create doubt and uncertainty.

Possible Selves

Possible selves is a term used to explain the future-oriented component of self-concept. Future expectations are important variables in goal setting and motivation (Lee & Oyserman, 2009). For example, a nursing student might think, "I can see myself becoming a nurse practitioner." Such thoughts help the novice nurse work harder to achieve professional goals. Blazer (2008) suggests self-perceptions of personal health and well-being may be as important as objective data for predicting health outcomes over time. Communication can provide important support for exploring positive possibilities for personal identity and for helping clients reframe or avoid the establishment of negative possible selves.

Negative concepts of possible selves can become a self-fulfilling prophecy (Markus & Nurius, 1986). For example, Martha receives a performance evaluation indicating a need for improved self-confidence. Viewing the criticism as a negative commentary on her "self," she performs awkwardly and freezes when asked questions in the clinical area.

Self-Concept/Environment Relationships

The social environment plays an important role in shaping a person's self-concept. Set factors such as poverty, dysfunctional parenting styles, loss of a parent, lack of educational opportunities, and level of parental literacy contribute to negative self-concepts. A stable home environment, sports, academic success, professional opportunities, praise for successful accomplishments, and supportive parents and mentors help to foster positive self-concepts. **Reflective appraisals** refer to the personalized messages received from others that help shape self-concepts and contribute to self-evaluations (Hybels & Weaver, 2008).

Understanding the interplay between person and environment in explaining self-concept has important implications for the nurse-client relationship. It is a reciprocal relationship in which the nurse's perceptions of self and other limit or enhance communication, and

EXERCISE 4-1	Who Am I?

Purpose: To help students understand some of the self-concepts they hold about themselves.

Procedure:
This exercise may be done as homework exercise and discussed in class. The class should sit face-to-face in a circle.

Fill in the blanks to complete the following sentences. There are no right or wrong answers.
The thing I like best about myself is _____.
The thing I like least about myself is _____.
My favorite activity is _____.
When I am in a group, I _____.
It would surprise most people if they knew _____.
The most important value to me is _____.
I like _____.
I most dislike _____.
I am happy when _____.
I feel sad when _____.

I feel most self-confident when I _____.
I am _____.
I feel committed to _____.
Five years from now I see myself as _____.

Discussion:
1. What were the hardest items to answer? The easiest?
2. Were you surprised by some of your answers? If so, in what ways?
3. Did anybody's answers surprise you? If so, in what ways?
4. Did anyone's answers particularly impress you? If so, in what ways?
5. What did you learn about yourself from doing this exercise?
6. How would you see yourself using this self-awareness in professional interpersonal relationships with clients?

support or diminish a client's sense of self-esteem. Identity (self-concept) is carved out from personal experiences of life, and forms the basis for behavioral expression and interpersonal reactions to the environment. A well-defined, accurate self-concept allows nurses to effectively communicate in most situations.

Self-awareness for nurses is just as critical as it is for clients. Although cognitive awareness of the self-concept is never fully complete, the Johari Window (Luft & Ingham, 1955) provides a disclosure/feedback model to help people learn more about their self-concept. The model consists of four areas:

- Open self (arena): what is known to self and others
- Blind self: what is known by others, but not by self
- Hidden self (façade): what is known by self, but not by others
- Unknown self: what is unknown to self and also unknown to others

The larger the open self box is, the more one knows about oneself and the more flexibility there is to realistically interpret and constructively cope with challenging health situations. Increasing the open area through asking for and receiving feedback (decreasing blind self), and using self-disclosure (decreasing the hidden self) leads to more authentic self-awareness. Decreasing the level of unknown area through self-discovery, new

observations by others, and mutual illumination of experiences increases the open area.

The basic goal of any constructive relationship is to help the participants enlarge self-knowledge and enhance their potential by integrating disowned, neglected, unrecognized, or unrealized parts of the self into the personality. Expected outcomes include enhanced self-esteem, greater productivity, and increased personal satisfaction.

THEORETICAL MODELS OF SELF CONCEPT

William James (1890) was among the first theorists to address the self-concept as an important idea in psychology. He makes a distinction between "the I and the me: the I is equated with the self-as-knower and the me is equated with the self-as-known" (Konig, 2009, p. 102). James believed that a person has as many different social selves as there are distinct groups of persons about whose opinion he or she cares.

George Mead approaches the self from a sociologic perspective, emphasizing the influence of culture, moral norms, and language in framing self-concepts through interpersonal interactions (symbolic interactionism). The self affects and is influenced by how people experience themselves in relation to others (Elliott, 2008).

Any threat to the self-system creates anxiety. Freud's ego defense mechanisms help explain how a person unconsciously protect the self against full awareness of potential and actual threats (see Chapter 20).

The self is a central construct in humanistic and psychodynamic theories of personality. Carl Rogers (1951) defined the self as "an organized, fluid, but consistent conceptual pattern of perceptions of characteristics and relationships or the 'I' or the 'me' together with values attached to these concepts" (p. 498).

Harry Stack Sullivan (1953) believed that self-concepts begin in infancy. He referred to each person's self-images as a self-system that people develop to help them in the following ways: (1) develop a consistent image of self, (2) protect themselves against feeling anxiety, and (3) maintain their interpersonal security. Sullivan asserted that the self develops out of social interactions with others, most notably the mother. During early childhood, people develop self-personifications of a good me (resulting from reward and approval experiences), a bad me (resulting from punishment and disapproval experiences), and a not me (resulting from anxiety-producing experiences that are dissociated by the person as not being a part of their self-concept). Therapeutic interpersonal interactions can correct and build a different sense of self.

ERIKSON'S THEORY OF PSYCHOSOCIAL DEVELOPMENT

Erik Erikson (1968, 1982) believed that personality develops and becomes more complex as a person recognizes and responds to evolving developmental challenges (psychosocial crises) that occur with regularity throughout the life cycle. If individuals receive encouragement and support, they are more likely to master each psychosocial challenge and move successfully into the next stage of ego development with a strong sense of self.

The first four stages of Erikson's psychosocial model of development serve as building blocks for the central developmental task of establishing a healthy ego identity (identity vs. identity diffusion). Working through the remaining stages of ego development refines and expands the ego identity established in late adolescence.

Successful resolution of developmental tasks in adulthood includes finding a meaningful occupation, establishing committed relationships and starting a family, contributing to the welfare of family and others, and sharing one's wisdom with the larger community. A well-lived life results in a sense of integrity about oneself and one's life at life's closing chapter. Failure to master previous developmental stages can leave a person feeling despair and regret. Mastering psychosocial tasks successfully throughout the life cycle helps people feel a sense of integrity and enthusiasm about the life they have led, with few regrets, even when confronting death. Failure to successfully complete tasks associated with a developmental stage results in a reduced capacity to effectively negotiate later stages and a weakened sense of self. Erikson believed that stage development is never final. People have the potential to successfully rework developmental stages at a later time.

Erikson's stages of ego development are outlined in Table 4-1. Nurses use Erikson's model as an important part of client assessment. Analysis of behavior patterns using this framework can identify age-appropriateness or arrested ego identity development. Exercise 4-2 focuses on applying Erikson's concepts to client situations.

Developing an Evidence-Based Practice

Rowland JH, Desmond KA, Meyerowitz BE, et al.: Role of breast reconstructive surgery in physical and emotional outcomes among breast cancer survivors, *J Natl Canc Inst* 92(17):1422–1429, 2000.

A self-report questionnaire was twice administered to 1957 breast cancer survivors to compare whether type of surgery influenced the psychosocial outcomes, including body image and feelings of attractiveness.

Results: Of women who had a mastectomy with reconstructive surgery, 45.4% reported that the breast cancer had a negative impact on their sex lives. These negative outcomes were far greater than for women whose breast cancer was treated with a lumpectomy (29.8%), and more even than the women who had a mastectomy without reconstruction (41.3%). However, beyond the first year after diagnosis, the women's quality of life was more likely to be influenced by her age and exposure to adjuvant therapy than by her type of breast surgery.

Application to Your Clinical Practice: More studies are needed on the effects of breast cancer surgical treatments on self-image, but based on results from this study, your counseling about treatment choices might need to consider age and surgical invasiveness as factors in the clients' decision-making process about treatment choices.

TABLE 4-1	Erikson's Stages of Psychosocial Development, Clinical Behavior Guidelines, and Stressors		
Stage of Personality Guidelines	**Ego Strength or Virtue**	**Clinical Behavior Guidelines**	**Stressors**
Trust vs. mistrust	Hope	Appropriate attachment behaviors Ability to ask for assistance with an expectation of receiving it Ability to give and receive information related to self and health Ability to share opinions and experiences easily Ability to differentiate between how much one can trust and how much one must distrust	Unfamiliar environment or routines Inconsistency in care Pain Lack of information Unmet needs (e.g., having to wait 20 minutes for a bedpan or pain injection) Losses at critical times or accumulated loss Significant or sudden loss of physical function (e.g., a client with a broken hip being afraid to walk)
Autonomy vs. shame and doubt	Willpower	Ability to express opinions freely and to disagree tactfully Ability to delay gratification Ability to accept reasonable treatment plans and hospital regulations Ability to regulate one's behaviors (overcompliance, noncompliance, suggest disruptions) Ability to make age-appropriate decisions	Overemphasis on unfair or rigid regulation (e.g., putting clients in nursing homes to bed at 7 p.m.) Cultural emphasis on guilt and shaming as a way of controlling behavior Limited opportunity to make choices in a hospital setting Limited allowance made for individuality
Initiative vs. guilt	Purpose	Ability to develop realistic goals and to initiate actions to meet them Ability to make mistakes without undue embarrassment Ability to have curiosity about health care Ability to work for goals Ability to develop constructive fantasies and plans	Significant or sudden change in life pattern that interferes with role Loss of a mentor, particularly in adolescence or with a new job Lack of opportunity to participate in planning of care Overinvolved parenting that does not allow for experimentation Hypercritical authority figures No opportunity for play
Industry vs. inferiority	Competence	Work is perceived as meaningful and satisfying Appropriate satisfaction with balance in lifestyle pattern, including leisure activities Ability to work with others, including staff Ability to complete tasks and self-care activities in line with capabilities Ability to express personal strengths and limitations realistically	Limited opportunity to learn and master tasks Illness, circumstance, or condition that compromises or obliterates one's usual activities Lack of cultural support or opportunity for training
Identity vs. identity diffusion	Fidelity	Ability to establish friendships with peers Realistic assertion of independence and dependence needs Demonstration of overall satisfaction with self-image, including physical characteristics, personality, and role in life	Lack of opportunity Overprotective, neglectful, or inconsistent parenting Sudden or significant change in appearance, health, or status Lack of same-sex role models

TABLE 4-1	Erikson's Stages of Psychosocial Development, Clinical Behavior Guidelines, and Stressors—cont'd		
Stage of Personality Guidelines	**Ego Strength or Virtue**	**Clinical Behavior Guidelines**	**Stressors**
Identity vs. isolation	Fidelity	Ability to express and act on personal values Congruence of self-perception with nurse's observation and perception of significant others	
Intimacy vs. isolation	Love	Ability to enter into strong reciprocal interpersonal relationships Ability to identify a readily available support system Ability to feel the caring of others Ability to act harmoniously with family and friends	Competition Communication that includes a hidden agenda Projection of images and expectations onto another person Lack of privacy Loss of significant others at critical points of development
Generativity vs. stagnation and self-absorption	Caring	Demonstration of age-appropriate activities Development of a realistic assessment of personal contributions to society Development of ways to maximize productivity Appropriate care of whatever one has created Demonstration of a concern for others and a willingness to share ideas and knowledge Evidence of a healthy balance among work, family, and self-demands	Aging parents, separately or concurrently with adolescent children Obsolescence or layoff in career "Me generation" attitude Inability or lack of opportunity to function in a previous manner Children leaving home Forced retirement
Integrity vs. despair	Wisdom	Expression of satisfaction with personal lifestyle Acceptance of growing limitations while maintaining maximum productivity Expression of acceptance of certitude of death, as well as satisfaction with one's contributions to life Lack of opportunity	Rigid lifestyle Loss of significant other Loss of physical, intellectual, and emotional faculties Loss of previously satisfying work and family roles

---

EXERCISE 4-2	Erikson's Stages of Psychosocial Development

Purpose: To help students apply Erikson's stages of psychosocial development to client situations.

Procedure:
This exercise may be done as a homework exercise with the results shared in class.

To set your knowledge of Erikson's stages of psychosocial development, identify the psychosocial crisis or crises each of the following clients might be experiencing:
1. A 16-year-old unwed mother having her first child
2. A 50-year-old executive "let go" from his job after 18 years of employment
3. A stroke victim paralyzed on the left side
4. A middle-aged woman caring for her mother, who has Alzheimer's disease
5. A 17-year-old high-school athlete suddenly paralyzed from the neck down.

Discussion:
1. What criteria did you use to determine the most relevant psychosocial stage for each client situation?
2. What conclusions can you draw from doing this exercise that would influence how you would respond to each of these clients?

SELF-CONCEPT AS A NURSING DIAGNOSIS

The self-concept is an essential starting point for understanding the behavior of clients in nurse-client relationships. Serious injury or illness inevitably challenges self-concept. As a person's perception of inner self-coherence is disturbed, the future becomes uncertain and unpredictable (Ellis-Hill & Horn, 2000). The following case example illustrates the extent of challenge.

Case Example

My values in life have changed completely. It was incredibly difficult to realize that as a 45-year-old man I was "good for nothing." I was the rock that everybody relied on. Suddenly, it was I who had to ask others for help. I'm prone to this disease and I know that one day I will fall ill again (Raholm, 2008, p. 62).

Four aspects of self-concept are particularly relevant to consider in nurse-client relationships: body image, personal identity, self-esteem, and spirituality. These issues are addressed in Gordon's (2007) functional health patterns under self-perception, self-concept patterns, and value-belief patterns. North American Nursing Diagnosis Association (NANDA International, 2009). Relevant to self-concept are nursing diagnoses related to body image, human dignity, personal identity, powerlessness, self-concept, and self-esteem. Disturbances in self-concept directly and indirectly influence role relationships, as discussed in Chapter 7.

BODY IMAGE

Body image is the physical dimension of self-concept. Our body image changes throughout life, influenced by the process of aging, the appraisals of others, cultural and social factors, and physical changes resulting from illness or injury.

Physical appearance and body image are not necessarily the same. Body image refers to how people perceive their physical characteristics. For example, individuals with an eating disorder may see themselves as a "fat" person despite being dangerously underweight.

The value individuals place on body image reflects sociocultural norms and media presentations. Different cultures characterize similar physical characteristics as positive and others as negative. In the United

States, a trim figure for women and a lean, muscular body for men are admired (Vartanian, 2009). In other cultures, obesity may be viewed as a sign of prosperity, fertility, or the ability to survive (Boston Women's Health Book Collection, 1998).

Body image is closely intertwined with personal identity such that any change in body function or physical appearance can affect personal identity and challenge a person's self-esteem. Hair loss with chemotherapy, moon face with high doses of prednisone, stroke limitations, removal of a breast or limb, burns, and loss of energy can all affect body image.

Physical appearance influences how people respond to a person (Rhode, 2009). Physically attractive people, appropriately dressed, and well groomed typically command more positive attention than those who are not. Individuals who deviate significantly from the norm in height, weight, or physical characteristics, and those who look considerably older or younger than their chronologic age often suffer discrimination (Williams, 2009). They speak of receiving subtle inequities, of being treated differentially, and as having intellectual and character shortcomings attributed to them solely on the basis of appearance.

Case Example

Anne has been obese since she was a small child. In adulthood, she weighs 275 pounds, and is very self-conscious about her weight. Although she has tried many diets, she has been unsuccessful in losing significant amounts of weight. Whenever she visits her in-laws, her mother-in-law serves her small portions, reminds her that she is overweight, and makes subtle suggestions about how her marriage would be more successful if she were thinner. Anne feels even worse about herself and dreads visiting. She clearly knows she is obese and doesn't need a reminder that she is overweight articulated in a family social situation.

Disturbances in body image can be long lasting. In a study of overweight adolescents, a primary theme that emerged was "a forever knowing of self as overweight" (Smith & Perkins, 2008).

HIDDEN BODY IMAGE DISTURBANCES

Although most people think of body image as describing visible differences in physical characteristics, subtle differences related to loss of body function apply. Medical conditions such as traumatic brain injury, infertility, impotence, loss of bladder or bowel function, and reliance on mechanical devices such as dialysis and pacemakers can create unseen body image disturbances. Loss of energy from cancer treatments can change a person's self-image as a person with zest and vigor, to one who is frail and vulnerable.

Alteration in control and loss of sensation also represent body image disturbance. Clients in pain from fibromyalgia and those subject to seizures, alcoholism, cardiac arrhythmias, or diabetic fluctuations in blood sugar may exhibit few obvious physical changes, but they can experience similar feelings of insecurity and uncertainty about their body image.

Assessment Strategies

The *meaning* of body image is an important dimension to assess as it differs from person to person. Some, like Ray Charles or Christopher Reeves frame a negative body image as a positive feature of who they are. Others let a physical deviation become their only defining feature.

Assessment data supportive of a nursing diagnosis related to a self-concept disturbance in body image might include one or more of the following behaviors:

- Verbal expression of negative feelings about the body
- No mention of changes in body structure and function, or preoccupation with changed body structure or function
- Reluctance to look at or touch a changed body structure
- Social isolation and loss of interest in friends after a change in body structure, appearance, or function
- Physical changes usually require significant psychosocial and role performance adjustment (Drench, Noonan, Sharby, & Ventura, 2006); a comprehensive assessment should include the client's strengths and limitations, expressed needs and goals, the nature and accessibility of the client's support oonansystem, and the impact of body image change on lifestyle

Supportive Nursing Strategies

Modeling acceptance starts with the nurse. Nurses see clients with serious body image changes on a regular basis; for the client, it is a unique and potentially horrifying experience. Showing the client that a physical change does not frighten the nurse reduces the fear that people will turn away. Anticipatory guidance with visitors to prepare them for dramatic changes in their family member's or friend's appearance helps promote acceptance.

Providing relevant information and creating opportunities for the client to ask questions make it acceptable for the client to explore changes in self-concept related to body image is an important nursing strategy. Validation checks, asking whether the client has any questions, and suggesting realistic responses can facilitate communication about alterations in body image.

Nurses can introduce adaptive functioning by helping clients anticipate and respond with dignity to the reactions of others. Clients often worry about how their physical or emotional changes will be accepted by others. Asking questions about what the client expects, providing coaching, and helping clients identify social supports is helpful. Talking with others, for example, having a Reach for Recovery volunteer visit with a mastectomy client, is a simple intervention that helps increase the client's adjustment and acceptance of body image disturbances.

PERSONAL IDENTITY

Karademas et al. (2008) describe **personal identity** as an intrapersonal psychological process consisting of a person's perceptions or images of personal abilities, characteristics, and potential growth potential. Personal identity is based on cognitive understandings of the self derived from perceptual and cognitive processing of personally relevant data about the self.

Each person's self-concept is anchored in self-descriptions advanced by the culture. A clear cultural identity is positively related to self-concept clarity and self esteem (Usborne and Taylor, 2010). Understanding fundamental differences in cultural worldview orientation helps nurses frame interventions in ways that support ethno-cultural variations. For example, Western cultures tend to be individualistic, whereas Asian cultures see the individual as part of a collective group. Oyserman and Markus (1998) note:

> From a North American perspective, a collective answer to the "who am I" question is that "I am a bounded, autonomous whole." The solution to this question from a Japanese perspective is "I am a member or a participant of a group." (p. 110)

Exercise 4-3 helps the nurse identify the contribution of life experiences that contribute to self-concept.

EXERCISE 4-3	Contribution of Life Experiences to Self-Concept

Purpose: To help students identify some of the many personal variations in lived experiences, contributing to self-concept. There are no right or wrong responses.

Procedure:
1. Pair off with another student, preferably one with whom you are not well acquainted.
2. Student A spends 5 minutes questioning Student B to collect a biography of facts, including such information as ethnic background, number of siblings, place of birth, job or volunteer experiences, unusual life experiences, types of responsibilities, and favorite leisure activities. The process is then reversed, and Student B interviews Student A.

3. Each student introduces the other to the class, using the information gained from the interview.

Discussion:
1. Were you surprised by any of the information you found out?
2. How did your perception of other students change in light of the information shared?
3. In what ways were your perceptions different from your initial impression of your partner after the interview portion of the exercise?
4. What did you learn about yourself from doing this exercise?
5. How do you think what you learned might apply to nursing practice?

The Challenge of Health Status Changes

Illness, genetic factors, pain, or injury affecting cognitive abilities can compromise or crush the sense of personal identity. For example, in a study of stroke victims, findings showed a more negative sense of self, reduced social activity, and lower self-esteem, even after rehabilitation (Ellis-Hill & Horn, 2000). Individuals with brain injury or dementia can suffer a complete loss of self. Although sensory images enter the psyche, the normal cognitive processes people use to interpret their meaning can't make sense of them. Without cognitive ability, people don't know who they are. People with dementia lose their ability to set realistic goals, implement coherent patterns of behavior, or control basic elements of their lives. As the disease progresses, they can no longer recognize significant others or retain a sense of their personal identity.

Perception and cognition play an important role in a person's recognition of personal identity and the ability to communicate who they are to other people. Any health change can challenge a person's stable sense of personal identity. People get used to other persons treating them in certain ways because of status, work, or personality characteristics. Heijmans et al. (2004) suggest that, in addition to accepting an illness with its accompanying personal needs, people may need to adapt to an altered social identity and find new ways to initiate and maintain social relationships. This requires an emotional appraisal and adjustment, because things are not the same for the client or for those with whom the person interacts. Renegotiating relationships can be awkward, and clients often need the nurse's help in how to respond.

Case Example

Linda is an RN working in a busy surgery center. Returning to work after a hospitalization for major depression, she was no longer allowed to be in charge of her unit. Other staff became highly protective of her. She was carefully watched to ensure that she was not going to relapse and given simpler tasks to avoid stressing her out. Linda couldn't understand why her coworkers didn't see her as the same person she was before. Her depression was in remission. But in the eyes of her coworkers, Linda had been reclassified as a mentally ill person. Their efforts were well-intentioned, but they had demoralizing effects on Linda's personal identity.

PERCEPTION

Perception is referred to as the gatekeeper of personal identity because it is the initial cognitive process through which a person transforms external sensory data into selected images of reality. Perception allows a person to cluster sensory images into a meaningful pattern. It is a cognitive process, not an emotional one. Consider the image in Figure 4-2. Depending on where your eyes focus, one can draw different conclusions about the image. The same is true about life: Reality lies in the eye of the beholder. Perceptions differ because people develop mindsets that automatically alter sensory data in personal ways. Messages perceived as being consistent with a person's self-concept are likely to be heard, whereas messages that are incompatible with self-images create emotional distress. Global perceptual distortions can occur as a result of delirium, psychosis, or psychoactive drug reactions.

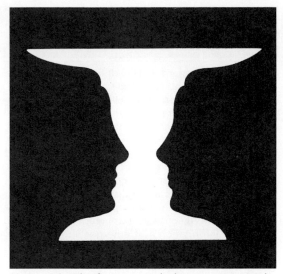

Figure 4-2 The figure-ground phenomenon. Are the figures presented in white against a black background or in black against a white background? Does it make a difference in your perception of the figures? *(From the Westinghouse Learning Corporation:* Self-instructional unit 12: perception, 1970. *Reprinted with permission.)*

Mental disorders such as depression and schizophrenia generate a distorted perceptual filter affecting perception and cognitive interpretations. Clients can distort the meaning of objective data, leading the person to engage in dysfunctional behaviors as a result. Validation of perceptual data is needed because the nurse and the client may not be processing the same reality. For example, others may perceive a person as being witty and interesting, whereas the individual internally views himself as dull and boring. Simple perceptual distortions can be challenged with compassionate questioning and sometimes, targeted humor.

Case Example

Grace Ann Hummer is a 65-year-old widow with arthritis, a weight problem, and failing eyesight. She looks older than she is chronologically. Admitted for a minor surgical procedure, Ms. Hummer tells the nurse she does not know why she came. Nothing can be done for her because she is too old and decrepit.

> *Nurse:* As I understand it, you came in today for removal of your bunions. Can you tell me more about the problem as you see it? *(Asking for this information separates the current situation from an overall assessment of ill health.)*

> *Client:* Well, I've been having trouble walking, and I can't do some of the things I like to do that require extensive walking. I also have to buy "clunky" shoes that make me look like an old woman.

> *Nurse:* So you are not willing to be an old woman yet? *(Taking the client's statement and challenging the cognitive distortion presented in her initial comments with humor allows the client to view her statement differently.)*

> *Client* (laughing): Right, there are a lot of things I want to do before I'm ready for a nursing home.

COGNITION

Cognition is a complex, creative, logical process that people use to make sense of perceptions. The cognitive aspects of self-concept are best characterized by the level, clarity, and logic of thinking. People with strong critical thinking skills tend to make good decisions. An example of a cognitive distortion is imagining the worst-case scenario when something minor goes wrong.

Assessment

Cognitive assessment is accomplished through client history, mental status examination, and assessment of functional capabilities. Clients or close significant others, or both, should be asked about the client's medical and psychiatric history, medications, and any significant changes in observed changes in memory, cognitive reasoning, or expressive language. Inquiring about functional abilities to perform activities of daily living is valuable. Client data are compared with the performance of others with similar demographic background and life experiences. Significant deviations, as well as defined changes in the quality and quantity of cognitive performance, are areas for concern. It is crucial for example, to differentiate between cognitive dysfunction as the result of medication adverse effects, delirium, or depression and a true dementia (Arnold, 2005).

Serious injury or illness creates major challenges to personal identity. Particularly devastating to one's self-concept is disease or injury affecting the brain because of their impact on processing information and communicating with others. They can erase memories, skills and the knowledge needed to conduct essential life tasks. Treating each client as a valued person, with relevant ideas, opinions, and feelings should underscore each specific treatment plan. With effort, it is usually possible to communicate even with cognitively compromised individuals in simple ways.

Planning and Intervention

Respect for the client perspective, active listening, and active involvement in collaborative planning strengthen a sense of personal identity through ownership and understanding of the treatment plan. Trying to understand the client as a valued person and the personalized meaning of the health disruption is an important common denominator in supporting the client's personal identity.

Case Example

Jenna was a professor at a major university when she was diagnosed with advanced metastatic breast cancer. All her life, Jenna had been a take-charge person, and relished her capacity to run her life effectively and efficiently. People responded to her with high regard and respect because of her position and her personality. Admitted to the hospital, Jenna brought her pre-illness self-image of being treated with deference and expected similar responsiveness from staff. Her health care providers, unfamiliar with her background and personal identity issues, expected compliance with no challenges to their authority. When she would become angry about her inability to have control about her medical situation, the staff considered her a difficult, obstinate client. Viewed from a "patient" context, her behavior seemed irrational; understood from the perspective of a having a sudden challenge to a lifelong self-concept of independence and deference, her seemingly "irrational" behavior made sense. Once the connection was made to Jenna's personal identity issues, a different dialogue emerged between staff and client, with a deeper respect for Jenna's set of expectations and interpersonal needs. Provision of needed support for information and collaborative interpersonal responses resulted in a positive change in Jenna's attitude, and full participation in her treatment.

Supportive Nursing Strategies

Interventions needed to strengthen personal identity in the face of major illness, injury, or death in clinical settings start with respecting individual preferences, values, and beliefs, and applying the simple axiom of treating each patient with the same respect as you would like to be treated in a similar situation. Box 4-1 presents guidelines to strengthen realistic perceptions and

| BOX 4-1 | Interventions to Enhance Personal Identity: Perceptions and Cognition |

- Take time to orient newly admitted clients to the unit, patient rights, and the normal care routine.
- Pay close attention to the client's "story" of the present health care experience, including concerns about coping, impact on self and others, and hopes for the future.
- Remember that each client is unique. Respect and tailor responses to support individual differences in personality, personal responses, intellect, values, and understanding of medical processes.
- Encourage as much client input as is realistically possible into diagnostic and therapeutic regimens.
- Provide information as it emerges about changes in treatment, personnel, discharge, and after care. Include family members whenever possible, particularly when giving difficult news.
- Explain treatment procedures including rationale, and allow ample time for questions and discussion.
- Encourage family members to bring in familiar objects or pictures, particularly if the client is in the hospital or care facility for an extended period.
- Encourage as much independence and self-direction as possible.
- Avoid sensory overload, and repeat instructions if the client appears anxious.
- Use perceptual checks to ensure you and the client have the same understanding of important material.

facilitate accurate cognitive processing of health care information.

Frequent perceptual checks and active listening are helpful interventions (see Chapter 10). When combined with well-thought-out inferences about the meaning of client behaviors, they enhance the quality of decision-making in the nurse-client relationship. Checking in with clients allows the nurse to use perceptual data in a conscious, deliberate way to facilitate the relationship process. Because the client feels heard and because communication focuses on matters of interest and concern to the client, mutuality occurs with greater frequency.

Successful outcomes related to a nursing diagnosis of personal identity disturbances include new adaptive coping skills, a richer appreciation of life and one's purpose, a reordering of priorities, and enriched relationships with family and friends. A positive reframing of personal identity in the face of serious illness can contribute to better treatment adherence and a stronger sense of well-being.

Responding to Cognitive Distortions. It is not so much what happens to us as it is how we interpret and respond to our circumstances that create problems. Box 4-2 identifies common cognitive distortions. Simple perceptual distortions can be challenged with compassionate questioning, new information, and simple targeted humor. Cognitive behavioral therapy (CBT), originally developed by Aaron Beck, is the treatment of choice for clients with significant perceptual/cognitive distortions. With CBT approaches, people are initially taught to recognize their cognitive distortions, when thoughts interact with inner emotions to control behavior. This awareness is followed with strategies designed to reframe negative thinking patterns. Providing additional information, using Socratic questioning, modeling cues to behavior, and coaching clients to challenge cognitive distortions through the use of positive self-talk, mindfulness, values exploration, and a present orientation are common techniques.

Self-talk is a cognitive strategy people can use to lessen cognitive distortions. When the thought carries a negative value, it can affect the individual as though the thought represented the whole truth about the person. The thought "I stuttered in the interview" becomes emotionally translated into "I know I probably won't get the job. I'm just no good." One feature of one interview suddenly becomes a major defining statement of self. The pervading thoughts create a decrease in self-esteem.

Supportive Nursing Strategies. Changing internal self-talk resets the thinking process. With positive self-talk as a therapeutic strategy, the person chooses the feeling he or she will have about a situation or person. Providing additional information, modeling cues to behavior, using Socratic questioning to challenge the validity of cognitive distortions, and coaching clients to use positive self-talk is helpful. Exercise 4-4 gives practice in recognizing and responding to cognitive distortions.

Combining self-talk strategies with social support forms the basis for a prevention plan designed to correct cognitive distortions. A thinking schema that allows the client to step back and view the situation as an objective observer might before beginning to resolve it is helpful. Enlisting the help of others for support and advice leads to more effective problem solving.

BOX 4-2	Examples of Cognitive Distortions

- "All or nothing" thinking—the situation is all good or all bad; a person is trustworthy or untrustworthy.
- Overgeneralizing—one incident is treated as if it happens all the time; picking out a single detail and dwelling on it.
- Mind reading and fortune-telling—deciding a person does not like you without checking it out; assuming a bad outcome with no evidence to support it.
- Personalizing—seeing yourself as flawed, instead of separating the situation as something you played a role in but did not cause.
- Acting on "should" and "ought to"—deciding in your mind what is someone else's responsibility without perceptual checks; trying to meet another's expectations without regard for whether it makes sense to do so.
- "Awfulizing"—assuming the worst; every situation has a catastrophic interpretation and anticipated outcome.

EXERCISE 4-4	Correcting Cognitive Distortions

Purpose: To provide students with practice in recognizing and responding to cognitive distortions.

Procedure:
This exercise may be done in small groups of four or five students. Using the definitions of cognitive distortions presented in the text, identify the type of cognitive distortion and the response you might make in each of the following situations:
1. I shouldn't feel anxious about making this presentation in class.
2. I am boring and people don't like to talk to me.
3. I shouldn't get upset when people don't approve of me.
4. If I hadn't been raised in a dysfunctional family, I would be a different person.
5. If I don't get high grades, my family will think less of me.
6. I can't experience true satisfaction unless I do things perfectly.

Discussion:
1. How do cognitive distortions affect behavior?
2. In what ways can you use this exercise to enhance your nursing practice and personal relationships?

Feedback and social support are powerful antidotes to cognitive distortions about responsibility. Although a plan to correct cognitive distortions is easier to articulate than to implement, these guidelines have proved useful in helping people to relinquish faulty thinking patterns and to take constructive action instead.

SELF-ESTEEM: EMOTIONAL ASPECTS OF PERSONAL IDENTITY

Self-esteem refers to the affective or emotional aspects of self (Huitt, 2004). Representing an emotional appraisal of a person's worth or value, **self-esteem** is defined as the emotional value a person places on his or her personal self-worth in relation to others and the environment. Self-esteem affects a person's ability to weather stress without major changes in self-perception. With a positive attitude about self, an individual is more likely to view life as a glass that is half full rather than half empty. People who view themselves as worthwhile and as being valuable members of society have high self-esteem. People with low self-esteem do not value themselves and do not feel valued by others.

Self-esteem mirrors a person's inner sense of self and adds an additional filter to perceptual and cognitive awareness of self. It also reflects cultural norms, genetic temperament, and supportive relationships. A key characteristic is the respect people have for themselves and their opinion of their conduct of life. Self-esteem can be related to either a specific dimension of self, "I am a good writer," or it may have a more global meaning, "I am a good person who is worth knowing."

People with high self-esteem have a strong emotional and intellectual conviction that they are worthy of respect and recognition, and believe that they have something unique and useful to offer to society. They respect and like who they are, and are generally satisfied with their looks, personality, skills, and ability to successfully negotiate their lives. They accept responsibility for their success and failures, and take calculated risks to achieve important personal goals. They are more likely to be motivated to make changes. Life's inevitable problems are viewed as challenges that one can learn and grow from.

Self-esteem is not something that happens suddenly. People who learn to set realistic standards for themselves and strive to meet them are more likely to experience higher self-esteem. They are able to manage feelings and emotions in a positive way. They know and like themselves, based on an accurate perception of their strengths and limitations. In this way, the emotional components of self-concept are joined together with perceptual and cognitive components of personal identity.

By contrast, people with low self-esteem do not hold a high opinion of themselves and feel that they are worth less than others. They tend to be defensive in relationships and seek constant reassurance from others because of their own self-doubt. Instead of taking actions that could raise self-esteem, they worry and see challenges as problems rather than as opportunities.

Self-esteem tends to be relatively stable over time and across situations, but the experience of success or failure can cause fluctuations in self-esteem (Crocker, Brook, & Niiya, 2006). Sources of situational challenges to self-esteem include loss of a job; loss of an important relationship; negative change in appearance, role, or status; and verbal or physical abuse, neglect, chronic illness, codependency, and criticism by significant others. These situations leave people feeling unvalidated and undervalued as good persons. Illness, injury, and other health issues challenge a person's self-esteem. Findings from a sizable number of research studies demonstrate an association between lower self-esteem in clients and changes in health status, functional abilities, and emotional dysfunction (Vartanian, 2009; Vickery, Sepehri, & Evans, 2008).

Situational self-esteem can be influenced by cognitive strategies to correct affective distortions in communication and maladaptive thinking patterns interfering with a person's self-worth. Self-esteem can be enhanced through personal choices to engage fully with life, trying new things and learning new skills. Encouraging relationships with family, friends, teachers, and successful participation in social activities and clubs promote the process of achieving self-esteem. Exercise 4-5 introduces the role of social support in building self-esteem.

Assessment Strategies

Self-esteem is closely linked to our emotions, particularly those that directly involve self-concepts such as pride or shame (Brown & Marshall, 2001). Verbal and nonverbal behaviors that indicate powerlessness, frustration, inadequacy, anxiety, anger, or apathy suggest low self-esteem. Factors that contribute to affective margins of distortion in communications with clients are presented in Figure 4-3. Exercise 4-6 provides practice with clarifying feelings.

EXERCISE 4-5 | Social Support

Purpose: To help students understand the role of social support in significant encounters.

Procedure:
1. Describe a "special" situation that had deep meaning for you.
2. Identify the person or people who helped make the situation meaningful for you.

3. Describe the actions taken by the people or person identified above that made the situation memorable.

Discussion:
1. What did you learn about yourself from doing this exercise?
2. What do you see as the role of social support in making memories?
3. How might you use this information in your practice?

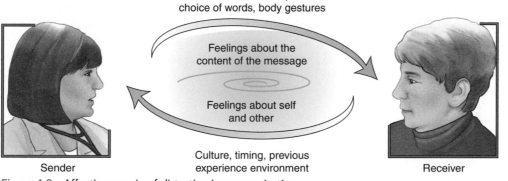

Tone of voice, facial expression
choice of words, body gestures

Feelings about the
content of the message

Feelings about self
and other

Culture, timing, previous
experience environment

Sender   Receiver

Figure 4-3   Affective margin of distortion in communication.

EXERCISE 4-6 | Clarifying Feelings

Purpose: To provide an opportunity to develop skill in recognizing underlying emotions and responding effectively to them.

Procedure:
This exercise should be done in small groups of three to five students.

A class has been assigned a group project for which all participants will receive a common group grade. Each group consists of six students. Develop a group understanding of the feelings experienced in each of the following situations, as well as a way to respond to each. Consider the possible consequences of your intervention in each case.
1. Don tells the group that he is working full time and will be unable to make any group meetings. There are so many class requirements that he also is not sure he can put much effort into the project,

although he would like to help and the project interests him.
2. Martha is very outspoken in group. She expresses her opinion about choice of the group project and is willing to make the necessary contacts. No one challenges her or suggests another project. At the next meeting, she informs the group that the project is all set up and she had made all the arrangements.
3. Joan promises she will have her part of the project completed by a certain date. The date comes and Joan does not have her part completed.

Discussion:
1. What are some actions the participants can take to move the group forward?
2. How can you use this exercise as a way of understanding and clarifying feelings in clinical work situations?

Nurses can help clients sort out and clarify the facts and emotions that get in the way of a person's awareness of his or her intrinsic value. Note how the client describes achievements. Does the client devalue accomplishments, project blame for problems on others, minimize personal failures, or make self-deprecating remarks? Does the client express shame or guilt? Does the client seem hesitant to try new things or situations, or express concern about ability to cope with events? Observe defensive behaviors.

| TABLE 4-2 | Behaviors Associated with High vs. Low Self-Esteem |
People with High Self-Esteem	People with Low Self-Esteem
Expect people to value them	Expect people to be critical of them
Are active self-agents	Are passive or obstructive self-agents
Have positive perceptions of their skills, appearance	Have negative perceptions of their skills, appearance, sexuality, and behaviors
Perform equally well when being observed as when not being observed	Perform less well when being observed
Are nondefensive and assertive in response to criticism	Are defensive and passive in response to criticism
Can accept compliments easily	Have difficulty accepting compliments
Evaluate their performance realistically	Have unrealistic expectations about their performance
Are relatively comfortable relating to authority figures	Are uncomfortable relating to authority figures
Express general satisfaction with life	Are dissatisfied with their lot in life
Have a strong social support system	Have a weak social support system
Have a primary internal locus of control	Rely on an external locus of control

Lack of culturally appropriate eye contact, poor hygiene, self-destructive behaviors, hypersensitivity to criticism, need for constant reassurance, and an inability to accept compliments are behaviors associated with low self-esteem. Table 4-2 identifies characteristic behaviors related to self-esteem.

Therapeutic Strategies

Armed with an understanding of the underlying personalized feelings as a threat to self-esteem, (e.g., intense fear, anguish about an anticipated loss, and lack of power in an unfamiliar situation), nurses provide the opening for the client to tell his or her story. The nurse might identify a legitimate feeling by saying, "It must be frustrating to feel that your questions go unanswered," and then saying, "How can I help you?" From a nonreactive position, the nurse can demonstrate caring about the client as a person by helping the client obtain needed information and seeking validation of legitimate client concerns.

When people have low self-esteem, they feel they have little worth and that no one really cares enough to bother with them. The nurse helps clients increase self-esteem by being psychologically present as a sounding board. Just the process of engaging with another human being who offers a different perspective can have the effect of enhancing self-esteem. The implicit message the nurse conveys with personal presence and interest, information, and a guided exploration of the problem is twofold. The first is

confirmation of the client: "You are important, and I will stay with you through this uncomfortable period." The second is the introduction of the possibility of hope: "There may be some alternatives you haven't thought of that can help you cope with this problem in a meaningful way." Once a person starts to take charge of his or her life, a higher level of well-being can result.

The nurse can use several strategies to help a client deepen self-esteem. Communication in the form of focused questions can assist clients in reflecting on their strengths and accomplishments. The nurse can give the client self-esteem–related feedback: "The thing that impresses me about you is. . ." or, "What I notice is that although your body is weaker, it seems as if your spirit is stronger. Is that your perception as well?" Such questions help the client focus on positive strengths. Exercise 4-7 strengthens the nurse's skill in this area.

Evaluation

Self-esteem behavior outcomes are evaluated by comparing the number of positive self-statements with those originally observed. Behaviors suggestive of enhanced self-esteem include the following:

- Taking an active role in planning and implementing self-care
- Verbalizing personal psychosocial strengths
- Expressing feelings of satisfaction with self and ways of handling life

EXERCISE 4-7	Positive Affirmations: Contributions to Self-Esteem

Purpose: To help students experience the effects of interpersonal comments on self-esteem.

Procedure:

This exercise may be done in a group or used as a homework assignment and later discussed in class.

1. List a positive affirming comment you received recently, something someone did or said that made you feel good about yourself.
2. List a disconfirming comment you received recently, something someone did or said that made you feel bad about yourself.

3. What have you done recently that you feel helped enhance someone else's self-esteem?

Discussion:

1. In general, what kinds of actions help enhance self-esteem?
2. What are some things people do or fail to do that diminish self-esteem?
3. What are some specific things you might be able to do in a clinical setting that might help a client develop a sense of self-worth?
4. What did you learn about yourself from doing this exercise?

SELF-EFFICACY

Self-efficacy is strongly associated with self-esteem, and the nursing diagnosis of powerlessness. People who believe that they can handle threatening situations value their competence and ability to succeed. They are less likely to harbor self-doubts or dwell on personal deficiencies when difficulties arise. **Self-efficacy** is a term originally developed by Albert Bandura (2007) in referring to a person's perceptual belief that he or she has the capability to perform general or specific life tasks successfully. Self-efficacy influences motivation and outcome expectancies. People need to believe that they can succeed in performing a task or coping with a difficult situation to actively try to master the tasks involved. People with a strong sense of self-efficacy can approach difficult tasks as challenging and master them. Self-efficacy helps them sustain their efforts in the face of temporary setbacks and decreases anxiety. Those with a weak sense of self-efficacy view difficult tasks as threatening and will not persist if obstacles or setbacks occur.

People develop self-efficacy through personal experience with mastering tasks, seeing others similar to themselves perform tasks successfully, and through verbal support. Breaking difficult tasks down into achievable steps and completing them constructs a resilient sense of self-efficacy.

Self-help and mutual support groups can be helpful adjuncts to treatment for clients having trouble with self-efficacy in managing their illness or injury. Discovering that others have similar issues and have found ways to cope with them successfully encourages clients and reinforces a sense of self-efficacy and hope that they too can achieve functional success. The understanding, social support, and reciprocal learning found in these groups provide opportunities for valuable information sharing and role modeling (Humphreys, 2004).

SPIRITUAL ASPECTS OF PERSONAL IDENTITY

Spiritual self-concepts, found in the innermost core of an individual, are concerned with a person's relationship with God or a higher power, and the vital life forces that support wholeness. When a person's body fails, or circumstances seem beyond one's control, it is often the spirit that sustains a person's sense of self-integrity and helps them maintain a more balanced equilibrium. Baldacchino and Draper (2001) note the presence of a spiritual force in a client's strong will to live, positive outlook, and sense of peace.

Spirituality is a unified concept, closely linked to a person's worldview, providing a foundation for a personal belief system about the nature of God or a Higher Power, moral-ethical conduct, and reality. Spirituality is a term often used synonymously with religion, but it is a much broader concept (Baldacchino & Draper, 2001). A key difference is that religion involves a formal acceptance of beliefs and values within an organized faith community, whereas spirituality describes self-chosen beliefs and values that give meaning to a person's life. It may or may not be associated with a particular faith (Tanyi, 2006).

Spirituality is associated with meaning and purpose in life (Sessanna, Finnell, & Jezewski, 2007; Tanyi, 2006). A number of research studies link spirituality to health, quality of life, and well-being (Molzahn & Sheilds, 2008).

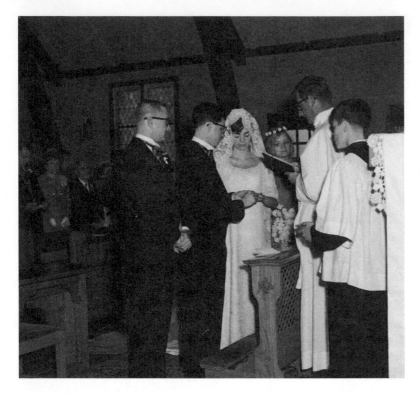

Spirituality plays a significant in personal identity.

Spirituality helps us answer vital questions about what it is to be human, which human events have depth and value, and what are imaginative possibilities of being. Over the course of a lifetime, spiritual beliefs change, deepen, or are challenged by circumstances that are beyond a person's control. Spiritual strength allows nurses and other health care professionals to willingly stand with others in darkness, and yet remain whole—to deal with the everyday challenges and stresses of nursing in a spirit of peace and hope. Spiritual aspects of self-concept can be expressed through:

- Membership in a specific religious faith community with a set of formal, organized beliefs
- Nature, meditation, or other personalized lifeways and practices linked with a higher purpose in life
- Cultural and family beliefs about forgiveness, justice, human rights, right and wrong learned in early childhood
- Crisis, or existential situations that stimulate a search for purpose, meaning, and values lying outside the self

Health crises can be a time of spiritual renewal, when one discovers new inner resources, strengths, and capacities never before tested. Or it can be a time of spiritual desolation, leaving the individual feeling powerless to control or change important life circumstances (Krebs, 2001).

Assessment

The Joint Commission (2004) mandates that health care agencies, including long-term hospice and home care services, must assess spiritual needs, provide for the spiritual care of clients and their families, and supply appropriate documentation of that care. Carson and Stoll (2008) refer to three areas of spiritual concern as a framework for nursing assessment: spiritual distress, spiritual needs, and spiritual well-being. Spiritual distress wears many faces: a lack of purpose and meaning in life, inability to forgive, loss of hope, and spirit of alienation. NANDA (2009) nursing diagnoses present specific nursing interventions for providing spiritual support: Risk for Spiritual Distress, Spiritual Distress, Readiness for Enhanced Hope, and Readiness for Enhanced Spiritual Well-being.

Assessment of spiritual needs should be approached with respect and sensitivity for the client's beliefs and values. Assessment questions might include evaluation of the client's

- Willingness to talk about personal spirituality or beliefs
- Belief in a personal God or Higher Power
- Relevance of specific religious practices to the individual
- Changes in religious practices or beliefs
- Areas of specific spiritual concern activated by the illness; for example, is there an afterlife?
- Extent to which illness, injury, or disability has had an effect on spiritual beliefs
- Sources of hope and support
- Desire for visitation from clergy or pastoral chaplain

A client's spiritual needs may be quite obvious and firmly anchored in positive relationships with clergy and a personal God, or defined philosophical understanding of life and one's place in it. Spiritual needs also can reveal evidence of conflict or anger toward a Higher Power, who is held responsible for a negative health situation. For example, the noted author C. S. Lewis (1976) calls his God "the cosmic sadist" as he experienced his personal grief following the death of his wife. Spiritual pain can be as severe as physical pain and often is closely accompanied by emotional pain. Asking about the effect an illness or health problem has had on spiritual beliefs yields useful information. Being able to talk freely about spiritual distress helps put it into perspective (McSherry, 2000).

Identifying a client's current religious affiliations and practices is important, and inquiring about religious rituals important to the client is essential. Josephson and Peteet (2007) suggest that the client's words can be an entry into a discussion of spirituality; for instance, if the client uses a phrase such as "By the grace of God, I passed the final examination," you might ask something like, "It sounds like God plays a role in your life, is that true?" (p. 186).

Spiritual rituals and practices can be used to promote hope, support, and peace for a client experiencing spiritual pain. You can inquire about current spiritual practices and preferences by asking, "Are there any spiritual practices that are particularly important to you now?" When assessing the client's current spiritual preferences, you should also consider past religious affiliations. It is not unusual for the religion listed on the client's chart to be different from the religious practices the client currently follows. In addition, people who have never committed to a strong sense of religion previously will seek religious support in times of crisis (Baldacchino & Draper, 2001). Spiritual assessment information should be documented in the client's record.

Spiritual well-being can be demonstrated through hopefulness in the face of adversity, compassion for self and others, and a sense of inner peace. Miller (2007) suggests, "Hope is central to life and specifically is an essential dimension for successfully dealing with illness and for preparing for death" (p. 12). Hope is critical in maintaining the "spirit" of a person in health care settings. How else can one explain the will to live or the complete serenity of some individuals in the face of life's most adverse circumstances? Hope does not guarantee a positive outcome. It simply helps a person stay connected with life. Lack of hope is expressed in feelings of powerlessness, hopelessness, and frustration. Useful assessment questions might consist of: "What do you see as your primary sources of strength at the present time?" and, "In the past, what have been sources of strength for you in difficult times?" Miller (2007) identified several hope-inspiring strategies found in the literature, for example, helping clients and families to develop achievable aims, realize a sense of interpersonal connectedness, live in the present, and find meaning in their illness/situation. Sharing uplifting memories, affirmation of worth, and unconditional caring presence can stimulate a sense of hopefulness.

Case Example

At age 16, Robert became a double amputee as a result of a skiing accident. One morning, Mrs. Johnson walked into Robert's room and found him crying. Her first response was to leave the room as she thought, "I can't handle this today." But she managed to stop herself, and she went over to Robert and touched his shoulder. He continued to sob and said, "What am I going to do? I wish I were dead. My whole life is sports. I would have qualified for an athletic scholarship if this hadn't happened. I feel like my life is over at 16."

Mrs. Johnson recognized the feelings of despair that Robert was expressing, and said to him, "It doesn't seem like life has any meaning at all. You are feeling that this is such an unfair thing to have happened to you. I agree with you, it is. But let's talk about it" (Carson & Koenig, 2008, pp. 140–141).

Exercise 4-8 helps in understanding spiritual responses to distress. Spirituality can be a powerful resource for families and it is important to incorporate

EXERCISE 4-8	Responding to Issues of Spiritual Distress

Purpose: To help students understand responses in times of spiritual distress.

Procedure:
Review the following case situations and develop an appropriate response to each.
1. Mary Trachter is unmarried and has just found out she is pregnant. She belongs to a fundamentalist church in which sex before marriage is not permitted. Mary feels guilty about her current status and sees it as "God punishing me for fooling around."
2. Linda Carter is married to an abusive, alcoholic husband. Linda reads the Bible daily and prays for her husband's redemption. She feels that God will

turn the marriage around if she continues to pray for changes in her husband's attitude. "My trust is in the Lord," she says.
3. Bill Compton tells the nurse, "I feel that God has let me down. I was taught that if I was faithful to God, He would be there for me. Now the doctors tell me I'm going to die. That doesn't seem fair to me."

Discussion:
1. Share your answers with others in your group.
2. Give and get feedback on the usefulness of your responses.
3. In what ways can you use this new knowledge in your nursing care?

questions about the family's spirituality if they are involved with the client. Each family's expression of spirituality and use of spiritual resources is unique. Tanyi (2006) suggests nurses can incorporate spiritual assessment with the family, using questions such as

What gives the family meaning in their daily routines?

What gives the family strength to deal with stress or crisis?

How does the family describe their relationship with God/Higher Power or the universe?

What spiritual rituals, practices, or resources do the family use for support?

Are their any conflicts between family members related to spiritual views, and if so, what might be the impact on the current health situation?

STRATEGIES

The compassionate presence of the nurse in the nurse-client relationship is the most important tool the nurse has in helping the client explore spiritual and existential concerns (Carson & Koenig, 2008). Providing opportunities for clients to be self-reflective about their spirituality helps people sustain their beliefs, values, and spiritual sense of self in the face of tragedy. Gordon and Mitchell (2004) write, "Spiritual care is usually provided in a one-to-one relationship, is completely person centered and makes no assumptions about personal conviction or life orientation" (p. 646).

Providing privacy and quiet times for spiritual activities is important. The support of "nursing presence" and unstructured time for helping clients cope with spiritual issues, combined with referrals to chaplains, is an important component of nursing intervention. Nurses can help individuals and families contact spiritual advisors or clergy, or act as their advocate in ensuring appropriate spiritual rituals are followed related to dietary restrictions, Sabbath activities, meditating or praying, and at end of life. For example, in some forms of the Jewish religion, turning lights on or off or adjusting the position on an electric bed is not permitted on the Sabbath. There is no rule against these tasks being accomplished by the nurse.

Philosophical discussion may not be necessary. Spiritual connections can provide comfort for the dying and their families through prayer or hymns. Thomas (2009) describes the impact of familiar spiritual songs as he reflects on spiritual moments spent with his wife at the end of her life.

Case Example

Susan and I would share the passing alone. An elderly, angelic, soul-wizened, African American nursing assistant (Eleanor) had been assigned to assist us. She reminded me of a well-experienced midwife at the opposite end of life.

In the middle of the night, Eleanor quietly began to sing the old religious hymns that Susan and I knew so well. I watched tension drain from Susan's skin. [Susan knew the words by heart.] The words are so comforting, relaxing, reassuring. I was softly humming along as

Susan was bathed in this blessing. This was an emotionally, spiritually perfect moment.

Just as I began to quietly tell Eleanor the story about the meaning of those songs to Susan, I observed Susan's hand come out from under the sheet, I was holding her foot at that point. Her index finger slowly, but firmly, wagged back and forth. DO NOT tell that story was the clear message. I continued to hum along softly. How did she know?

Here we are, deep into the night of September 14, 1999, and the same hymns are bathing, soothing, and reassuring us as they have generations of Believers. Susan knew, and I should have, that anything I said would cause this moment to evaporate. The precious, tender, delicate moment would be ruined (Thomas, 2009).

Prayer and Meditation

Praying with a client, even when the client is of a different faith, can be soothing for some patients. Nurses need to distinguish between their own spiritual orientation and needs, and that of their clients. It is not appropriate to impose a spiritual ritual on a client that would be at odds with his or her spiritual beliefs. There should be some evidence from the client's conversation that praying or reading the Bible with a client would be an acceptable support.

According to some researchers (Daaleman, Usher, Williams, Rawlings, & Hanson, 2008; Sulmasy, 2006), spiritual support can be effectively provided through indirect means such as recognizing the human value and dignity of clients, and respecting their autonomy in shared decision making, as by supporting them through prayer.

Evaluation

Client outcomes associated with successful resolution of spiritual distress, and/or spiritual well being include connecting, or reconnecting with God or a higher power, decreased guilt, forgiveness of others, expressions of hope, and evidence that the client finds meaning in his or her current situation. Thomas (2009) describes his spiritual process of journeying to a different place with grief as follows:

Twice walked into the Valley of the Shadow of Death with a dearly loved partner, lost that loved one to eternity, fell into the deeper Valley of Grief, and each time managed to climb out as a stronger, spiritually embraced person.

SUMMARY

Chapter 4 focuses on the self-concept as a key variable in the nurse-client relationship. Self-concept refers to an acquired constellation of thoughts, feelings, attitudes, and beliefs that individuals have about the nature and organization of their personality. Self-concepts are created through experiences with the environment and personal characteristics.

The four aspects of self-concept patterns most relevant to the practice of nursing and the nurse-client relationship are body image, personal identity, self-esteem, and spirituality. Disturbances in body image refer to issues related to changes in appearance and physical functions, both overt and hidden. Personal identity is constructed through cognitive processes of perception and cognition. Serious illnesses such as dementia and psychotic disorders threaten or crush a person's sense of personal identity. Self-esteem is associated with the emotional aspect of self-concept, and reflects the value a person puts on the personal self-concept and its place in the world. Assessment of spiritual needs and corresponding spiritual care is a Joint Commission requirement for quality care.

Understanding the dimensions of self-concept and the critical role it plays in directing behavior is key to working effectively with clients and families. It is always a core variable to consider in nurse-client relationships. Nurses play an important role in providing support and guidance for clients related to self-concept.

ETHICAL DILEMMA What Would You Do?

Sarah Best, a 16-year-old ice-skater, is brought into the emergency department after being in a car accident. The physician examines Sarah and determines that her right leg needs to be amputated below the knee. Sarah's parents are traveling in Europe and cannot immediately be located. Sarah refuses surgery. The physician asks Sarah's nurse, Ann, to get Sarah's consent. If you were in Ann's position, what would you do?

REFERENCES

Arnold E: Sorting out the 3 D's: Delirium, dementia, depression, *Holist Nurs Pract* 19(3):99–104, 2005.

Baldacchino D, Draper P: Spiritual coping strategies: a review of the literature, *J Adv Nurs* 34(6):833–841, 2001.

Bandura A: Self-efficacy in health functioning. In Ayers S, et al, editor: *Cambridge handbook of psychology, health & medicine*, ed 2, New York, 2007, Cambridge University Press, pp 191–193.

Boston Women's Health Book Collective: *Our bodies, ourselves for the new century*, New York, 1998, Touchstone Simon & Schuster.

Blazer D: How do you feel about. . .? Health outcomes late in life and self-perceptions of health and well-being, *The Gerontologist* 48(4): 415–422, 2008.

Brown J, Marshall M: Self-esteem and emotion: some thoughts about feelings, *Pers Soc Psychol Bull* 27(5):575–584, 2001.

Carson V, Koenig H: *Spiritual dimensions of nursing practice* (Revised ed.), West Conshohoeken, PA, 2008, Templeton Press.

Carson V, Stoll R: Spirituality: Defining the indefinable and reviewing its place in nursing. In Carson V, Koenig H, editors: *Spiritual dimensions of nursing practice* (Revised ed.), West Conshohoeken, PA, 2008, Templeton Press.

Crocker J, Brook AT, Niiya Y: The pursuit of self-esteem: contingencies of self-worth and self-regulation, *J Pers* 74(6):1749–1771, 2006.

Cunha C, Goncalves M: Commentary: Accessing the experience of a dialogical self: Some needs and concerns, *Culture & Psychology* 15(3): 120–133, 2009.

Daaleman TP, Usher BM, Williams SW, et al: An exploratory study of spiritual care at the end of life, *Ann Fam Med* 6(5):406–411, 2008.

Drench M, Noonan A, Sharby N, et al: *Psychosocial Aspects of Health Care*, 2006, Prentice Hall.

Elliott A: *Concepts of the self*, Malden, MA, 2008, Polity Press.

Ellis-Hill C, Horn S: Change in identity and self-concept: a new theoretical approach to recovery following a stroke, *Clin Rehabil* 14(3):279–287, 2000.

Erikson E: *Identity: youth and crisis*, New York, 1968, Norton.

Erikson E: *The life cycle completed: a review*, New York, 1982, Norton.

Gordon M: *Self-perception-self-concept pattern, Manual of nursing diagnoses*, ed 11, Chestnut Hill, MA, 2007, Bartlett Jones.

Gordon T, Mitchell D: A competency model for the assessment and delivery of spiritual care, *Palliat Med* 18(7):646–651, 2004.

Heijmans M, Rijken M, Foets M, et al: The stress of being chronically ill: from disease-specific to task-specific aspects, *J Behav Med* 27:255–271, 2004.

Huitt W: Self-concept and self-esteem, 2004: In *Educational psychology interactive*, Valdosta, GA, 2004, Valdosta State University. Available online: http://www.edpsycinteractive.org/col/regsys/self.html. Accessed November 26, 2009.

Humphreys K: *Circles of recovery: self-help organizations for addictions*, Cambridge, 2004, Cambridge University Press.

Hunter E: Beyond death: inheriting the past and giving to the future, transmitting the legacy of one's self, *Omega* 56(40):313–329, 2008.

Hybels S, Weaver R: *Communicating effectively*, ed 9, New York, 2008, McGraw-Hill.

James W: *The principles of psychology* (vol 1), New York, 1890, Henry Holt.

Joint Commission on the Accreditation of Health Care Organizations: *Comprehensive accreditation manual for hospitals: the official handbook*, Chicago, 2004, JCAHO. Available online: www.jcaho.org. Accessed April 15, 2009.

Josephson A, Peteet J: Talking with patients about spirituality and worldview: practical interviewing techniques and strategies, *Psychiatr Clin North Am* 30:181–197, 2007.

Karademas E, Bakouli A, Bastouonis A, et al: Illness perceptions, illness-related problems, subjective health and the role of perceived primal threat: Preliminary findings, *J Health Psychol* 13(8): 1021–1029, 2008.

Konig J: Moving experience: dialogues between personal cultural positions, *Culture & Psychology* 15(1):97–119, 2009.

Krebs K: The spiritual aspect of caring: an integral part of health and healing, *Nurs Adm Q* 25(3):55–60, 2001.

Lee SJ, Oyserman D: Possible selves theory. In Anderman E, Anderman L, editors: *Psychology of classroom learning: an encyclopedia*, Detroit, MI, 2009, Macmillan Reference.

Lewis CS: *A grief observed*, New York, 1976, Bantam Books.

Luft J, Ingham H: The Johari window, a graphic model of interpersonal awareness. In *Proceedings of the western training laboratory in group development*, Los Angeles, 1955, UCLA.

Markus H, Nurius P: Possible selves, *Am Psychol* 41:954–969, 1986.

McCormick M, Hardy K: *Re-visioning family therapy: race, culture and gender in clinical practice*, ed 2, New York, 2008, The Guilford Press.

McSherry W: *Making sense of spirituality in nursing practice*, New York, 2000, Harcourt.

Miller J: Hope: A construct central to nursing, *Nurs Forum* 42(1):12–19, 2007.

Molzahn A, Sheilds L: Why is it so hard to talk about spirituality? *Can Nurse* 10(4):25–29, 2008.

NANDA International: *Nursing Diagnosis: Definitions and Classification 2009–2011*, Ames, Iowa, 2009, J. Wiley and Sons.

Oyserman D, Markus H: Self as social representation. In Flick U, editor: *The psychology of the social*, Cambridge, United Kingdom, 1998, Cambridge University Press, pp 107–125.

Prescott A: *The concept of self in medicine and health care*, New York, 2006, Nova Science Publishers, Inc.

Raholm MB: Uncovering the ethics of suffering using a narrative approach, *Nurs Ethics* 15(1):62–72, 2008.

Rhode D: The injustice of appearance, *Stanford Law Rev* 61(5): 1033–1102, 2009.

Rogers C: *Client centered therapy*, New York, 1951, Houghton Mifflin.

Rowland JH, Desmond KA, Meyerowitz BE, et al: Role of breast reconstructive surgery in physical and emotional outcomes among breast cancer survivors, *J Natl Cancer Inst* 92(17):1422–1429, 2000.

Sessana L, Finnell D, Jezewski MA: Spirituality in nursing and health related literature: a concept analysis, *J Holist Nurs* 25(4):252–262, 2007.

Smith MJ, Perkins K: Attending to the voices of adolescents who are overweight to promote mental health, *Arch Psychiatr Nurs* 22(6): 391–393, 2008.

Sullivan HS: *The interpersonal theory of psychiatry*, New York, 1953, W.W. Norton & Co., Inc.

Sulmasy DP: Spiritual issues in the care of dying patients, *J Am Med Assoc* 296(11):1385–1392, 2006.

Tanyi R: Spirituality and family nursing: spiritual assessment and interventions for families, *J Adv Nurs* 53(3):287–294, 2006.

Thomas J: *My Saints Alive: A Journey of Life, Love, and Loss*. Unpublished manuscript, Charlottesville, VA, September 2010.

Usborne E, Taylor D: The role of cultural identity clarity for self-concept, clarity, self-esteem, and subjective well-being, *Pers Soc Psychological Bulletin* 36(7):883–897, 2010.

Vartanian L: When the body defines the self: Self-concept clarity, internalization, and body image, *J Soc Clin Psychol* 28(1):94–126, 2009.

Vickery C, Sepehri A, Evans C: Self-esteem in an acute stroke rehabilitation sample: a control group comparison, *Clin Rehabil* 22:179–187, 2008.

Williams N: Addressing negative attitudes to weight, *Pract Nurse* 37(3):33–34, 2009.

CHAPTER 5

The Nurse-Client Relationship

Elizabeth C. Arnold

OBJECTIVES

At the end of the chapter, the reader will be able to:

1. Define key concepts in the nurse-client relationship.
2. Describe the characteristics of therapeutic nurse-client relationships.
3. Discuss therapeutic use of self in nurse-client relationships.
4. Describe the four phases of a nurse-client relationship.
5. Discuss tasks in each of the four phases of the relationship.
6. Compare and contrast adaptations for short-term relationships.

This chapter focuses on the characteristics and structure of nurse-client relationships in clinical practice. Included in the chapter is a comprehensive discussion of the therapeutic relationship as the cornerstone of professional nursing practice (Carter, 2009). Characteristics of the helping relationship related to authenticity, presence, boundaries, and self-awareness are explored as essential components of effective therapeutic relationships. Developmental stages of relationship are identified, and strategies nurses can apply to long- and short-term relationships are addressed.

BASIC CONCEPTS

The Joint Commission (2001) affirms the role of the nurse in therapeutic relationships with clients and families: "Nearly every person's every health care experience involves the contribution of a registered nurse. Birth and death, and all the various forms of care in between, are attended by the knowledge, support and comforting of nurses" (p. 5). It is an awesome responsibility, and of particular importance as nursing moves into the community with shorter term, less structured therapeutic relationships between nurse and client/family.

KEY CONCEPTS IN THERAPEUTIC RELATIONSHIPS

DEFINITIONS

A **therapeutic relationship** is a professional, interpersonal alliance in which the nurse and client join together for a defined period to achieve health-related treatment goals. The time spent in the relationship may be short, spanning up to an 8-hour shift in a hospital, or it can be longer term, lasting weeks or months in a rehabilitation center. Because each nurse and client has a distinctive personality, the human interactions within each relationship are unique (Chauhan & Long, 2000). Regardless of the time spent, each relationship with a client can be meaningful and important to clients.

The term *client* can refer to any individual, family, group, or community with an identified health care need requiring nursing intervention. Nurses enter therapeutic relationships with a specialized body of knowledge, a genuine desire to help others, and an openness to the client's experience. Guiding principles (e.g., presence, purpose, mutuality, authenticity, empathy, active listening, confidentiality, and respect for the dignity of the client) strengthen the healing influence of a therapeutic relationship (McGrath, 2005). Box 5-1 identifies strategies to facilitate empathy.

The nurse-client relationship is an interdependent relationship. Martin Buber's (1958) I and Thou relation in which each is aware of and respects the other in building a shared reality forms the foundation for therapeutic conversations. He described an I-thou relationship as an equal relationship marked by respect, mutuality, and reciprocity. Neither is an "object" of study. Instead, there is a process of mutual discovery and each person feels free to be authentic. The essence of the I-thou relationship allows each person to be who he or she is as a unique human being worthy of respect even when the person is being difficult.

Buber's work forms a theoretical foundation for using confirming responses in which the helping person identifies an observable strength of another person and comments on it. He described this way of responding as follows: "Man wishes to be confirmed in his being by man and wishes to have a presence in the being of the other. Secretly and bashfully, he watches for a yes which allows him to be" (Buber, 1957, p. 104).

BOX 5-1	Suggestions for Facilitating Empathy

- Actively listen carefully to the client's concerns. (Use open-ended questions; avoid closed-ended questions).
- Tune in to physical and psychological behaviors that express the client's point of view.
- Do self-checks, often for stereotypes or premature understanding of the client's issues.
- Set aside judgments or personal biases.
- Be tentative in your listening responses and ask for validation frequently.
- Mentally picture the client's situation and ask appropriate questions to secure information about areas or issues you are not clear about.
- Give yourself time to think about what the client has said before responding or before asking the next question.
- Mirror the client's level of energy and language.
- Be authentic in your responses.

Modified from Egan G: *The skilled helper*, ed 7, Pacific Grove, CA, 2002, Brooks Cole Publishing, by permission.

With the current emphasis on team collaboration in health service care delivery, collaborative relationships with other professionals have become increasingly important. LaSala (2009) notes, "The core values of human dignity, respect, caring, and compassion are not only central to the care of patients but also to nurses' interactions with one another, members of the interdisciplinary team, and others" (p. 427).

CHARACTERISTICS OF THERAPEUTIC RELATIONSHIPS

Although therapeutic helping relationships share many characteristics of a social relationship, there are distinct structural and functional distinctions. Table 5-1 presents the differences between a therapeutic helping

TABLE 5-1	Differences Between Helping Relationships and Social Relationships

Helping Relationships	Social Relationships
Helper takes responsibility for the conduct of the relationship and for maintaining appropriate boundaries.	Both parties have equal responsibility for the conduct of the relationship.
Relationship has a specific purpose and a health-related goal.	Relationship may or may not have a specific purpose or goals.
Relationship terminates when the identified goal is met.	Relationship can last a lifetime or terminate without goal achievement.
Focus of the relationship is on needs of the helpee.	The needs of both partners should receive equal attention.
Relationship is entered through necessity.	Relationship is entered into spontaneously, accompanied by feelings of liking.
Choice of who to be in relationship is not available to either helper or helpee.	Behavior for both participants is spontaneous; people choose companions.
Self-disclosure is limited for the helper, encouraged for the helpee.	Self-disclosure for both parties in the relationship is expected.
Understanding should always be put into words.	Understanding does not necessarily need to be put into words.

relationship and a social relationship. The goal of a therapeutic relationship is ultimately promotion of the client's health and well-being. This is true even when the client is dying or is uncooperative.

Client Centered

A therapeutic relationship is client or patient centered. Client-centered approaches, first described by Carl Rogers (1958), are based on the belief that each person has within him or herself the capacity to heal, given support from a helping person who treats the client with the utmost respect and unconditional regard in a caring, authentic relationship (Anderson, 2001). Client-centered care includes the client's individual preferences, values, beliefs, and needs as a fundamental consideration in all nursing interventions.

In therapeutic relationships, clients are the personal experts on their life experiences; the nurse is the consultive expert on health care matters. The nurse's expertise derives from integrated empirical, personal, aesthetic, and ethical ways of knowing. This knowledge helps guide the client to reflect on and clarify what is important in the dialogue, and offers professional insights that the client may not have considered previously.

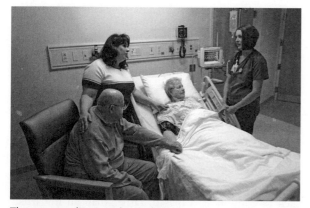

The nurse-client relationship is an interdependent relationship.

In recent decades, patient- or client-centered care has been acknowledged as a core value in service delivery. Its relevance as an essential component of quality health care measures was strongly stated in the Institute of Medicine (2001) published report "Crossing the Quality Chasm: A New Health System for the 21st Century." This document charged health care systems to

- Respect patients' values, preferences and expressed needs
- Coordinate and integrate care across boundaries of the system
- Provide the information, communication, and education that people need and want
- Guarantee physical comfort, emotional support, and the involvement of family and friends (pp. 52–53)

From a functional perspective, client-centered relationships require nurses to step back and compassionately listen to each individual client or family concerns. Keeping in mind that each person's experience is different, despite similarities in diagnosis, relevant questions are: "What is this person's human experience of living with this illness or injury" and "How can I as a health care professional help you at this point in time?"

From Mutuality to Partnership

Health care consumers are increasingly expected to be active partners in their own health care (McGrath, 2005; McQueen, 2000). Nurse-client relationships are designed to empower clients and families to assume as much responsibility as possible in self-management of chronic illness. Both nurse and client have responsibilities, and work toward agreed-on goals. Shared knowledge, mutual decision-making power, and respect for the capacities of client to actively contribute to his or her health care to whatever extent is possible are active components of the partnership required of client centered care. Exercise 5-1 looks at shared decision making.

A client-centered partnership honors the client's right to self-determination and gives the client and family maximum control over health care decisions. The client always has the right to choose personal goals and courses of action, even when they are at odds with the nurse's ideas. An effective collaborative partnership between nurse and client results in enhanced self-management, better health care utilization, and improved health outcomes (Hook, 2006).

Professional Boundaries

Emotional integrity in the nurse-client relationship is "reliant on maintaining relational boundaries" (LaSala, 2009, p. 424). **Professional boundaries** represent invisible structures imposed by legal, ethical, and professional standards of nursing that respect nurse and

EXERCISE 5-1	Shared Decision Making

Purpose: To develop awareness of shared decision making in treatment planning.

Procedure:
1. Read the following clinical situation.
    Mr. Singer, age 48 years, is a white, middle-class professional recovering from his second myocardial infarction. After his initial attack, Mr. Singer resumed his 10-hour workday, high-stress lifestyle, and usual high-calorie, high-cholesterol diet of favorite fast foods, alcohol, and coffee. He smokes two packs of cigarettes a day and exercises once a week by playing golf.
    Mr. Singer is to be discharged in 2 days. He expresses impatience to return to work, but also indicates that he would like to "get his blood pressure down and maybe drop 10 pounds."
2. Role play this situation in dyads, with one student taking the role of the nurse, and another student taking the role of the client.
3. Develop treatment goals that seem realistic and achievable, taking into account Mr. Singer's preferences and values, and health condition.
4. After the role-play is completed, discuss some of the issues that would be relevant to Mr. Singer's situation and how they might be handled. For example, what are some of the ways in which you could engage Mr. Singer's interest in changing his behavior to facilitate a healthier life style?

client rights, and protect the functional integrity of the alliance between nurse and client. Bruner and Yonge (2006) suggest that "rather than a line, boundaries represent a continuum with issues related to boundaries ranging from a lack of involvement to overinvolvement" (p. 39). Examples of relationship boundaries involve the setting, time, purpose, and length of contact, maintaining confidentiality, and use of appropriate professional behaviors.

Professional boundaries define how nurses should relate to clients as a helping person, that is, not as a friend, not as a judge, but as a skilled professional companion committed to helping the client achieve mutually defined health care goals (Briant & Freshwater, 1998). Maintaining appropriate professional behavior is a clear interpersonal boundary that makes the relationship safe for the client in much the same way as guardrails protect the public from falling into danger when observing a tourist attraction. Professional boundaries spell out the parameters of the health care relationship (Fronek, Kendall, Ungerer, Malt, Eugarde, & Geraghty, 2009). Nurses are ethically bound to observe the boundaries needed to make a relationship therapeutic (Sheets, 2001). When clients seek health care, they are in a vulnerable position and look to their health care providers as responsive guides to helping them achieve optimum health and well-being.

Boundary Violations and Crossings

The National Council of State Boards of Nursing (NCSBN, 2007) describes professional boundaries as the spaces between the nurse's position power and client vulnerability. The nurse, not the client, is responsible for maintaining professional boundaries. **Boundary violations** take advantage of the client's vulnerability and represent a conflict of interest that usually is harmful to the goals of the therapeutic relationship. Examples of boundary violations include sexual encounters with clients, excessive personal disclosures, personal or business relationships, and requests/acceptance of special favors or expensive gifts. Extensive following of a client after discharge is a common boundary violation. Boundary violations are ethically wrong.

Boundary crossings are less serious infractions. They give the appearance of impropriety but do not actually violate prevailing ethical standards. Hartley (2002) suggests, "With boundary crossings, context is everything. What is appropriate behavior in one context may not be in another" (p. 7). Examples of boundary crossings include meetings outside of the relationship or disclosing personal intimate details about aspects of the nurse's life that would not be common knowledge (Bruner & Yonge, 2006). Repeated boundary crossings such as continuing a biased, rather than an impartial, relationship with a client should be avoided.

Nurses need to carefully examine their behaviors, look for possible misinterpretations or unintended consequences, and seek supervision when boundary crossings occur. For example, suppose the client perceives your extra involvement as more than a responsive gesture. How will other clients or family members view the extra attention? Is reliance on the extra time or effort spent with a client likely to jeopardize that client's journey to independence (Hartley, 2002)?

LEVEL OF INVOLVEMENT

An important feature of a therapeutic relationship is the helping person's level of involvement. The term *involvement* relates to the degree of the nurse's attachment and active participation in the client's care. The level of involvement may fluctuate, depending on the needs of the client, but it should never exceed the boundaries of professional behavior (see Figure 5-1). It becomes problematic when the nurse limits the level of involvement to perfunctory tasks or becomes emotionally overinvolved in the client's care. To be effective, nurses must maintain emotional objectivity, whilst remaining human and present to clients. Heinrich (1992) notes that nurses constantly walk a thin line between having compassion for a client and developing a relationship that is too close, resulting in a friendship with potential serious complications for the client, as well as the nurse.

Overinvolvement can be associated with countertransference (O'Kelly, 1998), resulting from the nurse's unresolved feelings about previous relationships. It often occurs when the client is particularly needy, or feeds the nurse's ego by considering him or her as special, or the only one who understands.

Overinvolvement results in the nurse's loss of an essential objectivity needed to support the client in meeting health goals (Kines, 1999). In addition to its impact on the nurse-client relationship, overinvolvement can compromise the nurse's obligation to the service agency, a professional commitment to the treatment regimen, collegial relationships with other health team members, and professional responsibilities to other clients (Morse, 1991).

Warning signs that the nurse is becoming overinvolved include the following:

- Giving extra time and attention to certain clients
- Visiting clients in off hours
- Doing things for clients that the clients could do for themselves
- Discounting the actions of other professionals
- Keeping secrets with the client
- Believing that the nurse is the only one who understands the client's needs

The opposite of overinvolvement is *disengagement*, which occurs when nurses find themselves withdrawing from clients because of a client's behavior or the intensity of client suffering. Deaths and high stress levels on a unit can create compassion fatigue, which can lead to disengagement as a self-protective mechanism (Hofmann, 2009). Nurses tend to disengage from clients who are sexually provocative, complaining, hostile, or extremely anxious or depressed. Physical characteristics such as poor hygiene, marked physical disability, socially stigmatized illness, or an unusual or altered appearance can negatively affect the nurse's willingness to engage with a client.

Signs of disengagement include withdrawal, limited perfunctory contacts, minimizing the client's suffering, and defensive or judgmental communication. Regardless of the reason, the outcome of disengagement is that the client feels isolated and sometimes abandoned when care is mechanically delivered with limited human connection.

Maintaining a helpful level of involvement is always the responsibility of the professional nurse (see Figure 5-1). Carmack (1997) suggests that nurses can take the following actions to regain perspective:

- Assume full responsibility for the process of care while acknowledging that the outcome usually is not within your control.
- Focus on the things that you can change while acknowledging that there are things over which you have no control.
- Be aware and accepting of your professional limits and boundaries.
- Monitor your reactions, and seek assistance when you feel uncomfortable about any aspect of the relationship.
- Balance giving care to a client with taking care of yourself, without feeling guilty.

Debriefing after a highly emotional event helps nurses resolve and put strong feelings into perspective.

Every nurse-client relationship can be plotted on this continuum of professional behavior

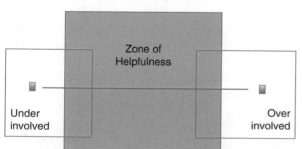

Figure 5-1   Levels of Involvement: A Continuum of professional Behavior. From: National Council of State Boards of Nursing (NCSBN) Professional Boundaries. www.ncsbn.org/Professional_Boundaries_2007_Web.pdf, 2007.

Support groups for nurses working in high-acuity nursing situations and mentoring of new nurses are recommended.

THERAPEUTIC USE OF SELF

The therapeutic relationship is not simply about what the nurse does, but who the nurse *is* in relation to clients and families. One of the most important tools nurses have at their disposal is the use of self. LaSala (2009) uses the words of Florence Nightingale, that a nurse achieves "the moral ideal" whenever he or she uses "the whole self" to form relationships with "the whole of the person receiving care" (p. 423) to explain the optimum involvement of self in the nurse-client relationship. The relationships that nurses establish with clients and their families and other practitioners in which "the whole self" is drawn into the process serves as the primary means for putting into action health treatments and healing interventions needed for client support and self-care.

Authenticity

Authenticity is a precondition for the therapeutic use of self in the nurse-client relationship. Authenticity requires recognizing personal vulnerabilities, strengths, and limitations, working within this knowledge in the service of the client, and seeking help when needed to further relationship goals. Self-awareness allows you to fully engage with a client, knowing that parts of the relationship may be painful, distasteful, or uncomfortable. Daniels (1998) suggests that when nurses recognize parts of themselves in their clients, they humanize the nurse-client relationship.

Nurses need to be clear about their personal values, beliefs, stereotypes, and personal perspectives because of their potential influence on client decisions (McCormack & McCance, 2006; Morse, Havens, & Wilson, 1997). There are some clients whom nurses simply don't like working with (Erlen & Jones, 1999). It is up to the nurse, not the client, to resolve interpersonal issues that get in the way of the relationship. Nurses need to acknowledge overinvolvement, avoidance, anger, frustration, or detachment from a client when it occurs. A useful strategy in such situations is to seek further understanding of the client as a person by acknowledging your knowledge deficit and seeking to correct it.

Authenticity requires admitting mistakes. For example, a nurse might promise a client to return

Case Example

Brian Haggerty is a homeless individual who tells the nurse, "I know you want to help me, but you can't understand my situation. You have money and a husband to support you. You don't know what it is like out on the streets." Instead of feeling defensive, the nurse might say, "You are right, I don't know what it is like to be homeless, but I would like to know more about your experiences. Can you tell me what it has been like for you?" With this listening response, the nurse invites the client to share his experience. The data might allow the nurse to appreciate and address the loneliness, fear, and helplessness the client is experiencing, which are universal feelings.

immediately with a pain medication and then forget to do so because of other pressing demands. When the nurse brings the medication, the client might accuse the nurse of being uncaring and incompetent. It would be appropriate for the nurse to apologize for forgetting the medication, and for the extra discomfort suffered by the client.

Presence

Nursing presence involves being with the client in the moment, in a manner that both nurse and client can recognize. McDonough-Means, Kreitzer and Bell (2004) describe presence as having two dimensions: "being there" and "being with" (p. S25). The sense of connectivity is simultaneously experienced by those involved in the process: nurse, client, family. Nursing presence is evidenced through active listening, relevant caring communication, and sharing of skills, knowledge, and competencies related to client-specific problems (McCormack & McCance, 2006; Morse et al., 1997). Presence involves the nurse's capacity to know when to provide help and when to stand back, when to speak frankly, and when to withhold comments because the client is not ready to hear them. The gift of presence enriches the sense of self, and life of both patient and nurse, in ways that are unique to each person and situation (Covington, 2003; Easter, 2000).

Self-awareness

Peplau (1997) notes that nurses must observe their own behavior, as well as the client's, with "unflinching self-scrutiny and total honesty in assessment of their behavior in interactions with patients" (p. 162). Self-awareness requires a reflective process that seeks to

BOX 5-2	Key Questions for Reflection in a Client-Centered Interaction

- Can I behave in some way that will be perceived by the other person as trustworthy and as dependable or consistent in some deep sense?
- Can I be expressive enough as a person that what I am will be communicated unambiguously?
- Can I let myself experience positive attitudes toward this other person—attitudes of warmth, caring, liking interest, and respect?
- Can I be strong enough as a person to be separate from the other?
- Can I let myself enter fully into the world of my client's feelings and personal meanings, and see these as he or she does?
- Can I act with sufficient sensitivity that my behavior will not be perceived as a threat in the relationship?
- Can I meet this other individual as a person who is in the process of becoming, or will I be bound by his or her past and by my past?

From Rogers C: The characteristics of a helping relationship. In Rogers C, editor: *On becoming a person*, Boston, 1961, Houghton-Mifflin.

understand one's personal values, feelings, attitudes, motivations, strengths, and limitations—and how these affect practice and client relationships. By critically and simultaneously examining the behaviors of the client and the nurse, and what is going on in the relationship, nurses can create a safe, trustworthy, and caring relational structure (Lowry, 2005). Questions developed by Carl Rogers (1958) that nurses can ask themselves to promote the professional self-awareness needed in nurse-client relationships are presented in Box 5-2.

Developing an Evidence-Based Practice

Sahlsten M, Larsson I, Lindencrona C et al.: Patient participation in nursing care, *Journal of Clinical Nursing* 14:35–42, 2005.

This qualitative study, using a grounded theory method, was designed to clarify the registered nurse's understanding of patient participation in nursing care by studying staff nurses' interpretations of patient participation and how it occurred. A purposive sample of 31 registered nurses providing inpatient nursing care in five different hospitals participated in focus groups.

Results: Study results revealed four different approaches and procedures involved with patient participation: interpersonal procedure (mutual interaction between nurse and patient), therapeutic approach (understanding and being understood, contact, respect), focus on resources (exchange of information and knowledge), and opportunities for influence (information, choices, decisions).

Application to Your Clinical Practice: As health consumers become active partners in their personal health care, their participation with nurses to achieve desired outcomes becomes an integral component of their nursing care. How would you see the factors identified in this study applied to your nursing care of clients?

APPLICATIONS

PHASES OF THE RELATIONSHIP

Peplau (1952) described four sequential phases of a nurse-client relationship, each characterized by specific tasks and interpersonal skills: preinteraction, orientation, working (problem identification and exploitation), and termination. The phases are overlapping and serve to broaden as well as deepen the emotional connection with clients (Reynolds, 1997). Although her theoretical model of relationships is better applied to long-term relationships, the concepts hold true for short encounters. Peplau identified six professional roles the nurse can assume during the course of the nurse-client relationship (Box 5-3).

BOX 5-3	Peplau's Six Nursing Roles

1. *Stranger* role: Receives the client the same way one meets a stranger in other life situations; provides an accepting climate that builds trust
2. *Resource* role: Answers questions, interprets clinical treatment data, gives information
3. *Teaching* role: Gives instructions and provides training; involves analysis and synthesis of the learner experience
4. *Counseling* role: Helps client understand and integrate the meaning of current life circumstances; provides guidance and encouragement to make changes
5. *Surrogate* role: Helps client clarify domains of dependence, interdependence, and independence, and acts on client's behalf as advocate
6. *Leadership* role: Helps client assume maximum responsibility for meeting treatment goals in a mutually satisfying way

TABLE 5-2	Interviewing and Relationship Skills		
Phase	**Stage**	**Purpose**	**Skills**
Orientation Phase			
Engagement, assessment	Gathering information, defining the problem, identifying strengths	To determine how the client views the problem and what client strengths might be used in their resolution	Basic listening and attending; open-ended questions, verbal cues, and leads
Working (Implementation) Phase			
Planning (identification component)	Determining outcomes: What needs to happen to reduce the self-care demand? Where does the client want to go?	To find out how the client would like to be; how things would be if the problems were solved	Attending and basic listening; influencing; feedback
Implementation (exploitation component)	Explaining alternatives and options	To work toward resolution of the client's self-care needs	Influencing; feedback balanced by attending and listening
Termination Phase			
Evaluation	Generalization and transfer of learning	To enable changes in thoughts, feelings, and behaviors; to evaluate the effectiveness of the changes in modifying the self-care need	Influencing; feedback; validation

Data Sources: Ivey A, Ivey M: Ivey's five stage model of interviewing. In Ivey A, editor, *Intentional interviewing and counseling*, Monterey, CA, 2002, Brooks/Cole; and Richmond V, McCroskey J, Payne S: *Nonverbal behavior in interpersonal relations*, Englewood Cliffs, NJ, 1987, Prentice Hall; Peplau H: Peplau's theory of interpersonal relations, *Nursing Science Quarterly* 10(4):162–167, 1997.

Peplau's developmental stages parallel the nursing process. The orientation phase correlates with the assessment phase of the nursing process. The identification component of the working phase corresponds to the planning phase, whereas the exploitation phase parallels the implementation phase. The final resolution phase of the relationship corresponds to the evaluation phase of the nursing process (see Chapter 2 for details on the nursing process). Table 5-2 identifies interviewing strategies associated with each phase of the nurse-client relationship.

PREINTERACTION PHASE

The preinteraction phase is the only one in which the client does not directly participate. Awareness of professional goals is important. Developing professional goals helps the nurse select concrete, specific nursing actions that are purposeful and aligned with individualized client needs.

Professional goals differ from client goals, having to do with the nurse's knowledge, competence, and control of role responsibilities in the nurse-client relationship. Although professional goals are not communicated

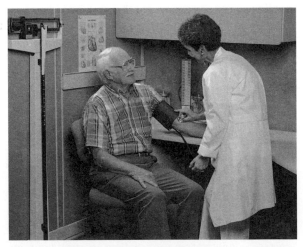

Concepts of the therapeutic relationship are present even in brief encounters.

directly to clients, they are present as professional behaviors in all aspects of nursing care.

Having an idea of potential client issues before meeting with the client is helpful. For example, a different approach is required for a client whose infant is in the neonatal intensive care unit, than for a client who is rooming in with a healthy infant.

If the relationship is to be ongoing, for example, in a subacute, rehabilitation, or psychiatric setting, it is important to share initial plans related to time, purpose, and other details with staff. This simple strategy helps avoid scheduling conflicts.

Creating the Physical Environment

Specific client needs dictate the most appropriate interpersonal setting. When the interview takes place at the client's bed in a hospital setting, the curtain should be drawn and the nurse can sit at an angle facing the client. One-on-one relationships with psychiatric clients commonly take place in a designated, noiseless room apart from the client's bedroom. In the client's home, the nurse is always the client's guest. A private space in which the nurse and client can talk without being uninterrupted is essential. Each time a nurse is sensitive to the environment in a nurse-client relationship, the nurse models thoughtfulness, respect, and empathy.

ORIENTATION PHASE

The nurse enters the relationship in the "stranger" role and begins the process of developing trust by providing the client with basic information about the nurse (e.g., name and professional status) and essential information about the purpose, nature, and time available for the relationship (Peplau, 1997). It can be a simple introduction: "I am Susan Smith, a registered nurse, and I am going to be your nurse on this shift." Nonverbal supporting behaviors of a handshake, eye contact, and a smile reinforce spoken words. Introductions are important even with clients who are confused, aphasic, comatose, or unable to make a cogent response because of mental illness or dementia. Introductions may need to be repeated, particularly for cognitively disabled clients.

Next, the nurse can ask the client, "How would you prefer to be addressed?" Assure the client that personal information will be treated as confidential (Heery, 2000). Explain that data will be shared with other members of the health care team as needed for making relevant clinical decisions and informing the client about the general composition of the health care team. Exercise 5-2 is designed to give you practice in making introductory statements.

Clarifying the Purpose of the Relationship

Clarity of purpose related to identifiable health needs is an essential dimension of the nurse-client relationship (LaSala, 2009). It is difficult to fully participate in any working partnership without understanding

EXERCISE 5-2	Introductions in the Nurse-Client Relationship

Purpose: To provide experience with initial introductions.

Procedure:
The introductory statement forms the basis for the rest of the relationship. Effective contact with a client helps build an atmosphere of trust and connectedness with the nurse. The following statement is a good example of how one might engage the client in the first encounter:

   "Hello, Mr. Smith. I am Sally Parks, a nursing student. I will be taking care of you on this shift. During the day, I may be asking you some questions about yourself that will help me to understand how I can best help you."

1. Role-play the introduction to a new client with one person taking the role of the client; another, the nurse; and a third person, an involved family member, with one or more of the following clients:
   a. Mrs. Dobish is a 70-year-old client admitted to the hospital with a diagnosis of diabetes and a question about cognitive impairment.
   b. Thomas Charles is a 19-year-old client admitted to the hospital after an auto accident in which he broke both legs and fractured his sternum.
   c. Barry Fisheis is a 53-year-old man who has been admitted to the hospital for tests. The physician thinks he may have a renal tumor.
   d. Marion Beatty is a 9-year-old girl admitted to the hospital for an appendectomy.
   e. Barbara Tangiers is a 78-year-old woman living by herself. She has multiple health problems including chronic obstructive pulmonary disease and arthritis. This is your first visit.

Discussion:
1. In what ways did you have to modify your introductions to meet the needs of the client or circumstances, or both?
2. What were the easiest and hardest parts of doing this exercise?
3. How could you use this experience in your clinical practice?

its purpose and expectations. Clients need basic information about the purpose and nature of the interview or relationship, including what information is needed and how the information will be used, how the client can participate in the treatment process, and what the client can expect from the encounter. To understand the importance of orientation information, consider the value of having a clear syllabus for your nursing courses.

The length of the relationship dictates the depth of the orientation. An orientation given to a client by a nurse assigned for a shift would be different from that given to a client when the nurse assumes the role of primary care nurse over an extended period. When the relationship is of longer duration, the nurse should discuss the parameters of the relationship (e.g., length of sessions, frequency of meetings, and role expectations of the nurse and client).

Initial meetings should have two outcomes: First, the client should emerge from the encounter with a better idea of the most relevant health issues; second, the client should feel that the nurse is interested in him or her as a person. At the end of the contact, the nurse should thank the client for his or her participation and indicate what will happen next.

Establishing Trust

Carter (2009) defines **trust** as "a relational process, one that is dynamic and fragile, yet involving the deepest needs and vulnerabilities of individuals" (p. 404). Starting with the first encounter, clients begin to assess the nurse's trustworthiness. Kindness, competence, and a willingness to become involved are communicated through the nurse's words, tone of voice, and actions. Does the nurse seem to know what he or she is doing? Is the nurse tactful and respectful of cultural differences? Data regarding the level of the nurse's interest and knowledge base are factored into the client's decision to engage actively in a therapeutic relationship. Confidentiality, sensitivity to client needs, and honesty strengthen the relationship.

The level of trust fluctuates with illness, age, and successful and unsuccessful encounters with others (Carter, 2009). Knowledge of the client's developmental level helps frame therapeutic conversations. For example, you would hold a different conversation with an adolescent client than you would with an elderly client. The acutely ill client will need short

contacts that are to the point and related to providing comfort and care. The client's current health situation is a good starting place for choice of topic.

Trusting the nurse is particularly difficult for the seriously mentally ill, for whom the idea of having a professional person care about them can be incomprehensible. Having this awareness helps the nurse look beyond the bizarre behaviors that these clients present in response to their fears about helping relationships. Many mentally ill clients will respond better to shorter, frequent contacts until trust is established. Schizophrenic clients often enter and leave the space occupied by the nurse, almost circling around a space that is within visual distance of the nurse. With patience and tact, the nurse engages the client slowly with a welcoming look and brief verbal contact. Over time, brief meetings that involve an invitation and a statement as to when the nurse will return help reduce the client's anxiety, as indicated in the following dialogue.

Case Example

Nurse (with eye contact and enough interpersonal space for comfort): Good morning, Mrs. O'Connell. My name is Karen Quakenbush. I will be your nurse today.

(Client looks briefly at the nurse and looks away, then gets up and moves away.)

Nurse: This may not be a good time to talk with you. Would you mind if I checked back later with you? (The introduction coupled with an invitation for later communication respects the client's need for interpersonal space and allows the client to set the pace of the relationship.)

Later, the nurse notices that Mrs. O'Connell is circling around the area the nurse is occupying but does not approach the nurse. She smiles encouragingly and repeats nondemanding invitations to the client until the client is more willing to trust. (Creating an interpersonal environment that places little demand on either party initially allows the needed trust to develop in the relationship.)

Identifying Client Needs

Therapeutic relationships should directly revolve around the client's needs and preferences. Each person's experience and individualized expression of them will be different. How clients perceive their health status, reasons for seeking treatment at this time, and expectations for health care are critical data, which you can begin to elicit by simply asking the client why he or she is seeking treatment at this time. Using questions that follow a logical sequence and asking only one question at a time help clients feel more comfortable, and is likely to elicit more complete data.

Client and family expectations can facilitate or hinder the treatment process. When health professionals treat elderly, adolescent, or physically handicapped clients as though they are mentally incapacitated in assessment interviews, it devalues them as a person. On the other hand, family members are sometimes reluctant to challenge a client's perceptions in front of the client and may need a private interview. Nurses need to include *both* perspectives for accurate assessment.

Similarities and differences between client and family perceptions of illness and treatment are important data. If there is reason to suspect the reliability of the client as a historian, interviewing significant others assumes greater importance. Family/client agreement or disagreement about diagnosis, treatment goals, or ways to provide care are critical data. For example, if a client has one perception about personal self-care abilities and family members have a completely different awareness, these differences can become a nursing concern.

Participant Observation

Peplau describes the role of the nurse in all phases of the relationship as being a participant observer. This means that the nurse simultaneously participates in and observes the progress of the relationship from the nurse and the client perspective. When validated with the client, observations about the client's behavior and words serve as guides for subsequent dialogue and actions in the relationship. According to Peplau,

observation includes self-awareness and self-reflection on the part of the nurse. This is as critical to the success of the relationship as is the assessment of the client's situation (McCarthy and Aquino-Russell, 2009).

Case Example

Terminally ill client (to the nurse): It's not the dying that bothers me as much as not knowing what is going to happen to me in the process.

Nurse: It sounds as though you can accept the fact that you are going to die, but you are concerned about what you will have to experience. Tell me more about what worries you.

By linking the emotional context with the content of the client's message, the nurse enters into the client's world and shows a desire to understand the situation from the client's perspective. Nurses need to be aware of the different physical and nonverbal cues clients give with their verbal messages. Noting facial expressions and nonverbal cues with "You look exhausted" or "You look worried" acknowledges the presence of these factors and normalizes them. Exercise 5-3 is designed to help you to critically observe a person's nonverbal cues.

Defining the Problem

Nurses act as a sounding board, asking questions about parts of the communication that are not understood and helping clients to describe their problems in concrete terms. The nurse asks for specific details to bring the client's needs into sharper focus, for example, "Could you describe for me what happened next," or "Tell me something about your reaction to (your problem)," or "how do you feel about. . ."? Time should

EXERCISE 5-3	Nonverbal Messages

Purpose: To provide practice in validation skills in a nonthreatening environment.

Procedure:
1. Each student, in turn, tries to communicate the following feelings to other members of the group without words. They may be written on a piece of paper, or the student may choose one directly from the following list.
2. The other students must guess what behaviors the student is trying to enact.

Pain	Anxiety	Shock	Disinterest
Anger	Disapproval	Disbelief	Rejection
Sadness	Relief	Disgust	Despair
Confidence	Uncertainty	Acceptance	Uptightness

Discussion:
1. Which emotions were harder to guess from their nonverbal cues? Which ones were easier?
2. Was there more than one interpretation of the emotion?
3. How would you use the information you developed today in your future care of clients?

be allowed between questions for the client to respond fully. Commonly, such questions are asked but not enough time is allowed for the client to respond.

Clients usually find it easier to talk about factual data related to a problem rather than to express the feelings associated with the issue. For example, saying "It sounds as if you feel _____ because of _____" helps the client to articulate the relationships between situational data and its emotional impact.

Once the nurse and client develop a working definition of the problem, they can begin to brainstorm the best ways to meet treatment goals. The brainstorming process occurs more easily when nurses are relaxed and willing to understand views different from their own. Brainstorming involves generating multiple ideas and suspending judgment until after all possibilities are presented. The next step is to look realistically at ideas that could work given the resources the client has available right now. Resistance can be worked through with empathetic reality testing. Peplau (1997) suggests that a general rule of thumb in working with clients is to "struggle with the problem, not with the patient" (p. 164). The last part of the process relates to determining the kind of help needed and who can best provide it. Assessment of the most appropriate source of help is an important but often overlooked part of the evaluation needed in the orientation phase.

Defining Goals

Unless clients are physically or emotionally unable to participate in their care, they should be treated as active partners in developing personal goals. Goals should have meaning to the client. For example, modifying the exchange lists with a diabetic adolescent's input so that they include substitutions that follow normal adolescent eating habits can facilitate acceptance of unwelcome dietary restrictions. The nurse conveys confidence in the client's capacity to solve his or her own problems by expecting the client to provide data, to make constructive suggestions, and develop realistic goals.

WORKING (EXPLOITATION/ACTIVE INTERVENTION) PHASE

With relevant treatment goals to guide nursing interventions and client actions, the conversation in the working phase turns to active problem solving related to assessed health care needs. Clients are able to discuss deeper, more difficult issues and to experiment with new roles and actions. Corresponding to the implementation phase of the nursing process, the working phase focuses on self-direction and self-management to whatever extent is possible in promoting the client's health and well-being.

Peplau (1997) has categorized the client role as dependent, interdependent, or independent, based on the amount of responsibility the client is willing or able to assume for his or her care. Nurses should provide enough structure and guidelines for clients to explore problem issues and develop realistic solutions, but no more than are needed (Ballou, 1998). Avoid taking more responsibility for actions than the client or situation requires. For example, it may seem more efficient to give a bath to a stroke victim than to watch the client struggle through the bathing process with the nurse providing coaching when the client falters. However, what happens when the client goes home if she has not learned to bathe herself?

Breaking a seemingly insoluble problem down into simpler chunks is a nursing strategy that makes doing difficult tasks more manageable. For example, a goal of eating three meals a day may seem overwhelming to a person suffering from nausea and loss of appetite associated with gastric cancer. A smaller goal of having applesauce or chicken soup and a glass of milk three times a day may sound more achievable, particularly if the client can choose the times.

In even the most difficult nursing situations, there are options, even if the choice is to die with dignity or to change one's attitude toward an illness or a family member. The client's right to make decisions, provided they do not violate self or others, needs to be accepted by the nurse, even when it runs contrary to the nurse's thinking. This protects the client's right to autonomy.

Case Example

LaSala (2009) presents a case example in which a client with lymphoma refused a blood transfusion after her first round of chemotherapy. Her physician was upset that she would not accept this logical treatment. The nurse in the situation said, "I explained to him what her beliefs were and why she refused blood. He continued to look confused, and I said, 'We may not understand it fully, but we have to respect her decision and not let our personal opinions impede our care.' He looked at me and said I was absolutely right" (p. 425).

Tuning in to Client Response Patterns

The art of nursing requires that nurses recognize differences in client response patterns. Elderly adults may need a slower pace, and people in crisis will need a simple structured level of support. Throughout the working phase, nurses need to be sensitive about whether the client is still responding at a useful level. Looking at difficult problems and developing strategies to resolve those problems is not an easy process, especially when resolution requires significant behavioral changes. If the nurse is perceived as inquisitive rather than facilitative, communication breaks down.

It is the responsibility of the nurse, not the client, to pace interactions in ways that offer support, as well as challenge. Deciding whether to proceed is a clinical judgment that should be based on the client's response and overall body language. Examples of warning signs that the pace may need adjustment include loss of eye contact, fidgeting, abrupt changes in subject, or asking to be left alone. At the same time, strong emotion should not necessarily be interpreted as reflecting a level of interaction stretching beyond the client's tolerance. Tears or an emotional outburst may reflect honestly felt emotion. A well-placed comment, such as, "I can see that this is difficult for you," acknowledges the feeling and may stimulate further discussion.

The working phase may produce uneven results, with two steps forward and one backward, even when the plan is appropriate. Mistakes are to be expected. They should be treated as temporary setbacks and new information requiring a modification in strategy. Developing alternative constructive coping mechanisms is as important to support as the actual plan. Coping with unexpected responses can strengthen the client's problem-solving abilities by compelling the person to consider alternative options (i.e., a Plan B) when the original plan does not bring about the desired results. Exercise 5-4 examines the role of brainstorming in generating alternative strategies.

As clients use the relationship to support coping with health-related situations, nurses can offer anticipatory guidance and role rehearsal for difficult aspects of this process. Sometimes, simply anticipating the worst-case scenario for a given action allows the client to see that even the worst possibility is manageable.

Defusing Challenging Behaviors

Challenging behaviors can sabotage the therapeutic relationship if they are not addressed early in the relationship process. There is no one way to approach a client, and no single interpersonal strategy that works equally well with every client. Some clients clearly are more emotionally accessible and attractive to work with than others. When a client seems unapproachable or uninterested in human contact, it can be quite disheartening for the nurse. It is not uncommon for the nurse to report the kind of initial contact with a client seen in the following case examples.

EXERCISE 5-4 | **Selecting Alternative Strategies**

Purpose: To help students develop a process for considering and prioritizing alternative options.

Procedure:
You have two exams within the next two weeks. Your car needs servicing badly. Because of all the work you have been doing, you have not had time to call your mother, and she is not happy. Your laundry is overflowing the hamper. Several of your friends are going to the beach for the weekend and have invited you to go along. How can you handle it all?
1. Give yourself 5 minutes to write down all the ideas that come to mind for handling these multiple responsibilities. Use single words or phrases to express your ideas. Do not eliminate any possibilities, even if they seem far-fetched.

2. In groups of three or four students, choose a scribe and then share the ideas you have written down.
3. Select the three most promising ideas.
4. Develop several small, concrete, achievable actions to implement these ideas.
5. Share the small-group findings with the class group.

Discussion:
1. In what ways were the solutions you chose similar or dissimilar to those of your peers?
2. Were any of your ideas or ways of achieving alternative solutions surprising to you or to others in your group?
3. What did you learn from doing this exercise that could help you and a client generate possible solutions to seemingly impossible situations?

Case Example ▬

"I tried, but he just wasn't interested in talking to me. I asked him some questions, but he didn't really answer me. So I tried to ask him about his hobbies and interests. It didn't matter what I asked him. He just turned away. Finally, I gave up because it was obvious that he just didn't want to talk to me."

Although, from the nurse's perspective, this client's behavior may represent a lack of desire for a relationship, in most cases, the rejection is not personal. It can reflect boredom, insecurity, or physical discomfort. Anxiety expressed as anger or unresponsiveness may be the only way a client can control fear in a difficult situation. Rarely does it have much to do with the personal approach used by the nurse unless the nurse is truly insensitive to the client's feelings or the needs of the situation. In this situation, the nurse might say, "It seems to me that you just want to be alone right now. But I would like to help you, so if you don't mind, I'll check back later with you. Would that be OK with you?" Most of the time, clients appreciate the nurse's willingness to stay involved.

For novice nurses, it is important to recognize that all nurses have experienced some form of client rejection at one time or another. The nurse needs to explore whether the timing was right, whether the client was in pain, and what other circumstances might have contributed to the client's attitude. Behaviors that initially seem maladaptive may appear quite adaptive when the full circumstances of the client's situation are understood.

Before confronting a client, the nurse should anticipate possible outcomes. The nurse needs to appreciate the impact of the confrontation on a client's self-esteem. Calling a client's attention to a contradiction in behavioral response is usually threatening. Constructive feedback involves drawing the client's attention to the existence of unacceptable behaviors or contradictory messages whereas respecting the fragility of the therapeutic alliance and the client's need to protect the integrity of the self-concept. To be effective, constructive confrontations should be attempted only when the following criteria have been met:

- The nurse has established a firm, trusting bond with the client.
- The timing and environmental circumstances are appropriate.
- The confrontation is delivered in a private setting, and in a nonjudgmental and empathetic manner.
- Only those behaviors capable of being changed by the client are addressed.
- The nurse supports the client's right to self-determination.

Case Example ▬

Mary Kiernan is 5 feet 2 inches tall and weigh 260 pounds. She has attended weekly weight management sessions for the past 6 weeks. Although she lost 8 pounds the first week, 4 pounds in week 2, and another 4 pounds in week 2, her weight loss seems to have hit a plateau. Jane Tompkins, her primary nurse, notices that Mary seems to be able to stick to the diet until she gets to dessert; then she cannot resist temptation. Mary is very discouraged about her lack of further progress.

Consider the effect of each response on the client.

Response A:
Nurse: You're supposed to be on a 1,200-calorie-a-day diet, but instead you're sneaking dessert. When you eat dessert when you are on a diet, you are kidding yourself that you will lose weight.

Response B:
Nurse: I can understand your discouragement, but you have done quite well in losing 16 pounds. It seems as though you can stick to the diet until you get to dessert. Do you think we need to talk a little more about what hooks you when you get to dessert? Maybe we need to find alternatives that would help you get back on track.

The first statement is direct, valid, and concise, but it is likely to be disregarded or experienced as unfeeling by the client. In the second response, the nurse reframes a behavioral inconsistency as a temporary setback. By first introducing an observed strength of the progress achieved so far, the nurse reaffirms trust in the client's resourcefulness. Both responses would require similar amounts of time and energy on the part of the nurse; however, the client is more likely to accept the nurse's second comment as more supportive.

Self-disclosure

Self-disclosure by the nurse refers to the intentional revealing of personal experiences or feelings that are similar to or different from those of the client. The purpose of self-disclosure is to deepen trust, to role-model self-disclosure as a beneficial mode of communicating for people who have trouble disclosing information about themselves. Appropriate self-disclosure can facilitate the relationship, providing the client with information that is both immediate and personalized (Deering, 1999).

Quality, not quantity, is a key characteristic of effective sharing in the working phase. Sharing should be solely for the clinical benefit of the client and never to meet the personal agenda of the nurse. Nurses should not share intimate details of their lives with their clients. The nurse, not the client, is responsible for regulating the amount of disclosure needed to facilitate the relationship. If the client asks a nonoffensive, superficial question, the nurse may answer briefly with a minimum of information and return to a client focus. Simple questions such as, "Where did you go to nursing school?" and "Do you have any children?" may represent the client's effort to establish common ground for conversation (Morse, 1991). Answering the client briefly and returning the focus to the client is appropriate. If the client persists with questions, the nurse may need to redirect the client by saying, "I'd like to spend this time talking about you," or simply indicate that personal questions are not relevant to understanding the client's health care needs.

Deering (1999) suggests the following guidelines for keeping self-disclosure at a therapeutic level: (a) use self-disclosure to help clients open up to you, not to meet your own needs; (b) keep your disclosure brief; and (c) don't imply that your experience is exactly the same as the client's. Exercise 5-5 provides an opportunity to explore self-disclosure in the nurse-client relationship.

TERMINATION PHASE

It is important to be clear from the beginning about how long a therapeutic relationship will last. During the course of the relationship, termination can be mentioned, and clients should be told well in advance of an impending termination date. In the termination phase, the nurse and client evaluate the client's responses to treatment, and explore the meaning of the relationship and what goals have been achieved. Discussing client achievements, how the client and nurse feel about ending the relationship, and plans for the future are an important part of the termination phase.

Termination is a significant issue in long-term settings such as skilled nursing facilities, bone marrow transplant units, rehabilitation hospitals, and state psychiatric facilities. Significant long-term relationships can and do develop in these settings. If the relationship has been effective, real work has been accomplished. Nurses need to be sufficiently aware of their own feelings so that they may use them constructively without imposing them on the client. It is appropriate for nurses to share some of the meaning the relationship held for them, as long as such sharing fits the needs of the interpersonal situation and is not excessive or too emotionally intense.

EXERCISE 5-5	Recognizing Role Limitations in Self-disclosure

Purpose: To help students differentiate between a therapeutic use of self-disclosure and spontaneous self-revelation.

Procedure:
1. Make a list of three phrases that describe your own personality or the way you relate to others, such as the following:
   I am shy.
   I get angry when criticized.
   I'm nice.
   I'm sexy.
   I find it hard to handle conflicts.
   I'm interested in helping people.
2. Mark each descriptive phase with one of the following:
   A = Too embarrassing or intimate to discuss in a group.
   B = Could discuss with a group of peers.

C = This behavior characteristic might affect my ability to function in a therapeutic manner if disclosed.
3. Share your responses with the group.

Discussion:
1. What criteria were used to determine the appropriateness of self-disclosure?
2. How much variation is there in what each student would share with others in a group or clinical setting?
3. Were there any behaviors commonly agreed on that would never be shared with a client?
4. What interpersonal factors about the client would facilitate or impede self-disclosure by the nurse in the clinical setting?
5. What did you learn from doing this exercise that could be used in future encounters with clients?

Termination of a meaningful nurse-client relationship in long-term settings should be final. To provide the client with even a hint that the relationship will continue is unfair. It keeps the client emotionally involved in a relationship that no longer has a health-related goal. This is a difficult issue for nursing students, who either see no harm in telling the client they will continue to keep in contact or who feel they have used the client for their own learning needs and to completely close the door is unfair. However, this perception underestimates the positive things that the client received from the relationship and denies the fact that good-byes, painful as they may be, are a part of life and certainly not new for the client or for the nursing student.

Termination behaviors the nurse may encounter include avoidance, minimizing of the importance of the relationship, anger, demands, or additional reliance on the nurse. When the client is unable to express feelings about endings, the nurse may recognize them in the client's nonverbal behavior.

Case Example

A teenager who had spent many months on a bone marrow transplant unit had developed a real attachment to her primary nurse, who had stood by her during the frightening physical assaults to her body and appearance that were occasioned by the treatment. The client was unable to verbally acknowledge the meaning of the relationship with the nurse directly, despite having been given many opportunities to do so by the nurse. The client said she couldn't wait to leave this awful hospital and that she was glad she didn't have to see the nurses anymore. Yet, this same client was found sobbing in her room the day she left, and she asked the nurse whether she could write to her. The relationship obviously had meaning for the client, but she was unable to express it verbally.

Gift Giving

Clients sometimes wish to give nurses gifts at the end of a constructive relationship because they value the care nurses have given to them. Gift giving is a delicate matter that does not lend itself to absolute dictums, but instead invites reflection and professional judgment. Nurses should consider: What meaning does the gift have for the relationship, and in what ways might accepting it change the dynamics of the therapeutic alliance? Would giving or receiving a gift present issues for other clients or their families?

There is no one answer about whether gifts should or should not be exchanged. In fact, if the nurse handled every situation in the same fashion, the nurse would be denying the uniqueness of each nurse-client relationship. Each relationship has its own character and its own strengths and limitations, so what might be appropriate in one situation would be totally inappropriate in another. Token gifts such as chocolates or flowers may be acceptable. In general, nurses should not accept money or gifts of significant material value. Should this become an issue, you might suggest making the gift to the health care agency or a charity. It is always appropriate to simply thank the client for their generosity and thoughtfulness (Lambert, 2009). Exercise 5-6 is designed to help you think about the implications of gift giving in the nurse-client relationship.

Evaluation

Objective evaluation of clinical outcomes achieved in the nurse-client relationship should focus on the following:

- Was the problem definition adequate and appropriate for the client?
- Were the interventions chosen adequate and appropriate to resolve the client's problem?
- Were the interventions implemented effectively and efficiently to both the client's and the nurse's satisfaction in the allotted time frame?
- Is the client progressing toward maximum health and well-being? Is the client satisfied with his or her progress and care received?
- If follow-up care is indicated, is the client satisfied and able to carry forward his or her treatment plan in the community?

ADAPTATIONS FOR SHORT-TERM RELATIONSHIPS

Hagerty and Patusky (2003) argue the need to reconceptualize the nurse-patient relationship to one of human relatedness, given the brevity of hospital stays in today's evolving health care arena. Driven by the economics of managed care, nurses must help clients determine what they need and how to develop solutions that fit their situation much more quickly than previously. Although nurses can and should follow the phases of the relationship, developing a therapeutic relationship in short-term care could be more accurately termed a working alliance with active support.

The same recommendations for self-awareness, empathy, therapeutic boundaries, active listening, competence,

EXERCISE 5-6	Gift-Giving Role-play

Purpose: To help students develop therapeutic responses to clients who wish to give them gifts.

Procedure:
Review the following situations and answer the discussion questions.

Situation:
Mrs. Terrell, a hospice nurse, has taken care of Mr. Aitken during the last 3 months of his life. She has been very supportive of the family. Because of her intervention, Mr. Aitken and his son were able to resolve a long-standing and very bitter conflict before he died. The whole family, particularly his wife, is grateful to Mrs. Terrell for her special attention to Mr. Aitken.
Role-play Directions for Mrs. Aitken
You are very grateful to Mrs. Terrell for all of her help over the past few months. Without her help, you do not know what you would have done. To show your appreciation, you would like her to have a $300 gift

certificate at your favorite boutique. It is very important to you that Mrs. Terrell fully understand how meaningful her caring has been to you during this very difficult time.
Role-play Directions for Mrs. Terrell
You have given the Aitken family high-quality care and you feel very good about it, particularly the role you played in helping Mr. Aitken and his son reconcile before Mr. Aitken's death. Respond as you think you might in this clinical situation, given the previous data.
Discussion:
1. Discuss the responses made in the role-playing situation.
2. Discuss the other possible responses and evaluate the possible consequences.
3. Would you react differently if a client gave you a gift of $200 or a hand-crocheted scarf? If so, why?
4. Are there gifts clients give a nurse that are intangible? How should these gifts be acknowledged?

---

mutual respect, partnership, and level of involvement hold true as key elements of brief therapeutic relationships.

Orientation Phase

The therapeutic alliance begins with the same type of introduction and description of purpose identified for long-term relationships, with a focus on the nurse and client working as partners to develop a shared understanding of the client's health problems. Establishing a working alliance where time is an issue requires a "here and now" focus on problem identification and an emphasis on quickly understanding the context in which it arose.

Begin your client assessment by asking the client the reason for seeking care. Eliciting the client's concerns and allowing the client to tell his or her story

conveys respect and interest. Listen for what is left out and pay attention to what the client's story elicits in you. Support and empathy help build trust quickly. Dealing with the client's feelings with a statement such as "Tell me more about. . ." (with a theme picked up from the client's choice of words, hesitancy, or nonverbal cues) keeps the conversation flowing.

As the nurse interacts with the client, there are opportunities to observe client strengths and to comment on them. Every client has healthy aspects of his or her personality, and personal strengths that can be drawn on to facilitate individual coping responses. Exercise 5-7 provides an opportunity to explore the value of acknowledging personal strengths.

An important component of brief therapeutic relationships is the rapid development of a central focus, which is developed during an initial client evaluation.

EXERCISE 5-7	Identifying Client Strengths

Purpose: To identify personal strengths in clients with serious illness.

Procedure:
Think about a client you have had or a person you know who has a serious illness.

What personal strengths does this person possess that could have a healing impact? Strengths can be courage, patience, fighting spirit, family, and so on.

Write a one-page description of the client and the personal strengths observed (this can include how

the client is coping with his or her medical or psychological condition).

Discussion:
1. If you hadn't had to write the description, would you have been as aware of the client's strengths?
2. How could you help the client maximize his or her strengths to achieve quality of life?
3. What did you learn from this exercise that you can use in your clinical practice?

Cappabianca, Julliard, Raso and Ruggiero (2009) suggest that a simple statement posed at the beginning of each shift, such as, "What is your most important need today?" or "What is the most important thing I can do for you today?" helps focus the relationship. This type of question demonstrates intent to understand and meet each client's unique needs in a shortened time frame. It helps client and nurse develop a shared understanding of what is uniquely important to the client in the present moment.

Because the time frame for a therapeutic relationship may be a few hours or days, nurses need to focus on what is absolutely essential, rather than what would be nice to know. Finding out how much the client already knows can save a lot of time. Developed from this discussion are treatment goals that can be realistically achieved, and are consistent with client goals, beliefs, and preferences.

Planning will be smoother if the nurse and client choose problems that are of interest to the client and that offer the best return on investment. Included in the planning should be the risks and cost/benefits for each targeted clinical outcome given the shortened time frame. Looking at the client's needs from a broader contextual perspective, one that takes into consideration which problems, if treated, would also help correct other health problems, has a double benefit in terms of client success and satisfaction. Engaging the client's family early in the treatment process is helpful.

As nurses increasingly move from a bedside role into a managerial coordination role, they become increasingly responsible for clarifying, integrating, and coordinating different aspects of the client's care, as part of an interdisciplinary team. An important component of this responsibility is ensuring that the client/family understands and is able to negotiate treatment initiatives with health care team providers.

Working Phase

Brief relationships need to be solution-focused right from the beginning. Giving clients your undivided attention and using concise active listening responses is absolutely essential to being able to frame issues in a solution focused way. A central focus, agreed on by nurse and client, allows for the small behavioral changes and related coping skills needed to meet client goals in short-term relationships. Finding ways to collaborate makes the most effective use of time, and confrontation should be avoided. Longer term

issues are not examined in depth and support beyond what is needed to stabilize the client. Clients respond best to nurses who appear confident and empathetic. An excellent way of helping clients discover the solutions that fit them best is by engaging the client in determining and implementing activities to meet therapeutic goals at every realistic opportunity. Conveying a realistically hopeful attitude that the goals developed with the client are likely to be achieved is important. Action plans should be as simple and specific as possible. Changes in the client's condition or other circumstances may require treatment modifications that should be expected in short term relationships. Keeping clients and families informed and working with them on alternative solutions is essential to maintaining trust in short term relationships.

Termination Phase

The termination phase in short-term relationships can include discharge planning, agency referrals, and arranging for follow-up appointments in the community for the client and family. Anticipatory guidance in the form of simple instructions or review of important skills also may be appropriate, depending on the circumstances. Interpersonal relationships with other health care disciplines, families, and communities to support positive client health changes should be the norm, not the exception with short-term therapeutic relationships.

The importance of the relationship, no matter how brief, should not be underestimated. Although the client may be one of several persons the nurse has taken care of during that shift, the relationship may represent the only interpersonal or professional contact available to a lonely and frightened person. Even if contact has been minimal, the nurse should endeavor to stop by the client's room to say good-bye. The dialogue in such cases can be simple and short: "Mr. Jones, I will be going off duty in a few minutes. I enjoyed working with you. Miss Smith will be taking care of you this evening." If you will not be returning at a later date, this information should be shared with the client.

SUMMARY

The nurse-client relationship represents a purposeful use of self in all professional relations with clients and other people involved with the client. Respect for the dignity of the client and self, person-centered communication, and authenticity in conversation are process threads underlying all communication responses.

Therapeutic relationships have professional boundaries, purposes, and behaviors. Boundaries keep the relationship safe for the client. They spell out the parameters of the therapeutic relationship and nurses are ethically responsible for maintaining them throughout the relationship. Effective relationships enhance the well-being of the client and the professional growth of the nurse. The professional relationship goes through a developmental process characterized by four overlapping yet distinct stages: preinteraction, orientation, working phase, and termination phase. The preinteraction phase is the only phase of the relationship the client is not part of. During the preinteraction phase, the nurse develops the appropriate physical and interpersonal environment for an optimal relationship, in collaboration with other health professionals and significant others in the client's life.

The orientation phase of the relationship defines the purpose, roles, and rules of the process, and provides a framework for assessing client needs. The nurse builds a sense of trust through consistency of actions. Data collection forms the basis for developing relevant nursing diagnoses. The orientation phase ends with a therapeutic contract mutually defined by nurse and client.

The working phase is the problem-solving phase of the relationship, paralleling the planning and implementation phases of the nursing process. As the client begins to explore difficult problems and feelings, the nurse uses a variety of interpersonal strategies to help the client develop new insights and methods of coping.

The final phase of the nurse-client relationship occurs when the essential work of the active intervention phase is finished. The ending should be thoroughly and compassionately defined early enough in the relationship that the client can process it appropriately. Primary tasks associated with the termination phase of the relationship include summarization and evaluation of completed activities, and referrals when indicated. Short-term relationships incorporate the same skills and competencies as traditional nurse-client relationships, but with a sharper focus on the here and now. The action plan needs to be as simple and specific as possible.

REFERENCES

Anderson H: Postmodern collaborative and person-centered therapies: what would Carl Rogers say? *Journal of Family Therapy* 23:339–360, 2001.

Ballou K: A concept analysis of autonomy, *J Prof Nurs* 14(2):102–110, 1998.

Briant S, Freshwater D: Exploring mutuality within the nurse-patient relationship, *Br J Nurs* 7(4):204–206, 1998.

Bruner K, Yonge O: Boundaries and adolescents in residential treatment centers: what clinicians need to know, *Journal of Psychosocial Nursing* 44(9):38–44, 2006.

Buber M: *I and thou* (Smith RG. translator). New York, 1958, Charles Scribner's.

Buber M: Distance and relation, *Psychiatry* 20:97–104, 1957.

Cappabianca A, Julliard K, Raso R, Ruggiero J: Strengthening the nurse-patient relationship: what is the most important thing I can do for you today, *Creat Nurs* 15(3):151–156, 2009.

Carmack B: Balancing engagement and disengagement in caregiving, *Image (IN)* 29(2):139–144, 1997.

Carter M: Trust, power, and vulnerability: a discourse on helping in nursing, *Nurs Clin North Am* 44:393–405, 2009.

Chauhan G, Long A: Communication is the essence of nursing care, 2: ethical foundations, *Br J Nurs* 9(15):979–984, 2000. Available online: http://www.cno.org/docs/prac/41033_Therapeutic.pdf.

Covington H: Caring presence: delineation of a concept for holistic nursing, *J Holist Nurs* 21(3):301–317, 2003.

Daniels L: Vulnerability as a key to authenticity, *Image J Nurs Sch* 30(2):191–193, 1998.

Deering CG: To speak or not to speak? Self-disclosure with clients, *Am J Nurs* 99(1 Pt 1):34–38, 1999.

Easter A: Construct analysis of four modes of being present, *J Holist Nurs* 18(4):362–377, 2000.

Egan G: *The skilled helper*, ed 7, Pacific Grove, CA, 2002, Brooks Cole Publishing.

Erlen JA, Jones M: The patient no one liked, *Orthop Nurs* 18(4):76–79, 1999.

Fronek P, Kendall M, Ungerer G, Malt J, Eugarde E, Geraghty T: Towards healthy professional-client relationships: the value of an interprofessional training course, *J Interprof Care* 23(10):16–29, 2009.

Hagerty B, Patusky K: Reconceptualizing the nurse-patient relationship, *J Nurs Scholarsh* 35(2):145–150, 2003.

Hartley S: Drawing the lines of professional boundaries, *Renalink* 3(2): 7–9, 2002.

Heery K: Straight talk about the patient interview, *Nursing* 30(6):66–67, 2000.

ETHICAL DILEMMA What Would You Do?

Kelly, age 20 years, has been admitted with a tentative medical diagnosis: rule out AIDS. John is a 21-year-old student nurse assigned to care for Kelly. He expresses concern to his instructor about the client's sexual orientation. The instructor notes that John spends the majority of his time with his only other assigned client, who is in for treatment of a minor heart irregularity. What conclusions might be drawn regarding the reason John spends so little time caring for Kelly? If you were John, what would be important to you in understanding and resolving your feelings?

Heinrich K: When a patient becomes too special, *Am J Nurs* 22(11): 62–64, 1992.

Hofmann P: Addressing compassion fatigue, *Health Care Executive* (Sept/Oct):40–42, 2009.

Hook M: Partnering with patients—A concept ready for action, *J Adv Nurs* 56(2):133–143, 2006.

Institute of Medicine: *Crossing the quality chasm: a new health system for the 21st century*, Washington, DC, 2001, National Academy Press.

Joint Commission, *The Health care at the crossroads: strategies for addressing the evolving nursing crisis*, Washington, DC, 2001, Author.

Kines M: The risks of caring too much, *Can Nurs* 95(8):27–30, 1999.

Lambert K: Gifts and gratuities for the case manager, *Professional Case Management* 14(1):53–54, 2009.

LaSala C: Moral accountability and integrity in nursing practice, *Nurs Clin North Am* 44:423–434, 2009.

Lowry M: Self-awareness: is it crucial to clinical practice? Confessions of a self-aware-aholic, *Am J Nurs* 105(11):72CCC–72DDD, 2005.

McCarthy C, Aquino-Russell CA: comparison of two nursing theories in practice: Peplau and Parse, *Nurs Sci Q* 22(1):34–40, 2009.

McDonough-Means MJ, Kreitzer, Bell I: Fostering a healing presence and investigating its mediators, *J Altern Complement Med* 10(Suppl 1): S25–S41, 2004.

McCormack B, McCance TV: Development of a framework for person-centred nursing, *J Adv Nurs* 56(5):472–479, 2006.

McGrath D: Healthy conversations: key to excellence in practice, *Holist Nurs Pract* 19(4):191–193, 2005.

McQueen A: Nurse–patient relationships and partnership in hospital care, *J Clin Nurs* 9(5):723–731, 2000.

Morse J: Negotiating commitment and involvement in the nurse-patient relationship, *J Adv Nurs* 16:455–468, 1991.

Morse JM, Havens GA, Wilson S: The comforting interaction: developing a model of nurse-patient relationship, *Sch Inq Nurs Pract* 11(4):321–343, 1997.

National Council of State Boards of Nursing (NCSBN): *Professional boundaries*, Chicago, 2007, Author. Available online: www.ncsbn.org/Professional_Boundaries_2007_Web.pdf. Accessed December 15, 2009.

O'Kelly E: Countertransference in the nurse-patient relationship: a review of the literature, *J Adv Nurs* 28(2):391–397, 1998.

Peplau HE: *Interpersonal relations in nursing*, New York, 1952, Putnam.

Peplau HE: Peplau's theory of interpersonal relations, *Nurs Sci Q* 10(4): 162–167, 1997.

Reynolds W: Peplau's theory in practice, *Nurs Sci Q* 10(4):168–170, 1997.

Rogers C: The characteristics of the helping relationship, *Personnel Guidance Journal* 37(1):6–16, 1958.

Sheets V: Professional boundaries: staying in the lines, *Dimens Crit Care Nurs* 20(5):36–40, 2001.

CHAPTER 6

Bridges and Barriers in the Therapeutic Relationship

Kathleen Underman Boggs

OBJECTIVES

At the end of the chapter, the reader will be able to:

1. Identify concepts that enhance development of therapeutic relationships: caring, empowerment, trust, empathy, mutuality, and confidentiality.
2. Describe nursing actions designed to promote trust, empowerment, empathy, mutuality, and confidentiality.
3. Describe barriers to the development of therapeutic relationships: anxiety, stereotyping, and lack of personal space.
4. Identify nursing actions that can be used to reduce anxiety and respect personal space and confidentiality.
5. Identify research-supported relationships between communication outcomes, such as client empowerment and improvements in self-care.
6. Discuss how findings from research studies can be applied to clinical practice.

This chapter focuses on the components of the nurse-client relationship, showing how nursing communication affects client health outcomes and satisfaction. Health communication is a multidimensional process and includes aspects from both the sender and the receiver of the message. Your communication skills influence outcomes such as anxiety, adherence to treatments, and satisfaction with care. To establish a therapeutic relationship, you need to understand and apply the concepts of respect, caring, empowerment, trust, empathy, and mutuality, as well as confidentiality and veracity (Figure 6-1). Additional bridges fostering the relationship are your ability to put into practice the ethical aspects of respecting the client's autonomy and treating your client in a just and beneficent manner. Understanding communication barriers in the relationship (e.g., anxiety, stereotyping, or violations of personal space or confidentiality) affects the quality of the relationship. Implementing actions that convey feelings of respect, caring, warmth, acceptance, and understanding to the client is an interpersonal skill that requires practice. Caring for others in a meaningful way improves with experience. Novice students may encounter interpersonal situations that leave them feeling helpless and inadequate. Feelings of sadness, anger, or embarrassment, although overwhelming, are common. Through discussion of these feelings in peer groups and experiential learning practice activities, you gain skill. The self-awareness strategies identified in Chapter 4 and the use of educational groups described in Chapter 12 provide useful guidelines for working through your feelings.

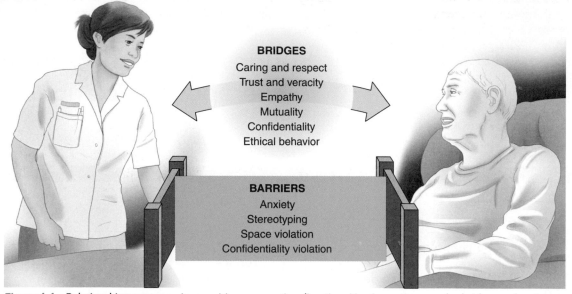

BRIDGES
Caring and respect
Trust and veracity
Empathy
Mutuality
Confidentiality
Ethical behavior

BARRIERS
Anxiety
Stereotyping
Space violation
Confidentiality violation

Figure 6-1   Relationships can move in a positive or negative direction. Nursing actions can be bridges or barriers to a good nurse-client interaction.

BASIC CONCEPTS

BRIDGES TO THE RELATIONSHIP

Nursing communication is crucial to efficient provision of quality care for your clients (Finke, 2008). Your communication skills affect client outcomes such as satisfaction with care, improved coping, adherence to treatment, adaptation to institutional care, peaceful death, and level of anxiety. Communication also affects us as providers in terms of our job satisfaction and stress levels (Sheldon & Ellington, 2008). The following concepts will help you improve your communication. Barriers to use of each concept are described.

RESPECT

Conveying genuine respect for your client assists in building a professional relationship with him or her. As your mutual goal is to maximize the client's health status, you convey respect for his values and opinions. Asking clients what they prefer to be called and always addressing them as such is a correct initial step. Of course, you avoid the sort of casual addresses portrayed in bad television shows, such as "How are you feeling, honey?" "Mom, hold your baby," or "How are we feeling today?" We try to remember that

hospitalized clients feel a loss of control in relation to interpersonal relationships with staff.

Barrier: Lack of Respect

In the Williams and Irurita study (2004), clients felt devalued when they perceived that staff were avoiding talking with them or were unfriendly; they felt comforted when a little "chitchat" was exchanged. Lack of respect among members of the team has also been often cited as a cause of adverse client outcomes. Lack of respect for the nurse by the physician has been cited as a factor leading to communication failures resulting in harm to the client (Sutcliffe, Leewton, & Rosenthal, 2004). Safety issues and communication is discussed in Chapter 22.

CARING

Caring is an intentional human action characterized by commitment and a sufficient level of knowledge and skill to allow you to support the basic integrity of your client. You offer caring to your client by means of the therapeutic relationship. Your ability to care develops from a natural response to help those in need, from the knowledge that caring is a part of nursing ethics, and from respect for self and others. As a caring nurse, you will involve clients in their struggle for health and well-being rather than simply doing things for your clients.

Provision of a caring relationship that facilitates health and healing is identified as an essential feature of contemporary nursing practice in the Social Policy Statement of the American Nurses Association (ANA, 1995). In the professional literature, the focus of the caring relationship is clearly placed on meeting the client's needs. A formal model is even titled "patient-centered care." It involves understanding the client's perceived needs and expectations for health. This is a shift away from the old "I am the provider of treatment for this disease" kind of thinking. The behavior of "caring" is not an emotional feeling. Rather, it is a chosen response to your client's need. You willingly give of yourself to another through your compassion, concern, and interest. Caring is an ethical responsibility that guides a health care provider to advocate for the client.

Clients want us to understand why they are suffering. We tend to speak in a language in medicine that values facts and events. Clients, in contrast, value associations and causes. To bridge this potential gap, you need to convey a sense that you truly care about your client's perspective. Caring has a positive influence on health status and healing. Clients can focus on accomplishing the goals of health care instead of worrying about whether care is forthcoming. The nurse gains from the caring relationship by experiencing satisfaction in meeting the client needs.

Families also need to experience a sense of caring from the nurse. Many families do not believe we have a clear understanding of the problems they are encountering while caring for their ill family member. This is especially true if the illness is not easily observable. One French study of effects of proactive communication with families of dying clients found that "caring" interventions in the form of longer conferences where family members could express emotions and talk with ethics and palliative care experts in conjunction with written materials did decrease their anxiety and depression (Lautrette et al., 2007).

Barrier: Lack of Caring

Although nursing has had a long-standing commitment to client-focused care, sometimes you may observe a situation in which you feel a nurse is apathetic, trying to meet her own needs rather than the client's needs. Some nurses develop a detachment that interferes with expressions of caring behaviors. At other times, a nurse can be so rushed to meet multiple demands that she seems unable to focus on the client. Exercise 6-1 will help you focus on the concept of caring.

EMPOWERMENT

Empowerment is assisting the client to take charge of his own life. We use the interpersonal process to provide information, tools, and resources that help our clients build skills to reach their health goals. Empowerment is an important aim in every nurse-client relationship, and is addressed by nursing theories such as Orem's view of the client as an agent of self-care. Studies demonstrate that the more involved a client is in his own care, the better the health outcome.

At a personal level, empowered clients feel valued, adopt successful coping methods, and think positively. Empowerment has to do with people power: In helping our clients to take control of their lives, we identify and build on their existing strengths.

Barriers

Empowerment is purposeful. It encourages clients to assume responsibility for their own health. This is in direct contrast with the paternalistic attitude formerly found in medicine and characterized by the attitude of "I know what is best for you or I can do it better." An Australian study showed that lack of information about giving care, managing medicines, or recognizing approaching crises was the major impediment to empowering family members to care for sick relatives

---

EXERCISE 6-1	Application of Caring

Purpose: To help students apply caring concepts to nursing.

a transparency on the overhead projector so the entire group can see.

Procedure:
Identify some aspect of caring that might be applied to nursing practice. Write each on the chalkboard or

Discussion:
In a large group, discuss examples of how this form of caring could be implemented in a nurse-client situation.

(Wilkes, White, & O'Riordan, 2000). Failure to allow our client to assume personal responsibility, or failure to provide him with appropriate resources and support, undermines empowerment.

TRUST

Establishing **trust** is the foundation in all relationships. The development of a sense of interpersonal trust, a sense of feeling safe, is the keystone in the nurse-client relationship. Trust provides a nonthreatening interpersonal climate in which the client feels comfortable revealing his needs. The nurse is perceived as dependable. Establishment of this trust is crucial toward enabling you to make an accurate assessment of your client's needs.

Trust is also the key to establishing workable relationships. Lack of trust in the workplace has detrimental effects for the organization and coworkers, undermining performance and commitment (Laschinger & Finegan, 2005). According to Erikson (1963), trust is developed by experiencing consistency, sameness, and continuity during care by a familiar caregiver. Trust develops based on past experiences. In the nurse-client relationship, maintaining an open exchange of information contributes to trust. For the client, trust implies a willingness to place oneself in a position of vulnerability, relying on health providers to perform as expected. Honesty is a basic building block in establishing trust. Studies show that clients or their surrogates want "complete honesty" and most prefer complete disclosure (Evans et al., 2009). Box 6-1 lists interpersonal strategies that help promote a trusting relationship.

Barrier: Mistrust

Mistrust has an impact not only on communication but on healing process outcomes. Trust can be replaced with mistrust between nurse and client. Just as some agency managers treat employees as though they are not trustworthy, some nurses treat some clients as though they are misbehaving children. Such would be the case if a client fails to follow the treatment regimen and is labeled with the nursing diagnosis of "noncompliant." In other examples, the community health nurse who is inconsistent about keeping client appointments or the pediatric nurse who indicates falsely that an injection will not hurt are both jeopardizing client trust. It is hard to maintain trust when one person cannot depend on another. Energy that should be directed toward coping with health problems is rechanneled into

BOX 6-1	Techniques Designed to Promote Trust

- Convey respect.
- Consider the client's uniqueness.
- Show warmth and caring.
- Use the client's proper name.
- Use active listening.
- Give sufficient time to answer questions.
- Maintain confidentiality.
- Show congruence between verbal and nonverbal behaviors.
- Use a warm, friendly voice.
- Use appropriate eye contact.
- Smile.
- Be flexible.
- Provide for allowed preferences.
- Be honest and open.
- Give complete information.
- Provide consistency.
- Plan schedules.
- Follow through on commitments.
- Set limits.
- Control distractions.
- Use an attending posture: arms, legs, and body relaxed; leaning slightly forward.

assessing the nurse's commitment and trustworthiness. Having confidence in the nurse's skills, commitment, and caring allows the client to place full attention on the situation requiring resolution. Clients can also jeopardize the trust a nurse has in them. Sometimes clients "test" a nurse's trustworthiness by sending the nurse on unnecessary errands or talking endlessly on superficial topics. As long as nurses recognize testing behaviors and set clear limits on their roles and the client's role, it is possible to develop trust. Exercise 6-2 is designed to help students become more familiar with the concept of trust.

EMPATHY

Empathy is the ability to be sensitive to and communicate understanding of the client's feelings. It is a crucial characteristic of a helping relationship. Empathy is an important element of effective communication and is associated with improved client satisfaction and adherence to treatments (Morse et al., 2008). The American Academy of Pediatrics has a policy statement emphasizing the need to communicate empathy to clients and family (Levetown, 2008). An empathetic nurse perceives and *understands* the client's emotions *accurately*. Empathy is the ability to put oneself into the

EXERCISE 6-2	Techniques That Promote Trust

Purpose: To identify techniques that promote the establishment of trust and to provide practice in using these skills.

Procedure:
1. Read the list of interpersonal techniques designed to promote trust (Box 6-1).
2. Describe the relationship with your most recent client. Was there a trusting relationship? How do you know? Which techniques did you use? Which ones could you have used?

or

In triads, have one learner interview a second to obtain a health history, whereas the third observes and records trusting behaviors. Rotate so that everyone is an interviewer. Interviews should last 5 minutes each. At the end of 15 minutes, each observer shares findings with the corresponding interviewer.

Discussion:
Compare techniques.

---

client's position. Some nurses might term this as *compassion*, which has been identified by staff nurses as being crucial to the nurse-client relationship. Communication skills are used to convey respect and empathy. Although expert nurses recognize the emotions a client feels, they hold on to their objectivity, maintaining their own separate identities. As a nurse, you should try not to overidentify with or internalize the feelings of the client. If internalization occurs, objectivity is lost, together with the ability to help the client move through his or her feelings. It is important to recognize that the client's feelings belong to the client, not to you.

Communicate your understanding of the meaning of a client's feelings by using both verbal and nonverbal communication behaviors. Maintain direct eye contact, use attending open body language, and keep a calm tone of voice. Acknowledge your client's message about his feelings by restating what you understand him to be conveying. Then, have him validate that this is accurate. If you need more information about his feelings, ask him to expand on his message, perhaps asking, "Are there other things about this that are bothering you?" Now that you have full information, you can directly make interventions to address his needs. Armed with accurate data, you can communicate your client's feelings to other providers if necessary.

Barrier: Lack of Empathy

Failure to understand the needs of clients may lead you to fail to provide essential client education or to provide needed emotional support. The literature indicates that major barriers to empathy exist in the clinical environment, including lack of time, lack of trust, lack of privacy, or lack of support. Several studies suggest that lack of empathy will affect the quality of care, result in less favorable health outcomes, and

lower client satisfaction (Levetown, 2008). However, providers can be taught to express empathy.

MUTUALITY

Mutuality basically means that the nurse and the client agree on the client's health problems and the means for resolving them, and that both parties are committed to enhancing the client's well-being. This is characterized by mutual respect for the autonomy and value system of the other. In developing mutuality, you maximize your client's involvement in all phases of the nursing process. Mutuality is collaboration in problem solving and "drives" the communication at the initial encounter (Feldman-Stewart & Brundage, 2008). Evidence of mutuality is seen in the development of individualized client goals and nursing actions that meet a client's unique health needs. Exercise 6-3 gives practice in evaluating mutuality.

Nurses need to respect interpersonal differences. We involve clients in the decision-making process. We accept their decisions even if we do not agree with them. Effective use of values clarification as described in Chapter 3 assists clients in decision making. Clients who clearly identify their own personal values are better able to solve problems effectively. Decisions then have meaning to the client. There is a greater probability he will work to achieve success. When a mutual relationship is terminated, both parties experience a sense of shared accomplishment and satisfaction.

VERACITY

As described in Chapters 2 and 3, legal and ethical standards mandate specific nursing behaviors, such as confidentiality, beneficence, and respect for client autonomy. These behaviors are based on professional nursing values that stem from the ethical principles.

EXERCISE 6-3	Evaluating Mutuality

Purpose: To identify behaviors and feelings on the part of the nurse and the client that indicate mutuality.

Procedure:
Complete the following questions by answering yes or no after terminating with a client; then bring it to class. Discuss the answers. How were you able to attain mutuality, or why were you unable to attain it?
1. Was I satisfied with the relationship?
2. Did the client express satisfaction with the relationship?
3. Did the client share feelings with me?
4. Did I make decisions for the client?
5. Did the client feel allowed to make his or her own decisions?
6. Did the client accomplish his or her goals?
7. Did I accomplish my goals?

Discussion:
In a large group, discuss mutuality.

By adhering to these "rules," nurses build their therapeutic relationships with individual clients. *Veracity* contributes to the establishment of a therapeutic relationship. When the client knows he can expect the truth, the development of trust is promoted and helps build the relationship.

OTHER BARRIERS TO THE RELATIONSHIP

A few additional barriers that affect the development of the nurse-client relationship include anxiety, stereotyping, and lack of personal space. Barriers inherent in the health care system are also commonly discussed in the professional literature. Under managed care, barriers often reflect cost-containment measures. Such barriers include lack of consistent assignment of nurse to client and increased use of temporary staff such as agency nurses or "floats." Lack of time can result from low staff/client ratios or early discharge. The primary care literature describes agency demand for minimal appointment time with clients. Primary care providers such as nurse practitioners are often constrained to focus just on the chief complaint to maximize the number of clients seen, leading to "the 15-minute office visit." Other system barriers include communication conflicts with other health professionals, conflicting values, poor physical arrangements, and lack of value placed on caring by for-profit agencies. These system barriers limit the nurse's ability to develop substantial rapport with clients. Adequate time is essential to develop therapeutic communication to achieve effective care responsive to client needs. Try Exercise 6-4.

Anxiety

Anxiety is a vague, persistent feeling of impending doom. It is a universal feeling; no one fully escapes it. The impact on the self is always uncomfortable. It occurs when a threat (real or imagined) to one's self-concept is perceived. Lower satisfaction with communication is associated with increased client anxiety. Anxiety is usually observed through the physical and behavioral manifestations of the attempt to relieve the anxious feelings. Although individuals experiencing anxiety may not know they are anxious, specific behaviors provide clues that anxiety is present Exercise 6-5 identifies behaviors associated with anxiety. Table 6-1 shows how an individual's sensory

EXERCISE 6-4	Building Communication Bridges Simulation

Purpose: To evaluate current communication skills.

Directions:
In small groups, one student role-plays a client telling the nurse her story of some past unpleasant medical experience; one student is the nurse conversing with the client; the rest of the group is listeners.

Discussion:
1. What aspects of the interaction demonstrated empathy, respect, caring, etc.?
2. Listeners should give the following feedback:
   a. Comment on positive aspects observed.
   b. Offer constructive criticism only after making a positive comment.
   c. Identify any behaviors that served as barriers.
   d. Suggest alternative strategies the nurse could use.
   e. Think about times when you used bridges or barriers.

EXERCISE 6-5	Identifying Verbal and Nonverbal Behaviors Associated with Anxiety

Purpose: To broaden the learner's awareness of behavioral responses that indicate anxiety. Procedure: List as many anxious behaviors as you can think of. Each column has a few examples to start. Discuss the lists in a group and then add new behaviors to your list.	Verbal Quavering voice Rapid speech Mumbling Defensive words	Nonverbal Nail biting Foot tapping Sweating Pacing

TABLE 6-1	Levels of Anxiety with Degree of Sensory Perceptions, Cognitive and Coping Abilities, and Manifest Behaviors

Level of Anxiety	Sensory Perceptions	Cognitive/Coping Ability	Behavior
Mild	Heightened state of alertness; increased acuity of hearing, vision, smell, touch	Enhanced learning, problem solving; increased ability to respond and adapt to changing stimuli; enhanced functioning*	Walking, singing, eating, drinking, mild restlessness, active listening, attending, questioning
Moderate	Decreased sensory perceptions; with guidance, able to expand sensory fields	Loss of concentration; decreased cognitive ability; cannot identify factors contributing to the anxiety-producing situation; with directions can cope, reduce anxiety, and solve problems; inhibited functioning	Increased muscle tone, pulse, respirations; changes in voice tone and pitch, rapid speech, incomplete verbal responses; engrossed with detail
Severe	Greatly diminished perceptions; decreased sensitivity to pain	Limited thought processes; unable to solve problems even with guidance; cannot cope with stress without help; confused mental state; limited functioning	Purposeless, aimless behaviors; rapid pulse, respirations; high blood pressure; hyperventilation; inappropriate or incongruent verbal responses
Panic	No response to sensory perceptions	No cognitive or coping abilities; without intervention, death is imminent	Immobilization

*Functioning refers to the ability to perform activities of daily living for survival purposes.

perceptions, cognitive abilities, coping skills, and behaviors relate to the intensity and level of anxiety experienced.

A mild level of anxiety heightens one's awareness of the surrounding environment, and fosters learning and decision making. Therefore, it may be desirable to allow a mild degree of anxiety when health teaching is needed or when problem solving is necessary. It is not prudent, however, to prolong even a mild state of anxiety.

Greater levels of anxiety decrease perceptual ability. The anxious state is accompanied by verbal and nonverbal behaviors that inhibit effective individual functioning. For example, anxiety causes you to hold your breath, which can lead to even greater levels of anxiety (Puetz, 2005). Moderate-to-severe anxiety on the part of either nurse or client hinders the development of the therapeutic relationship. To accomplish goals and attain mutuality, greater levels of anxiety must be reduced. Once the presence of anxiety has been identified, the nurse needs to take appropriate action. Strategies to reduce anxiety are listed in Box 6-2.

Severe anxiety requires medical and psychiatric intervention to alleviate the stress. A prolonged panic state is incompatible with life. It is such an extreme level of anxiety that, without immediate medical and psychiatric assistance, suicide or homicide may ensue. Some of these interpersonal strategies used to reduce moderate

BOX 6-2	Nursing Strategies to Reduce Client Anxiety

- Active listening to show acceptance
- Honesty; answering all questions at the client's level of understanding
- Clearly explaining procedures, surgery, and policies, and giving appropriate reassurance based on data
- Acting in a calm, unhurried manner
- Speaking clearly, firmly (but not loudly)
- Giving information regarding laboratory tests, medications, treatments, and rationale for restrictions on activity
- Setting reasonable limits and providing structure
- Encouraging clients to explore reasons for the anxiety
- Encouraging self-affirmation through positive statements such as "I will" and "I can"
- Using play therapy with dolls, puppets, and games
- Drawing for young clients
- Using therapeutic touch, giving warm baths, back rubs
- Initiating recreational activities such as physical exercise, music, card games, board games, crafts, and reading
- Teaching breathing and relaxation exercises
- Using guided imagery
- Practicing covert rehearsal

From Gerrard B, Boniface W, Love B: *Interpersonal skills for health professionals*, Reston, VA, 1980, Reston Publishing.

anxiety also are used during severe anxiety and panic attacks as part of a team approach to client care.

Choosing from various strategies to reduce client anxiety can be difficult. Not all methods are appropriate or work equally well with all clients. If a nurse attempting to build trust pushes a client too fast into revealing what he is not yet ready to discuss, this can increase anxiety. You need to accurately identify your client's level of anxiety. You should also identify and reduce your own anxiety. Anxiety can cloud your perceptions and interfere with relationships.

Stereotyping and Bias

Stereotyping is the process of attributing characteristics to a group of people as though all persons in the identified group possessed them. People may be stereotyped according to ethnic origin, culture, religion, social class, occupation, age, and other factors. Even health issues can be the stimulus for stereotyping individuals. For example, alcoholism, mental illness, and sexually transmitted diseases are fertile grounds for the development of stereotypes. Stereotypes have been shown to be consistent across cultures and somewhat across generations, although the value placed on a stereotype changes.

Stereotypes are learned during childhood and reinforced by life experiences. They may carry positive or negative connotations. For example, Harding, North, and Perkins (2008) suggest that our culture has stereotyped an image of men as less feeling than women. We all have personal biases, usually based on unconscious past learning. As nurses, we may act on these unknowingly. Stereotypes negate empathy and erode the nurse-client relationship. As nurses, we must work to develop insight into our own expectations and prejudgments about people. Telenurses in Hoglund and Holmstrom's (2008) study revealed distrust in fathers' competence to provide care for ill children, an example of stereotyping by nurses. Stewart and Payne's (2008) study showed that mentally making an intentional resolution to avoid a stereotype enables one to change.

Stereotypes are never completely accurate. No attribute applies to every member of a group. All of us like to think that our way is the correct way, and that everyone else thinks about life experiences just as we do. The reality is that there are many roads in life, and one road is not necessarily any better than another.

Emotions play a role in the value we place on negative stereotypes. Stereotypes based on strong emotions are called prejudices. Highly emotionally charged stereotypes are less amenable to change. In the extreme, this can result in discrimination. Discrimination as a legal statute refers to actions in which a person is denied a legitimate opportunity offered to others because of prejudice. In the United States, federal laws prohibit workplace discrimination based on age, creed, gender, sexual preference, disability, race, religion, or genetics.

Everyone has biases. If nurses bring their biases with them to the clinical situation, they will distort their perception, prevent client change, and disrupt the provider-client relationship. Nurses need to make it a goal to reduce bias. We do this by recognizing a client as a unique individual, both different from and similar to self. Acceptance of the other person needs to be total. This unconditional acceptance, as described by Carl Rogers (1961), is an essential element in the helping relationship. It does not imply agreement or approval; acceptance occurs without judgment. Mr. Fred Rogers, the children's television show host, ended his programs by telling his audience, "I like

EXERCISE 6-6	Reducing Clinical Bias by Identifying Stereotypes

Purpose: To identify examples of nursing biases that need to be reduced. Practice in identifying professional stereotypes and in how to reduce them is one component of maintaining high-quality nursing care.

Procedure:
Each of the following scenarios indicates a stereotype. Identify the stereotype and how it might affect nursing care. As a nurse, what would you do to reduce the bias in the situation? Are there any individuals or groups of people for whom you would not want to provide care (e.g., homeless women with foul body odor and dirty nails)?
Situation A
Mrs. Daniels, an obstetric nurse who believes in birth control, comments about her client, "Mrs. Gonzales is pregnant again. You know, the one with six kids already! It makes me sick to see these people on

welfare taking away from our tax dollars. I don't know how she can continue to do this."
Situation B
Mrs. Brown, a registered nurse on a medical unit, is upset with her 52-year-old female client. "If she rings that buzzer one more time, I'm going to disconnect it. Can't she understand that I have other clients who need my attention more than she does? She just lies in bed all day long. And she's so fat; she's never going to lose any weight that way."
Situation C
Mrs. Waters, a staff nurse in a nursing home, listens to the daughter of a 93-year-old resident, who says, "My mother, who is confused most of the time, receives very little attention from you nurses, while other clients who are lucid and clear-minded have more interaction with you. It's not fair! No wonder my mother is so far out in space. Nobody talks to her. Nobody ever comes in to say hello."

you just the way you are." How wonderful if we, as nurses, could convey this type of acceptance to our clients through our words and actions. Exercise 6-6 examines ways of reducing clinical bias.

Overinvolvement as a Barrier

Objectivity is important if you are to provide competent, professional care. This may be more likely to occur in a long-term relationship. Sharing too much information about yourself, your job problems, or about your other clients can become a barrier if your client becomes unclear about his role in your relationship. Many of us enjoy warm relationships with our clients, but if we are to remain effective, we need to be alert to the disadvantages of overinvolvement.

Violation of Personal Space

Personal space is an invisible boundary around an individual. The emotional personal space boundary provides a sense of comfort and protection. It is defined by past experiences, current circumstances, and our culture.

Proxemics is the study of an individual's use of space. Optimal territorial space needed by most individuals living in Western culture: 86 to 108 square feet of personal space. Other research has found that 60 square feet is the minimum needed for each client in multiple-occupancy rooms, and 80 square feet is the minimum for private rooms in hospitals and institutions. Critical care units offer even less square footage.

Among the many factors that affect the individual's need for personal distance are cultural dictates. In some cultures, people approach each other closely, whereas in others, more personal space is required. In most cultures, men need more space than women do. People generally need less space in the morning. The elderly need more control over their space, whereas small children generally like to touch and be touched by others. Although the elderly appreciate human touch, they generally do not like it to be applied indiscriminately. Situational anxiety causes a need for more space. Persons with low self-esteem prefer more space, as well as some control over who enters their space and in what manner. Usually people will tolerate a person standing close to them at their side more readily than directly in front of them. Direct eye contact causes a need for more space. Placing oneself at the same level (e.g., sitting while the client is sitting, or standing at eye level when the client is standing) allows the nurse more access to the client's personal space because such a stance is perceived as less threatening.

Hospitals are not home. Many nursing care procedures are a direct intrusion into your client's personal space. Commonly, procedures that require tubes (e.g., nasal gastric intubation, administration of oxygen, catheterization, and intravenous initiation) restrict the mobility of the client and the client's sense of control over personal territory. When more than one health professional is involved, the impact of the intrusion on the client may be even stronger. In many instances, personal space requirements are an integral part of a person's self-image. When clients lose control over personal space, they may experience a loss of identity and self-esteem. It's recommended you maintain a social physical body distance of 4 feet when not actually giving care. Consider the issue of respect for personal space in the clinical examples presented in Box 6-3.

When institutionalized clients are able to incorporate parts of their rooms into their personal space, it

increases their self-esteem and helps them to maintain a sense of identity. This feeling of security is evidenced when a client asks, "Close my door, please." Freedom from worry about personal space allows the client to trust the nurse and fosters a therapeutic relationship. When invasions of personal space are necessary while performing a procedure, you can minimize impact by explaining why a procedure is needed. Conversation with clients at such times reinforces their feelings that they are human beings worthy of respect and not just objects being worked on. Advocating for the client's personal space needs is an aspect of the nursing role. This is done by communicating your clients preferences to the members of the health team and including them in their care plan.

Home is not quite home when the home health nurse, infusion nurse, or other aides invade the client's personal space. Some modification of "take-charge" behavior is required when giving care in a client's home.

BOX 6-3   Clinical Examples of Personal Space Issues for Clients

- The nurse places the client on the bedpan without drawing the curtain on a postpartum unit. When the client protests, the nurse states, "Well, we're all girls here."
- The chief resident comes in with an entourage of residents and medical students. They draw the curtain and the chief resident, standing close to the client, informs the client that his cancer is terminal. The entourage moves on to the next client.
- Miss Jones has just been brought to the emergency department as a rape victim. Because of the circumstances, she is unable to change her clothes until she has been examined. It is an unusually busy night in the emergency department, and the policy is to practice triage and treat the most serious cases first. Because Miss Jones is not considered an emergency case, it will be some time before she is examined.
- Dr. Michaels has had an auto accident for which he is receiving emergency treatment by a multidisciplinary team. He is conscious, but no one calls him by name or seems to notice his wife standing outside the door.
- Barbara Burk has just been admitted to a psychiatric unit. The policy on the unit is to keep all valuables, razors, hand mirrors, and money locked up in the nurses' station. All clients must strip and shower under supervision soon after they arrive on the unit. It was not Barbara's choice to seek inpatient treatment, and she is very scared.
- Mr. Novack is admitted to the coronary care unit. He is hooked up to a cardioscope so his cardiac condition can be monitored continuously, and nasal oxygen is applied. The defibrillator is located close to his bed. His family is allowed to come in one at a time for 5 minutes once every hour as long as the visits do not interfere with nursing care or necessary treatment procedures.

Cultural Barriers

Cross-cultural communication is discussed extensively in Chapter 11. Every interaction encounters a basic challenge of communicating between the culture of a client and the medical culture of the health professional (Teal & Street, 2009). Cultural background and level of health literacy may have a powerful influence on communication practices. For example, Gordon and associates (2006) found lower levels of participation in cancer communication by ethnic minority clients. It is important to identify any cultural issues that will influence how your client or their family responds to your type of health communication. In some cultures, the sick role is no longer valid after symptoms disappear, so when your client's diabetes is under control, he and his family may no longer see the need for special diet or medication (Chang & Kelly, 2007). As we move into a more multicultural society, all health care providers need to work to become culturally competent communicators.

Cultural competence requires us to become aware of the arbitrary nature of our own cultural beliefs. *Culturally competent communication* is characterized by a willingness to try to understand and respond to your client's beliefs. Knowledge of the client's cultural preferences helps you avoid stereotyping and allows you to adapt your communication (Ngo-Metzger, August, Srinivasan, Liao, & Meyskens, 2008; Teal & Street, 2008).

Gender Differences

Gender is defined as the culture's attributions of masculine or feminine. Recently, more attention has been given to gender role, communication barriers, and health inequalities. In Hoglund and Holmstrom's (2008) study, phone calls by male clients to female telenurses revealed expressions of disrespect related to the nurse's gender, as well as her professional advice. Earlier studies seemed to show little communication or outcome difference relevant to the gender of the care provider. But Harding and coauthors' (2008) more recent study indicated that male nurses' touching of clients is problematic. This is because although our culture equates female touch with caring, being touched by a male individual is perceived as sexual. Women traditionally were considered to be better communicators, but some studies found no differences. Although results are mixed, it appears that gender need not be a factor in developing therapeutic communication with clients.

Developing an Evidence-Based Practice

Rask MT, Jensen ML, Andersen J, Zachariae R: Effects of an intervention aimed at improving nurse-patient communication in an oncology outpatient clinic, *Cancer Nursing*, 32(1):E1–E11, 2009.

This Danish study evaluated the effects of a 2-day training program for nurses working in a cancer treatment clinic. The hypothesis was that the training would improve nurse empathy and attentiveness, and client perception of their own mood and self-efficacy. Nurses (N = 24) and clients (N = 413) were randomly assigned to treatment and control groups. Outcomes were measured at baseline entry into this study, then at 1 week, and again at 3 months after the workshop.

Results: The hypothesis was not supported. The researchers gave many explanations including study design weaknesses, brevity of the skills training, the baseline already high levels of nurse competencies (all nurses were very experienced with more than 5 years' working time), and high client satisfaction; thus, there was not much room for improvement. At baseline, 21.7% of the nurses reported feeling "burned out," and although this improved at the 1-week measurement, the improvement did not persist (i.e., a "treatment effect"). Interestingly, the only measure of difference between control group and treatment group nurses was that control nurses reported greater frequency of stress related to conflicts with other nurses. Total stress scores for both groups were stable over time. Clients rated nurses they knew as having higher empathy than those having their first contact with the nurse. Clients were satisfied (99.8%) with nurse interpersonal and professional skills.

Application to your practice: Nurses dealing with clients who are being treated for cancer have a relatively high level of job-related stress. You and your coworkers need to be aware of indications of stress and develop some stress reduction strategies. You need to monitor peer interactions for conflict and actively use conflict reduction strategies. Assignments should allow for the client to be cared for by a familiar nurse as often as possible.

The researchers support the need for communications training for nurses and suggest that it takes a longer time than was available in this workshop to master nurse-client communication skills such as clarification, use of open-ended questions, empathy, listening, self-disclosure, and confrontation. They state that nurses need to tailor their communication to meet the needs and preferences of their clients, and suggest that there is a need to determine what type of communication is expected by clients in cancer outpatient settings.

APPLICATIONS

Many nursing actions recommended here are mandated by the American Nurses Association Code of Ethics for Nurses discussed in Chapter 2. The actions specified include confidentiality, autonomy, beneficence, veracity, and justice. Mutuality is addressed in the ANA position statement on human rights. Providers with good communication skills have greater professional satisfaction and experience less job-related stress (Maguire & Pitceathly, 2002; Rask et al., 2009). Studies of client perceptions generally show a correlation between good nurse communicators and good quality of care (Jha, Orav, & Zheng, 2008), although not all do so (Rask et al., 2009). Practice exercises provide you with opportunities to improve your skills. Part of any simulation exercise to strengthen nursing communication is the offering of feedback (Kim, Heerey, & Kols, 2008).

STEPS IN THE CARING PROCESS

Several articles identify four steps to help you communicate C.A.R.E. to your client:

C = First *connect* with your client. *Offer your attention.* Here you introduce your purpose in developing a relationship with your client (i.e., meeting his health needs). Use his formal name, and avoid terms of endearment such as "sweetie." Show an intent to care. Attentiveness is a part of communication skill training that is probably decreased by work-related stress, time constraints, and so forth.

A = The second step is to *appreciate* the client's situation. Although the health care environment is familiar to you, it is a strange and perhaps frightening situation for your client. Acknowledge his point of view and express concern.

R = The third step is to *respond* to what your client needs. What are his priorities? Expectations for health care?

E = The fourth step is to *empower* the client to problem-solve with you. Here he gains strength and confidence from interactions with providers enabling him to move toward achievement of goals.

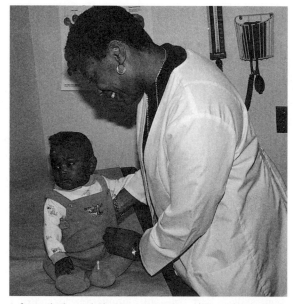

Infants lack verbal communication skills. The nurse's comforting touch and pleasant vocal tone help overcome this barrier. (Courtesy Adam Boggs.)

The ability to become a caring professional is influenced by your previous experiences. A person who has received caring is more likely to be able to offer it to others. Caring should not be confused with caretaking. Although caretaking is a part of caring, it may lack the necessary intentional giving of self. Self-awareness about feelings, attitudes, values, and skills is essential for developing an effective, caring relationship.

STRATEGIES FOR EMPOWERMENT

Your goal is to assist the client to assume more responsibility for their health conditions by teaching them new roles and skills to manage their illnesses (Sullivan, 2008). We may never fully understand the decisions some clients make, but we support their right to do so. Your method for empowering should include the following key strategies:

- *Accept* your clients as they are by refraining from any negative judgments.
- Assess their level of understanding, *exploring their perceptions and feelings* about their conditions and discussing issues that may interfere with self-care.
- Establish mutual goals for client care by forming an alliance, *mutually deciding* about their care.
- Find out how much information your clients want to know.
- Reinforce the client *autonomy,* for example, by allowing them to choose the content in your teaching plan.
- *Offer information* in an environment that enables them to use it.
- Make sure your clients *actively participate* in their care plan.
- Encourage clients to network with a support group.
- Clarify with your clients that they hold the major *responsibility* for both the health care decisions they make and their consequences.

APPLICATION OF EMPATHY TO LEVELS OF NURSING ACTIONS

Nursing actions that facilitate empathy can be classified into three major skills: (a) recognition and classification of requests, (b) attending behaviors, and (c) empathetic responses.

Processing requests: Two types of requests are for information and action. These requests do not involve interpersonal concerns and are easier to manage. Another form of request is for understanding involvement, which entails the client's need for empathetic understanding. This type of request requires greater interpersonal skills. It can be misinterpreted as a request for action or information. The nurse may have to clarify whether the client needs only what he or she specifically asks for, or whether further exploration of the meaning of the need is necessary.

Use attending behaviors: *Attending behaviors* facilitate empathy and include an attentive, open posture; responding to verbal and nonverbal cues through appropriate gestures and facial expressions; using eye contact; and allowing client self-expression. Verbally acknowledging nonverbal cues shows you are attending. As does offering time and attention, showing interest in the client's issues, offering helpful information, and clarifying problem areas. These responses encourage clients to participate in their own healing.

Make empathetic responses: You communicate *empathy* when you show your client that you understand how he is feeling. This helps him identify emotions that are not readily observable and connect them with the current situation. For example, observing nonverbal client cues such as worried facial expression and verbalizing this reaction with an empathetic comment, such as "I understand that this is very difficult for you," validates what your client is feeling and tells him you understand him. Using the actions listed in Table 6-2, the nurse applies attending behaviors and nursing actions to express empathy. Verbal prompts such as "Hmm," "Uh-huh," "I see," "Tell me more," and "Go on" facilitate expression of feelings. The nurse uses open-ended questions to validate perceptions. Using informing behaviors listed in Table 6-2 enlarges the database by providing new information and gives feedback to your client. If your client's condition prevents use of familiar communication strategies to demonstrate empathy, the nurse can use alternative techniques such as touch (refer to Chapter 17).

REDUCTION OF BARRIERS IN NURSE-CLIENT RELATIONSHIPS

Recognition of barriers is the first step in eliminating them, and thus enhancing the therapeutic process. Practice with exercises in this chapter should increase your recognition of possible barriers. Findings from many studies (Evans et al., 2009) emphasize the crucial importance of honesty, cultural sensitivity, and caring, especially in listening actively to suggestions and complaints from client and family. Refer to

TABLE 6-2		Levels of Nursing Actions
Level	**Category**	**Nursing Behavior**
1	Accepting	Uses client's correct name
		Maintains eye contact
		Adopts open posture
		Responds to cues
2	Listening	Nods head
		Smiles
		Encourages responses
		Uses therapeutic silence
3	Clarifying	Asks open-ended questions
		Restates the problem
		Validates perceptions
		Acknowledges confusion
	Informing	Provides honest, complete answers
		Assesses client's knowledge level
		Summarizes
4–5	Analyzing	Identifies unknown emotions
		Interprets underlying meanings
		Confronts conflict

BOX 6-4	Tips to Reduce Relationship Barriers

- Establish trust.
- Demonstrate caring and empathy.
- Empower the client.
- Recognize and reduce client anxiety.
- Maintain appropriate personal distance.
- Practice cultural sensitivity and work to be bilingual.
- Use therapeutic relationship-building activities such as active listening.
- Avoid medical jargon.

Box 6-4 for a summary of strategies to reduce barriers to the nurse-client relationship.

RESPECT FOR PERSONAL SPACE

Before providing care, you need to assess your client's personal space needs. A comprehensive assessment includes cultural and developmental factors that affect perceptions of space and reactions to intrusions. (Discuss Exercise 6-7.) To increase your client's sense of

| EXERCISE 6-7 | Personal Space Differences |

Purpose: To identify individual needs for personal space among different client populations.

Procedure:
Following is a list of factors that affect personal space. Each has a clinical example. Write another example (clinical or personal) for each factor.
1. Culture
   Mrs. Hopi, a Native American who is in the intensive care unit for a heart attack, is surrounded by her family and tribe members throughout her stay in the hospital. Would your family insist on being with you?
2. Sex
   Mr. Smith, a retired steel worker, greets his community health nurse with a smile and a gesture to enter his apartment. His ailing wife greets the nurse with outstretched arms and a kiss. If Mr. Smith greeted you this way, would your response be different?
3. Degree of acquaintance
   The nurse meets Mrs. Parker at the prenatal clinic for the first time. They maintain a distance of 5 feet during the initial interview. How far away would you sit?
4. Situational anxiety
   Mrs. Cook just returned from a brain scan, and she is quite anxious about the results. As the nurse attempts to comfort Mrs. Cook by placing her hand on Mrs. Cook's arm, Mrs. Cook snatches her arm away and retorts, "Just leave me alone."

Discussion:
1. What is your own preferred space distance? To what do you attribute this preference?
2. Under what circumstances do your needs for personal space change?

personal space, you can decrease close, direct eye contact. Instead, sit beside the client or position the chairs at angles for counseling or health teaching. Clients in intensive care units, where there are many intrusive procedures, benefit from decreased eye contact during certain times, such as when being bathed or during suction, wound care, and changing of dressings. At the same time, it is important for you to talk gently with your client during such procedures and to elicit feedback, if appropriate.

To minimize the loss of a sense of personal space, we should demonstrate regard for our client's dignity and privacy. Closed doors for private rest and periods of uninterrupted relaxation are respected. Personal belongings are arranged and treated with care, particularly with very old and very young clients, for whom personal items may be highly significant as a link with a more familiar environment. Elderly clients can become profoundly disoriented in unfamiliar environments because their internal sensory skill in processing new information is often reduced. Encouraging persons in long-term facilities to bring pictures, clothing, and favorite mementos is an important nursing intervention with such clients.

RESPECT FOR PERSONAL SPACE IN HOSPITAL SITUATIONS

Obviously, there is a discrepancy between the minimum amount of space an individual needs and the amount of space hospitals are able to provide in multiple-occupancy rooms. Actions to ensure private space and show respect include:

- Providing privacy when disturbing matters are to be discussed
- Explaining procedures before implementing them
- Entering another person's personal space with warning (e.g., knocking or calling the client's name) and, preferably, waiting for permission to enter
- Providing an identified space for personal belongings
- Encouraging the inclusion of personal and familiar objects on the client's nightstand
- Decreasing direct eye contact during hands-on care
- Minimizing bodily exposure during care
- Using only the necessary number of people during any procedure
- Using touch appropriately

VIOLATIONS OF CONFIDENTIALITY

Discussing private information casually with others is an abuse of confidentiality. Nursing reports and interdisciplinary team case conferences are examples of acceptable forums for the discussion of privileged communication. This information is not discussed outside what is needed for nursing or medical care; to do so would undermine the basis for your therapeutic relationship with your client. Federal confidentiality regulations are discussed in Chapter 2.

AVOIDING CROSS-CULTURAL DISSONANCE

The ANA's statement on cultural diversity in nursing practice highlights the importance of recognizing intracultural variation and assessing each client as an individual (ANA, 1991). Becoming culturally sensitive includes avoiding barriers to communication that occur when generalizing about our client's beliefs based on his membership, rather than taking the time to learn personal preferences. Identify your client's health values, beliefs, health practices, or family factors that may affect his communication with you (Neuhauser & Kreps, 2008).

SUMMARY

This chapter focuses on essential concepts needed to establish and maintain a therapeutic relationship in nursing practice: caring, empowerment, trust, empathy, mutuality, and confidentiality. Respect for the client as a unique person is a basic component of each concept.

Caring is described as a commitment by the nurse that involves profound respect and concern for the unique humanity of every client and a willingness to confirm the client's personhood.

Empowerment is assisting the client to take charge of his or her own health.

Trust represents an individual's emotional reliance on the consistency and continuity of experience. The client perceives the nurse as trustworthy, a safe person with whom to share difficult feelings about health-related needs.

Empathy is the ability to perceive accurately another person's feelings and to convey their meaning to the client. Nursing behaviors that facilitate the development of empathy are accepting, listening, clarifying and informing, and analyzing. Each of these behaviors implicitly recognizes the client as a unique individual worthy of being listened to and respected.

Mutuality includes as much shared communication and collaboration in problem solving as the client is capable of providing. To foster mutuality within the relationship, nurses need to remain aware of their own feelings, attitudes, and beliefs.

Barriers that affect the development of the nurse-client relationship, such as anxiety, stereotyping, overfamiliarity, or intrusion into personal space, are described. High levels of anxiety decrease perceptual ability. The nurse needs to use anxiety- and stress-reduction strategies when clients demonstrate moderate anxiety levels. Stereotypes are generalizations representing an unsubstantiated belief that all individuals of a particular social group, race, or religion share the same characteristics. No allowance is made for individual differences. Developing a nonjudgmental, neutral attitude toward a client helps the nurse reduce clinical bias in nursing practice. Personal space, defined as an invisible boundary around an individual, is another conceptual variable worthy of attention in the nurse-client relationship. The emotional boundary needed for interpersonal comfort changes with different conditions. It is defined by past experiences and culture. Proxemics is the term given to the study of humans' use of space. To minimize a decreased sense of personal space, you demonstrate a regard for your client's dignity and privacy.

ETHICAL DILEMMA What Would You Do?

There are limits to your professional responsibility to maintain confidentiality. Any information that, if withheld, might endanger the life or physical and emotional safety of the client or others needs to be communicated to the health team or appropriate people immediately.

Consider the teen who confides his plan to shoot classmates. Can you breach confidentiality in this case? How about the 5-year-old child in whom you notice genital warts (human papillomavirus) on his anus, but who shows no other signs of sexual abuse?

REFERENCES

American Nurses Association: *Cultural diversity in nursing practice* [position statement], Washington, DC, 1991, Author.

American Nurses Association: *Nursing's social policy statement*, Washington, DC, 1995, Author. Available online: http://nursingworld.org. Accessed November 2004.

Chang M, Kelly AE: Patient education: addressing cultural diversity and health literacy issues, *Urol Nurs* 27(5):411–417, 2007.

Erikson E: *Childhood and society*, ed 2, New York, 1963, Norton.

Evans LR, Boyd EA, Malvar G, et al: Surrogate decision-makers' perspectives on discussing prognosis in the face of uncertainty, *Respiratory & Critical Care Medicine* 179(1):48–53, 2009.

Feldman-Stewart D, Brundage MD: A conceptual framework for patient-provider communication: a tool in the PRO research tool box, *Quality Life Res* 18:109–114, 2008.

Finke EH, Light J, Kitko L: A systematic review of the effectiveness of nurse communication with patients with complex communication needs with a focus on the use of augmentive and alternative communication, *J Clin Nurs* 17(16):2102–2115, 2008.

Gordon HS, Street RL, Sharf BF, et al: Racial differences in doctors' information giving and patients' participation, *Cancer* 107(6):1313–1320, 2006.

Harding T, North N, Perkins R: Sexualizing men's touch: male nurses and the use of intimate touch in clinical practice, *Res Theory for Nurs Pract* 22(2):88–102, 2008.

Healthy People 2010. Health Communication. . . [Chapter 11]. http://web.health.gov/healthypeople/.

Hoglund AT: Holmstrom I: 'It's easier to talk to a woman': aspects of gender in Swedishtelenursing, *J Clin Nurs* 17:2979–2986, 2008.

Jha AK, Orav EJ, Zheng J, Epstein AM: Patients' perceptions of hospital care in the United States, *N Engl J Med* 359(18):1921–1931, 2008.

Kim YM, Heerey M, Kols A: Factors that enable nurse-patient communication in a family planning context: a positive deviance study, *Int J Nurs Stud* 45(10):1411–1421, 2008.

Laschinger HK, Finegan J: Using empowerment to build trust and respect in the workplace: a strategy for addressing the nursing shortage, *Nurs Econ* 23(1):6–13, 2005.

Lautrette A, Darmon M, Megarbane B, et al: A communication strategy and brochure for relatives of patients dying in the ICU, *N Engl J Med* 356(5):459–478, 2007.

Levetown M: American Academy of Pediatrics Committee on Bioethics: Communicating with children and families: from everyday interactions to skill in conveying distressing information, *Pediatrics* 121(5):e1442–e1460, 2008.

Maguire P, Pitceathly C: Key communication skills and how to acquire them, *Br Med J* 325:697–700, 2002.

Morse DS, Edwardson EA, Gordon HS: Missed opportunities for interval empathy in lung cancer communications, *Arch Intern Med* 168(17):1853–1858, 2008.

Neuhauser L, Kreps GL: Online cancer communication: meeting the literacy, cultural and linguistic needs of diverse audiences, *Patient Educ Couns* 71:365–377, 2008.

Ngo-Metzger Q, August KJ, Srinivasan M, Liao S, Meyskens FL: End-of-life care: guidelines for patient-centered communication, *Am Fam Physician* 77(2):167–174, 2008.

Puetz BE: The winning job interview, *Am J Nurs* (Career Guide 2005 Supp):30–32, 2005.

Rask MT, Jensen ML, Andersen J, Zachariae R: Effects of intervention aimed at improving nurse-patient communication in an oncology outpatient clinic, *Cancer Nurs* 32(1):E1–E11, 2009.

Rogers C: *On becoming a person*, Boston, 1961, Houghton-Mifflin.

Sheldon LK, Ellington L: Application of a model of social information processing to nursing theory: how nurses respond to patients, *J Adv Nurs* 64(4):388–398, 2008.

Stewart BD, Payne BK: Bringing automatic stereotyping under control: implementation intensions as efficient means of thought control, *Pers Soc Psychol Bull* 34(10):1332–1345, 2008.

Sullivan CF: Cybersupport: empowering asthma caregivers, *Pediatr Nurs* 34(3):217–224, 2008.

Sutcliffe KM, Leewton E, Rosenthal MM: Communication failures: an insidious contributor to medical mishaps, *Acad Med* 79(2):186–194, 2004.

Teal CR, Street RL: Critical elements of culturally competent communication in the medical encounter: a review and model, *Soc Sci Med* 68(3):533–543, 2009.

Wilkes L, White K, O'Riordan L: Empowerment through information, *Austrian Journal of Rural Health* 8(1):41–46, 2000.

Williams AM, Irurita VF: Therapeutic and non-therapeutic interpersonal interactions: the patient's perspective, *J Clin Nurs* 13(7):806–815, 2004.

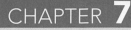

CHAPTER 7

Role Relationship Patterns

Elizabeth C. Arnold

OBJECTIVES

At the end of the chapter, the reader will be able to:

1. Define role as a framework for role performance and role relationships.
2. Discuss the professional roles of the nurse.
3. Describe the components of professional role socialization in professional nursing education.
4. Describe interprofessional education.
5. Discuss professional role development as a registered nurse.
6. Identify factors needed to create supportive work environments for nurses.
7. Discuss professional role relationship behaviors with colleagues.
8. Describe professional role behaviors supporting nurse-client relationships.
9. Discuss the advocacy role in nurse-client relationships.
10. Discuss role performance as a nursing diagnosis.

This chapter explores the concept of role and role relationships in nursing practice from two perspectives: (a) professional nursing role; and (b) role as a functional health pattern, and nursing diagnosis. Key concepts of professional socialization, professional communication, and professional development are addressed.

BASIC CONCEPTS

ROLE

Role is defined as the traditional pattern of behavior and self-expression performed by or expected of an individual within a given society. People develop social and professional roles throughout life. Some are conferred at birth (ascribed roles) and some are attained (acquired roles) during a lifetime. People can have several social roles at the same time (Chaudhary & Sriram, 2001). For example, Marge is a professional nurse, a mother, a wife, a daughter, a lay minister in her church, and president of the parent-teacher association at her children's school. Each role carries different expectations. When the expectations of one role interfere with the discharge of other important life roles, conflict, burnout, or both can occur.

ROLE RELATIONSHIPS

Roles have performance and relationship dimensions that affect how people relate to one another. Social customs and expected professional standards of practice reinforce the performance aspect of role relationships. For example, consider the different professional role expectations of a lawyer, a physician, and a dentist. Each profession has a different set of skills and professional role competencies based on their education and training.

Behavioral expectations in role relationships are reciprocal as role perceptions and expectations influence communication content and delivery. Consider your own "role" as a nursing student and how it has influenced your relationships and communication with clinical instructors, your clients, professional peers, your friends, and other significant people in your life. What do others expect of you, simply because you are now a nursing student?

Roles provide guides for behavior that are in part socially regulated and in part individually determined. Standards for individual role performance reflect personal, social, cultural, gender, institutional, and family expectations. Role relationships are recognizable through membership in a community or through differences in work responsibilities, cooperative activities, education, and social affiliations. Stronger role expectations may be held for people in public roles, for example, elected politicians, ministers, and teachers because of the trust people have in them as a function of their role. Changes in social circumstances such as marriage, widowhood, retirement, job promotions, or birth of a child can alter personal and societal interpretations of individual and professional roles. Exercise 7-1 is designed to help you focus on the complexity of different life roles.

PROFESSIONAL NURSING ROLES

Nursing roles are developed from and linked to the discipline of nursing. The criteria (Box 7-1) for describing a professional discipline, originally developed by Flexner (1915), still hold true today. In their seminal work on nursing as a discipline, Donaldson and Crowley (1978) identify three key themes that distinguish and delimit the discipline of professional nursing:

1. Concern with principles and laws that govern the life processes, well-being, and optimum functioning of human beings

BOX 7-1	Flexner's Criteria of a Professional Role

- Members share a common identity, values, attitudes, and behaviors.
- A distinctive specialized substantial body of knowledge exists.
- Education is extensive, with both theory and practice components.
- Unique service contributions are made to society.
- There is acceptance of personal responsibility in discharging services to the public.
- There is governance and autonomy over policies that govern activities of profession members.
- There is a code of ethics that members acknowledge and incorporate in their actions.

2. Concern with the patterning of human behavior in interaction with the environment in critical life situations
3. Concern with the processes by which positive changes in health status are affected (p. 113)

Willis, Grace, and Roy (2008) identify a similar unifying focus for the discipline related to facilitating meaning, choice, quality of life, humanization, and healing through nursing interventions. The robustness of nursing as a professional discipline is evidenced in the fact that its core descriptors as a discipline are as salient today as they were elegantly described in 1978. Clearly, the nursing role is much more complex than it was in 1978. Evidence for expanded roles is found in the transition of nursing education from the hospital training to increasing levels of educational preparation and practice certifications required of professional nurses. Nursing content and skill sets necessarily change in relation to new and different health

EXERCISE 7-1	Understanding Life Roles

Purpose: To expand students' awareness of the responsibilities, stressors, and rewards of different life roles.

Procedure:
1. Think of all the roles you assume in life.
2. Write a description of the specific responsibilities, stressors, and rewards related to each role.
3. Share some of your roles and their descriptions. (Share only what you feel comfortable revealing.)

Discussion:
As a group, discuss how these different aspects of life roles affect a person's overall functioning.

1. How can this help you to understand your clients better?
2. Discuss what would happen with these roles if you were incapacitated?
3. How might such a situation affect your coping ability?
4. How might it affect others?
5. What roles do you hold in common with other participants in this exercise?
6. What does this exercise suggest about possible role overload or conflict?

care situations; the fundamental essence of nursing as a discipline remains constant.

ROLE BEHAVIORS IN PROFESSIONAL NURSING

Anthony and Landeen (2009) note, "Nursing education has a history of tension and inter-reliance with historical events that encompasses nursing practice, human and social needs, geo- and socio-political processes" (p. 2). At no time in recent history has there been such a complex accumulation of historical events directly and indirectly impacting health care delivery and nursing education. Professional nursing roles have evolved and expanded to reflect the increasing complexities of health care, globalization, changing client demographic characteristics and diversity, and the exponential growth of health information technology (Hegarty, Condon, Walsh, & Sweeney, 2009). With the rapid changes in health care, there is no single role descriptor to explain how professional nursing roles fit in to the health care hierarchy, or will do so in the future. Figure 7-1 identifies the evolving role

competencies required of contemporary nurses, identified by the Institute of Medicine (2003).

Types of Professional Roles

The significance of the professional nurse's role is emphasized in the Joint Commission's first white paper, entitled *Health Care at the Crossroads* (2002), which states, "... in the end, nurses are the primary source of care and support for patients at the most vulnerable points in their lives" (p. 4). Clinical skills related to health promotion, risk reduction, and collaboration with clients and health care providers in primary care are recognized as modern hallmarks of clinical role competence. As providers of care, nurses delegate and supervise related care activities for allied professional staff. Nurses provide leadership and coordination in health care improvement through advocacy and education, and participate in research. Proficiency in biotechnology and health information technology has become an expected competency required of professional nurses (American Association of Colleges of Nursing [AACN], 2008; Gugerty, 2007). Regardless

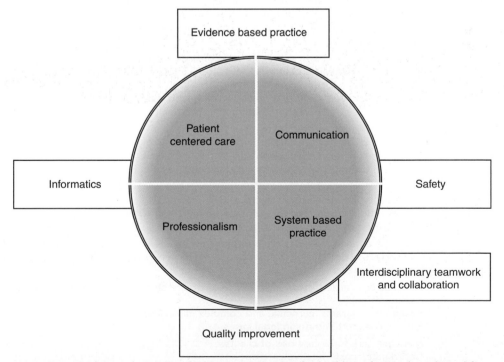

Figure 7-1 **Professional nursing role: core competencies for health professionals.** *Adapted from Institute of Medicine (IOM): Health professions education: a bridge to quality (pp. 45–46). Washington, DC, 2003, National Academies Press, 2003.*

of setting, nurse-client relationships and professional communication provide a primary means through which nurses implement professional roles in providing quality health care and contribute to shaping the health care delivery system.

Table 7-1 identifies the many different types of roles associated with professional nursing practice. Nursing roles are adapted for practice in prisons, schools, home care, shopping malls, and faith-based settings. Nurses provide care individually and as part of multidisciplinary health care teams with the military, during disasters, in the juvenile justice system, with the homeless, in the fields with migrant workers, and in clinics for the uninsured.

Increasingly, nurses are assuming active advocacy roles to inform policy makers, educators, other health care providers and consumers to increase and protect the funding, accessibility, and availability of quality health services. Exercise 7-2 is designed to help you look at the different role responsibilities of practicing nurses.

Advanced Practice Roles

Advanced practice nurses are registered nurses with a baccalaureate degree in nursing and an advanced degree in a selected clinical nursing specialty with relevant clinical experience. Certification and state licensing requirements vary according to state for practice in

TABLE 7-1	Professional Nursing Roles with Associated Responsibilities
Role	**Role Responsibilities**
Caregiver	Uses the nursing process to: a. Provide complete or partial compensatory care for clients who cannot provide these self-care functions for themselves b. Implement supportive/educative actions to promote optimum health c. Reinforce the natural, developmental, and healing processes within a person to enhance well-being, comfort, function, and personal growth
Teacher	Provides health teaching to individual clients and families. Develops and implements patient education programs to promote/maintain healthful practices and compliance with treatment recommendations. Guides individuals in their human journey toward wholeness and well-being through psychoeducation.
Client advocate	Protects client's right to self-determination. Motivates individuals and families to become informed, active participants in their health care. Mediates between client and others in the health care environment. Acts as client's agent in coordinating effective health care services.
Manager	Coordinates staff and productivity. Delegates differentiated tasks to appropriate personnel. Facilitates communication within and among departments. Serves on committees to improve and maintain quality of care. Makes decisions and directs relevant changes to ensure quality care.
Evaluator	Sets quality assurance/care standards. Reviews records and monitors compliance with standards. Makes recommendations for improvement.
Researcher	Develops and implements research/grant proposals to broaden understanding of important issues in clinical practice and validate nursing theories as a basis for effective nursing practice.
Consultant	Provides specialized knowledge/advice to others on health care issues (requires advanced preparation). Evaluates programs, curricula, and complex clinical data. Serves as expert witness in legal cases.
Case manager	Manages care for a caseload of clients. Coordinates cost-effective care options. Monitors client progress toward expected behavioral outcomes. Collaborates with other professionals to ensure quality care across health care settings.

EXERCISE 7-2	Professional Nursing Roles

Purpose: To help students explore different nursing roles.

Procedure:
Conduct an occupational interview with a practicing nurse about the different responsibilities involved in his or her job, the training and credentials required for the position, the client population encountered, the difficult and rewarding aspects of the job, and why the nurse chose a particular area or role in nursing. Write your findings in a short, descriptive summary. Questions you might ask are listed below, but you are also encouraged to create your own explorative questions.
- What made you decide to pursue nursing?
- What kinds of clients do you work with?

- What do you like best about your job?
- What would you do in an average workday?
- What is the most difficult aspect of your job?
- What kinds of preparation or credentials does your position require?
- What is of greatest value to you in your role as a professional nurse?

Discussion:
1. Were you surprised by any of your interviewee's answers? If so, in what ways?
2. What similarities and differences do you see in the results of your interview compared with those of your classmates?
3. In what ways can you use what you learned from doing this exercise in your future professional life?

BOX 7-2	Advanced Practice Roles

Nurse practitioners (NPs) provide first-line health care services across the health-illness continuum in a variety of primary and acute care settings. They may practice either as an independent practitioner or in collaboration with a physician, depending on state laws. NPs can diagnose and treat common medical conditions and injuries, conduct physical examinations and provide preventive care, and medically manage common chronic health problems in the community such as diabetes and high blood pressure. Acute care and specialty NPs (such as neonatal, pediatric, psychiatric, and geriatric NPs) use advanced clinical skills, diagnostic reasoning, and direct skilled management of specialized health care needs. Nurse practitioners can have prescriptive authority in most states, in conjunction with a statutorily mandated written agreement with a designated collaborating physician, approved by the state Board of Nursing.

Certified nurse-midwives provide a wide variety of first-line and clinical management of prenatal and gynecologic care to normal, healthy women. They perform uncomplicated delivery of babies in hospitals, private homes, and birthing centers, and continue with follow-up postpartum care. Certified nurse-midwives also have prescriptive authority under a mandated agreement with a designated collaborating physician, approved by the state Board of Nursing.

Clinical nurse specialists provide care and consultation in a specialty area, such as cardiac, oncology, neonatal, pediatric, obstetric/gynecologic, medical-surgical, or psychiatric nursing. In some states, clinical specialists in psychiatric nursing have limited prescriptive authority. Clinical nurse specialists also perform indirect clinical nursing roles such as staff development, nursing education, administration, and informatics.

Certified registered nurse anesthetists administer anesthesia and conscious sedation in more than one third of the hospitals in the United States.

advanced practice roles. Box 7-2 identifies the four categories of advanced practice nursing in contemporary health care.

Expanded advanced practice roles can include "entrepreneur, recruiter, editor, publisher, ethicist, labor relations expert, nurse anesthetist, lobbyist, [and] culture broker" (Roberson, 1992, p. 4). Many advanced practice nurses (nurse practitioners and some clinical specialists) have prescriptive authority. In addition to clinical roles, advanced practice nurses function in research, educational, and administrative roles. Each expanded role requires specialized competency training to manage care independently in an advanced specialty role. Exercise 7-3 helps you to explore the different specialty areas available for professional nurses in advanced practice.

NURSING EDUCATION AND PROFESSIONAL ROLE PERFORMANCE

The nursing profession has evolved from a primarily apprenticeship model to one with sophisticated educational models and multiple training options. All

| EXERCISE 7-3 | Exploring Advanced Practice Roles in Nursing Practice |

Purpose: To explore different specialty areas in nursing.

Procedure:

1. Select a specialty area about which you have an interest in learning more and obtain the American Nurses Association standards of practice for that specialty.
2. Interview a nurse in that specialty area.

3. Write a summary of your impressions of the practice of nursing in that specialty area, describing aspects that are especially important to you.

Discussion:
Students or student groups can present their summaries and discuss aspects of the specialty area that impress them the most. Do you see common threads across clinical specialties?

registered nurses currently are educationally prepared in colleges and universities, at associate's degree, baccalaureate, master's, and doctoral levels (Erickson & Ditomassi, 2005). Educational career ladders are available for nurses to advance from bedside nurses to advanced practice levels involved with research, clinical expertise, consultation, education, and administration. Hegyvary (2007) asserts that there is no form of self-investment more significant than education for realizing one's full potential as a nurse.

NEW MODELS IN NURSING EDUCATION

In 2003, the American Association of Colleges of Nursing (AACN) introduced two new models of professional education. They were developed in response to expanded clinical roles in nursing practice, the Institute of Medicine's Report on Medical Errors, and to offset nursing faculty shortages. The clinical nurse leader (CNL) role prepares students with a baccalaureate degree in another field to become an advanced nurse generalist. An accelerated generalist nursing curriculum combines baccalaureate and master's level courses, which emphasize clinical leadership skills, and training in health care systems management at the clinical unit level. The CNL "designs, implements, and evaluates client care by coordinating, delegating and supervising the care provided by the health care team, including licensed nurses, technicians, and other health professionals" (AACN, 2003, paragraph 2). Students who satisfactorily complete program requirements are awarded a generic master's degree. Graduates can sit for the NCLEX professional nursing licensing examination and are eligible for certification as a CNL. To practice as an advanced practice nurse in a clinical specialty, the CNL must complete master's-level preparation in an advanced practice specialty.

A second professional role, Doctor of Nursing Practice (DNP), represents a terminal degree in advanced clinical nursing practice. It is designed for nurses who want a clinical rather than research-focused doctorate. The curriculum combines advanced nursing practice competencies with a solid foundation in clinical science, evidence-based practice methods, system leadership, information technology, health policy, and interdisciplinary collaboration (American Association of Colleges of Nursing, AACN, 2004). According to Mundinger (2005), the DNP degree will expand and complement current master's specialty education and roles.

Interprofessional education

The Institute of Medicine (2003), in its landmark report, *Health Professions Education: A Bridge to Quality*, calls for health professionals to develop competencies in working together in interdisciplinary teams. The report identifies "working in interdisciplinary teams" as one of five core competencies needed in today's health care delivery. Promoting interdisciplinary education and providing shared learning opportunities is an important way to develop the respect and integration students need to function in interdisciplinary health care teams.

Interprofessional education is defined as "occasions when two or more professions learn from and about each other to improve collaboration and the quality of care" (Oandasan & Reeves, 2005, p. 24). This does not mean that nursing and other health care professional roles are interchangeable. Nursing, medicine, dentistry, pharmacy and social work are distinct health disciplines that prepare clinicians to assume different practice roles using discipline specific practice standards. Helping students understand the natural interdependence between professions required for today's interdisciplinary care, whereas at the same time recognizing the unique knowledge and skill set of each discipline, is a critical foundation for interprofessional training. Students gain firsthand understanding of the professional values held by other disciplines and collectively identify with important health care issues. In the process of sharing knowledge and experience, students learn the tools of collaborative problem solving (Fronek et al., 2009).

The goal of interprofessional education is to provide students with the knowledge, skills, and attitudes needed to effectively collaborate and improve the quality of health care through interdisciplinary problem solving. Skills to enhance teamwork and to clarify roles in providing client-centered care are important in both discipline-specific and interprofessional learning (Pecukonis, Doyle, & Bliss, 2008).

The impetus for interprofessional education comes from many sources. The Pew Health Professions Commission (1993) recommends revision of health professions curricula to include shared interprofessional learning in academic settings, and the AACN (2008) recently identified "interprofessional communication and collaboration for improving patient health outcomes" (p. 3) as one of nine essential outcomes expected of nursing graduates. The Joint Commission suggests that safe, effective clinical care requires an interdisciplinary collaborative team approach (Walsh, Gordon, Marshall, Wilson, & Hunt, 2005).

Introducing interprofessional courses as part of the basic nursing curriculum helps students articulate their own professional roles, and understand how collaboration and teamwork can more effectively resolve complex issues to enhance clinical outcomes (Margalit, Thompson, Visovsky, et al., 2009). Students can learn trust and respect for each discipline's competencies, and the team building collaborative skills through direct experience with each other's clinical practices. Collaborative interactions modeled by interdisciplinary faculty add to the learning experience.

Learning about Interdisciplinary Collaboration

Rodts and Lamb (2008) state that "any new role requires an understanding of what it is and what it is not" (p. 131). An interdisciplinary, collaborative role is no different. Nursing students must have a solid understanding of their own discipline's specific roles and responsibilities so that they can articulate them clearly to professionals in other disciplines. To maintain nursing's integrity as a profession, the profession must retain control of its knowledge base, skills, and accountability for practice. At the same time, nurses must be willing to work collaboratively with other professionals as part of an interdisciplinary team. Figure 7-1 identifies core competencies needed in today's health care delivery system.

Although interdisciplinary collaboration is still in its infancy as an integral part of professional curriculums, shared elective classes involving interdisciplinary education for two or more disciplines are increasing at the baccalaureate and graduate level (Herbert, 2005). Frequent topics covered in interprofessional electives include ethics, death and dying, emergency preparedness, gerontology, and legal issues. In preparing courses, Aveyard, Edwards, and West (2005) suggest topics need to be "both enhanced by an interdisciplinary approach and not hindered by a lack of detailed attention to field-specific content" (p. 64). As student nurses, you have a unique opportunity to help make the nursing discipline visible as a key player and carve out nursing's role in the evolution of interdisciplinary collaboration as a primary care strategy.

NURSING VALUES AND ROLE SOCIALIZATION

Although the core values and fundamental features of professional nursing remain constant, the scope of practice and implementation of associated professional nursing roles continues to evolve as we enter the 21st century.

PROFESSIONAL ROLE SOCIALIZATION
Essential Values and Professional Behaviors
The AACN (1986) first published examples of the essential values, attitudes, personal qualities, and professional behaviors associated with the profession of nursing and later refined them in 2008 (see Table 7-2). Key elements of the professional nursing role include the acquisition, development, and integration of health-related psychomotor, social, and cognitive skills, and the achievement of a sense of self as a professional nurse within an ethical, competency-based framework.

Role socialization refers to the process through which a student nurse learns the professional norms, values, and skills associated with the professional nursing role, and acquires identity features of the

TABLE 7-2	**Values and Qualities of Professionalism in Nursing**	
Essential Values	**Examples of Attitudes and Personal Qualities**	**Examples of Professional Behaviors**
1. Altruism Concern for the welfare and well-being of others	Caring Commitment Compassion Generosity Perseverance	Demonstrates understanding of cultures, beliefs, and perspectives of others Advocates for clients, particularly the most vulnerable Takes risks on behalf of clients and colleagues Mentors other professionals
2. Autonomy Right to self-determination Capacity to exercise choice	Confidence Hope Independence Openness Self-direction Self-discipline	Plans care in partnership with clients Honors the right of patients and families to make decisions about health care Provides information so patients can make informed choices
3. Human dignity Respect for the inherent worth and uniqueness of individuals and populations	Consideration Empathy Humaneness Kindness Respectfulness Trust	Safeguards the individual's right to privacy Addresses individuals as they prefer to be addressed Maintains confidentiality of clients and staff Treats others with respect regardless of background or personal characteristics Shows respect for colleagues Designs and provides culturally competent care
4. Social justice Uses moral and legal principles to promote fair treatment	Courage Objectivity Acceptance Assertiveness Fairness Self-esteem	Acts as a health care advocate to encourage legislative policies favorable to quality health care Allocates resources fairly Treats all clients fairly regardless of background or personal characteristics Interacts with other providers in a nondiscriminatory manner
5. Integrity Faithfulness to fact or reality	Accountability Honesty Inquisitiveness Rationality Reflectiveness	Documents nursing care accurately and honestly Incorporates the American Nurses Association Code of Ethics in care provision and demonstrates accountability for actions Seeks to remedy errors made by self or others Participates in professional efforts to protect the public from misinformation about nursing

Adapted from American Association of College and University Education for Professional Nursing: *Final report*, Washington, DC, 1986, American Association of Colleges of Nursing; and American Association of Colleges of Nursing: *Essentials of baccalaureate nursing education for professional nursing practice* (pp. 27–28), Washington, DC, 2008, Author.

profession. It is an interactive developmental process that starts when students enter a nursing program and begin to learn the "pure" form of nursing knowledge. Initially, nursing students are absorbed in learning the basic knowledge required of the professional role. They are dependent on textbooks and their instructor to help them find the one "right answer" to health care problems. As students become comfortable with foundational nursing knowledge, they begin to consider multiple options as they integrate professional judgment into clinical care planning. Students are able to apply scientific knowledge to practice in a realistic manner and "to relate new material to their previous knowledge base" (Cohen, 1981, p. 18).

The next phase involves internalizing the culture, that is, the values, standards, and role behaviors associated with professional nursing. Pecukonis, Doyle, and Bliss (2008) note that "each discipline possesses its own professional culture that shapes the educational experience; determines curriculum content, core values, dress, salience of symbols" (p. 417). Student nurses are accountable for presenting themselves as professionals to other health providers and the public. For example, professional appearance is important. Although a common dress code for professional nurses is "scrubs," attire should be neat, clean, and properly fitted. The professional "image" of the nurse is an unspoken factor in how others perceive the profession.

Nursing faculty and clinical preceptors serve as important socializing agents, helping students learn the values, traditions, norms, and competencies of the nursing profession (Neil et al., 1998). A clinical preceptor is an experienced nurse, chosen for clinical competence and charged with supporting, guiding, and participating in the evaluation of student clinical competence (Paton, Thompson-Isherwood, & Thirsk, 2009). Clients/families, mentors, and peers serve as informal socializing agents in ways that can contribute to a student's understanding of the professional nursing role. As preceptors, other nurses and clinical faculty model desirable nursing role behaviors; students begin to identify with them and learn the normative expectations associated with the professional nursing role.

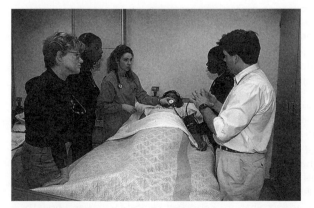

Nurses learn behavioral standards from instructors, nursing staff, and other students.

The last phase of the socialization process focuses on an internalization of professional norms and values as an integral part of self. With increasing clinical experience, nursing students become self-directed and committed to the role of professional nurse.

PROFESSIONAL ROLE DEVELOPMENT AS A REGISTERED NURSE

Professional role development does not end with graduation and licensure as a registered nurse. After graduation, standard means of continued professional development include continuing education, staff development, conference attendance, academic education, specialized training, and research activities. Professional learning occurs through informal means such as consultation, professional reading, experiential learning, giving presentations, and self-directed activities. At advanced practice levels, nurses are required to complete a certain level of continuing education activities within designated time frames to maintain their specialty certification.

From Novice to Expert: Process of Skill Acquisition

Patricia Benner (1984, 2000; Norman, 2008) describes five developmental stages of increasing proficiency associated with the professional nursing role: novice, advanced beginner, competence, proficiency, and expert. The first developmental stage is referred to as the *novice stage*. With limited nursing experience, novice nurses need structure and tend to compare clinical findings with the textbook picture because they lack the practice experience to do otherwise. Theoretical knowledge and confidence in the expertise of more practiced nurses serve as guides to practice. Veteran nurses can re-experience the novice stage any time that nurse makes a career change and enters a new clinical area or specialty, never having had experience with a particular client population (Thomas, 2003).

In stage 2, the advanced beginner stage, nurses understand the basic elements of practice and can organize and prioritize clinical tasks. Although clinical analysis of health care situations occurs at a higher level than strict association with the textbook picture, the advanced beginner is only able to partially grasp the unique complexity of each client's situation.

Stage 3, the competence stage, occurs 1 to 2 years into nursing practice. The competent nurse is able to easily "manage the many contingencies of clinical nursing" (Benner, 1984, p. 27). Nurses in this stage begin to practice the "art" of nursing. The nurse views the clinical picture from a broader perspective and is more confident about his or her role in health care.

Stage 4, the proficiency stage, occurs 3 to 5 years into practice. Nurses in this stage are self-confident about their clinical skills and perform them with competence, speed, and flexibility. The proficient nurse sees the clinical situation as a whole, has well-developed psychosocial skills, and knows from experience what needs to be modified in response to a given situation (Benner, 1984). Stage 5, expert, is marked by a high level of clinical skill and the capacity to respond authentically and creatively to client needs and concerns. Expert nurses can recognize the unexpected and work with it creatively. They demonstrate mastery of technology, sensitivity in interpersonal relationships, and specialized nursing skills in all aspects of their caregiving. Being an expert nurse is not an end point; nurses have the professional and ethical responsibility to continuously upgrade and refine their clinical skills through professional development and clinical skill training. Table 7-3 identifies behaviors associated with different levels of Benner's model (Norman, 2008).

Mentoring. Expert or seasoned nurses often serve as mentors for their less-experienced colleagues. Mentoring is defined as a special type of professional relationship in which an experienced nurse or clinician (mentor) assumes a role responsibility for guiding the professional growth and advancement of a less-experienced person (protégé). Yonge, Billay, Myrick, and Luhanga (2007) make several distinctions between mentorship and preceptorship. A mentoring relationship can last over several months or years, whereas the assigned relationship between a preceptor and less experienced nurse is a short-term relationship with a defined end date focused on clinical teaching and role modeling. The mentor relationship is broader and more personal. Nurses choose a mentor rather than having one assigned.

Each mentoring experience is unique because of the people and situations involved. Excellent mentors demonstrate role expertise and model the highest levels of personal professionalism. They share values

TABLE 7-3	Benner's Stages of Clinical Competence
Nurse Competency Level	**Description of Behaviors**
Advanced Beginner	• Enters clinical situations with some apprehension • Sees task requirements as central to the clinical context, whereas other aspects of the situation are seen as background • Requires knowledge application to meet clinical realities • Perceives each clinical situation as a personal challenge • Are typically dependent on standards of care, unit procedures
Competent	• Focuses more on clinical issues in contrast to tasks • Can handle familiar situations • Expects certain clinical trajectories on the basis of the experience with particular patients • Searches for broader explanations of clinical situations • Has enhanced organizational ability, technical skills • Focuses on managing patients' conditions
Competent Proficient	• Responds to particulars of clinical situations in a broader way • Requires an experiential base with past patient populations • Understands patient transitions over time • Learns to gauge involvement with patients/families to promote appropriate caring
Expert	• Has increased intuition regarding what are important clinical factors and how to respond to these • Engages in practical reasoning • Anticipates and prepares for situations while remaining open to changes • Performs care in "fluid, almost seamless" manner • Bonds emotionally with patients/families depending on their needs • Sees the big picture, including the unexpected • Works both with and through others

From Norman V: Uncovering and recognizing nurse caring from clinical narratives, *Holistic Nursing Practice* 22(6):324, 2008, by permission.

and tips for success, and provide support, structure, and challenges to the mentee or protégé. In many instances, they help facilitate contacts with significant people. Benefits to the mentor include satisfaction in seeing the achievements of the mentee and expansion of clinical excellence through interacting others. Hoffman, Harris, and Rosenfield (2008) suggest that mentoring of students in interprofessional education should contain the following elements:

- Engagement in students' own values
- Guidance reflecting principles of self-directed learning
- Creation of awareness for opportunities that facilitate self-discovery and maturation (p. 103)

Networking. Networking is an essential component of personal role development, and ultimately of advancing the status of professional nursing roles in health care delivery systems. Professional networking is defined as "establishing and using contacts for information, support, and other assistance in order to achieve career goals" (Puetz, 2007, p. 577). Nurses can use networking when they are in the market for a new job, need a referral, want to receive or share information about an area of interest, or need assistance with making a career choice. For example, if you want to write an article, you might want to discuss your ideas and get guidance from someone who is published.

Networking contacts can be with peers from as close as the nursing unit on the floor below, or people you meet at an international professional conference. Participating in activities of nursing organizations or continuing education events provides fertile opportunities for networking. Having business cards with you and following up with a thank-you e-mail or note is helpful.

Networking can offer professional opportunities for developing new ideas and receiving feedback that might not otherwise be available. Through networking contacts, nurses can communicate their expertise and share their ideas while gathering information from their contacts. This give and take of information is often the bridge to developing or strengthening collaborative relationships with others in the field. For example, extensive networking among oncology nurses was the impetus for the formation of the Oncology Nursing Society. Networking is closely associated with coordination and collaboration activities, and is destined to become increasingly important in determining the future impact of advanced practice nursing.

Developing an Evidence-Based Practice

Foley BJ, Minick P, Kee C: Nursing advocacy during a military operation, Western Journal of *Nursing Research* 22(4):492–507, 2000.

This qualitative phenomenologic study was designed to explore the advocacy role experiences of military nurses and to provide a rich description of the common meanings of their advocacy practices. A purposive sample of 24 military nurses was interviewed and data analysis completed using a constant comparison methodology.

Results: Themes revealed one constitutive pattern associated with the concept of advocacy, namely, safeguarding, with four related themes described as being the patient's voice, protecting, attending the whole person, and preserving the patient's personhood. A recommendation from this study is the need to coach nurses in how to relate to other members of the health team as the patient's advocate.

Application to Your Clinical Practice: As a profession, nurses need to develop research evidence and implement relevant study findings to advocate for the health and well-being of their clients. What themes do you associate with client advocacy in your clinical setting? Would these themes be the same or different in a community setting?

APPLICATIONS

PROFESSIONAL ROLE BEHAVIORS WITH COLLEAGUES

Developing productive role relationships with other professionals does not just happen. Professional role behaviors and strong relationships with nursing and other professional colleagues include full acceptance of one's fair share of the workload. Masters (2005) asserts that if nurses are to engage in interprofessional work relationships, they must be able to clearly articulate professional nursing values. Development of supportive, dependable relationships with coworkers—with those you dislike as well as with those you can work with easily—is essential. Maintaining zero tolerance for gossip and criticism helps establish you as a professional with ethical integrity and worthy of trust.

Respecting the views of other disciplines and communicating in an organized, thoughtful manner has an impact on how practitioners from other disciplines perceive the nurse's role and value as competent health care professionals. Using critical thinking, focused communication skills, and professional behaviors in interactions with professional colleagues is just as important as it is with clients and their families.

How nurses present their ideas in writing and speaking is critical. If you use e-mails to communicate, remember that your e-mail is a reflection of you as a professional person. Use complete, well-thought-out sentences, and check punctuation, grammar, and spelling. Likewise, voice-mail messages should be professional in content and delivery.

VERBAL COMMUNICATION WITH PROFESSIONAL COLLEAGUES

When communicating with professional colleagues, it is important to remain sensitive to the tasks at hand, and to develop an understanding of how the work of different disciplines affects the nurse's work and contributes to overall treatment goals. Collaboration in joint decision making and coordination of care with colleagues requires knowing when to hold and when to let go of ideas and opinions. Most of the time, decisions are not either/or processes, but it is easy to lose sight of alternative options. Placing issues in order of priority is a useful organizing strategy for assessing, defining, and clarifying problems. Persistence and a good sense of humor are essential characteristics of honest interpersonal relationships with professional peers.

E-mail or memos can provide quick routine information that does not require discussion. Face-to-face interaction or telephone conversations are preferred for communicating in the professional environment about difficult or emotional issues that could be misinterpreted. Serving as an informed resource to other providers helps build rapport and encourages others to work with you to achieve relevant treatment and organizational goals.

SELF-AWARENESS

Self-awareness is an essential aspect of effective professional relationships with colleagues and a necessary antecedent to the full development of the professional role in nursing. Malloch and Porter-O'Grady (2005) assert that "knowing from the internal self what needs to be done and living those beliefs and values in the real world marks the leader's journey" (p. 101).

Professional self-awareness promotes recognition of the need for continuing education, the acceptance of accountability for one's own actions, the capacity to be assertive with professional colleagues, and the capability of serving as a client advocate when the situation warrants it, even if it is uncomfortable to do so. Exercises 7-4 and 7-5 are designed to help you explore the use of personal strengths in professional role development.

PROFESSIONAL RIGHTS

All health professionals, including nurses, have rights as well as significant responsibilities in interprofessional relationships with colleagues. Box 7-3 lists the American Nurses Association (2002) Bill of Rights for Registered Nurses. Rights carry with them corresponding responsibilities. Think about your professional collegial relationships and your dual professional commitment to self and others. Think about the professional values identified in this textbook, and reexamine the components of professionalism. Each of those components is basically a professional responsibility. Add your ideas for rights next to those responsibilities. Exchange ideas about professional rights and responsibilities with others.

EXERCISE 7-4	Incorporating Personal Strengths in Role Development

Purpose: To help highlight the use of personal strengths as skills or assets in role development.

Procedure:
1. Pair up with another student.
2. Share a personal strength that you have observed about your assigned partner related to implementation of the professional nursing role and describe the behavior that supports your assessment. (Examples might be persistence, sense of humor, balanced approach, energetic, thoughtful, caring, inquisitive, take charge, laid-back, etc.)

Discussion:
1. Discuss how personal strengths can be used to enhance the professional role.
2. Compare and contrast what different students envisioned as personal strengths.
3. Did doing this exercise help you to learn something about the value of personal strengths?
4. Did anything surprise you about doing this exercise?
5. How can you use this information in your own role development?

EXERCISE 7-5	Looking at My Development as a Professional Nurse

Purpose: To help students focus on their self-development as professional nurses.

Procedure:
Write the story of how you chose to become a nurse in a one- or two-page essay (may be done as a homework assignment). There are no right or wrong answers; this is simply your story. You may use the following questions as guides in developing your story.
1. What are your reasons for choosing nursing as a profession?
2. What factors influenced your decision (e.g., people, circumstances, or situations)?
3. What does being a nurse mean to you?
4. What fears do you have about your ability to function as a professional nurse?

5. How do you think being a nurse will affect your personal life?
6. What type of nursing do you want to pursue?

Discussion:
1. In what ways is your story similar to or different from those of your classmates?
2. As you wrote your story, were you surprised by any of the data or feelings?
3. Students can discuss some of the realistic difficulties encountered as nursing students, both professionally and personally, and ways to handle them. Through discussion, explore the following:
   a. The practices nursing students will need to follow to achieve their vision
   b. The types of supports nurses need to foster their ongoing professional development

BOX 7-3	The American Nurses Association's Bill of Rights for Registered Nurses

- Nurses have the right to practice in a manner that fulfills their obligations to society and to those who receive nursing care.
- Nurses have the right to practice in environments that allow them to act in accordance with professional standards and legally authorized scopes of practice.
- Nurses have the right to a work environment that supports and facilitates ethical practice, in accordance with the Code of Ethics for Nurses and its interpretive statements.

- Nurses have the right to freely and openly advocate for themselves and their patients, without fear of retribution.
- Nurses have the right to fair compensation for their work, consistent with their knowledge, experience, and professional responsibilities.
- Nurses have the right to a work environment that is safe for themselves and their patients.
- Nurses have the right to negotiate the conditions of their employment, either as individuals or collectively, in all practice settings.

Reprinted from American Nurses Association: Know your rights: ANA's Bill of Rights arms nurses with critical information. *American Nurse* 34(6), 16, 2002, by permission.

CREATING SUPPORTIVE WORK ENVIRONMENTS

A responsive work environment that values nurses and is committed to quality client-centered care attracts nurses and improves clinical outcomes for clients. Likewise, nurses who are enthusiastic, competent, dependable, adaptable, and responsible are key variables in creating a satisfying, quality work environment. In a study of what types of environmental support create satisfaction for professional nurses, Kramer and Schmalenberg (2002) uncovered the following factors chosen by the majority of the nurses surveyed:

- Working with other nurses who are clinically competent

- Good nurse-physician relationships and communication
- Nurse autonomy and accountability
- Supportive nurse manager-supervisor
- Control over nursing practice and practice environment
- Support for education (in-service, continuing education, etc.)
- Adequate nurse staffing
- Paramount concern for the patient

In an effort to develop and support work environments favorable to nurses, the American Nurses Association, through its American Nurses Credentialing Center (ANCC), developed the Magnet Recognition Program in 1993. Over the years, magnet recognition has become "the global standard for excellence in nursing practice" (Morgan, 2009, p. 105).

MAGNET RECOGNITION

The **magnet recognition program** recognizes nursing excellence in health care institutions and agencies, and identifies them as work environments that act as a "magnet" for professional nurses desiring to work there because of the institutions' excellence (American Nurses Credentialing Center [ANCC] 2004). In 2008, the magnet model was redesigned to include five interactive elements known to support excellence in nursing practice work environments (see Figure 7-2). Characteristics of a magnet culture include:

- Active support of education
- Clinically competent nurses
- Positive interdisciplinary professional relationships
- Control over and autonomy in nursing practice
- Client-centered care for clients and families
- Adequate staffing and nurse-manager support (ANCC, 2006).

A magnet health care facility is characterized as one in which nurses have a high level of job satisfaction and lower staff nurse turnover, exemplary professional practice, and demonstrate commitment at every nursing level to effective, efficient, quality care (American Nurses Credentialing Center). Nurses in a magnet work environment are valued and have a strong

voice in decision making about care delivery. They are encouraged and rewarded for involvement in shaping research-based nursing practice. Staffing ratios are viewed as appropriate, and the hospital demonstrates excellent treatment outcomes and client satisfaction. Communication among health professionals is open, and there is an appropriate mix of health care personnel to ensure quality care. Exercise 7-6 can help you think about how you would see yourself in the professional nursing role in the future.

BECOMING KEY PLAYERS IN A GLOBAL HEALTH CARE ARENA

Malloch and Porter-O'Grady (2005) suggest that we are living in an information-based societal infrastructure that is primarily relational and that functions horizontally in a global world without boundaries. Professional nursing requires an expanded set of skill competencies in the 21st century, as presented in Table 7-4.

Making the role of the professional nurse visible in the 21st century is a task that nurses must undertake to strengthen the public's recognition of the nursing profession in an interdisciplinary health care delivery system. Although nurses are the largest professional group in the health care workforce (Hassmiller & Cozine, 2006), their role is not as visible as it

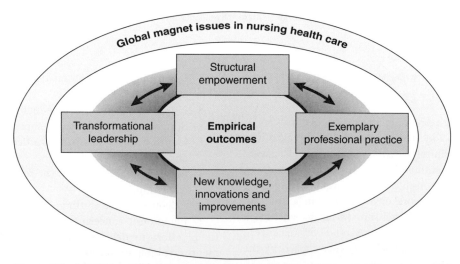

Figure 7-2   **Magnet model components.** *(Developed from Morgan S: The magnet (TM) model as a framework for excellence,* Journal of Nursing Care Quality *24(2):105–108, 2009 (p. 106).*

EXERCISE 7-6	Envisioning the Future

Purpose: To help students think about the nursing role they would like to aspire to in the future. Envisioning the future helps nurses to develop focused career goals.

Procedure:
1. Envision your career 5 years after graduation.
2. Write a detailed narrative of what you would be doing and what your career would be like as you might describe it to a classmate at your 5-year reunion.
3. Have one student take the role of the storyteller and the other the role of the classmate at the reunion. The person taking the role of the classmate should ask questions to clarify any aspects of the speaker's career vision that are not clear.
4. Reverse positions and repeat.

Discussion:
1. How difficult was it for you to think about what you want to do in the future?
2. What steps will you have to take to achieve your goal?
3. How will you go about finding out more about the career path you see yourself taking?

TABLE 7-4	Old versus New Skill Sets for Professional Nurses in the 21st Century

Employee	Knowledge Worker
Functional analysis	Conceptual synthesis
Manual dexterity	Competent integrated care
Fixed skill set	Mobile skill set
Process, value-based practice	Outcome-based practice
Individual practice	Interdisciplinary team performance

Modified from Mallach K, Porter-O'Grady T: A new vessel for leadership: new rules for a new age. In *The quantum leader: applications for the new world of work,* Sudbury, MA, 2005, Jones and Bartlett.

should be. Neither physicians nor nurses seem to fully appreciate the depth of the nurse's contribution to health care delivery (Coombs, 2004). In some ways, the work of the nurse is invisible until a crisis such as the nursing shortage brings the work of nurses to the forefront of people's attention. Individual nurses and nursing organizations need to work together to strengthen the professional nursing role.

In addition to defining our professional roles in ways that are understandable, nurses need to project a positive activist image of the professional nursing role within their communities by

- Developing partnerships with clients, health care professionals, policy makers, and community agencies in the care of vulnerable populations
- Reflecting on and documenting what nurses do and the broad scope of services they provide for the public

- Participating as members of interdisciplinary teams and multidisciplinary groups with defined expertise as nurses to address significant health care issues from a nursing perspective
- Maintaining competence and acting in a professional manner
- Advocating for systems of care that provide adequate accessible health care for all people
- Developing and participating in continuing education programs to ensure continued competence as a professional nurse
- Promoting the public and professional understanding of the professional nursing role
- Contributing to ethical discussions that support principled practices in clinical settings

PROFESSIONAL ROLE BEHAVIORS IN NURSE-CLIENT RELATIONSHIPS

A nurse's first professional role responsibility is to the client. Acting in a professional manner at all times is essential to maintaining the integrity of nursing as a profession. Expected professional role behaviors in nurse-client relationships emphasize the following qualities:

- An ability to view clients as individual, holistic beings
- Respect for the basic human dignity of all clients, regardless of differences from oneself
- An attitude of cultural openness and tolerance for divergent ways of thinking
- Sensitivity to individual clients' ability to access health care and adhere to prescribed regimens
- An understanding of the impact that illness and/or disability may have on clients
- Adherence to nursing standards of care

- Use of research evidence to improve nursing practice (Masters, 2005, pp. 156–157)

Role relationships with a client can affect the quality of nursing care in the nurse-client relationship when the worth of the client as a person, for example, is judged on the basis of socioeconomic status, level of education, ethnicity, health state, or level of consciousness. Perceptions of role relationships can affect effective treatment decision making. For example, roles become important when questioning a health care provider's professional judgment is not considered an appropriate behavior in the client's culture, or when the family, rather than the client, is culturally expected to make important health care decisions.

Professional performance behaviors in the nurse-client relationship include much more than simple caring; they require a sound knowledge base, as well as specific technical and interpersonal competencies. On a daily basis, nurses must collect and process multiple, often indistinct pieces of behavioral data. Nurses work creatively with clients and families to come up with workable solutions that are realistic and in tune with the client's beliefs, values, and preferences. Through words and behaviors in relationship with other health care providers and agencies, nurses consistently serve as advocates for their clients and family members.

Today's nurse functions in a high-tech, managed health care environment in which the human caring aspects of nursing are easier to overlook. Unique challenges to the nurse-client relationship include shorter client contacts, decreased continuity, technology, and lower levels of trust in relation to these factors. Yet, the nurse-client relationship will become increasingly important in helping clients feel cared for in a health care environment that sometimes neglects the psychosocial needs of clients in favor of cost-effectiveness and efficient use of time.

Case Example

Marilyn describes her experience with her husband's nurse:

"It was truly amazing. Whenever she came into the room, she always washed her hands, while asking me how the day had gone, and how I was doing. She made direct eye contact, and seemed genuinely interested in hearing from me directly about the day's events, rather than simply reading the chart. It was such a simple thing, but it made all the difference." (O'Connell, 2009)

In today's health care environment, clients are expected to take an active role in self-management of their condition to whatever extent is possible. The expectation is for an equal partnership, with clients having shared power and authority as joint decision makers in their health care. With a client-centered model of health care delivery, the client's thoughts, concerns, and questions are welcomed and encouraged. Every decision related to the client's diagnosis and treatment should be a shared determination made with the medical team based on combined input and joint responsibility for implementing the recommendations. This use of the client's self-knowledge and inner resources allows nurses to more effectively respond to client needs.

Client Rights and Responsibilities

The American Hospital Association (AHA, 2003) has developed a brochure outlining the rights and responsibilities of patient care partnership in lieu of its former Patient's Bill of Rights. It is accessible in multiple languages on the AHA Web site. Hospitals today have copies of comprehensive patient rights posted on their Web site. Written copies are given to clients on admission. A sample listing of common patient rights and responsibilities is provided in Box 7-4.

ADVOCACY ROLES IN THE NURSE-CLIENT RELATIONSHIP

Merriam-Webster's Dictionary (2009) defines advocate as "one that pleads the cause of another; one that supports or promotes the interests of another." Nurses are advocates for clients every time they protect, defend, and support a client's rights, and/or intervene on behalf of clients who cannot do so for themselves. The ANA (2001) affirms advocacy as an essential role in its Code of Ethics for Nurses, stating, "The nurse promotes, advocates for, and strives to protect the health, safety and rights of the patient."

Clients who benefit from advocacy fall into two categories: those who need advocacy because of vulnerability caused by their illness, and those who have trouble successfully navigating the health care system. Nursing actions that constitute client advocacy include facilitating access to essential health care services for clients, ensuring quality care, protecting client rights, and acting as a liaison between clients and the health care system to procure quality care.

BOX 7-4	Patient Rights and Responsibilities

All clients have the following rights:

- Impartial access to the most appropriate treatment regardless of race, age, sexual preference, national origin, religion, handicap, or source of payment for care
- To be treated with respect, dignity, and personal privacy in a safe, secure environment
- Confidential treatment of all communication and other records related to care or payment, except as required by law or signed insurance contractual arrangements (all clients should receive Notice of Privacy Practices)
- Active participation in all aspects of decision making regarding personal health care
- To know the identity and professional status of each health care provider
- To have treatments and procedures explained to them in ways they can understand
- To receive competent interpreter services, if required to understand care or treatment

- To refuse treatment, including life-saving treatment, after being told of the potential risks associated with such refusal
- To receive appropriate pain management
- To express grievances regarding any violation of patient rights internally and/or to the appropriate agency

All clients have the following responsibilities:
- To treat their care providers with respect and courtesy, including timely notification for appointment cancellations
- To provide accurate, complete information about all personal health matters
- To follow recommended treatment plans
- To assume responsibility for personal actions, if choosing to refuse treatment
- To follow hospital regulations regarding safety and conduct

Sources: The patient care partnership: rights and responsibilities. Available at: http://www.aha.org/aha/issues/Communicating-With-Patients/pt-care-partnership.html. and President's Advisory Commission on Consumer Protection and quality in the health care industry (1997). Available at: www.hcqualitycommission.gov/final/append_a.html.

A key means of employing client advocacy is the nurse-client relationship (Negarandeh, Oskouie, Fhmadi, Nikravesh, & Hallberg, 2006). Within the relationship, nurses listen carefully to clients, help them foresee potential difficulties, answer questions honestly, and apply the clinical knowledge and skills identified in Box 7-5 for the benefit of the client.

The goal of advocacy support is to empower clients and to help them attain the services they need for self-management of health issues. Examples of individuals needing advocacy include survivors of domestic violence, chronically mentally ill clients, pregnant teenagers, the homeless, frail elders—in fact, virtually anyone unable to act cogently on their own behalf. As health care services in the public sector become scarcer because of economic considerations, advocacy becomes an even greater emphasis. Several authors (Welchman and Griener, 2005; Mahlin, 2010) argue that nursing's professional organizations need to take up the gauntlet to collectively advocate for resolution of systemic client care issues in health care settings. For more information on nurse involvement in advocacy at the community level, see Chapter 24.

BOX 7-5	Knowledge Base Needed for Client Advocacy

- Knowledge of the client's values, beliefs, and preferences, and alignment with treatment goals
- Knowledge of informed consent procedures, current third-party payment policies, institutional policies
- Awareness of one's own personal, professional, and cultural biases, and the ways they might impact client advocacy
- Awareness of potential power or recognition needs that could compromise the integrity of the client advocacy process
- Knowledge of print materials and online resources relevant to the client's needs

- Knowledge of organizational system variables related to service delivery
- Knowledge of current laws, policies, and regulations that affect service delivery
- Knowledge of community resources including referral processes, eligibility and access requirements
- Effective communication strategies for consultation and collaboration needed for advocacy of the client's issues
- Knowledge of required documentation, management, and interpretation of client records needed for effective advocacy

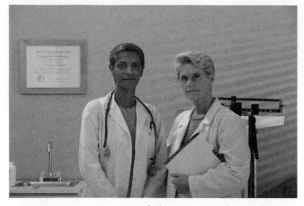

An important component of the nurse's role is advocacy for clients.

Advocacy should support client autonomy. Zomorodi and Foley (2009) note the importance of differentiating advocacy strategies from paternalism in which the nurse decides what is best for the client. Clients need to be in control of their own destiny, even when the decision reached is not what you as the nurse would recommend for the client's health and well-being. You need to recognize when to speak for the client and when to encourage the client to speak up. In general, encouraging clients to take responsibility to speak on their own behalf is more effective.

To be effective, the nurse's advocacy efforts should be systematically implemented and related to client identified needs, beliefs and values, and preferences. Questions you might ask include: (a) What does the client believe is the most pressing problem? (b) What supports (e.g., family, minister, rabbi, social services) are in place? (c) What health or social services is the client familiar with or resistant to considering? A client's sense of powerlessness can decrease when the answers to these questions become the starting points for developing realistic solutions to difficult problems. When advocacy efforts include referrals to community resources, factors to be considered include compatibility with the client's expressed need, financial resources, accessibility (time as well as place), and ease of contact.

Client advocacy sometimes provides a connective link between ethics and the law. Nurses must be willing and able to take a stand in situations involving poor medical management of a client. This is not easy, when risk to employment or possibility of censure is associated with this form of client advocacy.

On the other hand, being too cautious or having misplaced loyalties to colleagues that interfere with appropriate protective advocacy can become a legal as well as an ethical issue. Sometimes, the only person willing to defend or promote the cause of the client is the nurse.

In the following case example, a client admitted to postanesthesia care unit (PACU) suddenly had a significant change in his vital signs. The nurse called the operating room (OR), but the surgeon was scrubbing for the next operation and said he would call her later.

Case Example

The PACU nurse said to tell the surgeon that he needed to break scrub and come to PACU immediately to check his patient. So he quickly came. When he checked the patient, he asked for OR to bring a tray so that he could open the incision to take a quick look and let it drain. "No," the PACU nurse responded. "You need to take her back to the OR, where anesthesia can keep watch on her airway." As the patient returned to the PACU, the surgeon approached the PACU nurse and thanked her for her assertiveness on behalf of the patient (Odom, 2002, p. 76).

Exercise 7-7 provides a clinical situation in which the nurse's advocacy role is in conflict with traditional nursing and medical advice. Sometimes the nurse serves as dual advocate for the client and a family member. For example, in a child abuse situation, nurses act as an advocate of the child by taking the steps necessary to provide a protective and safe environment for the child, including reporting abuse situations. The same nurse can be an advocate for the parents by referring them to appropriate community resources and helping them develop more productive methods for coping with situational stressors.

ROLE PERFORMANCE AS A NURSING DIAGNOSIS

Role performance disturbance has been designated by NANDA (2009) as a nursing diagnosis. *Healthy People 2010* identifies quality of life as a priority goal. Quality of life and role performance are interconnected. How effectively a person is able to function within expected roles influences his or her reputation within society and affects his or her sense of self-esteem. That role relationships and performance matter to people as essential elements of their well-being is evidenced in the emergence of symptoms of depression, feelings of

| EXERCISE 7-7 | Client Advocate Role-play |

Purpose: To understand the nurse advocacy role in difficult and conflict-filled clinical situations.

Procedure:
1. Read the following clinical situation and answer the questions in writing.
2. Have one student play the role of the client and another play the role of the nurse.
3. After the role-play, examine your written answers. See whether there are any changes you would like to make.
4. Finally, make up a situation and give it to your colleague with the same questions. Role-play the situation with your colleague, this time taking the role of the client.

Situation:
A 65-year-old man has been a client on the medical unit for 10 days, and you are assigned to care for him for the next 4 days. Diagnostic workup and tests reveal that he has cancer of the larynx. Surgery is indicated and has been scheduled. The doctor discusses his diagnosis and prognosis with him in your presence.

During the next 2 days, the client becomes increasingly withdrawn and introspective. Subsequently, he requests to speak with you and the physician. He states that he does not wish to have any surgery performed and no medication given, that he "has lived a good life" and would like you and the health team to accept his decision to die. He asks that no tube feedings or intravenous fluids be given. He asks that you cooperate and support his wishes.

Discussion:
1. What would your reaction be in this situation?
2. What does the statement "death with dignity" mean to you?
3. Do you think the client has the right to refuse treatment that may be life-sustaining?
4. What nursing care should you provide for this man as he continues to refuse food and fluids (keeping in mind that the client is an equal partner in his care)?
5. What conflicts does this situation pose for you? How would you see yourself dealing with them?
6. How can you, as a nurse, respect the integrity of a client's decision when it conflicts with promoting maximum client health functions?
7. Does the client's age influence your acceptance of his decision?
8. How will you support the client when faced with other health care professionals who disapprove of the client's decision?
9. What risks will you be taking in supporting the client?

Adapted from Uusral D: Values clarification in nursing: application to practice, *American Journal of Nursing* 78:2058–2063, 1978.

emptiness, and even suicidal thoughts when a significant personal or professional role ceases to exist. Examples of lost role relationships include job loss, divorce, retirement, death of a significant person, and a chronic or debilitating illness.

For clients, significant changes in their behavioral ability to function in expected roles as a result of illness, disability, or other life changes can be devastating. Alterations in normal roles, compromised role performance, and changes in role relationships are common sources of frustration and emotional pain to clients and families. The effects of alteration in role performance and role relationships within the family and work environment are such an important dimension of self-concept that they warrant a nursing diagnosis: ineffective role performance.

Nurses need to be sensitive to the changes in role relationships that even a minor illness or injury produces. An altered health status can change an individual's social role from one of independent self-sufficiency to one of vulnerability and dependence on others. For example,

when lack of physical stamina after a heart attack prevents a woman from fulfilling her customary caregiving roles in the home, she can experience a loss of self-confidence and personal value that can affect her rehabilitation (Arnold, 1997).

Most people do not assume the sick role voluntarily. At the hospital door, the client forsakes, either temporarily or permanently, recognized social roles in the family, work situation, and community. Regardless of how competent the person may be in other life roles, questions about role performance inevitably arise when illness strikes. Often, clients must learn new role behaviors that are unfamiliar and unsettling to previously held self-concepts. Illness or disability, whether actual or perceived, also strain family equilibrium and coping abilities. Sometimes alterations in role performance are intimately associated with the illness and will never be regained.

Clients and their families need the compassionate support of the nurse to incorporate the meaning of role changes occasioned by their illness or disability

Case Example

Dan was diagnosed with dementia in his mid-50s. He was a man of many talents who headed a large accounting firm before his illness. His wife had never worked outside of the home. Dan handled all of the finances, and his wife generally deferred to him for decisions. His son is in his first year of college on a 4-year scholarship, and there is one younger child in the home. The progression of the disease has been swift and incapacitating. Dan had not yet invested in long-term care insurance. He is too young for Social Security and is functional enough to not qualify for disability retirement. His illness creates significant changes for his wife, who now must take over running the household finances. His son is not sure whether he should come home or continue his studies. The younger child is robbed of a normal childhood role because of his father's illness. Dan himself feels depressed and unsure of what roles he can still fulfill. If you were Dan's nurse, what suggestions might you have for Dan and his family related to role relationships?

into an otherwise basically healthy self-concept. Asking open-ended, focused questions about the client's family relationships, work, and social roles helps the nurse to accurately assess potential alterations in role relationships in personal, social, and work relationships (Box 7-6). The questions should

| BOX 7-6 | Sample Assessment Questions Related to Role Relationships |

Family
- "What changes do you anticipate as a result of your illness (condition) in the way you function in your family?"
- "Who do you see in your family as being most affected by your illness (condition)?"
- "Who do you see in your family as being supportive of you?"

Work
- "What are some of the concerns you have about your job at this time?"
- "Who do you see in your work situation as being supportive of you?"

Social
- "How has your illness affected the way people who are important to you treat you?"
- "To whom do you turn for support?"
- "If _____ is not available to you, who else might provide social support for you?"

be asked in a conversational manner at a pace the client can tolerate.

With shortened hospital stays, potential role changes should be addressed as part of discharge planning or follow-up in the community, or both. Nurses working in long-term rehabilitation settings can help their clients look at transferable skills and personal strength they may possess that could be used in a different way, for example, good communication skills, persistence, patience, and so on. Many times clients are not aware of transferable skills that can be put to good use when previous capabilities are no longer available to them. Exercise 7-8 can help you understand the nature of transferable skills.

Health is a value-laden concept for many people. Preconceived notions of role disruption for an ill or disabled person occur more commonly when the illness is protracted, recurrent, or seriously role disruptive. Even when the person is fully capable of resuming previous role responsibilities after a documented extended illness, it is not uncommon for them to find that they are being "laid off" when they return to work.

Nurses need to help clients learn how to respond to subtle and not-so-subtle discriminatory actions associated with people's lack of understanding of the client's health situation.

SUMMARY

How nurses perceive their professional role and how they function as a nurse in that role has a sizable effect on the success of interpersonal communication in the nurse-client relationship. The professional nursing role should be evidenced in every aspect of nursing care, but nowhere more fully than in the nurse-client relationship. A professional nurse's first role responsibility is to the client. Because hospitals no longer are the primary settings for nursing practice, nurse practice roles take place in nontraditional and traditional community based health care settings. Advanced practice roles include the nurse practitioner, clinical nurse specialist, certified nurse-midwife, and nurse anesthetist. Two new roles, the CNL and the DNP, were introduced in 2003. A new concept in nursing education is interdisciplinary course

Nurses learn professional role behaviors through the process of professional role socialization. Professional development as a nurse is a lifelong commitment. Benner's five developmental stages of increasing proficiency

EXERCISE 7-8	Transferable Skills

Purpose: To help students understand the nature of transferrable skills that can be used in other situations.

Procedure:

1. Think of the one achievement of which you are most proud.
2. List the strengths or personal actions that went into this accomplishment. For example, "I was a good swim instructor" can be recast into personal strengths, such as "I was a good swim instructor because I was dependable, organized, patient, and persistent; I am able to relate easily to children; and I was compassionate with slow learners and able to inspire others."
3. Identify the physical, psychological, and psychosocial characteristics that contributed to the accomplishment (e.g., athletic ability, being raised in a large family, ethnic origin).
4. Share your achievement with your classmates.

Discussion:

1. How many different aspects of yourself were you able to identify as being a part of your accomplishment?
2. What physical, psychological, and psychosocial characteristics contributed to your achievement?
3. As you listened to the other students' reports, did you think of any other factors present in your situation?
4. Do you see any of these talents or strengths as "transferable skills" you might use in other situations?
5. What did you learn about yourself from this exercise?
6. How might you apply what you learned in this exercise to working therapeutically with clients?

describe the nurse's progression from novice to expert. Mentorship and continuing education assist nurses in maintaining their competency and professional role development. Interdisciplinary collaboration and health care teams have stimulated the development of shared elective classes involving two or more disciplines, for example, nursing and medicine or pharmacy.

Role performance disturbance has been designated by NANDA (2009) as a nursing diagnosis. Quality of life and role performance are interconnected. Examples of lost role relationships include job loss, divorce, retirement, death of a significant person, and a chronic or debilitating illness. Clients and their families need the compassionate support of the nurse to incorporate the meaning of role changes occasioned by their illness or disability into an otherwise basically healthy self-concept. Nurses can help clients and families identify and use transferable skills learned in previous roles in different ways.

ETHICAL DILEMMA	What Would You Do?

Bishop and Scudder (1996) said that nurses have a professional obligation not only to provide efficient, effective, and attentive care, but to do so in the context of a caring relationship. What do you think they meant by this statement? What does this statement have to do with the nurse's role? Why is this an ethical issue?

REFERENCES

American Association of Colleges of Nursing: *Values, qualities, and behaviors associated with professionalism in nursing practice,* Washington, DC, 1986, Author.

American Association of Colleges of Nursing: *The essentials of baccalaureate education for professional nursing practice,* Washington, DC, 2008, Author.

American Association of Colleges of Nursing: *Working paper on the role of the clinical nurse leader,* 2003. Available online: http://www.aacn.nche.edu/Publications/WhitePapers/ClinicalNurseLeader.htm. Accessed August 28, 2009.

American Association of Colleges of Nursing: *AACN position statement on the practice doctorate in nursing,* Washington, DC, 2004, American Association of Colleges of Nursing. Available online: http://www.aacn.nche.edu/DNP/DNPPositionStatement.htm. Accessed August 28, 2009.

American Hospital Association: *The patient care partnership; understanding expectations, rights and responsibilities,* Atlanta, 2003, Author. Available online: http://www.aha.org/aha/issues/Communicating-With-Patients/pt-care-partnership.html. Accessed December 30, 2009.

American Nurses Association: Know your rights: ANA's Bill of Rights arms nurses with critical information, *Am Nurse* 34(6):16, 2002.

American Nurses Association: *Code of ethics for nurses with interpretive statements,* Silver Spring, MD, 2001, American Nurses Publishing.

American Nurses Credentialing Center: *Magnet recognition program: recognizing excellence in nursing services: application manual,* Silver Spring, MD, 2004, Author.

American Nurses Credentialing Center: Objectives of the magnet recognition program. In *ANCC Magnet Recognition Program,* revised April 6, 2006. Available online: http://www.nursingworld.org/ancc/magnet/index.html.

Anthony S, Landeen J: Evolution of Canadian nursing curricula: a critical retrospective analysis of power and caring, *Int J Nurs Educ Scholarsh* 6(1, Article 18):1–14, 2009.

Arnold E: The stress connection: women and coronary heart disease, *Crit Care Nurs Clin North Am* 9(4):565–575, 1997.

Aveyard H, Edwards S, West S: Core topics of health care ethics: the identification of core topics for interprofessional education, *J Interprof Care* 19(1):63–69, 2005.

Benner P: *From novice to expert: excellence and power in clinical nursing practice*, Menlo Park, CA, 1984, Addison-Wesley.

Benner P: *From novice to expert: excellence and power in clinical nursing practice*, comm ed, New York, 2000, Prentice Hall.

Bishop AH, Scudder JR Jr: *Nursing ethics: therapeutic caring presence*, Boston, 1996, Jones and Bartlett.

Chaudhary N, Sriram S: Dialogues of the self, *Culture & Psychology* 7(3):379–392, 2001.

Cohen H: *The nurse's quest for a professional identity*, Menlo Park, CA, 1981, Addison-Wesley.

Coombs MA: *Power and conflict between doctors and nurses: breaking through the inner circle in clinical care*, London, 2004, Routledge.

Donaldson SK, Crowley DM: The discipline of nursing, *Nurs Outlook* 26(2):113–120, 1978.

Erickson J, Ditomassi M: The clinical nurse leader: new in name only, *J Nurs Edu* 44(3):99–100, 2005.

Flexner A: Is social work a profession?. In *Proceedings of the National Conference on Social Work*, New York, 1915.

Fronek P, Kendall M, Ungerer G, Malt J, Eugard E, Geraghty T: Towards healthy professional-client relationships: the value of an interprofessional training course, *J Interprof Care* 23(1):16–29, 2009.

Gugerty B: Nursing at a crossroads—education, research, training, and informatics, *J Healthc Inf Manag* 21(1):12–14, 2007.

Hassmiller S, Cozine M: Addressing the nurse shortage to improve the quality of patient care, *Health Aff* 25(1):268–274, 2006.

Hegarty J, Condon C, Walsh E, Sweeney J: The undergraduate education of nurses: looking to the future, *Int J Nurs Educ Scholarsh* 6(1, Article 17):1–11, 2009.

Hegyvary S: An agenda for nursing as a means to improve health, *J Nurs Scholarsh* 39(2):103–104, 2007.

Herbert C: Changing the culture: interprofessional education for collaborative patient centered practice in Canada, *J Interprof Care* (Suppl 1):1–4, 2005.

Hoffman S, Harris A, Rosenfield D: Why mentorship matters: students, staff and sustainability in interprofessional education, *J Interprof Care* 22(1):103–105, 2008.

Institute of Medicine (IOM): *Health professions education: a bridge to quality*, Washington, DC, 2003, National Academies Press.

Joint Commission: *The Health care at the crossroads: addressing the evolving nursing crisis*, Washington DC, 2002, Author.

Kramer M, Schmalenberg C: Staff nurses identify essentials of magnetism. In McClure M, Hinshaw AS, editors: *Magnet hospitals revisited: attraction and retention of professional nurses*, Washington, DC, 2002, American Nurses Publication.

Mahlin M: Individual patient advocacy, collective responsibility and activism within professional organizations, *Nurs Ethics* 17(2):247–254, 2010.

Malloch K, Porter-O'Grady T: *The quantum leader: applications for the new world of work*, Sudbury, MA, 2005, Jones and Bartlett.

Margalit R, Thompson S, Visovsky C, et al: From professional silos to interprofessional education: campuswide focus on quality of care, *Qual Manag Health Care* 18(3):165–173, 2009.

Masters K: *Role development in professional nursing practice*, Sudbury, MA, 2005, Jones and Bartlett.

Merriam-Websters Dictionary: Available online: http://www.merriam-webster.com/dictionary/advocate. Accessed December 30, 2009.

Morgan S: The magnet (TM) model as a framework for excellence, *J Nurs Care Qual* 24(2):105–108, 2009.

Mundinger M: Who's who in nursing: bringing clarity to the doctor of nursing practice: 2005, *Nurs Outlook* 53(4):173–176, 2005.

NANDA Nursing diagnosis 2009–2011: *Definitions and classification (NANDA nursing diagnosis)*, Ames Iowa, 2009, John Wiley & Sons Ltd.

Negarandeh R, Oskouie F, Fhmadi F, Nikravesh M, Hallberg IR: Patient advocacy: barriers and facilitators, *BMC Nursing* (5):3, 2006. Available online: http://www.biomedcentral.com/1472-6955/5/3. Accessed September 9, 2009.

Neil K, McCoy A, Parry C, et al: The clinical experiences of novice students in nursing, *Nursing Education* 23(4):16–21, 1998.

Oandasan I, Reeves S: Key elements for interprofessional education. Part I: The learner, the educator and the learning context, *J Interprof Care* 19:21–38, 2005.

O'Connell M: *Personal communication*, June, 2009.

Odom J: The nurse as patient advocate, *J Perianesth Nurs* 17(2):75–76, 2002.

Paton B, Thompson-Isherwood R, Thirsk L: Preceptors matter: an evolving framework, *J Nurs Educ* 48(4):213–216, 2009.

Pecukonis E, Doyle O, Bliss D: Reducing barriers to interprofessional training: Promoting interprofessional cultural competence, *J Interprof Care* 22(4I):417–428, 2008.

Pew Health Professions Commission: *Health professions education for the future: schools in service to the nation*, San Francisco, 1993, Pew Commission.

Puetz B: Networking, *Public Health Nurs* 24(6):577–579, 2007.

Roberson M: Our diversity gives us strength: comment and opinion, *Am Nurse* 24(5):4, 1992.

Rodts M, Lamb K: Transforming your professional self: encouraging lifelong personal and professional growth, *Orthop Nurs* 27(2):125–131, 2008.

Thomas J: Changing career paths: from expert to novice, *Orthop Nurs* 22(5):332–334, 2003.

Walsh CL, Gordon MF, Marshall M, Wilson F, Hunt T: Interprofessional capability: a developing framework for interprofessional education, *Nurse Educator Practitioner* 5:230–237, 2005.

Welchman J, Griener G: Patient advocacy and professional associations: individual and collective responsibilities, *Nurs Ethics* 12(3):296–304, 2005.

Willis DG, Grace PJ, Roy C: A central unifying focus for the discipline: facilitating humanization, meaning, choice, quality of life, and healing in living and dying, *Adv Nurs Sci* 31(1):E28–E40, 2008.

Yonge O, Billay D, Myrick F, Luhanga F: Preceptorship and mentorship: not merely a matter of semantics, *Int J Nurs Educ Scholarsh* 4(1, Article 19):1–13, 2007.

Zomorodi M, Foley BJ: The nature of advocacy vs. paternalism in nursing: clarifying the 'thin line', *J Ad Nurs* 65(8):1746–1752, 2009.

CHAPTER 8

Losses and Endings: Communication Skills at End of Life

Elizabeth C. Arnold

OBJECTIVES

At the end of the chapter, the reader will be able to:

1. Describe the concept of loss.
2. Describe the stages of death and dying.
3. Discuss the concept of palliative care.
4. Discuss theory-based concepts of grief and grieving
5. Define grief and describe common patterns of grieving.
6. Describe the nurse's role in palliative care.
7. Discuss key issues and approaches in end-of-life (EOL) care.
8. Identify cultural and spiritual needs in EOL care.
9. Describe supportive strategies for children.
10. Discuss strategies to help clients achieve a good death.
11. Identify stress issues for nurses in EOL care.

This chapter examines the nurse-client relationship in the context of palliative and EOL care. The chapter identifies theory frameworks related to the stages of dying and the process of grief and grieving. The Application section discusses the process of identifying and responding to client and family needs in EOL care. This chapter spotlights the communication issues in the care nurses provide to dying clients and as they meet the needs of grieving families. Helping clinicians recognize and cope with the high stress of providing quality EOL care is also addressed.

BASIC CONCEPTS

THE CONCEPT OF LOSS

Corless (2001) defines **loss** as "a generic term that signifies absence of an object, position, ability or attribute" (p. 352). Important losses occur as part of everyone's personal experience. Anything or anyone in whom we invest time, energy, or a part of ourselves can be experienced as a loss. When people *suffer the loss of* someone or something important to them, there is a loss of their sense of "wholeness" and a break in the person's expected life story (Attig, 2004). The loss remains in that person's mind, even with the passage of time (Levine, 2005). When a fresh loss occurs, previous losses are remembered. Consider the theme of loss in each of the following normal life experiences:

- A wife loses a 35-year-old marriage through divorce
- A cherished family pet dies
- A couple loses their dream home through foreclosure
- A woman suffers a miscarriage
- A parent dies

The feelings associated with loss differ only in the intensity with which one experiences them. Mark Twain noted: "Nothing that grieves us can be called little; by the eternal laws of proportion a child's loss of a doll and a king's loss of a crown are events of the same size" (Mark Twain Quotations, 2002). Some losses are unfinished; others occur simultaneously or sequentially.

Multiple losses occurring over a short period intensify the experience. Older adults will experience the deaths of friends and family members with greater frequency. One loss can precipitate multiple losses. For example, the client with Alzheimer's disease doesn't simply lose memory. Accompanying cognitive loss are profound losses of role, communication, independence, and loss of identity. Lifestyle changes are required to accommodate for the cognitive loss.

Multiple losses complicate the grieving process and usually take longer to resolve. Helping people focus on one relationship at a time instead of trying to address the losses together is helpful. Acknowledgment of the differences between single and multiple loss helps put the enormity of multiple losses into perspective (Mercer & Evans, 2006). Exercise 8-1 is designed to help you understand the dimensions of personal loss.

DEATH: THE FINAL LOSS

Death is associated with loss; it signals the end of all that life holds on this earth: successes, failures, relationships, careers, laughter, and pain. More than a biological event, dying has spiritual, social, and cultural features that help people make sense of its meaning. Dobratz (2002) describes a human life pattern in dying patients that is "shaped by self-integration, inner cognition, creation of personal meanings, and connection to others and a higher being" (p. 139).

Silveira and Schneider (2004) suggest that "planning for the end of life is planning for the unknown" (p. 349). Although death is a necessary part of the circle of life, dying is often feared, even if people believe in an afterlife. As Chenitz (1992), a nurse dying of AIDS noted, "Like many people with AIDS, I am not afraid of death. I am afraid of dying. The dying process and how that will be handled is of great concern to me" (p. 454).

When asked, most clients identify fear of pain and of experiencing their last phase of life unaccompanied as their two principal fears (Pashby, 2010). Clients and families need to know that help is always available from someone knowledgeable, who cares about them, and is willing to anticipate and respond to their personal care needs as they appear.

Nurses are not immune from these fears. It is often difficult for nurses to maintain a balance between their own sensitivity to death and well-being, and providing the empathy and support needed by clients and families. This is why self-awareness about death and dying issues is so important in providing palliative care.

THEORETICAL FRAMEWORK: STAGES OF DYING

Elisabeth Kübler-Ross (1969) provides a five-stage framework for understanding the process of dying. Not every person experiences each stage.

DENIAL

Kübler-Ross (1969) characterizes denial stage as the "No, not me" stage. Nurses should be sensitive to the client's need for denial. Some people remain in the denial stage throughout their illness; their right to do so should be respected.

EXERCISE 8-1	The Meaning of Loss

Purpose: To consider personal meaning of losses.

Procedure:
Consider your answers to the following questions:
- What losses have I experienced in my life?
- How did I feel when I lost something or someone important to me?
- How was my behavior affected by my loss?
- What helped me the most in resolving my feelings of loss?
- How has my experience with loss prepared me to deal with further losses?
- How has my experience with loss prepared me to help others deal with loss?

Discussion:
1. In the larger group, discuss what gives a loss its meaning.
2. What common themes emerged from the group discussion about successful strategies in coping with loss?
3. How does the impact of necessary losses differ from that of unexpected, unnecessary losses?
4. How can you use in your clinical work what you have learned from doing this exercise?

ANGER

Kübler-Ross (1969) refers to anger as the "Why me?" stage, associated with feelings about the unfairness of life, or anger with God. Feelings get projected on those closest to the client. The client lashes out at family, friends, and staff members. Those closest to the client may need support in recognizing that the anger is not a personal attack.

BARGAINING

Kübler-Ross (1969) refers to the bargaining stage as the "Yes, me, but . . . I need just a little more time." The bargaining stage involves pleading for time extension or special consideration. Bargaining is not a futile exercise. Sometimes the extra energy a person gets by trying to postpone death can provide a meaningful moment for client and family; consider the father, wanting to stay alive for his daughter's wedding. By supporting hope and avoiding challenges to the client's reality, the nurse facilitates the process of living while dying.

DEPRESSION

Kübler-Ross (1969) characterizes the depression stage as the "Yes, me" stage, accompanied by depressive feelings. Mood swings and depressive feelings are hard for families to tolerate, but very common. Nursing strategies in this stage include helping clients to accept depression as being a normal response, and being present to clients and families as an empathetic, listening witness to their experience.

ACCEPTANCE

Pashby (2010) notes that the theoretical stages seem to mirror the physiologic decline experienced at the EOL.

Clients who are weak and bedridden with declining consciousness as death approaches come more readily to the final stage of acceptance. The acceptance stage is characterized by an acknowledgment of the inevitable EOL. As the client approaches death, there is a gradual detachment from the world, and the person is almost "void of feeling" (Kübler-Ross, 1969, p. 124). Because of this, there can be a sense of peace.

PALLIATIVE CARE

Palliative care is defined as "a clinical approach designed to improve the quality of life for clients and families coping with a life threatening illness" (Davies & Higginson, 2004, p. 14). It is recognized as a philosophy of care and as an emerging practice discipline. The dimensions of palliative care identified by the World Health Organization (WHO) are presented in Box 8-1.

Clients are admitted to palliative care services when the client has a life-limiting disease with care needs that will go beyond traditional modes of medical intervention (Galanos, 2004; Morrison & Meier, 2004). Palliative care is unique in that it includes involved family members and the client with the life-limiting disease as one integrated unit of care. Clients initially admitted to palliative care services may still be receiving active treatment for their disease process to control symptoms and improve quality of life (McIlfatrick, 2007). Palliative care can augment treatment with attention directed to providing the secondary psychosocial, practical, and spiritual support services and assistance people need regarding EOL decisions and care. As the disease or disability progresses, palliative

---

BOX 8-1	Dimensions of Palliative Care

- Provides relief from pain and other distressing symptoms
- Affirms life and regards dying as a normal process
- Intends neither to hasten nor postpone death
- Integrates the psychological and spiritual aspects of patient care
- Offers a support system to help patients live as actively as possible until death
- Offers a support system to help the family cope during the patients illness and in their own bereavement

- Uses a team approach to address the needs of patients and their families, including bereavement counselling, if indicated
- Will enhance quality of life, and may also positively influence the course of illness
- Is applicable early in the course of illness, in conjunction with other therapies that are intended to prolong life, such as chemotherapy or radiation therapy, and includes those investigations needed to better understand and manage distressing clinical complications

From World Health Organization: *WHO Definition of Palliative Care*, 2008; available online: http://www.who.int/cancer/palliative/definition/en/. Accessed February 28, 2009.

TABLE 8-1	Quality Measures for Palliative and End-of-Life Care by Domain

Domain	Quality Measure
Patient and family-centered decision making	1. Assessment of the patient's decisional capacity 2. Documentation of a surrogate decision maker within 24 hours 3. Documentation of the presence and, if present, contents of advance directives 4. Documentation of the goals of care
Communication within the team, with clients and family	5. Documentation of timely physician communication with the family 6. Documentation of a timely interdisciplinary clinician-family conference
Continuity of care	7. Transmission of key information with transfer of the patient out of the intensive care unit (ICU) 8. Policy for continuity of nursing services
Emotional and practical support for patient and family	9. Open visitation policy for family members 10. Documentation that psychosocial support has been offered
Symptom management and comfort care	11. Documentation of pain assessment 12. Documentation of pain management 13. Documentation of respiratory distress assessment 14. Documentation of respiratory distress management 15. Protocol for analgesia/sedation in terminal withdrawal of mechanical ventilation 16. Appropriate medications available during withdrawal of mechanical ventilation
Spiritual support for patients and family	17. Documentation that spiritual support was offered
Emotional and organizational support for clinicians	18. Opportunity to review experience of caring for dying patients by ICU clinicians

From Mularski R, Curtis J, Billings J et al: Proposed quality measures for palliative care in the critically ill: a consensus from the Robert Wood Johnson Foundation care group, *Critical Care Medicine* 34(11 suppl):S406, 2006.

care still supports living while dying, but the focus becomes symptom management and movement toward achieving a good death, rather than active treatment. Table 8-1 identifies proposed quality measures for palliative care in the critically ill.

Palliative care strategies are designed to help clients and families understand the dying process as a part of life and to assist terminally ill clients to achieve the best quality of life in the time left to them. The basic axiom for palliative EOL care is to follow what clients actually want for themselves (Silveira & Schneider, 2004). Palliative care is dedicated to supporting families as resources and as units of care themselves. After the client's death, palliative care offers grief support for family members.

Palliative care and hospice are related concepts. A fundamental difference between the two approaches is that the palliative care team can admit and serve patients still receiving curative treatment, with no time restrictions regarding prognosis. Hospice clients must have a prognosis of 6 months or less, and cannot be

receiving active medical treatment. Hospice is considered part of the continuum of palliative care; it offers a quality care environment in the last segment of life.

NURSING INITIATIVES

Nurses have taken a leadership role in developing guidelines for quality EOL care through national initiatives. Nationally recognized nursing experts, funded by the American Association of Colleges of Nursing (AACN) and the City of Hope, have developed the End-of-Life Nursing Education Consortium (ELNEC), a national education initiative to improve EOL care in the United States. The ELNEC project targets undergraduate and graduate nursing faculty, continuing education providers, staff development educators, and pediatric and oncology specialty nurses in EOL care (AACN, 2006). Specific EOL training allows nurses to teach others and to enter into the lives of many more people facing EOL as skilled, compassionate professionals with specialized care tools (Malloy, Paice, Virani, Ferrell, & Bednash, 2008).

CONCEPTS OF GRIEF AND GRIEVING

The concept of **grief** describes the personal emotions and adaptive process a person goes through in recovering from loss. Common feelings include sadness and an acute awareness of the void accompanied by recurring, wavelike feelings of sadness and loss. Certain situations, time alone, holidays, and anniversaries allow grief feelings to resurface.

Case Example

"I would think I was doing okay, that I had a handle on my grief. Then without warning, a scent, a scene on television, an innocuous conversation would flip a switch in my mind, and I would be flooded with memories of my mother. My eyes would fill up with tears as my fragile composure dissolved. My grief lay right under the surface of my awareness and ambushed me at times and in places not of my choosing" (Anonymous).

THEORY-BASED FRAMEWORKS OF GRIEVING

Lindemann's Work on Grief

Eric Lindemann (1944/1994) pioneered the concept of grief work based on interviews with bereaved persons suffering a sudden tragic loss. He described patterns of grief, and the physical and emotional changes that accompany significant losses. Lindemann observed that grief can occur immediately after a loss, or it can be delayed. He summarized three components of support: (a) open, empathetic communication; (b) honesty; and (c) tolerance of emotional expression as being important in grieving. When the symptoms of grief are exaggerated or absent, it is considered pathologic or complicated grief. People experiencing complicated grief may require psychological treatment to resolve their grief and move into life again.

Engel's Contributions

George Engel's (1964) concepts built on Lindemann's work. He described three sequential phases of grief work: (a) shock and disbelief, (b) developing awareness, and (c) restitution.

In the shock and disbelief phase, a newly bereaved person may feel alienated or detached from normal— "literally numb with shock; no tears, no feelings, just absolute numbness" (Lendrum & Syme, 1992, pp. 24–25). Seeing or hearing the lost person, or sensing his or her presence is a normal, temporary altered sensory experience related to the loss, which should not be confused with psychotic hallucinations.

In the immediate aftermath of death, families and friends surround a person with support and opportunities to talk. This support diminishes over time. The developing awareness phase occurs slowly as the void created by the loss fully enters consciousness. There is a loss of energy, not the kind that requires sleep, but rather a desire to accomplish things without having either the organizational capacity or energy to follow through with related tasks.

Case Example

"Throughout the year following my mother's death, I was aware of a persistent feeling of heaviness—not physical heaviness, but emotional and spiritual. It was as if a dark cloud hung over my heart and soul. I tired easily, with little energy to do anything but the most essential activities, and even those frequently received perfunctory attention. My usual pattern of 'sleeping like a log' was disrupted, and in its place I experienced uneasy rest that left me feeling as if I had never closed my eyes" (Anonymous).

Listening, identifying feelings, and having an empathetic willingness to repeatedly hear the client's story without needing to give advice or interpretation are helpful nursing interventions (Jeffries, 2005).

The *restitution phase* is characterized by adaptation to a new life without the deceased. There is a resurgence of hope and a renewed energy to fashion a new life. With successful grieving, the loss is not forgotten, but the pain diminishes, and is replaced with memories that enrich and give energy to life. John Thomas (2010) describes his sense of new beginnings:

I want to be known as one who

- Has one foot planted firmly in this life and the other seeking a firm footing in the spiritual realm
- Is identified with life and love rather than loss and grief
- Walks with the stride of renewal rather than the shuffle of grief; a vigorous man with an appreciation for beauty and quality
- Is confident about the future without needing a tangible GPS
- Can still embrace life knowing that the pain of loss is intense
- Can be alone without being lonely

- Faced grief head-on and reached a deeper core of self and spirituality
- Has much to give in many arenas living a life that honors my past and sharing the blessing derived from it

CONTEMPORARY MODELS OF GRIEVING

Florczak (2008) states, "The newer worldview considers loss to be a unique, intersubjective process in which the individual maintains connections with the absent and the meaning of the experience continually changes" (p. 8). The past is not forgotten, and there is a continuous spiritual connection with the deceased, which illuminates different features of self and possibilities for fuller engagement with life. Features of past experiences with the loved one are rewoven into the fabric of a person's life in a new form. Contemporary authors Neimeyer (2001) and Attig (2001) emphasize meaning construction as a central issue in grief work.

PATTERNS OF GRIEVING

ACUTE GRIEF

Acute grief occurs as "somatic distress that occurs in waves with feelings of tightness in the throat, shortness of breath, an empty feeling in the abdomen, a sense of heaviness and lack of muscular power, and intense mental pain" (Lindemann, 1994, p. 155). Sudden traumatic deaths are more likely to stimulate acute grief reactions.

When the death is untimely (as with an accident or fatal heart attack), out of normal sequence (as in the case of a child's death), or complicated by stigma (as with death from addiction or suicide), the challenge for the family is greater. Survivors feel more guilt, anger, and helplessness.

Suicide survivors are at a disadvantage. Survivors typically overestimate their ability to influence the suicidal behavior or outcome. They are reluctant to discuss death details because of shame or perceived stigma. Survivors usually need more support. Often they get less because people don't know how to talk to them about suicides (Harvard Women's Health Watch, 2009). Suicide survivor support groups can offer the specialized help that many survivors need after a suicide (Felgelman, 2008).

Anticipatory Grief

Anticipatory grief is an emotional response that occurs before the actual death around a family member with a degenerative or terminal disorder. It also is experienced by a person anticipating his or her own death. Symptoms can be similar to those experienced after death and can be colored by ambivalent feelings.

Case Example

Marge's husband, Albert, was diagnosed with Alzheimer's disease 5 years ago. Albert is in a nursing home, unable to care for himself. Marge grieves the impending loss of Albert as her mate. At the same time, she would like a life of her own. Her "other feelings" of wishing it could all be over cause her to feel guilty. Exercise 8-2 helps you explore personal thoughts about grief.

Chronic Sorrow

Chronic sorrow is an ill-defined form of grief, occurring while a person is still alive, in relation to a limiting disease, or as an ongoing loss of potential in a loved one (Bowes, Lowes, Warner, & Gregory, 2009). It has been identified in parents of disabled or mentally ill children, spouses of dementia victims, and adults with a permanent disability or severe chronic illness.

EXERCISE 8-2	A Personal Grief Inventory

Purpose: To provide a close examination of one's history with grief.

Procedure:

Complete each sentence and reflect on your answers:

The first significant experience with grief that I can remember in my life was _____.

The circumstances were _____.

My age was _____.

The feelings I had at the time were_____.

The thing I remember most about that experience was _____.

I coped with the loss by _____.

The primary sources of support during this period were _____.

What helped most was _____.

The most difficult death for me to face would be _____.

I know my grief over a loss is resolved when _____.

Adapted from Carson VB, Arnold EN: *Mental health nursing: the nurse-patient journey* (p. 666), Philadelphia, 1996, WB Saunders.

Chronic sorrow is an intermittent grief process. In between, there are periods of emotional neutrality and positive emotions. It presents as a recurring sadness, particularly during exacerbations of symptoms, or comparisons with healthy people. Key distinctions between chronic sorrow and other forms of grieving include an inability to achieve closure and its discontinuous nature. Clients and family members may not be aware that they are grieving because they don't recognize having an ongoing incomplete loss as a legitimate loss to be grieved (Lafond, 2002). Providing timely support for families when there is a resurgence of symptoms can reduce stress.

Complicated Grieving

Complicated grieving represents a form of grief, distinguished by being unusually intense, significantly longer in duration, or incapacitating. A history of depression, substance abuse, death of a parent or sibling during childhood, prolonged conflict or dependence on the deceased person, or a succession of deaths within a short period predispose a person to complicated grief. Statements such as "I never recovered from my son's death," or "I feel like my life ended when my husband died" may indicate the presence of complicated grief.

Symptoms can appear as an absence of grief in situations where it would be expected, for example, a marine who displays no emotion over the deaths of war comrades. When deaths and important losses are not mourned, the feelings don't just disappear; they reappear in unexpected ways sometimes years later. Subsequent losses trigger an extreme reaction to a current loss. Complicated grief can result in clinical symptoms such as depression or anxiety disorders that require professional help. Exercise 8-3 provides a personal opportunity to reflect on the grieving process.

Developing an Evidence-Based Practice

Beckstrand R, Callister L, Kirchhoff K: Providing a "good death": critical care nurses' suggestions for improving end-of-life care, *American Journal of Critical Care* 15(1):38–45, 2006.

This survey study was part of a larger national study designed to elicit critical care nurses' views (N = 861) of EOL care in intensive care units. The goal of this report, consistent with the Institute of Medicine's recommendation to strengthen the knowledge base on EOL care, was to elicit suggestions on ways to improve EOL care.

Results: Study results indicated a common commitment of study subjects to helping clients achieve a good death, one marked with dignity and peace. Ways to achieve this goal were described as managing pain and discomfort, eliciting and following the clients' wishes for EOL care, facilitating family presence at time of death, and communicating effectively with other members of the health care team. Barriers were identified as time constraints, staffing patterns, and treatment decisions that did not reflect the clients' needs or wishes.

Application to Your Clinical Practice: As people live longer and the trajectory between time of diagnosis and time of death lengthens, palliative care becomes increasingly important. How could you, as a nurse, effectively help clients to die with dignity in a hospital setting? In a home setting?

EXERCISE 8-3   Reflections on the Grieving Process

Purpose: To provide students with an opportunity to see how putting into words the meaning a person had for you could facilitate the grieving process.

Procedure:
1. Write a letter to someone who has died or is no longer in your life. Before writing the letter, reflect on the meaning this person had for you and the person you have become.
2. In the letter, tell the person what they meant to you and why it is that you miss them.
3. Tell the person what you remember most about your relationship.
4. Tell the person anything you wished you had said but didn't when the person was in your life.

With a partner, each student should share his or her story without interruption. When the student finishes his or her story, the listener can ask questions for further understanding.

Discussion:
1. What was it like to write a letter to someone who had meaning in your life and is no longer available to you?
2. Were there any common themes?
3. In what ways was each story unique?
4. How could you use this exercise in your care of clients who are grieving?

NURSING ROLES IN PALLIATIVE CARE

IMPLEMENTING PALLIATIVE CARE CONCEPTS

Palliative care operates as a 24-hour resource, providing comprehensive, holistic services to clients and families in hospitals, people's homes, nursing homes, and outpatient settings. Ideally, palliative services are integrated at all levels of care, and are adapted to a client's specific cultural, social, and economic circumstances. Palliative care can be used concurrently with disease-modifying care, with the level of comfort care increasing according to client need (Savory & Marco, 2009).

The palliative care team is interdisciplinary, consisting of physicians, nurses, social workers, psychologists, and clergy specially trained in palliative care. In addition to supportive care for clients and families, team members provide education and consultation about EOL care for hospital staff. The treatment focus of palliative care is on pain control, physical symptom management, and easing the secondary psychosocial and spiritual distress experienced by clients with a terminal illness. If the client has had a special relationship with a physician, before admission to palliative care, the client or nurse can contact them. In some cases, the physician will stay involved; this can be a major source of comfort for clients and families.

Nurses play a pivotal role as professional coordinators, direct providers of care, and advocates for client autonomy and control in EOL care. They are in a key position to help families maintain family integrity, and to support their efforts in managing the process of living until death and in preparing for the death of their loved one. Quality indicators for EOL care are displayed in Figure 8-1.

Nurses must be aware of their own EOL experiences, including attitudes, expectations, and feelings about death and the process of dying. Miller (2001) notes, "As you become more clear about who you are and why you do what you do, you will become more receptive to whomever you are with" (p. 23). Exercise 8-4 is designed to promote self-awareness.

KEY ISSUES AND APPROACHES IN END-OF-LIFE CARE

TRANSPARENT DECISION MAKING

Clients and families face difficult, irreversible decisions in the last phase of life. Decisions related to discontinuation of fluids, antibiotics, blood transfusions, and ventilator support require a clear understanding of a complex care situation. Thelan (2005) defines **end-of-life decision making** as "the process that healthcare providers, patients and patients' families go through when considering what treatments will or will not be used to treat a life threatening illness" (p. 29).

EOL decisions should be transparent, meaning that all parties involved in the decision should fully

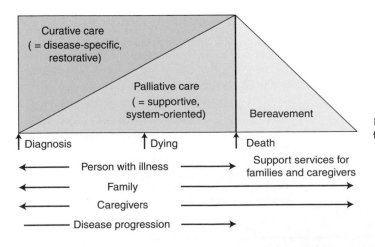

Figure 8-1   Model of curative and palliative care for progressive illness.

EXERCISE 8-4	Self Awareness about Death: A Questionnaire

Purpose: To explore students' feelings about death.

Procedure:

Answer the following questions.

1. Who died in your first personal involvement with death?
   a. Grandparent or great-grandparent
   b. Parent
   c. Brother or sister
   d. Other family member
   e. Friend or acquaintance
   f. Stranger
   g. Public figure
   h. Animal

2. To the best of your memory, at what age were you first aware of death?
   a. Younger than 3 years
   b. 3–5 years
   c. 5–10 years
   d. 10 years or older

3. When you were a child, how was death talked about in your family?
   a. Openly
   b. With some sense of discomfort
   c. Only when necessary, and then with an attempt to exclude the children
   d. As though it were a taboo subject
   e. Do not recall any discussion

4. Which of the following most influenced your present attitudes toward death?
   a. Death of someone else
   b. Specific reading
   c. Religious upbringing
   d. Introspection and meditation
   e. Ritual (e.g., funerals)
   f. Television, radio, or motion pictures
   g. Longevity of my family
   h. My health or physical condition
   i. Other

5. How often do you think about your own death?
   a. Very frequently (at least once a day)
   b. Frequently
   c. Occasionally
   d. Rarely (no more than once a year)
   e. Very rarely or never

6. What does death mean to you?
   a. The end; the final process of life
   b. The beginning of a life after death; a transition; a new beginning
   c. A joining of the spirit with a universal cosmic consciousness
   d. A kind of endless sleep; rest and peace
   e. Termination of this life, but with survival of the spirit
   f. Do not know

7. If you had a choice, what kind of death would you prefer?
   a. Tragic, violent death
   b. Sudden, but not violent death
   c. Quiet, dignified death
   d. Death in the line of duty
   e. Death after a great achievement
   f. Suicide
   g. Homicide victim
   h. There is no "appropriate" kind of death

8. If it were possible, would you want to know the exact date on which you are going to die?
   a. Yes
   b. No

9. If your physician knew that you had a terminal disease and a limited time to live, would you want him or her to tell you?
   a. Yes
   b. No
   c. It would depend on the circumstances

10. What efforts do you believe ought to be made to keep a seriously ill person alive?
    a. All possible efforts should be made (e.g., transplantation, kidney dialysis)
    b. Efforts should be made that are reasonable for that person's age, physical condition, mental condition, and pain
    c. After reasonable care, a natural death should be permitted
    d. A person with dementia should not be kept alive by artificial methods

11. If or when you are married, would you prefer to outlive your spouse?
    a. Yes, I would prefer to die second and outlive my spouse
    b. No, I would rather die first and have my spouse outlive me
    c. Undecided or do not know

12. What effect has this questionnaire had on you?
    a. It has made me somewhat anxious or upset
    b. It has made me think about my own death
    c. It has reminded me how fragile and precious life is
    d. Other effects

understand the implications of their decision. For example, to make an informed decision about use of life supports for terminal clients, clients and families need to know whether further treatments will enhance or diminish quality of life, their potential impact on life expectancy, whether the treatment is known to be effective or is an investigative treatment, and what types of adverse effects the client is likely to experience.

When the client is fully competent, he or she should make all treatment decisions. Ideally, EOL care choices should be made before a life-threatening illness occurs, or as early as possible after diagnosis (Kirchhoff, 2002). The nurse's role is to provide the client with full information, and to serve as his or her advocate in support of the person's right to make decisions about treatment and care (ANA, 1991; Erlen, 2005). Box 8-2 provides guidelines for talking with families about care options at EOL when an advance directive or durable power of attorney is not in effect.

USING ADVANCE DIRECTIVES

Miscommunication is a common underlying theme in creating confusion and delaying appropriate decisions about EOL care (Lang & Quill, 2004). Preferences are best expressed in advance directives (see Chapter 2), with discussions taking place in a compassionate, gentle manner, paced at the client/family's pace and level of understanding. Studies of family use of advance directives demonstrate significantly lower stress in families using them (Davis et al., 2005). In the hospital, advance directives should be kept in the front of the client's chart.

PAIN CONTROL AND MANAGEMENT

Pain control and management is an essential component of quality EOL care. Standards for pain management established by the Joint Commission (2010) require that every inpatient be routinely assessed for pain, with documentation of appropriate monitoring, and pain management. The American Pain Society (APS), Joint Commission, and Veteran's Administration have identified pain as the fifth vital sign with a nursing expectation of pain evaluation together with the standard vital signs (temperature, pulse, respiration, and blood pressure).

Pain is a subjective assessment, assessed verbally with the client and/or observed in client behavior. Routine assessments can identify previously unreported incidences of pain symptoms (Morrison & Meier, 2004).

Assessment questions include:
- Onset and duration of pain
- Location of the pain
- Character of the pain (sharp, dull, burning, persistent, changes with movement, direct or referred pain)
- Intensity—using a 0 to 10 numerical rating scale, with 0 being no pain and 10 being unbearable pain; assess children and clients having limited English with the Wong–Baker FACES Pain Rating Scale (Figure 8-2).
- History of substance dependence (crossover tolerance)

Behavioral indicators include abrupt changes in activity, crying, inability to be consoled, listlessness

---

| **BOX 8-2** | Talking with Families about Care Options at End of Life |

If neither durable power of attorney nor written directive is in effect:
- Determine who should be approached to make the decisions about care options.
- Determine whether any key members are absent. (Try to keep those who know the client best in the center of decision making.)
- Find a quiet place to meet where each family member can be seated comfortably.
- Sit down and establish rapport with each person present. Ask about the relationship each person has with the client and how each person feels about the client's current condition.

- Try to achieve a consensus about the patient's clinical situation, especially prognosis.
- Provide a professional observation about the client's status and expected quality of life—survival vs. quality of life. Ask what each person thinks the client would want.
- Should the family choose comfort measures only, assure the family of the attention to patient comfort and dignity that will occur.
- Seek verbal confirmation of understanding and agreement.
- Attention to the family's emotional responses is appropriate and appreciated.

Adapted from Lang F, Quill T: Making decisions with families at the end of life, *American Family Physician* 70(4):720, 2004.

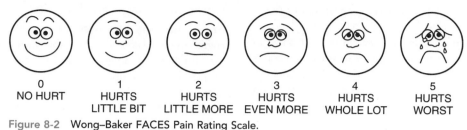

0
NO HURT

1
HURTS
LITTLE BIT

2
HURTS
LITTLE MORE

3
HURTS
EVEN MORE

4
HURTS
WHOLE LOT

5
HURTS
WORST

Figure 8-2   Wong–Baker FACES Pain Rating Scale.

or unwillingness to move, rubbing a body part, wincing, or facial grimacing (Atkinson, Chesters, & Heinz, 2009).

Having appropriate pain control for moderate-to-severe pain usually requires the use of opioids. Misperceptions about pain-relieving opioids are a major, unnecessary barrier to adequate pain control. Families will attribute signs and symptoms of approaching death such as increased lethargy, confusion, and declining appetite to side effects of opioids. With or without pain medication, actively dying clients become less responsive as death approaches. Although clients may experience drowsiness with initial dosing, this side effect quickly disappears.

Nurses should educate the family and client about the differences between disease progression and adverse effects related to opioids (Pashby, 2010). Essential information includes action, dosing intervals, side effects, and role pain control in client comfort and quality of life.

A second unfortunate barrier is fear of addiction (Clary & Lawson, 2009). All clients, including addicts, are entitled to appropriate and adequate pain management of severe pain. People do not become addicted from taking legally prescribed opioid medications for pain associated with terminal illness. There is a fundamental difference between taking essential medication for pain control on a prescribed scheduled basis and addictive uses. Addicted clients may require larger doses of pain medication because of cross-tolerance. Once the family understands the mechanisms and goals of pain control, and is assured that the client will not die or become addicted from its *appropriate* use, most will support its use in EOL care.

Clients approaching death can experience "breakthrough" pain, which occurs episodically as severe pain spikes. When breakthrough pain occurs, rescue medications, which are faster acting, can be used.

Touch and light massage are helpful adjuncts for pain relief.

COMMUNICATION IN END-OF-LIFE CARE

Curtis (2004) suggests that communication skill is equal to or supersedes clinical skill in EOL care. Everyone experiences a death differently; it is the uniqueness of each person's experience that the nurse attempts to tap into and facilitate through conversation. Conversations with clients and families provide nurses with insights about personal values and preferences regarding EOL care, and provide a forum to answer difficult questions in a supportive environment.

The quality of the relationship between nurse, patient, and family members is a key factor in how the last phase of life is experienced and negotiated (Mok & Chiu, 2004; Olthuis et al., 2006). EOL interactions help people find meaning, achieve emotional closure, and provide the best means for helping clients and families make complex life decisions. Listening and responding to clients as they cope with difficult issues around dying is easier said than done (Larson & Tobin, 2000). The challenge for nurses is to remain in a relationship with clients and families even when one feels inadequate to the task.

Schim and Raspa (2007) believe that the process of dying is a narrative: "Life-altering happenings are expressed through stories" (p. 202). Personal reflections are critical sources of assessment data. Once rapport is established, Pashby (2010) suggests nurses can ask clients how they learned of their diagnosis. She notes that a terminal diagnosis is usually a "Technicolor Moment" that the person remembers vividly and appreciates talking about. Other questions such as "What has changed for you since the diagnosis?" or "What is it like for you now?" provide additional data. Giving voice to the experience helps clients to consider its personal meaning and provides the nurse with a more complete picture of each person's distinctive concerns and goals.

Although most dying clients know that they are dying, it is not unusual for a client to ask in the course of conversation, "Am I going to die?" Before answering, find out more about the origin of the question. A useful listening response is, "What is your sense of it?" Box 8-3 provides guidelines for communicating with terminally ill clients.

Morgan (2001) suggests using a basic social process between nurse and client in palliative care, which she labeled protective coping and adjustment. The process involves nursing interactions that protect, maintain, and safeguard the integrity of clients, whereas at the same time helping them to determine and act on actions that are in their own best interests.

Communicating with Families

Family members have different levels of readiness to engage in discussions about the dying process. It is "normal" for an impending death to have a different impact on each family member, because each has had a unique relationship with the dying person. Conversations with families need not be long in duration, but regularity is important. Box 8-4 identifies family communication needs at EOL.

Common concerns include discontinuing life support; conflicts among family members about care; tensions between the client, family, and/or physician and family about treatment; where death should occur (home, hospital, hospice); if/when hospice should be engaged; and other concerns. Active listening can produce a creative outcome.

BOX 8-3 Guidelines for Communicating with Dying Clients

- Avoid automatic responses and trite reassurances.
- Each death is a unique, deeply personal experience for the client and should be treated as such.
- Avoid destroying hope. Reframe hope to what can happen in the here and now.
- Let the client lead the discussion about the future. Be comfortable with focusing on the here and now. (This discussion is not a one-time event; openings for discussion should be encouraged as the client's condition worsens.)
- Relate on a human level. Show humor, as well as sorrow.
- Use your mind, eyes, and ears to hear what is said, as well as what is not said.
- Respect the individual's pattern of communication and ways of dealing with stress. Support the client's desire for control of his or her life to whatever extent is possible.

- Maintain a sense of calm. Use eye contact, touch, and comfort measures to communicate.
- Do not force the client to talk. Respect the client's need for privacy and be sensitive to the client's readiness to talk, and let him or her know that you will be available to listen.
- Humility and honesty are essential. Be willing to admit when you do not know the answer.
- Be willing to allow the client to see some of your fears and vulnerabilities. It is much easier to open up to someone who is "human and vulnerable" than to someone who appears to have all the answers.
- Provide short, frequent times for family members to be with the dying client (without overtiring the client). Let them provide simple comfort measures if they desire to do so.

BOX 8-4 Family Communication Needs at End of Life

- Honest and complete answers to questions; repetition and further explanation if needed
- Updates about the client's condition and changes as they occur
- Clear, understandable explanations, delivered with empathy and respect
- Frequent opportunities to express concerns and feelings in a supportive, unhurried environment
- Information about what to expect—physical, emotional, spiritual—as death approaches
- Discussion of whom to call, legal issues, memorial or funeral planning

- Appreciation of the conflicts that families experience when the illness dictates that few options exist; for example, a frequent dilemma at EOL is whether life support measures are extending life or prolonging the dying phase.
- Short private times to be present and/or minister to the client
- Permission to leave the dying client for short periods with the knowledge that the nurse will contact the family member if there is a change in status

Case Example

The baby kind of started to dwindle real early in the morning. Mom was there by herself and all of a sudden wanted everything done . . . she was changing her mind. Once you started to talk to them further, and talk to the grandma, what her real problem was is that she didn't want that baby to die while she was there by herself. She wanted her mom to be there . . . so that changed the whole story quite a bit. We were like, "Yeah, we can keep this baby going for an hour until your mom gets here" (Lee & Dupree, 2008, p. 988).

Creating Family Memories

Clients and families need to talk about things other than the disease process and treatments. Nurses can help make this happen. There are spiritual stories, cultural stories, funny stories, developmental stories, narratives of advocacy, and family stories. Each reinforces the bonds and affirms the depth of meaning a family holds with a dying person. The moments of laughter, foibles, and shared experiences are connections that need to be remembered.

Case Example

Evelyn was an 83-year-old woman diagnosed with terminal lung cancer. During a guided imagery exercise, the nurse asked her to recall a time when she felt relaxed and happy. Evelyn described in vivid detail being with her family at a picnic near a lake many years ago. When her family came to visit that night, Evelyn related the story again, and the entire family talked about their parts in the remembered event. How they all laughed, what fun they had! It was one of their last conversations; one that reinforced family bonds in the initial telling and later as her family remembered Evelyn after her death. Her adult daughter made a special point of letting the nurse know how important sharing this story was to the client and family.

Providing Information

Nurses are key informants about client status and changes in the client's condition. There are fundamental differences in the level of information an individual or family will desire. The response of the client should determine the content and pace of sharing information. Talking with families about care details and potential outcomes should happen often, but even more frequently when the client's health status begins to decline or show a change.

Ideally, one nurse serves as the primary contact for the client and family, and acts as a liaison between providers and clients. This nurse keeps other health team members informed of new issues, and shares their input into planning and evaluation of care with the family. Using precise language, giving full and truthful information about the client's condition, and admitting to uncertainty, when it exists, are important dimensions of EOL information giving.

Family Conferences

Family conferences are effective tools to alleviate family anxiety about the dying process, reduce unnecessary conflict between family members, and assist family members with important decision-making processes. Principles related to EOL care, as presented in Box 8-5, offer guidelines for discussions. Gavrin (2007) notes, "the analog of informed consent is informed refusal" (p. S86). This concept becomes important to clients and families as a component of decision making related to withdrawing or withholding life support in EOL care. Although a physician commonly leads the discussion, nurses often present data and answer questions. Data sharing should be

---

| **BOX 8-5** | Principles Guiding End-of-Life Care |

- Discussions of medical futility with patients and family will be more effective if they include concrete information about treatment, its likelihood of success, and the implications of the intervention and nonintervention decisions.
- Effective decision making at the end of life can be improved with the use of advance directives and surrogate decision makers.
- Ethnic and cultural traditions and practices influence the use of advance directives and health care decision-making surrogates.

- Taking the time to explore the client's perceptions about quality of life at the end of life is a core component of clinical assessment and is essential to ensuring optimal outcomes.
- The cost of failing to offer clients and families a full range of end-of-life care options, services, and settings is an incalculable toll in terms of quality of life and utilization of appropriate health care resources at the end of life.

Modified from Bookbinder M, Rutledge DN, Donaldson NE et al.: End-of-life care series: part I: principles, *Online Journal of Clinical Innovations* 4(4):1–30, 2001, by permission. © 2001, Cinahl Information Systems.

compassionate, accurate, and presented in language understandable to the family. Contradictory recommendations and incomplete information add to a family's confusion and cause unnecessary distress (Wright, Wurr, Tomlinson, & Miller, 2009). A coordinated approach prevents fragmentary and inconsistent care.

Curtis (2004) recommends that there be a higher ratio of family member–to–health care provider speaking time, and that there be follow-up communication using a consistent physician-nurse team approach. Helping clients and families understand the importance of advance directives and do not resuscitate (DNR) orders can prevent later conflicts when tensions arise near the time of death (Boyle, Miller, & Forbes-Thompson, 2005). Nurses are invaluable resources in clarifying meanings with clients or individual family members after the conference.

ADDRESSING CULTURAL AND SPIRITUAL NEEDS IN END-OF-LIFE CARE

CULTURAL DIFFERENCES

Different cultures have distinctive communication and care standards for clients with life-threatening conditions, some of which are identified in Box 8-6 (Searight & Gafford, 2005). Other distinctions include: (a) type of care that provides comfort to the dying person; (b) understanding of the causes of illness and death; (c) appropriate care of the body and burial rites; and (d) expression of grief responses (Doolen & York, 2007; LaVera et al., 2002).

Asking clients/families directly about their cultural values and issues as a starting point helps ensure cultural safety for clients and families. A simple question such as "Can you tell me about how your family/culture/spiritual beliefs views serious illness or treatment?" provides a framework for discussion. When cultural differences are considered, it is important to avoid stereotyping, as each person's interpretation of their culture is unique. Once cultural needs are identified, every effort should be taken to honor their meaning to clients and families by incorporating them in care.

SPIRITUAL NEEDS

Glass, Cluxton, and Rancour (2001) note, "The transition from life to death is as sacred as the transition experienced at birth" (p. 49). The dying process, grief, and death itself herald a spiritual crisis—a crisis of faith, hope, and meaning for many people. Spiritual pain occurs when a person's sense of purpose is challenged or one's existence is threatened (Millspaugh, 2005).

Case Example

As I was assessing her, she burst into tears and told me that she thinks "God is punishing her for something and that this is why she has cancer." This was not the first time I heard this from a patient (LaPorte Matzo & Witt-Sherman, 2006, p. 1).

Spirituality becomes a priority for many people at EOL (Williams, 2006). It is not unusual for clients who have previously declined spiritual interventions to desire them as they move into the final phase of life. Spiritual beliefs and religious rituals provide a tangible vehicle for individuals and families to express and experience meaning and purpose. Religious practices and rituals relevant to EOL can be important to clients even if the person no longer formally practices the religion. Facilitating these practices touches the client's inner core and helps the person move toward a peaceful death (Bryson, 2004).

BOX 8-6	Cross-Cultural Variations in End-of-Life Care
• Emphasis on autonomy vs. collectivism • Attitudes toward advance directives • Decisions making about life support, code status guidelines • Preference for direct vs. indirect disclosure of information • Individual vs. family-based decision making about treatment	• Disclosure of life-threatening diagnoses • Provider's choice of words in verbal exchanges • Reliance on physician as the ultimate authority • Specific rituals or practices performed at time of death • Role of religion and spirituality in coping and afterlife • Views about suffering

Adapted from Searight H, Gafford J: Cultural diversity at the end of life: issues and guidelines for family physicians, *American Family Physician* 71(3):515–522, 2005.

Most people welcome an inquiry about their spiritual well-being (Morrison & Meier, 2004). People having a strong relationship with God and/or religious beliefs will usually indicate this connection. To elicit more information about its nature, an appropriate question is: "Is there anything I should know about your spiritual or religious views?" The answer can tell you what is important related to their current circumstances. Steinhauser et al. (2006) suggest that using the probe "Are you at peace?" is a useful way to ask the client about spiritual concerns without being intrusive. Nurses can ask the client and/or family if they would like a visit from an appropriate clergy or hospital chaplain, facilitate the initial contact if the answer is yes and provide essential information about the client's condition and/or family concerns (Barclay & Lie, 2007).

Not all people attach their concept of spirituality to a particular belief system. Instead, they define their spirituality from an existential perspective. Attig (2001) describes this sense of spirituality as follows:

> That within us that reaches beyond present circumstances, soars in extraordinary experiences, strives for excellence and a better life, struggles to overcome adversity, and searches for meaning and transcendent understanding. (p. 37)

When individuals frame their spirituality from an existential perspective, it is appropriate to explore spirituality sources in terms of meaningful relationships. Asking a question such as "Can you tell me about the relationship you had with someone whom you loved who has died?" helps start the conversation. A follow-up question relates to how the client feels about the person now. The value of this intervention is that it emphasizes that the person's life held meaning for this other person. This line of questioning indirectly tells the person that they too will be remembered after death (Pashby, 2010).

People benefit from telling stories about how they view their life and validate its meaning. A life review helps people consider the deeper values and purpose of their lives, the experience of joy and sorrow. As one person stated, "I lived my life as best I could. I have no regrets." A follow-up listening response to help the person put into words what he or she reflect on the meaning of a life well lived might be: "Tell me more about this." Whatever form spiritual distress takes, it is essential for the nurse to address it. Spiritual issues that trouble clients relate to forgiveness, unresolved guilt issues, expressions of love, saying good-bye to important people, and existential questions about the meaning of life, the hereafter, and concern for their family.

Clary and Lawson (2009) suggest that the EOL offers a final opportunity for people to experience spiritual growth. The most important intervention nurses can provide is to actively and respectfully listen to each client's search for clarity about their spirituality with compassion and a desire to understand. Helping clients think through spiritual preferences and assisting them to identify resources that can give them strength, courage, purpose, and encouragement to cope with their situation is highly valued. Providing explicit attention to inclusion of appropriate spiritual advisors, prayer, and scripture reading can be helpful to faith-based clients and families coping with a terminal condition.

Nurses need to take an honest look at their own spirituality. Self-awareness allows nurses to enter their client's spiritual world from an authentic position, without imposing personal values and beliefs. Exercise 8-5 is designed to help nurses understand the value of reflecting on a purposeful life.

SUPPORTIVE STRATEGIES FOR CHILDREN

When a child is diagnosed with a terminal illness or condition, the effect on parents is devastating and can last a lifetime. It can influence role functioning, friendships, and treatment of siblings (Hinds, Schum, Baker, & Wolfe, 2005). Children are such an integral part of their parent's identity that issues of parental protectiveness, guilt, caregiving, balancing family demands, and helplessness must be addressed in the course of providing direct care for the child. When caring for children, there are always two clients to consider: the parent(s) and the child.

Parents are the major anchoring force for most children, so supporting them as primary caregivers for their child is important. They need to be recognized as the expert and primary advocate for their child. Some may not feel they are up to the task, but with appropriate support surprise themselves. Critical to parent satisfaction is knowledge that everything possible was done for their child; that they received accurate, timely information and support; and that preventable suffering was not permitted.

EXERCISE 8-5 | Blueprint for My Life Story

Purpose: To view life as a whole, integrated process.

Procedure:

This is a two-part exercise. First, make a single life line across a blank sheet of paper, beginning with your birth. Identify the significant events in your life and then insert on your worksheet the age that you were when the event or moment occurred. When you are finished, answer the following questions:

Childhood

1. What was your happiest time as a child?
2. What were your saddest times?
3. What did you hope to become when you grew up?
4. Who were your companions as a child?
5. How did you view your mother? Your father? Your grandparents?
6. How did you feel about your home? Your neighborhood?
7. As a child, who was your most important relationship with?
8. Were boys and girls treated alike in school? In the family?
9. Where was your favorite space?
10. Where did you live as a child?

Adolescence

1. What subjects did you like best in school?
2. How and when did you get your first job?
3. Who were your companions as an adolescent, and what did you do with them?
4. Who was your first girlfriend or boyfriend?
5. Who had the most significant influence on you as an adolescent? In what ways?
6. What was most important to you as an adolescent?

Adulthood

1. What was the best job you ever had? The worst?
2. If you could choose your career again, what would you choose?
3. If you could relive any part of your life, what would it be?
4. What parts of your life are you particularly proud of?
5. Look back over your life. When were you happiest? Saddest?
6. What have you learned about life from the process of living?
7. What was the most exciting part of your life?
8. Who has influenced your life most as an adult?
9. If you could make three wishes, what would they be?

Record your answers in whatever way seems most appropriate to you. Spend some time thinking about the events you have identified on your lifeline and the answers you have provided in the narrative. Reflect on your life as a whole, with you as the primary actor, producer, and director. Think about ways in which you could write the remaining chapters of your life so they have special meaning for you.

Discussion:

In the larger group, discuss your lifeline.

1. In what ways were you surprised or comforted by the events that emerged from your lifeline?
2. As you contrast your lifeline with those of your classmates, do common themes emerge?
3. How could you use common themes as the basis for discussion with clients?

Parents often maintain hope for the child's survival even with a terminal diagnosis. This is because of a belief that it is not the natural order of things for a child to die, and because terminal symptom profiles for children are less predictable. Nurses can help identify situations in which there is a mismatch between a child's condition and a parent's understanding of that condition (Field & Behrman, 2002). They can help decrease parental anxiety by explaining changes in the child's appearance, and observing signs of distress in parents and siblings related to the child's progressive deterioration. If the child or family requires additional counseling to reduce stress, nurses can make appropriate referrals. Table 8-2 identifies common goals and provides examples of supportive care for children.

TALKING WITH CHILDREN ABOUT DEATH

Developmental level is a key factor in the child's attitude toward death. A child younger than 5 years has no clear concept of what death means. As a child matures, the finality of death becomes more real. Death is difficult for children because they don't have the cognitive development and life experiences to process them completely. Until children reach the formal operations stage of cognitive development, they can have fantasies about the circumstances surrounding the death, and their part in it.

Children don't express their grief in the same way as adults. Acting out, anger, fear, and crying are common responses, which appear spontaneously. One minute the child may be playing, the next he or she

TABLE 8-2	Common Goals and Examples of Supportive Care for Children
Goal	**Examples of Care**
Physical comfort	Using medications and behavioral interventions to prevent or relieve a child's pain, fatigue, or other symptoms Providing physical therapy to improve function and relieve pain
Emotional comfort	Providing psychotherapy including verbal and play techniques Arranging art, music, or other expressive therapies Encouraging visits from family and friends
Normal life	Informing the child and involving him or her in decisions (consistent with intellectual and emotional maturity) Planning with teachers and administrators for a child's return to school Organizing travel or camp experiences
Family functioning	Helping parents make special time for siblings Arranging respite for parents
Cultural or spiritual values	Accommodating religious rituals and traditional customs Encouraging continuation or adaptation of family holiday traditions
Preparing for death	Planning for parents, siblings, and others to be with the child at and after death Planning for remembrances or legacies of the child's life including pictures, videos, locks of hair, and handprints or hand molds

From Field M, Behrman R: *When children die: improving palliative and end of life care for children and their families* (p. 128). Washington DC, 2002, National Academies Press.

is angry or withdrawn. Preschoolers may repeatedly ask when someone close to them will be coming home even if parents tell them the person has died. Developmentally, they don't understand the permanence of death. Elementary school children accept the permanence of death, but view it in a concrete manner. Adolescents are aware of death as a final act.

Case Example

A short time after 5-year-old Aidan's grandfather died, he asked his grandmother where his grandfather had gone. His grandmother told him that grandpa had died, and was in heaven, to which Aidan said, "Oh no, grandma, he's in that brown box in the ground."

Regardless of age, parents can help their children understand the impending death or loss of a relative by explaining in a concrete, direct way what has happened, using clear, concrete language suitable to the child's developmental level. Children should be encouraged to talk about changes in the health of a parent or the impending death of a central person in their lives. Questions should be answered directly and honestly at the child's developmental level of comprehension. Check in with the child to find out how the child is coping at regular intervals.

The National Cancer Institute (2010) identifies three key concerns of children:

1. Did I cause the death to happen?
2. Is it going to happen to me?
3. Who is going to take care of me?

Parents can anticipate that these will be issues for children, and create opportunities for children to ask these questions. For example, if a child around the same age or a sibling dies, a child may be fearful that something similar will happen to him or her. Maintaining daily routines in the child's life after the death of a parent or primary caregiver is critical. Children need to know that they are safe and will be taken care of by the remaining adults in their life. If changes are needed, children should have ample time to make the adjustment rather than have a sudden move thrust on them without discussion. Children need physical contact, reassurance, and relevant discussions about the person who has died. If parents are unable to provide the level of communication a child needs, nurses can help them with appropriate referrals.

Sometimes a family will want to exclude young children from contact with or knowledge about a person who is likely to die soon. Usually children are aware of what is happening (Loomis, 2009). Encouraging family members to talk with children about changes in their relative's condition using clear, simple terms and allowing them to express their feelings freely is important. Drawing a picture or sending a note can be a useful way for the child to connect with a critically ill relative, if direct contact is not advised. With preparation, adolescents can benefit from being allowed to visit with the client.

Case Example

Brendan and his grandfather had a close relationship. Earlier in life, they would stroke each other's thumbs as part of a "special handshake." Now, at 15, his grandfather was close to death and unresponsive. As Brendan sat next to him, stroking his thumb in the remembered way, he felt sure that his grandfather had squeezed his hand more than once. This was a meaningful connection for Brendan.

HELPING CLIENTS ACHIEVE A GOOD DEATH

The Institute of Medicine (1997) defines a **good death** as "one that is free from unavoidable distress and suffering for patients, families and caregivers; in general accord with patients' and families' wishes; and reasonably consistent with clinical, cultural, and ethical standards" (p. 82). Death is a deeply personal experience. In a study of what constitutes a good death from the perspective of families, clients, and professionals, Steinhauser et al. (2000) identified six elements:

- Pain and symptom relief
- Transparent decision making
- Preparation for what to expect
- Achieving a sense of completion
- Contributing to others
- Receiving affirmation as a whole person

Maintaining a sense of control over what happens during the dying process and who is present at the end, having access to spiritual, emotional, and knowledgeable supports and being afforded hope, dignity, and privacy are also client/family values associated with a good death (Côté & Peplar, 2005; Kirchhoff, 2002; Smith, 2000). Exercise 8-6 provides you with the opportunity to personally think about what constitutes a good death.

SIGNS OF APPROACHING DEATH

As death approaches, there are subtle but significant changes in a person's behavior. With some people, changes are progressive and swift. With others, there is gradual downward spiral. Common symptoms include long periods of sleeping or coma, decreased urinary output, changes in vital signs, disorientation, restlessness and agitation, severe dyspnea (breathlessness), skin temperature, and color. Dying clients experience profound weakness such that they cannot independently complete even basic hygiene.

The process of watching someone die is frightening to families. Family members feel increasingly helpless in being able to properly meet client needs. They need anticipatory guidance about what to expect and concrete suggestions about ways to connect with their loved one. The American Cancer Society Web site offers an excellent description of typical changes in the client when death is near and a clear outline of what caregivers can do to provide comfort to the client. The Internet is an invaluable resource for general information and for family-to-family support. Recommended sites should be carefully screened for accuracy and appropriateness.

Direct comfort care is essential. Practical suggestions for care and availability are critical components of care as clients approach death. Nurses can recommend simple

EXERCISE 8-6	What Makes for a Good Death

Purpose: To help students focus on defining the characteristics of a good death.

Procedure:
1. In pairs or small groups, think about, write down, and then share briefly examples of a "good" and a "not-so-good" death that you have witnessed in your personal life or clinical setting.

2. What were the elements that you thought contributed to its being a "good" or "not-so-good" death?

Discussion:
Were there any common themes found in the stories as to what constitutes a "good" death? How could you use the findings of this exercise in helping clients achieve a "good" death?

care measures such as positioning, mouth and hygiene care, and so forth, to support family member efforts. They can provide immediate assessment data and explain its meaning. Nurses can encourage out-of-town family to visit, refer caregivers to support groups, and offer resource referrals for respite care. Most important, they can listen.

A common concern is the client's loss of appetite and interest in food. Most stop eating. Explaining that this is a natural process that occurs as the body begins to shut down in preparation for death helps with family understanding (Reid, McKenna, Fitsimons, & McCance, 2009). As death approaches, clients become increasingly unresponsive to voice and stimulus. Because hearing is the last sense to go, talking with the dying person in a soft voice, playing calming music, and using gentle touch can soothe the client in a meaningful way.

Creating a care environment in which the dying person feels valued, comforted, and treated as a unique individual (Volker & Limerick, 2007) is vital, even when the client is no longer cognizant of what is happening. Flexibility in allowing family and/or significant others open access to the client, while taking care that the visits are not taxing for the client, reduces family anxiety and can be comforting for all concerned. As clients weaken, they typically want to engage with fewer family and friends. Nurses can act as gatekeepers in helping clients balance their own needs for relationship with the needs of others, and helping everyone concerned to engage with each other in a meaningful way.

COMMUNICATION STRATEGIES

Presence is an important form of communication with dying clients and families. Casarett, Kutner, and Abrahm (2001) assert that simply by being with a family and bearing witness to the family's expression of grief, health care providers provide important emotional and practical support.

Case Example

"I remember standing next to my mom's bed. We had gone to her room to pay our last respects. A young nurse stood near to me and reached out gently and touched my shoulder. Softly she said, 'I'll just stay here with you in case you need something.' When I looked at her I saw eyes brimming with tears and a profound sadness on her face. Her presence meant so much; I was grateful for her open expression of sorrow. It confirmed the pain we were all experiencing" (Anonymous).

Most families find it difficult to leave a dying client, even for a short period. Assuring family members that the nurse will check on the client frequently, and will call the family immediately if change occurs, gives families permission to take a brief respite from the client.

CARING OF THE CLIENT AFTER DEATH

Respect for the dignity of the client continues after death. If the family is present at time of death, allowing uninterrupted private time with the client, before initiating postmortem care is important. If the family is not present, all excess equipment and trash should be removed from the room. You can offer presence and emotional support as you escort the family into the room. Some families will want privacy; others will appreciate having the presence of the nurse or chaplain. Family preference should be honored.

If the family is not immediately present, the client's belongings should be placed in a bag and given to the family after the visitation. Provide soft lighting, chairs for the family, and tissues. The client's head should be elevated at a 30-degree angle, in a natural position. Hair should be combed, exposed body parts cleaned, and dentures replaced, if possible. The tone of the room and the positioning of the client should "give a sense of peace for the family" (Marthaler, 2005, p. 217). It is important for the nurse to allow the family as much time as they need with the client. The nurse can obtain signatures to release the client to the funeral home after the family has spent some time with the client.

Nurses can offer healing presence for the family after death.

Case Example

"A nurse washes the body of a stillborn child, then wraps and brings the baby to the mother and father. She models for them the naturalness of holding their child as they say their goodbyes. She stays close for a while, then she recedes, allowing their privacy. Later she is quietly available as parents make plans for what they will do next. That is healing presence" (Miller, 2001, p. 11).

STRESS ISSUES FOR NURSES IN PALLIATIVE CARE SETTINGS

Nurses deeply invest themselves in the care and comfort of clients and families facing death, and can experience grief when the client dies. **Disenfranchised**

grieving is a term applied to the grief nurses can experience after the death of a client with whom they have had an important relationship (Brosche, 2007; Rushton et al., 2006). Unacknowledged grieving in professional nurses can be cumulative. Unlike their clients, who live through one loss at a time, nurses can experience several losses a week while caring for terminally ill clients and their families (Brunelli, 2005).

Nurses can experience **compassion fatigue**, a syndrome associated with serious spiritual, physical, and emotional depletion related to caring for clients that can affect the nurse's ability to care for other clients (Worley, 2005). Unrelieved compassion fatigue can result in burnout and a nurse's decision to leave nursing.

Case Example

Barbara was a new graduate, selected as a nursing intern on a research oncology unit, providing care for seriously ill pediatric oncology clients. She had a degree in another field and an excellent job, but always wanted to pursue nursing. Her original preceptor left the hospital and was replaced by an efficient nurse without much empathy. The stress of weekly deaths, severe symptomatology, and lack of empathetic support led Barbara to leave nursing entirely after less than a year. She returned to her former position.

Another source of stress is the moral distress associated with helping clients and families resolve conflicts about EOL care (Rushton et al., 2006). For example, the use of technology and life support, and use of phase I or II clinical trial drugs with terminally ill clients can create significant ethical dilemmas for nurses caring for these clients. Support groups in which nurses can successfully address and resolve the secondary stress of continuously caring for terminally ill clients and some of the ethical issues involved with that care are helpful to nurses.

SUMMARY

This chapter describes the stages of death and dying, and theory frameworks of Eric Lindeman and George Engel for understanding grief and grieving. Palliative care is discussed as a philosophy of care and an emerging discipline focused on making EOL care a quality life experience. A good death is defined as a peaceful death experienced with dignity and respect; one that wholly honors the client's values and wishes at the EOL. Nurses can offer compassionate communication, presence, and anticipatory guidance to ease the grief of loss. Seven domains of quality indicators for palliative and EOL care are identified as pain and symptom control, transparent decision making, communication, emotional and practical support, spiritual support, and continuity of care.

Nursing strategies are designed to help clients cope with the secondary psychological and spiritual aspects of having a terminal illness such that they achieve the best quality of life in the time left to them. Talking with clients about advance directives is a professional responsibility of the nurse, and it reduces unnecessary conflict among family members at this critical time in a person's life.

Talking with children about terminal illness and death in a relative, or in coping with a terminal diagnosis themselves should take into consideration the child's developmental level. Questions should be answered honestly and empathetically. Nurses can help families understand the behavioral changes signaling the body's natural shutdown of systems as death approaches. Providing support for clinicians is considered a quality indicator in EOL care. When not addressed, the disenfranchised grief that nurses experience with providing EOL care to multiple clients can lead to compassion fatigue, burnout, and moral distress.

ETHICAL DILEMMA   What Would You Do?

Francis Dillon has been on a ventilator for the past 3 weeks. Although there is virtually no chance of recovery, his family is reluctant to take him off the ventilator. What do you see as the ethical issues, and how would you, as the nurse, address this problem from an ethical perspective?

REFERENCES

American Association of Colleges of Nursing: *End-of-Life Nursing Education Consortium (ELNEC) fact sheet, updated March 2006*, Washington, DC, 2006, Author Available online: http://www.aacn.nche.edu/ELNEC/about.htm, Accessed July 25, 2020.

American Nurses Association: ANA position statements: nursing and the patient self determination acts, *ANA Nursubg World* 1991. Available online: www.nursingworld.org/readroom/position/ethics/etsdet.html.

Atkinson P, Chesters A, Heinz P: Pain management and sedation for children in the emergency department, *Br Med J* 339:b4234, 2009.

Attig T: Relearning the world: making and finding meanings. In Neimeyer R, editor: *Meaning reconstruction and the experience of loss*, Washington, DC, 2001, American Psychological Association, pp 33–53.

Attig T: Meanings of death seen through the lens of grieving, *Death Stud* 28:341–360, 2004.

Barclay L, Lie D: New guidelines issued for family support in patient-centered ICU, *Crit Care Med* 37:605–622, 2007.

Bowes S, Lowes L, Warner J, et al: Chronic sorrow in parents of children with type 1 diabetes, *J Adv Nurs* 65(5):992–1000, 2009.

Boyle D, Miller P, Forbes-Thompson S: Communication and end-of-life care in the intensive care unit, *Crit Care Nurs Q* 28(4):302–316, 2005.

Brosche T: A grief team within a healthcare system, *Dimens Crit Care Nurs* 26(1):21–28, 2007.

Brunelli T: A concept analysis: the grieving process for nurses, *Nurs Forum* 40(4):123–128, 2005.

Bryson KA: Spirituality, meaning, and trancendence, *Palliat Support Care* 2(3):321–328, 2004.

Casarett D, Kutner J, Abrahm J: Life after death: a practical approach to grief and bereavement, *Ann Intern Med* 134(3):208–215, 2001.

Chenitz WC: Living with AIDS. In Flaskerud JH, Ungvarski PJ, editors: *HIV/AIDS: a guide to nursing care*, Philadelphia, 1992, WB Saunders.

Clary P, Lawson P: Pharmacologic pearls for end of life care, *Am Fam Physician* 79(12):1059–1065, 2009.

Corless I: Bereavement. In Ferrell B, Coyle N, editors: *Textbook of palliative nursing*, New York, 2001, Oxford University Press.

Côté J, Peplar C: A focus for nursing intervention: realistic acceptance or helping illusions, *Int J Nurs Pract* 11:39–43, 2005.

Curtis JR: Communicating about end-of-life care with patients and families in the intensive care unit, *Crit Care Clin* 20:363–380, 2004.

Davies E, Higginson J, editors: *Palliative care: the solid facts*, Milan, 2004, European Office of the World Health Organization.

Davis B, Burns J, Rezac D, et al: Family stress and advance directives: a comparative study, *Am J Hosp Palliat Care* 7(4):219–229, 2005.

Dobratz M: The pattern of becoming: self in death and dying, *Nurs Sci Q* 15(2):137–142, 2002.

Doolen J, York N: Cultural differences with end of life care in the critical care unit, *Dimens Crit Care Nurs* 26(5):194–198, 2007.

Engel G: Grief and grieving, *Am J Nurs* 64(7):93–96, 1964.

Erlen J: When patients and families disagree, *Orthop Nurs* 24 (4):279–282, 2005.

Felgelman B, et al: Surviving after suicide loss: the healing potential of suicide survivor support groups, *Illness, Crisis and Loss* 16 (4):285–304, 2008.

Field M, Behrman R: *When children die: improving palliative and end of life care for children and their families*, Washington, DC, 2002, The National Academies Press.

Florczak K: The persistent yet everchanging nature of grieving a loss, *Nurs Sci Q* 21(1):7–11, 2008.

Galanos A: Hospital-based palliative care units: answering a growing need, *N C Med J* 65(4):217–220, 2004.

Glass E, Cluxton D, Rancour P, et al: Principles of patient and family assessment. In Ferrell B, Coyle N, editors: *Textbook of palliative nursing*, New York, 2001, Oxford University Press.

Gavrin J: Ethical considerations at the end of life in the intensive care unit, *Crit Care Med* 35(2):L S85–S94, 2007.

Harvard Womens Health Watch: *Left behind after suicide*, July 2009. Available at: www.health.harvard.edu.

Hinds P, Schum L, Baker J, et al: Key factors affecting dying children and their families, *J Palliat Med* 8(Suppl 1):S70–S78, 2005.

Institute of Medicine: Field MJ, Cassel CK, editors: *Approaching death: improving care at the end of life*, Washington: DC, 1997, National Academy Press.

Jeffries J: *Helping grieving people: a handbook for care providers*, New York, 2005, Brunner-Routledge.

Joint Commission: *The Approaches to pain management: an essential guide for clinical leaders*, ed 2, Oakbrook Terrace, IL, 2010, Joint Commission Resources.

Kirchhoff KT: Promoting a peaceful death in the ICU, *Critical Care Clinics of North America* 14:201–206, 2002.

Kübler-Ross E: *On death and dying: What the dying have to teach doctors, nurses, clergy, and their own families*, New York, 1969, Scribner.

Lafond V: *Grieving mental illness: a guide for patients and their caregivers*, ed 2, Toronto, 2002, University of Toronto Press.

Lang F, Quill T: Making decisions with families at the end of life, *Am Fam Physician* 70(4):719–723, 2004.

LaPorte Matzo M, Witt-Sherman D, editors: *Palliative care nursing: quality care to the end of life*, ed 2, New York, 2006, Springer.

Larson D, Tobin D: End-of-life conversations: evolving practice and theory, *JAMA* 284(12):1573–1578, 2000.

LaVera M, Crawley M, Marshall P, et al: Strategies for culturally effective end of life care, *Ann Intern Med* 136(9):673–677, 2002.

Lee KJ, Dupree C: Staff experiences with end-of-life care in the pediatric intensive care unit, *J Palliat Med* 11(7):986–990, 2008.

Lendrum S, Syme G: *Gift of tears: a practice approach to loss and bereavement counseling*, London, 1992, Routledge.

Levine S: *Unattended sorrow: recovering from loss and reviving the heart*, Emmaus, PA, 2005, Rodale.

Lindemann E: Symptomatology and management of acute grief, *Am J Psychiatry* 151(6 sesquicentennial Suppl):155–160, 1994. (Originally published in 1944).

Loomis B: End of life issues: difficult decisions and dealing with grief, *Nurs Clin North Am* 44:223–231, 2009.

Malloy P, Paice J, Virani R, et al: End of life-nursing education consortium: 5 years of educating graduate nursing faculty in excellent palliative care, *J Prof Nurs* 24(6):352–357, 2008.

Mark Twain Quotations, Newspaper Collections, & Related Resources, 2002. Available online: www.twainquotes.com.

Marthaler MT: End of life care: practical tips, *Dimens Crit Care Nurs* 24(5):215–218, 2005.

McIlfatrick S: Assessing palliative care needs: views of patients, informal carers and healthcare professionals, *J Adv Nurs* 57(1):77–86, 2007.

Mercer D, Evans J: The impact of multiple losses on the grieving process: an exploratory study, *Journal of Loss and Trauma* 11:219–227, 2006.

Miller J: *The art of being a healing presence*, Ft. Wayne, IN, 2001, Willowgreen Publishing.

Millspaugh D: Assessment and response to spiritual pain: part I, *J Palliat Med* 8(5):919–923, 2005.

Mok E, Chiu P: Nurse-patient relationships in palliative care, *J Adv Nurs* 48(5):475–483, 2004.

Morgan A: A grounded theory of nurse-client interactions in palliative care nursing, *J Clin Nurs* 10(4):583–584, 2001.

Morrison RS, Meier DE: Palliative care, *N Engl J Med* 350:2582–2590, 2004.

Mularski R, Curtis J, Billings A, et al: Proposed quality measures for palliative care in the critically ill: a consensus from the Robert Wood Johnson Foundation Critical Care Workgroup, *Crit Care Med* 34: S404–S411, 2006.

National Cancer InstituteNational Institutes of Health: Children and grief. Available online: http://www.cancer.gov/cancertopics/pdq/supportivecare/bereavement/Patient/page9. Accessed January 9, 2010.

National Consensus Project for Quality Palliative Care: *Clinical practice guidelines for quality palliative care*, 2004. Available online: http://www.nationalconsensusproject.org.

Neimeyer RA, editor: *Meaning reconstruction and the experience of loss*, Washington, DC, 2001, American Psychological Association.

Olthuis G, Dekkers W, Leget C, et al: The caring relationship in hospice care: an analysis based on the ethics of the caring conversation, *Nurs Ethics* 13(1):29–40, 2006.

Pashby N (Expert Hospice Nurse): Personal Communication, Odenton, MD, January 15, 2010.

Reid J, McKenna H, Fitsimons D, et al: Fighting over food: patient and family understanding of cancer cachexia, *Oncol Nurs Forum* 36(4):439–445, 2009.

Rushton CH, Reder E, Hall B, et al: Interdisciplinary interventions to improve pediatric palliative care and reduce health care professional suffering, *J Palliat Med* 9:922–933, 2006.

Savory E, Marco C: End of life issues in the acute and critically ill patient, *Scandanavian Journal of Trauma Resuscitation Emergency Medicine* 17:21, 2009.

Schim S, Raspa R: Cross disciplinary boundaries in end-of-life education, *J Prof Nurs* 23(4):201–207, 2007.

Searight H, Gafford J: Cultural diversity at the end of life: issues and guidelines for family physicians, *Am Fam Physician* 71(3):515–522, 2005.

Silveira M, Schneider C: Common sense and compassion: planning for the end of life, *Clinics Family Practice* 6(2):349–368, 2004.

Smith R: A good death, *BMJ* 320:129–130, 2000.

Steinhauser KE, Clipp EC, McNeilly M, et al: In search of a good death: observations of patients, families, and providers, *Ann Intern Med* 132(10):825–832, 2000.

Steinhauser KE, Voils C, Clipp E, et al: Are you at peace?: one item to probe spiritual concerns at the end of life, *Arch Intern Med* 166(1):101–105, 2006.

Thelan M: End of life decision making in intensive care, *Crit Care Nurse* 25(6):28–37, 2005.

Thomas J: *My Saints Alive: A Journey of Life, Loss, and Love*, Unpublished Manuscript, Charlottesville, VA, September 2010.

Volker D, Limerick M: What constitutes a dignified death? The voice of oncology advanced practice nurses, *Clin Nurse Spec* 21(5):241–247, 2007.

Williams AL: Perspectives on spirituality at the end of life: a metasummary, *Palliat Support Care* 4:407–417, 2006.

World Health Organization: *WHO definition of palliative care*, 2008. Available online: http://www.who.int/cancer/palliative/definition/en/. Accessed February 28, 2009.

Worley CA: The art of caring: compassion fatigue (from the editor), *Dermatol Nurs* 17(6):416, 2005.

Wright B, Wurr K, Tomlinson H, et al: Clinical dilemmas in children with life-limiting illnesses: decision making and the law, *Palliat Med* 23:238–247, 2009.

CHAPTER 9

Communication Styles

Kathleen Underman Boggs

OBJECTIVES

At the end of the chapter, the reader will be able to:

1. Describe the component systems of communication.
2. Discuss influence of gender and culture on professional communication.
3. Identify five communication style factors that influence the nurse-client relationship.
4. Discuss how metacommunication messages may affect client responses.
5. Cite examples of body cues that convey nonverbal messages.
6. Discuss application of research studies for evidence-based clinical practice.

This chapter explores styles of communication that serve as a basis for communications in the nurse-client relationship. Effective communication has been shown to produce better health outcomes, greater client satisfaction, and increased client understanding. Style is defined as the manner in which one communicates. Verbal style includes pitch, tone, and frequency. Nonverbal style includes facial expression, gestures, body posture and movement, eye contact, distance from the other person, and so on. These nonverbal behaviors are clues clients provide to us to help us understand their words. Sharpening our observational skills helps us gather data needed for nursing assessments and interventions. Both the client and the nurse enter their relationship with their own specific style of communication. Some individuals depend on a mostly verbal style to convey their meaning, whereas others rely on nonverbal strategies to send the message. Some communicators emphasize giving information; others have as a priority the conveying of interpersonal sensitivity. Longer nurse-client relationships allow each person to better understand the other person's communication style.

BASIC CONCEPTS

METACOMMUNICATION

Communication is a combination of verbal and nonverbal behaviors integrated for the purpose of sharing information. Within the nurse-client relationship, any exchange of information between two individuals also carries messages about how to interpret the communication.

Metacommunication is a broad term used to describe all of the factors that influence how the message is perceived (Figure 9-1). It is a message about how to interpret what is going on. Metacommunicated messages may be hidden within verbalizations or be conveyed as **nonverbal** gestures and expressions. The following case example should clarify this concept.

Case Example

Some studies find greater compliance to requests when they are accompanied by a metacommunication message that demanded a response about the appropriateness of this request:

Continued

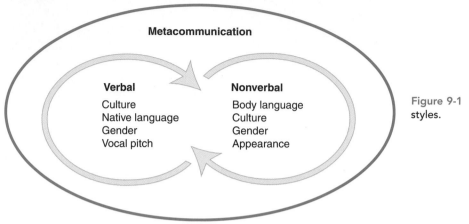

Metacommunication

Verbal
Culture
Native language
Gender
Vocal pitch

Nonverbal
Body language
Culture
Gender
Appearance

Figure 9-1   Factors in communication styles.

Case Example—cont'd

Student (smiling): We nursing students are trying to encourage community awareness in promoting environmental health and are looking for people to hand out fliers. Would you be willing?

(Metacommunication): I realize that this is a strange request, seeing that you do not know who I am, but I would really appreciate your help. I am a nice person.

In this metacommunicated message about how to interpret meaning, the student nurse used both verbal and nonverbal cues. She conveyed a verbal message of caring to her white, middle-class client by making appropriate, encouraging responses, and a nonverbal message by maintaining direct eye contact, presenting a smooth face without frowning, and using a relaxed, fluid body posture without fidgeting.

In a professional relationship, verbal and nonverbal components of communication are intimately related. A student studying American Sign Language for the deaf was surprised that it was not sufficient merely to make the sign for "smile," but rather she had to actually show a smile at the same time. This congruence helped convey her message. You can nonverbally communicate your acceptance, interest, and respect for your client.

VERBAL COMMUNICATION

Words are symbols used by people to think about ideas and communicate with others. Choice of words is influenced by many factors (e.g., your age, race, socioeconomic group, educational background, and sex) and by the situation in which the communication is taking place.

The interpretation of the meaning of words may vary according to the individual's background and experiences. It is dangerous to assume that words have the same meaning for all persons who hear them. Language is useful only to the extent that it accurately reflects the experience it is designed to portray. Consider, for example, the difficulty an American has communicating with a person who speaks only Vietnamese, or the dilemma of the young child with a limited vocabulary who is trying to tell you where it hurts. Our voice can be a therapeutic part of treatment.

Case Example

For weeks while giving care to Mrs. Garcia, a 42-year-old unconscious woman, her nurse used soothing touch and conversation. She also encouraged the client's husband to do the same. When the woman later regained consciousness, she told the nurse that she recognized her voice.

MEANING

There are two levels of meaning in language: denotation and connotation. Both are affected by one's culture. **Denotation** refers to the generalized meaning assigned to a word; **connotation** points to a more personalized meaning of the word or phrase. For example, most people would agree that a dog is a four-legged creature, domesticated, with a characteristic vocalization referred to as a bark. This would be the denotative, or explicit, meaning of the word. When the word is used in a more personalized way, it reveals the connotative level of meaning. "What a dog" and "His bark is worse than his bite" are phrases some people use to describe personal characteristics of human beings, rather than a four-legged creature. We need to be aware that many communications convey only a part of the intended meaning. Don't assume that the meaning of a message is the same for the sender and the receiver until mutual understanding is verified. To be sure you are getting your message across, ask for feedback.

CULTURE

Some people speaking English as a second language say the most difficult aspect is trying to translate the many slang terms and phrases that have double meanings. Extra time is needed when clients are experiencing stress or with clients who speak English as a second language. Use planned spaces of silence, which allows time to understand your meaning and to prepare a response. Verify to make sure that nuances of communication do not get lost.

Culture affects the pitch and tone clients use. For example, the tone of voice used to express anger varies according to culture and family. It may be difficult for you to tell when someone from another culture is angry because their vocalization of strong emotion may be more controlled. By contrast, you might interpret loud conversation with rapid vocalization as conveying anger when it is just a culturally acceptable way to convey emotional intensity. Chapter 11 discusses cultural communication in detail.

VERBAL STYLE FACTORS THAT INFLUENCE NURSE-TO-CLIENT PROFESSIONAL COMMUNICATION

The following six styles of communication are summarized in Table 9-1:

1. *Moderate pitch and tone in vocalization.* The oral delivery of a verbal message, expressed through tone of voice, inflection, sighing, and so on, is referred to as **paralanguage.** It is important to understand this component of communication because it affects how the verbal message is likely to be interpreted. For example, you might say, "I would like to hear more about what you are feeling" in a voice that sounds rushed, high-pitched, or harsh. Or you might make this same statement in a soft, unhurried voice that expresses genuine interest. In the first instance, the message is likely to be misinterpreted by the client, despite your good intentions. Your caring intent is more apparent to the client in the second instance. Voice inflection (pitch and tone), loudness, and fast rate either supports or contradicts the content of the verbal message. Ideas may be conveyed merely by emphasizing different portions of your statement (LeFebvre, 2008). When the tone of voice does not fit the words, the message is less easily understood and is less likely to be believed. A message conveyed in a firm, steady tone is more reassuring than one conveyed in a loud, abrasive, or uncertain manner. In contrast, if you speak in a flat, monotone voice when you are upset, as though the matter is of no consequence, you confuse the client, making it difficult for him to respond appropriately.

2. *Vary vocalizations.* In some cultures, sounds are punctuated, whereas in other cultures, sounds have a lyrical or singsong quality. We need to orient ourselves to the characteristic voice tones associated with other cultures.

3. *Encourage client involvement.* Professional styles of communication have changed over time. We now partner with our clients in promoting

TABLE 9-1	Styles That Influence Professional Communications in Nurse-Client Relationships
Verbal	**Nonverbal**
Moderates pitch and tone	Allows therapeutic silences
Varies vocalizations	Uses congruent nonverbal behaviors
Encourages client involvement	Uses facilitative body language
Validates client's worth	Uses touch appropriately
Advocate for client as necessary	Proxemics
Appropriately provides needed information	Attends to client's nonverbal cues

their optimal health. We expect and encourage our clients to assume responsibility for their own health. Consequently, provider-client communication has changed. Paternalistic, "I'll tell you what to do" styles are no longer acceptable.

4. *Validate client's worth.* Styles that convey "caring" send a message of individual worth that sustains the relationship with the client. For example, clients prefer providers who use a "warm" communication style to show caring, give information, and to allow them time to talk about their own feelings.

   Confirming responses validate the intrinsic worth of the person. These are responses that affirm the right of the individual to be treated with respect. They also affirm the client's autonomy (i.e., his or her right, ultimately, to make his or her own decisions). Disconfirming responses, in contrast, disregard the validity of feelings by either ignoring them or by imposing a value judgment. Such responses take the form of changing the topic, offering reassurance without supporting evidence, or presuming to know what a client means without verifying the message with the client. More-experienced nurses use more confirming communication. These communication skills are learned.

5. *Advocate for client when necessary.* Our personalities affect our style of social communication; some of us are naturally shy. But in our professional relationships, it often becomes necessary that we take on an assertive style of communicating with other health providers or agencies to obtain the best care or services for our client.

6. *Provide needed information appropriately.* Providing accurate information to our client in a timely manner in understandable amounts is discussed throughout this book. In our social conversations there often is a rhythm: "you talk—I listen," then "I get to talk, you listen." However, in professional communications, the content is more goal focused. Self-disclosure from the nurse needs to be limited. Telling a client your problems is not appropriate.

NONVERBAL COMMUNICATION

The majority of person-to-person communication is nonverbal. Think of the most interesting lecturer you ever had. Did this person lecture by making eye

contact? Using hand gestures? Moving among the students? Learners generally are most interested in lecturers whose nonverbal actions convey enthusiasm. The function of nonverbal communication is to give us cues about what is being communicated. Skilled use of nonverbal communication through (therapeutic) silences, use of congruent nonverbal behaviors, body language, touch, proxemics, and attention to client nonverbal cues such as his facial expression can improve your relationship and build rapport with a client (Kacperek, 1997).

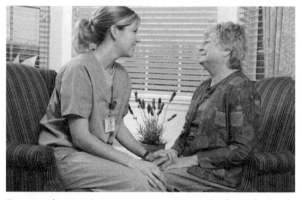

Emotional meanings are communicated through body language, particularly facial expression.

NONVERBAL STYLE FACTORS THAT INFLUENCE NURSE-TO-CLIENT PROFESSIONAL COMMUNICATION

We need to be aware of the position of our nonverbal messages as we talk to our client. Awareness of the position of our hands, the look on our face, and our body movements gives cues to our client (LeFebvre, 2008; Levy-Storms, 2008). It is important to use attending behaviors to convey to the client that his conversation is worth listening to. Think of the last time an interviewer kept fidgeting in his seat, glancing frequently at his wall clock or shuffling papers. How did this make you feel? What nonverbal message was being conveyed? Table 9-1 summarizes the following six nonverbal behaviors of a competent nurse:

1. *Allow silences.* In our social communications, we often become uncomfortable if conversation lags. There is a tendency to rush in to fill the void. But in our professional nurse-client communication, we use silence therapeutically, as

described in Chapter 10, giving our clients needed time to think about things.

2. *Use congruent nonverbal behaviors.* Nonverbal behavior should be congruent with the message and reinforce it. If you knock on your instructor's office door to seek help, do you believe her when she says she'd love to talk if you see her grimace and roll her eyes at her secretary? In another example, if you smile while telling your nurse-manager that your assignment is too much to handle, the seriousness of the message is negated.

Try to give nonverbal cues that are congruent with the message you are verbally communicating (Stovis, 2008). When nonverbal cues are incongruent with the verbal information, messages are likely to be misinterpreted. When your verbal message is inconsistent with the nonverbal expression of the message, the nonverbal expressions assume prominence and are generally perceived as more trustworthy than the verbal content.

You need to comment on any incongruences to help your client. For example, when you enter a room to ask Mr. Sala if he is having any postoperative pain, he may say "No," but he grimaces and clutches his incision. After you comment on the incongruent message, he may admit he is having some discomfort. Can you think of a clinical situation in which you changed the meaning of a verbal message by giving nonverbal "don't believe what I say" cues?

3. *Use facilitative body language. Kinesics* is an important component of nonverbal communication. Commonly referred to as **body language**, it is defined as involving the conscious or unconscious body positioning or actions of the communicator. Words direct the content of a message, whereas emotions accentuate and clarify the meaning of the words. Some nonverbal behaviors such as tilting your head or facing your client promote communication.

- **Posture.** Leaning forward slightly communicates interest and encourages your client to keep the conversation going. Keep your knees unlocked and body loose, not tight and tense.
- **Facial expression.** Six common facial expressions (surprise, sadness, anger, happiness/joy, disgust/contempt, and fear) represent global,

generalized interpretations of emotions common to all cultures. Facial expression either reinforces or modifies the message the listener hears. The power of the facial expression far outweighs the power of the actual words. So try to maintain an open, friendly expression without being boisterously cheerful. Avoid furrowed forehead or a distracted or bored expression.

- **Eye contact.** Making direct eye contact with your client generally conveys a positive message. Most clients interpret direct eye contact as an indication of your interest in what they have to say, although there are cultural differences.
- **Gestures.** Some gestures such affirmative head nodding help facilitate conversation by showing interest and attention. Use of open-handed gestures can also facilitate your nurse-client communication. Avoid folding arms across chest or fidgeting.

4. *Touch.* Touching a client is one of the most powerful ways you have to communicate nonverbally. Within a professional relationship, affective touch can convey caring and reassurance. In studies, nurses' touching clients has been reported to be perceived both positively as an expression of caring and negatively as threat (Harding, North, & Perkins, 2008; Inoue, Chapman, & Wynaden, 2006). Care must be taken to abide by the client's cultural proscriptions about the use of touch. This varies across cultures. An example would be the proscription some Muslim men and Orthodox Jewish men follow against touching women outside of family members. They might be uncomfortable shaking the hand of a female health care provider. In another example, some Native Americans use touch in healing, so that casual touching may be taboo.

All nurses caring directly for clients use touch to assess and to assist. We touch to help our client walk, roll over in bed, and so on. However, just as you are careful about invading the client's personal space, you are careful about when and where on his body you touch your clients. Gender of the nurse nuances the client's perception of the meaning of being touched. Harding et al.'s (2008) findings suggest that in our culture, whereas a woman's touch is seen as a normal expression of caring, we have sexualized male touching. This is a potential problem for male nurses. Therapeutic touch is discussed in Chapter 10.

5. *Proxemics.* We can use physical space to improve our interactions with clients (Buetow, 2009). Proxemics refers to a client's perception of what is a proper distance to be maintained between him and others. Use of space communicates messages. You've heard the phrase "Get out of my face" used when someone stands too close, often interpreted as an attempt to intimidate.

   • Each culture proscribes expectations for appropriate distance depending on the context of the communication. For example, the Nonverbal Expectancy Violations Model defines "proper" social distance for an interpersonal relationship as 1.5 to 4 feet in Western cultures. Americans feel crowded if someone stands closer than 3 feet (Stuart, 2009). The interaction's purpose determines appropriate space, so that appropriate distance in space for intimate interaction would be zero distance, with increased space needed for personal distance, social distance, and public distance. In almost all cultures, zero distance is shunned except for loving or caring interaction. In giving physical care, nurses enter this "intimate" space. Care needs to be taken when you are at this closer distance, lest the client misinterpret your actions. Violating the client's sense of space can be interpreted as threatening.

6. *Attend to Client's Nonverbal Body Cues.*

   • *Posture.* Often, the emotional component of a message can be indirectly interpreted by observing the client's body language. Rhythm of movement and body stance may convey a message about the speaker. For example, when a client speaks while directly facing you, this conveys more confidence than if he turns his body away from you at an angle. A slumped, head-down posture and slow movements might give you an impression of lassitude or low self-esteem, whereas his erect posture and decisive movements suggest confidence and self-control. Rapid, diffuse,

agitated body movements may indicate anxiety. Forceful body movements may symbolize anger. Bowing his head or seeing him slump his body after receiving bad news conveys his sadness. Can you think of other cues your client's body posture might give you?

   • *Facial expression.* Facial characteristics such as frowning or smiling add to the verbal message conveyed. Almost instinctively, we use facial expression as a barometer of another person's feelings, motivations, approachability, and mood. From infancy, we respond to the expressive qualities of another's face, often without even being aware of it. Therefore, assessing our client's facial expression together with his other nonverbal cues may reveal vital information that will affect the nurse-client relationship. Observing your client's facial expressions can signal his feelings. For example, a worried facial expression and lip biting may suggest an anxious client. Absence of a smile in greeting or grimacing may convey a message about how ill the client feels.

   • *Eye contact.* Research suggests that individuals who make direct eye contact while talking or listening create a sense of confidence and credibility, whereas downward glances or averted eyes signal submission, weakness, or shame. In addition to conveying confidence, maintaining direct eye contact communicates honesty (Puetz, 2005). Failure to maintain eye contact, known as *gaze aversion*, is perceived by adults and children as a nonverbal cue meaning that the person is lying to you. If your client's eyes wander around during a conversation, you may wonder if he is being honest. Even 6- and 9-year-olds in Einav and Hood's (2008) study were more likely to attribute lying to those who avert their gaze.

   • *Gestures.* Movements of his extremities may give cues about your client. Making a fist could convey how angry he is, just as use of stabbing, abrupt hand gestures may suggest distress or hugging arms (self-embracing gestures) might suggest fear.

Assessing the extent to which the client uses these nonverbal cues to communicate emotions helps you communicate better. Studies repeatedly show us that failure to acknowledge nonverbal cues is often associated with inefficient communication by the health provider (Mauksch, Dugdale, Dodson, & Epstein, 2008; Uitterhoeve et al., 2008).

It is best if we verify our assessment of the meaning of our client's nonverbal behaviors. Body cues, although suggestive, are imprecise. When communication is limited by the client's health state, pay even closer attention to nonverbal cues. Pain, for example, can be assessed through facial expression even when the client is only partially conscious.

Case Example

A client smiles but narrows his eyes and glares at the nurse. An appropriate comment for the nurse to make might be, "I notice you are smiling when you say you would like to kill me for mentioning your fever to the doctor. It seems that you might be angry with me."

EFFECTS OF SOCIOCULTURAL FACTORS ON COMMUNICATION

Communication is also affected by such factors as gender, cultural background, ethnicity, age, social class, and location.

GENDER

Communication patterns are integrated into gender roles defined by an individual's culture. Gender differences in communication studies have been shown to be greatest in terms of use and interpretation of nonverbal cues. This may reflect gender differences in intellectual style, as well as culturally reinforced standards of acceptable role-related behaviors. Of course, there are wide variations within the same gender.

We are now questioning whether traditional ideas about male and female differences in communication are as prevalent as previously thought. Is there really a major difference in communication according to gender? Not according to many reports. Some studies suggest different styles may be more greatly associated with social status differences in the two communicators rather than being a function of their gender (Helweg-Larsen et al., 2004).

What is factual and what is stereotype? More health care communication studies need to be done before we will really know. Because traditional thinking about gender-related differences in communication content

and process in both nonverbal and verbal communication are being revised, consider critically what you read.

Traditionally, female individuals in most cultures were said to tend to avoid conflict and to want to smooth over differences. They were said to demonstrate more effective use of nonverbal communication and to be better decoders of nonverbal meaning. Feminine communication was thought to be more person centered, warmer, and more sincere. Studies show that women tend to use more facial expressiveness, smile more often, maintain eye contact, touch more often, and nod more often. Women have a greater range of vocal pitch and also tend to use different informal patterns of vocalization than men. They use more tones signifying surprise, cheerfulness, and unexpectedness. Women tend to view conversation as a connection to others.

Traditionally, male individuals in Western cultures were thought to communicate in a more task-oriented, direct fashion, demonstrate greater aggressiveness, and boast about accomplishments. They also have been viewed as more likely to express disagreement. Studies show that men prefer a greater interpersonal distance between themselves and others, and that they use gestures more often. Men are more likely to maintain eye contact in a negative encounter, though overall they maintain less direct eye contact; they use less verbal communication than women in interpersonal relationships. Men are more likely to initiate an interaction, talk more, interrupt more freely, talk louder, disagree more, use hostile verbs, and talk more about issues.

Gender Differences in Communication in Health Care Settings

It has been suggested that more effective communication occurs when the provider of the care and the client are of the same gender, although this was not found to be true in some studies. In professional health care settings, women have been noted to use more active listening, using encouraging responses such as "Uh-huh," "Yeah," and "I see," and to use more supportive words.

CULTURE

Although there is clear evidence that effective communication is related to better client health outcomes, greater client satisfaction, and better compliance, there is less evidence showing how cultural competency directly affects health outcomes. However, there is anecdotal information indicating our communication is perceived through the filter of our client's cultural beliefs. For this reason, our health information is not always relevant to the client. Do you feel skillful in communicating with culturally diverse clients? To communicate as a culturally competent professional, you need to develop an awareness of the values of a specific client's culture and adapt your style and skills to be compatible with that culture's norms. Chapter 11 deals in depth with intercultural communication concepts.

LOCATION

A few studies, such as the one by Wallace et al. (2008), indicate that clients in urban areas report poorer communication by their health care providers. One factor that might affect these results is that rural clients tend to be cared for by the same "usual" providers. In a clinic or other busy location, lack of privacy certainly affects the style, as well as the content of your communication.

Developing an Evidence-Based Practice

Ness SM: Pain expression in the perioperative period: insights from a focus group of Somali women, *Pain Manage Nurs* 10 (2):65–75, 2009.

The verbal and nonverbal expression of pain varies across cultural groups. Expression of pain has not previously been studied in groups of Somali clients treated in the United States. This qualitative research study design used a focus group of four English-speaking postsurgical Somali immigrants to answer the research question: "How do Somali women express and communicate pain?"

Results: These adult women agreed that it was culturally acceptable to verbalize about their pain to anyone, describing it with words like "bad" or "huge," after staff nurses inquired if they were all right with expressing feeling pain (though they stated that only Allah really understands and, therefore, needs to be asked for help). Nonverbally, they believed they needed to be very quiet and make minimal body movements to avoid pain. They reported using sad facial expressions and eye-rolling movements. One very interesting common theme was their feeling of fear, because "in Somalia surgery is only performed for very severe problems ... and then you usually die."

Application to your clinical practice: Because of the small size and methodology of this study, it is difficult to make generalizations to all Somalis. The author believes it is important to communicate before surgery what to expect in the postoperative experience. She recommends that family members be part of this education, both because of the common fear of death and the fact that these women felt bad that they could not carry out their usual duties during their

recovery period. Results support findings from many other studies that indicate that pain needs to be understood within your client's cultural perspective, reflecting its subjective meaning to this person—its psychological, social, and spiritual significance.

APPLICATIONS
KNOWING YOUR OWN COMMUNICATION STYLE

The style of communication you use can influence your client's behavior and his compliance with treatment. According to Milton (2008), evidence suggests clients are dissatisfied with poor communication more than other aspects of their care. Exercises in prior chapters should give you basic skills used in the nurse-client relationship, but you bring your own communication style with you, as does your client. Because we differ widely in our personal communication styles, it is important for you to identify your style and to understand how to modify it for certain clients. Experienced nurses adapt their innate social style so their professional communication fits the client and the situation. Personality characteristics influence your style. For example, would you be described as more shy or assertive? One nurse might be characterized as "bubbly," whereas another is thought of as having a "quiet" manner. Similarly, clients have various styles. You need to make modifications so your style is compatible with client needs. Think about the potential for incompatibility in the following case.

Case Example

Nurse (in a firm tone): Mr. Michaels, it is time to take your medicine.
Mr. Michaels (complaining tone): You are so bossy.

Recognize how others perceive you. Consider all the nonverbal factors that affect a client's perception of you. Your gender, manner of dress, appearance, skin tone, hairstyle, age, role as a student, gestures, or confident mannerisms may make a difference. Exercise 9-1 may increase your awareness of gender bias.

The initial step in identifying your own style may be to compare your style with that of others. Ask yourself, "What makes a client perceive a nurse either as authoritarian or as accepting and caring?" The Exercise 9-2 video may help you to compare your style with that of others. The next step is to develop an awareness of alternative styles that you can

EXERCISE 9-1	Gender Bias

Purpose: To create discussion about gender bias.

Procedure:
In small groups, read and discuss the following comments that are made about care delivery on a geriatric psychiatric unit by staff and students: "Male staff tend to be slightly more confident and to make quicker decisions. Women staff are better at the feeling things, like conveying warmth."

Discussion:
1. Were these comments made by male or female staff?
2. How accurate are they?
3. Can you truly generalize any attribute to all male and female individuals?

EXERCISE 9-2	Self-Analysis of Video Recording

Purpose: To increase awareness of students' own style.

Procedure:
With a partner, role-play an interaction between nurse and client. Video record or use the video capacity of your cell phone to record a 1- to 2-minute interview with the camera focused on you. The topic of the

interview could be "identifying health promotion behaviors" or something similar.

Discussion:
What posture did you use? What nonverbal messages did you communicate? How did you communicate them? Were your verbal and nonverbal messages congruent?

comfortably assume if the occasion warrants. Next, it is important to figure out whether some other factors influence whether your style is appropriate for a particular client. How might their age, race, socioeconomic status, or gender affect their response to you?

INTERPERSONAL COMPETENCE

As early as 1984, Kasch proposed that nurse-client communication processes are based on the nurse's interpersonal competence. **Interpersonal competence** develops as the nurse comes to understand the complex cognitive, behavioral, and cultural factors that influence communication. This understanding, together with the use of a broad range of communication skills, helps you interact with your client as he or she attempts to cope with the many demands placed on him or her by the environment. Good communication skills are associated with competency. Competent communication skills are identified as one of the attributes of expert nurses who were perceived as having clinical credibility (Smith, 2005). In dealing with the client in the sociocultural context of the health care system, two kinds of abilities are required: social cognitive competency and message competency.

Social cognitive competency is the ability to interpret message content within interactions from the point of view of each of the participants. By embracing the client's perspective, you begin to understand how the client organizes information and formulates goals. This is especially important when your client's ability to communicate is impaired by mechanical barriers such as a ventilator. Clients who recovered from critical illnesses requiring ventilator support reported fear and distress during this experience.

Message competency refers to the ability to use language and nonverbal behaviors strategically in the intervention phase of the nursing process to achieve the goals of the interaction. Communication skills are used as a tool to influence the client to maximize his adaptation. When your instructor responds to your answer with a smile and affirmative head nod, saying, "Great answer," doesn't this make you feel successful?

STYLE FACTORS THAT INFLUENCE RELATIONSHIPS

The establishment of trust and respect in an interpersonal relationship with client and family is dependent on open, ongoing communication style. Having

BOX 9-1	Suggestions to Improve Your Communication Style

- Adapt yourself to your client's cultural values.
- Use nonverbal communication strategies, such as:
  - Maintain eye contact.
  - Display pleasant, animated facial expressions.
  - Smile often.
  - Nod your head to encourage the client to continue talking.
  - Maintain attentive, upright posture and sit at his or her level, leaning forward toward the client slightly.
  - Attend to proper proximity and increase space if client shows signs of discomfort, such as gaze aversion, leg swinging, or rocking.
  - Use touch with client if appropriate to the situation.
- Use active listening and respond to client's cues.
- Use verbal strategies to engage your client.
  - Use humor, but avoid gender jokes.
  - Attend to proper tone and pitch, avoiding being overly loud.
  - Avoid using jargon.
  - Use nonjudging language and open-ended questions.
  - Listen and avoid jumping in too soon with problem solving.
- Verbalize respect for client.
  - Ask permission before addressing client by his first name.
  - Convey caring comments.
- Use confirming, positive comments.

knowledge of communication styles is not sufficient to guarantee successful application. You need to understand how the materials discussed in this chapter interrelate. For example, providers who sit at client's eye level, at optimal distance (proxemics), without furniture between them (special configuration) will likely have more eye contact and use more therapeutic touching (Gorawara-Bhat, Cook, & Sachs, 2007). Box 9-1 contains suggestions to improve your own professional style of communicating.

SLANG AND JARGON

Different age groups even in the same culture may attribute different meanings to the same word. For example, an adult who says, "That's cool," might be referring to the temperature, whereas a teenager might convey his satisfaction by using the same phrase. In health care, the "food pyramid" is understood by nurses to represent the basic nutritional food groups needed for health; however, the term may have limited meaning for individuals not in the health professions.

MEDICAL JARGON

Beginning nursing students often report confusion while learning all the medical terminology required for their new role. Remembering our own experiences, we can empathize with clients who are attempting to understand their own health care. Careful explanations help clients overcome this communication barrier. For successful communication, words used should have a similar meaning to both individuals in

the interaction. An important part of the communication process is the search for a common vocabulary so that the message sent is the same as the one received. Consider the oncology nurse who develops a computer databank of cancer treatment terms. When admitting Mr. Michaels as a new client, the nurse uses an existing template model on her computer to create an individualized terminology sheet with just the words that would be encountered by him during his course of chemotherapy treatment.

RESPONSIVENESS OF PARTICIPANTS

How responsive the participants are affects the depth and breadth of communication. Reciprocity affects not only the relationship process, but also client outcomes (Sheldon & Ellington, 2008). Some clients are naturally more verbal than others. It is easier to have a therapeutic conversation with extroverted clients who want to communicate. You will want to increase the responsiveness of less verbal clients and enhance their communication responsiveness. Verbal and nonverbal approval encourages clients to express themselves. Elsewhere, we discuss skills that promote responsiveness such as active listening, demonstration of empathy, and acknowledgment of the content and feelings of messages. Sometimes acknowledging the difficulty your client is having expressing certain feelings, praising efforts, and encouraging use of more than one route of communication helps. Such strategies demonstrate interpersonal sensitivity. Studies show that listening to the care experience of a client, responding to verbal or nonverbal cues, and not

EXERCISE 9-3	Confirming Responses

Purpose: To increase students' skills in using confirming communication.

Procedure:
Change these disconfirming, negative messages into positive, confirming, caring comments.
1. "Three of your 14 blood sugars this week were too high. What did you do wrong?"

2. "Your blood pressure is dangerously high. Are you eating salty foods again?"
3. "You gained five pounds this week. Can't you stick to a simple diet?"

Discussion:
Was it relatively easy to send a positive, confirming message?

"talking down" empowered open speaking (Sadler, 2008; Uitterhoeve et al., 2008). A responsive care provider has been shown to improve compliance with the treatment regimen in multiple studies. Exercise 9-3 will help you practice using confirming responses.

ROLES OF PARTICIPANTS

Paying attention to the role relationship of the communicators may be just as important as deciphering the content and meaning of the message. The relationships between the roles of the sender and of the receiver influence how the communication is likely to be received and interpreted. The same constructive criticism made by a good friend and by one's immediate supervisor is likely to be interpreted differently, even though the content and style are quite similar. Communication between subordinates and supervisors is far more likely to be influenced by power and style than by gender. When roles are unequal in terms of power, the more powerful individual tends to speak in a more dominant style. This is discussed in Chapter 23.

CONTEXT OF THE MESSAGE

Communication is always influenced by the environment in which it takes place. It does not occur in a vacuum but is shaped by the situation in which the interaction occurs. Taking time to evaluate the physical setting and the time and space in which the contact takes place, as well as the psychological, social, and cultural characteristics of each individual involved, gives you flexibility in choosing the most appropriate context.

INVOLVEMENT IN THE RELATIONSHIP

Relationships generally need to develop over time because communication changes with different phases of the relationship. Uitterhoeve and colleagues (2008) validated prior research showing that nurses respond

to less than half of client concerns, and tend to focus on physical care whereas ignoring client's social emotional care. In these days of managed care, nurses working with hospitalized clients have less time to develop a relationship, whereas community-based nurses may have greater opportunities. To begin to explore ethical problems in your nursing relationships, consider the ethical dilemma provided.

ADVOCATE FOR CONTINUITY OF CARE

DeVoe et al.'s (2008) study showed that client's perception of positive health care communication is higher when the same individuals provide their care. These providers were more likely to listen to them, to explain things clearly, to spend enough time with them, and to show them respect. Because physicians and nurses communicate differently with clients, it is crucial that these professionals pool their information.

SUMMARY

Communication between nurse and client or nurse and another professional involves more than the verbalized information exchanged. Suggestions for improving your communication style are provided. Professional communication, like personal communication, is subtly altered by changes in pitch of voice and use of accompanying facial expressions or gestures. This chapter explores factors related to effective styles of verbal and nonverbal communication. Cultural and gender differences associated with each of these three areas of communication are discussed. For professionals, maintaining congruence is important. Style factors that affect the communication process include the responsiveness and role relationships of the participants, the types of responses and context of the relationships, and the level of involvement in the relationship. Confirming responses acknowledge the value of a person's communication, whereas disconfirming responses discount the validity of a person's feelings. More nonverbal strategies to facilitate nurse-client communication are discussed in later chapters.

ETHICAL DILEMMA   What Would You Do?

Katy Collins, RN, is a new grad who learns that a serious error has occurred on her unit that harmed a client. She realizes that if staff continue to follow the existing protocol, there is a risk this error will occur again. In a team meeting lead by an administrator, Katy raises this issue in a tentative manner. The leader speaks in a loud, decisive voice and states he wants input from the staff nurses. However, he glances at the clock, gazes over her head, and maintains a bored expression. Katy gets the message that the administration wants to smooth over the error, bury it, and go on as usual, rather than using resources and time to correct the underlying problem.

1. What ethical principle is being violated in this situation?
2. What message does the administrator's behavior convey?
3. Is his verbal and nonverbal message congruent?
4. What would you do if you were in Katy's place?

REFERENCES

Buetow SA: Something in nothing: negative space in the clinician-patient relationship, *Ann Fam Med* 7(1):80–83, 2009.

DeVoe JE, Wallace LS, Pandhi N, Solotaroff R, Fryer GE: Comprehending care in a medical home: a usual source of care and patient perceptions about healthcare communication, *J Am Board Fam Med* 21(5):441–450, 2008.

Einav S, Hood BM: Tell-tale eyes: children's attribution of gaze aversion as a lying cue, *Dev Psychol* 44(6):1655–1667, 2008.

Gorawara-Bhat R, Cook MA, Sachs GA: Nonverbal communication in doctor-elderly patient transactions [NDEPT]: development of a tool, *Patient Educ Couns* 66(2):223–234, 2007.

Harding T, North N, Perkins R: Sexualizing men's touch: male nurses and the use of intimate touch in clinical practice, *Res Theory Nurs Pract* 22(2):88–102, 2008.

Helweg-Larsen M, Cunningham SJ, Carrico A, et al: To nod or not nod: an observational study of nonverbal communication and status in female and male college students, *Psychol Women Q* 28(4):358–362, 2004.

Inoue M, Chapman R, Wynaden D: Male nurses' experiences of providing intimate care for women clients, *J Adv Nurs* 55(5):559–567, 2006.

Kacperek L: Non-verbal communication: the importance of listening, *Br J Nurs* 6(5):275–279, 1997.

Kasch CC: Communication in the delivery of nursing care, *Adv Nurs Sci* 6:71–88, 1984.

LeFebvre KB: Strengthen your verbal and nonverbal communication, *ONS Connect* 23(9):21, 2008.

Levy-Storms L: Therapeutic communication training in long-term institutions: recommendations for future research, *Patient Educ Couns* 73:8–21, 2008.

Mauksch LB, Dugdale DC, Dodson S, Epstein R: Relationship, communication, and efficiency in the medical encounter, *Arch Intern Med* 168(13):1387–1395, 2008.

Milton C: Boundaries: ethical implications for what it means to be therapeutic in the nurse-person relationship, *Nurs Sci Q* 21(1):18–21, 2008.

Puetz BE: The winning job interview, *Am J Nurs* (Career Guide 2005 Supp):30–32, 2005.

Sadler C: Listen and learn, *Nurs Stand* 22(28):22–23, 2008.

Sheldon LK, Ellington L: Application of a model of social information processing to nursing theory: how nurses respond to patients, *J Adv Nurs* 64(4):388–398, 2008.

Smith CS: Identifying attributes of clinical credibility in registered nurses, *Nurs Adm Q* 29(2):188–191, 2005.

Stovis TL: The art of communication: strategies to improve patient and information flow: radiology perspective, *Pediatr Radiol* (Suppl 4):S651–S654, 2008.

Stuart GW: *Principles and practice of psychiatric nursing*, ed 9, St. Louis, 2009, Mosby/Elsevier.

Uitterhoeve R, de Leeuw J, Bensing J, et al: Cue-responding behaviors of oncology nurses in video-simulated interviews, *J Adv Nurs* 61(1):71–80, 2008.

Wallace LS, DeVoe JE, Bennett IM, Roskos SE, Fryer GE: Perceptions of healthcare providers' communication skills: do they differ between urban and nonurban residents? *Health Place* 14:653–660, 2008.

CHAPTER 10

Developing Therapeutic Communication Skills

Elizabeth C. Arnold

OBJECTIVES

At the end of the chapter, the reader will be able to:

1. Discuss the concept of therapeutic communication.
2. Describe the characteristics of client-centered communication.
3. Apply communication strategies and skills in client-centered relationships.
4. Discuss active listening responses used in therapeutic communication.
5. Discuss the use of verbal responses as a communication strategy.
6. Describe other forms of communication used in nurse-client relationships.

Communication is an important cornerstone of all clinical encounters. This chapter focuses on therapeutic communication skills and strategies that nurses need to support, educate, and empower people to effectively cope with their health-related issues. The chapter reviews the purpose and components of therapeutic communication, using a client-centered focus. Applications describe active listening responses, verbal communication strategies, and other communication techniques applicable in nurse-client relationships.

BASIC CONCEPTS

THERAPEUTIC COMMUNICATION

Therapeutic communication, a term first coined by Jurgen Ruesch in 1961, refers to an interactive dynamic process entered into by nurse and client for the purpose of achieving identified health-related goals. It takes place within the context of a healing conversation, and encompasses both verbal and nonverbal components. Therapeutic communication skills serve as fundamental building blocks for the development of effective therapeutic relationships.

It differs from "social chit chat" in that it promotes the client's personal development (Peplau, 1960, p. 964). Therapeutic communication is the primary means through which nurse and client exchange information about health matters, plan treatment approaches, reach consensus about treatment decisions, conduct treatment activities, and evaluate clinical outcomes. It is the basis for developing the working partnerships between client and health providers needed to support improved treatment outcomes.

Each therapeutic conversation is unique because the people holding them are different (Caughan & Long, 2000). Communication techniques are similar to those used spontaneously in social situations, with notable modifications. Therapeutic conversations have a specific health related purpose. They take place within a defined health care format and are time limited. These conversations are subject to federal guidelines and professional standards regarding confidentiality and protected information. Characteristics of therapeutic communication are displayed in Figure 10-1. Therapeutic communication is client centered and uses a deliberate, health-focused dialogue. Direct interaction comes to an end

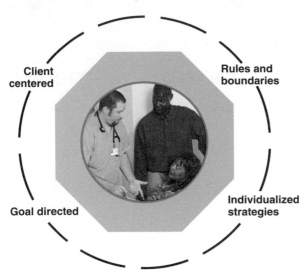

Figure 10-1   Characteristics of therapeutic communication.

when health goals are achieved, clients are discharged, or clients are referred to a different care setting.

PURPOSE OF THERAPEUTIC COMMUNICATION

Therapeutic conversations offer a safe, empathetic way for clients to explore the meaning of their illness experience and to learn the best ways of coping with it. Therapeutic conversations tell the story of a personal illness, with nurse and client both contributing to the telling of it.

Quality clinical communication is essential to achieving positive health outcomes and client satisfaction. Interpersonal communication skills influence the completeness of diagnostic information, compliance with treatment, and client satisfaction with care. "Good" clinical experiences typically involve human communication encounters in which human needs are respected and the humanity of the clinician is transparent. With "negative" clinical encounters, clients experience disconnects with the knowledge and interpersonal care the client or family expects from the provider. Poor communication is implicated as a key factor in clinical safety errors and malpractice allegations.

ESSENTIAL COMPONENTS

Fundamental components of communication—sender, receiver, message, channels, and context—are also applied to therapeutic communication. Therapeutic communication is a reciprocal process that begins

with active listening (Bush, 2001). Active listening combines verbal and nonverbal components of a message into an integrated, meaningful whole.

Active listening is a dynamic process in which a nurse hears a client's message, decodes its meaning, asks questions for clarification, and provides feedback to the client. Active listening allows people to offer presence and to bear witness to one another (Kagan, 2008). Attentive listening for the client's perspective without making judgments and also using listening responses increase understanding.

The goal of active listening is to fully understand what the client is trying to communicate through his or her story. As you ask clarifying questions and share your own thinking process about what you are hearing, you are developing a more in-depth understanding of the health care situation from the client's perspective.

Included in each participant's communicated message are important nonverbal instructions (**metacommunication**) about the interpretation of the message. If a nurse sits down in a relaxed position with good eye contact and actively listens, the verbal and nonverbal message of interest is congruent. The same verbal message, delivered while looking at the clock or a watch, provides a nonverbal message that the nurse doesn't have time to listen. When verbal and the nonverbal messages are congruent, the message is credible. If the two are incongruent, it creates doubt in the mind of the listener, and the message is suspect. If you notice nonverbal behaviors that seem to contradict words, or the client seems sad or distracted, you might want to call the client's attention to the discrepancy with a simple statement, such as, "You seemed quite animated yesterday; I notice that you seem a little subdued today. Is something going on that we should talk about?"

Verbal responses refer to the spoken words people use to communicate with each other. Unlike the written word, they cannot be erased, although they can be explained, or modified. Words are the primary means through which nurse and client will organize data about problems, explore different options, make meaning of experiences, and dialogue with each other. The meaning of words resides in the person who uses them, not in the words themselves. When languages or word connotations differ, meaning changes. Nurses should pay close attention to the client's verbal expression and forms of language (Kettunen, Poskiparta, & Liimatainen, 2001) and mirror them, when possible. Verbal responses should be clear, complete, and easily understandable. Choice of words is important. Words should neither overstate nor understate the situation. Words are not the sole source of meaning. Nadzam (2009) notes, "Communication is not just about what a person says, but how he or she says it" (p. 184). Nurses also need to be sensitive to what is left out of the message, as well as to what is included. How words are used should not cast doubt on the implications of the message. Straightforward messages are trustworthy. Vague messages are not.

Both words and nonverbal behaviors are subject to misinterpretation. Nurses need to check in with clients to ensure the accuracy of their perceptions. You can simply say, "I'd just like to check in with you to make sure that I understand. Are you saying that...?"

FACTORS THAT AFFECT COMMUNICATION
Personal Factors

Readiness to engage in therapeutic relationships is influenced by personal and environmental factors that the nurse should take into consideration when relating to clients and families. Eye contact, genuine respect for the client, and clear, concise messages are fundamental tools. Words that respect a person's culture, spiritual beliefs, and educational level capture the client's attention. Conversely, words that disregard or dismiss the fundamental personhood of the client or family as being less important than that of the health care provider cause unnecessary damage.

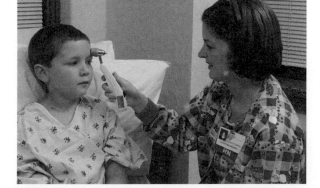

Whether you are sitting or standing, your posture should be relaxed, with the upper part of your body inclined slightly toward the client.

People communicate nonverbally through body language, eye contact, and level of attention. The nurse consciously uses body language, gestures, and minimal verbal cues to encourage further communication. Physical cues are used to accentuate words or connect with people nonverbally, as well as verbally (Box 10-1).

Communication breaks down when the nurse or client do not share the same understanding of messages. Barriers to effective communication occur in clients when they are:

- Preoccupied with pain, physical discomfort, worry, or contradictory personal beliefs
- Unable to understand the nurse's use of language or terminology
- Struggling with an emotionally laden topic
- Feeling defensive, insecure, or judged
- Confused by the complexity of the message—too many issues, tangential comments
- Deprived of privacy, especially if the topic is a sensitive one
- Have hearing or cognitive deficits that compromise receiving accurate messages

Barriers within the nurse occur when the nurse is not fully engaged with the client for the following reasons:

- Preoccupation with personal agendas
- Being in a hurry to complete physical care
- Making assumptions about client motivations
- Cultural stereotypes
- Defensiveness or personal insecurity about being able to help the client
- Thinking ahead to the next question
- Client emotionality or aggressiveness

Exercise 10-1 is designed to help students identify difficult communication issues in nursing practice.

PROFESSIONAL SELF-AWARENESS

Client-centered communication requires greater self-awareness. Nurses must become aware of their behaviors and responses, and recognize the sometimes unintentional effects these may have on the communication process.

Knowing your own biases and values is critical. Communication can be limited by a nurse's standards concerning, for example, different sexual preferences, alcoholism, and teenage pregnancy. Nurses may feel intimidated by clients who have higher social status, education, or influence, and respond in subtle ways to these differences. Caring for clients who refuse to comply with treatment or who have given up can be a communication challenge for the nurse.

| BOX 10-1 | Physical Behavioral Cues |

Emblems: Gestures or body motions having a generalized verbal interpretation (e.g., handshaking, baby waving bye-bye, sign language).

Illustrators: Actions that accompany and exemplify the meaning of the verbal message. Illustrators are used to emphasize certain parts of the communication (e.g., smiling, a stern facial expression, pounding the fist on a table). Illustrators usually are not premeditated.

Affect displays: Facial presentation of emotional affect. Similar to the illustrators just discussed, the sender has more control over their display (e.g., a reproving look, an alert expression, a smile or a grin, a sneer). Affect displays seem to be more pervasive nonverbal expressions of the client's emotional state. They have a larger range of meaning and act to support or contradict the meaning of the verbal message. Sometimes the generalized affect is not related to a specific verbal message (e.g., a depressed client may have a retarded emotional

affect throughout the relationship that has little to do with the communicated message).

Regulators: Nonverbal activities that adjust the course of the communication as the receiver gives important information to the sender about the impact of the message on the sender. Regulators include nodding, facial expressions, some hand movements, and looking at a watch.

Adaptors: Characteristic, repetitive, nonverbal actions that are client specific and of long duration. They give the nurse information about the client's usual response to difficult emotional issues. Sample behaviors include a psychogenic tic, nervous foot tapping, blushing, and twirling the hair.

Physical characteristics: Nonverbal information about the client that can be gleaned from the outward appearance of the person (e.g., skin tone, descriptions of height and weight and relation to body shape, body odor, physical appearance [dirty hair, unshaven, teeth missing or decayed]).

Adapted from Blondis M, Jackson B: *Nonverbal communication with patients: back to the human touch* (pp. 9–10), ed 2, New York, 1982, Wiley.

| EXERCISE 10-1 | Identifying Difficult Communication Issues |

Purpose: To help students identify common complicated communication issues with clients.

Procedure:
In groups of three to five students:
1. In round robin fashion, each student should share an elevator version of a nursing experience that illustrates a challenging communication encounter you have had or witnessed in a nurse-client encounter.
2. Identify what qualities made it difficult.

3. Describe what you did or would do next time to make it a positive experience for the client, nurse, or both.

Discussion:
1. Were there any common themes that your group found in the identified communication challenges?
2. Explore the insights you gained from doing this exercise.
3. How could you use what you learned from doing this exercise in your future nursing practice?

Self-awareness of personal prejudices and stereotypes allows nurses to separate the person from the behavior or problem, and to maintain the patience, neutrality, and understanding needed for therapeutic communication. Nurses have an ethical and professional responsibility to resolve personal issues so that countertransference feelings do not affect communication.

ENVIRONMENTAL FACTORS

Privacy, space, and timing are important factors that nurses need to consider. Clients need privacy, free from interruption and elimination of noise for meaningful conversations. "Noise" refers to any distraction,

which interferes with being able to pay full attention to the discussion (Weiten, Lloyd, Dunn & Hammer, 2009). For example, TV or music can be distracting.

People require different amounts of personal space for conversation (Hall, 1959). Therapeutic conversations typically take place within a social distance (3–4 feet is optimal). Culture, personal preference, nature of the relationship, and the topic will influence personal space needs. Clients experiencing high anxiety may need more physical space, whereas clients experiencing a sudden physical injury or undergoing a painful procedure appreciate having the nurse in closer proximity. Sitting at eye level with bedridden clients is helpful.

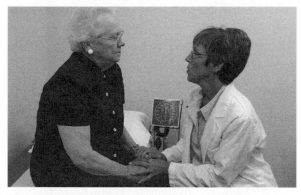

Most conversations take place within a social distance.

Timing is critical. Planning communication for periods when the client is able to participate physically and emotionally is both time-efficient and respectful of the client's needs. Clients must be given enough time to absorb material, to share their impressions, and to ask questions.

Client behavior can cue the nurse about emotional readiness and available energy. The presence of pain or variations in energy levels, anger, or anxiety will require extra time to inquire about the change in the client's behavior and its meaning, before proceeding with the health care dialogue.

CLIENT-CENTERED COMMUNICATION

CHARACTERISTICS

Client-centered care and collaborative partnerships in current health care deliverables require a broader span of communication skills. In the past, healing relationships were important sources of clinician information and expertise, which was shared with clients. Today, clients are viewed as equally important informational resources and collaborators in health care. Clients expect emotional support and guidance to assume greater personal responsibility for their health care. They not only require their clinicians to be technically competent; they expect them to be sensitive and accommodating of their concerns and treatment preferences. Clients want to be listened to, involved in their own care, and able to choose between treatment options. Epstein and Street (2007) identify six core, overlapping functions of patient-centered communication needed to achieve beneficial health outcomes.

- Fostering healing relationships
- Exchanging information
- Responding to emotions

- Managing uncertainty
- Making decisions
- Enabling patient self-management (p. 17)

Client-centered communication is an interactive reciprocal exchange of ideas in which nurses try to understand what it is like to be *this* person in *this* situation with *this* illness. Each client and family has its unique set of values, patterns of behavior, and preferences that must be taken into account. How clients communicate with the nurse varies, based on culture and social background factors. Client readiness to learn, personal ways of relating to others, physical and emotional conditions, life experiences, and place in the life cycle are related factors in planning and implementing contemporary care through therapeutic communication.

Client-centered conversations are structured to be person focused rather than problem focused. They include discussions needed for collaborative decision making and teaching clients self-management skills. Talking about complex health problems with a trained health professional allows clients and families to hear themselves, as they put health concerns into words. The feedback provided by the health professional ideally helps clients realistically sort out priorities and determine the actions they want to take in effectively coping with their health circumstances.

ACTIVE LISTENING IN CLIENT-CENTERED CONVERSATIONS

Active listening is an intentional form of listening, which contributes to fewer incidents of misunderstanding, more accurate information, and stronger health relationships (Straka, 1997). Listening responses in a client-centered health environment ask about *all* relevant client health concerns, and take into account the client's values, preferences, and expectations related to treatment goals, priorities, and attitudes about treatment suggestions. Queries might include open-ended questions such as "What is important to you now?" or "What are you hoping will happen with this treatment?" Sufficient information to support client decision-making and self-management of health problems is expected. Validation of client preferences might consist of asking the client, "How does the idea of _____ sound to you?" or "How easy will it be for you to learn to use your crutches?" Adding these questions may seem time consuming. If the answers lead to greater compliance and client satisfaction, then it may be more time efficient.

Developing an Evidence-Based Practice

McCabe C: Nurse-patient communication: an exploration of patients' experiences, *J Clin Nurs* 13:41–49, 2004.

This qualitative study was designed to elicit patient experiences of how nurses communicate. The study used a hermeneutic phenomenologic methodology to analyze data from unstructured interviews. A purposive sample of eight patients in a general hospital was interviewed. The researcher used a reflective process of describing and interpreting themes and subthemes, and yielded four themes related to the patient's experience of how nurses communicated with them.

Results: Identified were lack of communication, attending, empathy, and friendly nurses. The lack of communication perceived by patients related to nurses making assumptions about their concerns and needs.

Application to Your Clinical Practice: As a profession, nurses need to develop patient-centered communication, which involves letting patients know the nurse recognizes their feelings. What steps could you take to ensure that your patients feel heard?

APPLICATIONS
APPLYING CONCEPTS OF CLIENT-CENTERED COMMUNICATION

BUILDING RAPPORT

A client-centered communication process starts with the first encounter. Your initial presentation of yourself will influence the communication that follows. Your client should have your full attention. Entering the client's space with an open, welcoming facial expression, respectful tone, and direct eye contact declares your interest and intent to know this person.

Communication involves the whole self. Your posture immediately gives a message to the client, either inviting trust or conveying disinterest. Whether you are sitting or standing, your posture should be relaxed, facing the client and leaning slightly forward.

Introduce yourself and identify the client by name before beginning conversation. Introductions are important, especially if many health professionals are involved in the client's care (Van Servellen, 2009). When more than the client is involved in a discussion, expand the introductions if you are meeting other people for first time. It is important to center your attention on the client, but not ignore other family members. Speak directly to the client, but include family members with eye contact, physical cues, and so forth. Eye contact is an important inclusive gesture.

Keep in mind that clients will vary in their ability to effectively communicate their feelings, preferences, and concerns (Epstein & Street, 2007). Even their willingness to treat their clinicians as partner rather than absolute authority can reflect personality features, communication style, socioeconomic status, previous life experiences, and education level. Considering these factors allows you to phrase questions and interpret answers in meaningful ways.

Being fully present, providing relevant information, and listening to client concerns help build rapport through personalized communication. Clients who feel safe, accepted, and validated by their nurses find it easier to collaborate with them. Although rapport building begins with the initial encounter, it continues as a thread throughout the nurse-client relationship. Remember that clients are looking to you for not only competence, but for sincerity and genuine interest in them as individuals.

A client-centered communication process seeks to understand critical links between the client's life experiences and values, and their current health problems. Nurses should strive to understand the *whole* person, including information from and about family members affected by the client's illness.

The goal of client-centered communication is to find common ground related to identification of client problems, priorities, and treatment goals. Nurses need to understand what aspects of care are most important to a client and family, and what helps or hinders their capability to self-manage their health problems. Clients need to understand the full range of therapeutic choices available to them in treating and self-managing their illness.

The idea of health care as a shared partnership in which the client is an *equal* stakeholder and communicator in ensuring quality health care is relatively new. Building rapport requires:

- Empathetic objectivity, which allows you to experience clients as they are, not the way you would like them to be
- A "here and now" focus on the current issues and client concerns
- Demonstration of respect, and asking questions about cultural and social differences that can influence treatment

- Authentic interest in the client and a confident manner that communicates competence
- The capability to consider competing goals and alternative ways to meet them

Exercise 10-2 is designed to increase the student's understanding of communication strategies using a client-centered focus.

OBSERVATION

There are different "channels" of nonverbal communication (e.g., facial expressions, vocal tones, gestures and body positions, body movements, touch, and personal space). Take note of whether cues such as the client's facial expression, body movements, posture, and breathing rate support or negate the meaning of the spoken message.

Burgoon, Guerrero, & Floyd (2009) note up to 65% of interpersonal communication is nonverbal. Clients cannot always put their concerns into words. Some are not aware of them. Others experience powerful emotions that make verbalizing personal concerns difficult. Watch for nonverbal cues from the client. Changes in body language and nonverbal cues noted when the nurse or clinician is speaking can indicate discomfort with the message. The client who declares that he is ready for surgery and seems calm may be sending a different message through the tense muscles the nurse accidentally touches. This body language cue suggests that the client may be worried about the surgery. Environmental cues such as a half-eaten lunch or noncompliance with treatment can provide nonverbal evidence that a client is in distress. Calling attention to conflicting verbal and nonverbal responses is useful if done in a spirit of tentative inquiry. You might note that the client seems nervous or is not paying attention to what you are saying. Inquire about your perception: "I'm wondering what you are feeling right now, about what I am saying," or "I noticed when I mentioned _____, your expression changed." (Weiten, Lloyd, Dunn, & Hammer, 2009). Nonverbal behaviors and signals are culture bound so they may mean different things in different cultures (Samovar, Porter, & McDaniel, 2009). Exercise 10-3 provides practice with observing and interpreting the meaning of nonverbal behaviors.

ASKING QUESTIONS

A client-centered interview begins with encouraging clients to tell their story in an authentic way (Platt & Gaspar, 2001). Applicable questions are a primary means of helping clients tell their story, obtaining relevant information, and reducing misunderstandings. There are different ways of asking questions. Questions fall into three categories: open ended, closed ended, and circular.

Open-Ended Questions

Open-ended questions encourage the client to take the initiative. An open-ended question is similar to an essay question on a test. It is open to interpretation and cannot be answered by "yes," "no," or a one-word response. Questions are designed to permit the client to express the problem or health need in his or her own

---

EXERCISE 10-2	Using Client-Centered Communication Role-Play

Purpose: To use client-centered communication strategies.

Procedure:
1. Develop a one-paragraph scenario of a client situation that you are familiar with before class.
2. Pair off as client and nurse.
3. Conduct an initial *client-centered* 15-minute assessment interview using one of the scenarios, with the author of the paragraph taking the role of the nurse and the other student taking the client role.
4. Reverse roles and repeat with the second student's scenario.

Discussion:
1. In what ways were client-centered communication strategies used in this role-play?
2. How awkward was it for you in the nursing role to incorporate queries about the client's preferences, values, and so on?
3. What parts of the interview experience were of greatest value to you when you assumed the client role?
4. If you were conducting an assessment interview with a client in the future, what modifications might you make?
5. How could you use what you learned from doing this exercise in future nurse-client interviews?

EXERCISE 10-3	Observing for Nonverbal Cues

Purpose: To develop skill in interpreting nonverbal cues.

Procedure:
1. Watch a dramatic movie (that you haven't seen before) with the sound off for 15 minutes.
2. As you watch the movie, write down the emotions you see expressed, the associated nonverbal behavior, and your interpretations of the meaning and the other person's response.

Discussion:
In a large group, share your observations and interpretations of the scenes watched. Discussion should focus on the variations in the interpretations of the nonverbal language. Discuss ways in which the nurse can use observations of nonverbal language with a client in a therapeutic manner to gain a better understanding of the client. Time permitting, the movie segment could be shown again, this time with the sound. Discuss any variations in the interpretations without sound versus with verbal dialogue. Discuss the importance of validation of nonverbal cues.

words. They usually begin with words such as "what," "why," "how," "can you describe for me…" etc. Telling the story of an illness rather than listing discrete facts helps the client and nurse link the context of a health disruption with symptoms and provides more complete information. Open-ended questions ask the client to think and reflect on their situation. They help connect relevant elements of the client's experience (e.g., relationships, impact of the illness on self or others, environmental barriers, potential resources). Open-ended questions are used to elicit the client's thoughts and perspectives without influencing the direction of an acceptable response. For example,

"Can you tell me what brought you to the clinic (hospital) today?"
"What has it been like for you since the accident?"
"Where would you like to begin today?"
"What can I do to help you?"

These questions are general, rather than specific, and open to a variety of answers. An open-ended question

is usually just the introduction, requiring further dialogue about relevant topics. Ending the dialogue with a general open-ended question, such as "Is there anything else that is concerning you right now?" can provide relevant information that might otherwise be overlooked. Look for tone of voice, body movements, and so on as clues to the level of anxiety. Exercise 10-4 provides an opportunity to practice the use of open-ended questions.

Focused Questions

Focused questions require more than a yes or no answer, but place limitations on the topic to be addressed. Emergencies or other circumstances requiring immediate answers involve the use of focused or closed-ended questions. Focused questions can clarify the timing and sequence of symptoms, and concentrate on details about a client's health concerns, for example, when symptoms began, what other symptoms the client is having, or what the client has done to date to

EXERCISE 10-4	Asking Open-Ended Questions

Purpose: To develop skill in the use of open-ended questions to facilitate information sharing.

Procedure:
1. Break up into pairs. Role-play a situation in which one student takes the role of the facilitator and the other the sharer. (If you are in the clinical area, you may want to choose a clinical situation.)
2. As a pair, select a topic. The facilitator begins asking open-ended questions.
3. Dialogue for 5 to 10 minutes on the topic.
4. In pairs, discuss perceptions of the dialogue and determine what questions were comfortable and open ended. The student facilitator should reflect

on the comfort level experienced with asking each question. The sharing student should reflect on the efficacy of the listening responses in helping to move the conversation toward his or her perspective.

Discussion:
As a class, each pair should contribute examples of open-ended questions that facilitated the sharing of information. Compile these examples on the board. Formulate a collaborative summation of what an open-ended question is and how it is used. Discuss how open-ended questions can be used sensitively with uncomfortable topics.

resolve the problem. Clients with limited verbal skills sometimes respond better to focused questions because they require less interpretation. Examples include:

"Tell me more about the pain in your arm."

"Can you give me a specific example of what you mean by. . . ?"

Focused questions can be used to help clients prioritize immediate concerns; for example, "Of all the concerns we have talked about today, which is the most difficult for you?"

Circular questions are a form of focused questions that give attention to the interpersonal context in which an illness occurs. They identify differences in the impact of an illness on individual family members or changes in relationship brought about by the health circumstances (see Chapter 13).

Closed-Ended Questions

Closed-ended questions narrow the focus of the question to a single answer, for example, yes, no, or simple phrase answer. They are useful in emergency situations, when the goal is to obtain information quickly, and the context or client's emotional reactions are of secondary importance in the immediate situation. Examples of closed-ended questions include:

"Does the pain radiate down your left shoulder and arm?"

"When was your last meal?"

WHAT THE NURSE LISTENS FOR
Themes

Box 10-2 identifies what the nurse listens for in client-centered conversations. Therapeutic communication involves both intrapersonal and interpersonal processes. As Myers (2000) suggests, "Any actual dialogue has an inner, subjectively experienced component" (p. 151). Intrapersonal communication refers to the internal processing that goes on within a person about the underlying feeling or core idea associated with the verbal message. It is not usually intentionally expressed.

Listening for themes requires observing and understanding what the client is not saying, as well as what the person actually reveals. Identifying the underlying themes presented in a therapeutic conversation can relieve anxiety and provide direction for individualized nursing interventions. For example, the client may say to the nurse, "I'm worried about my surgery tomorrow." This is one way of framing the problem. If the same client presents his concern as "I'm not sure I will make it through the surgery tomorrow," the underlying theme of the communication changes from a generalized worry to a more personal theme of survival. Alternatively, a client might say, "I don't know whether my husband should stay tomorrow when I have my surgery. It is going to be a long procedure, and he gets so worried." The theme (focus) expresses her concern about her relationship with her husband. In each communication, the client expresses a distinct theme of concern related to a statement, but the emphasis in each requires a different response.

Emotional objectivity in making sense of client themes is essential. "Objectivity here refers to seeing what an experience is for another person, not how it fits or relates to other experiences, not what causes it, why it exists, or what purposes it serves. It is an attempt to see attitudes and concepts, beliefs and values of an individual as they are to him at the moment he expresses them—not what they were or will become" (Moustakas, 1974, p. 78). Exercise 10-5 provides practice in listening for themes.

BOX 10-2	Guidelines to Effective Verbal Expressions in the Nurse-Client Relationship
• Define unfamiliar terms and concepts. • Match content and delivery with each client's developmental and educational level, experiential frame of reference, and learning readiness. • Keep messages clear, concrete, honest, and simple to understand. • Put ideas in a logical sequence of related material. • Relate new ideas to familiar ones when presenting new information. • Repeat key ideas. • Reinforce key ideas with vocal emphasis and pauses.	• Keep language as simple as possible; use vocabulary familiar to the client. • Focus only on essential elements; present one idea at a time. • Use as many sensory communication channels as possible for key ideas. • Make sure that nonverbal behaviors support verbal messages. • Seek feedback to validate accurate reception of information.

EXERCISE 10-5	Listening for Themes

Purpose: To help students identify underlying themes in messages.

Procedure:

1. Divide into groups of three to five students.
2. Take turns telling a short story about yourselves—about growing up, important people or events in your life, or significant accomplishments (e.g., getting your first job).
3. As each student presents a story, take mental notes of the important themes. Write them down so you will not be tempted to change them as you hear the other students. Notice nonverbal behaviors accompanying the verbal message. Are they consistent with the verbal message of the sharer?
4. When the story is completed, each of the other people in the group shares his or her observations with the sharer.

5. After all students have shared their observations, validate their accuracy with the sharer.

Discussion:

1. Were the underlying themes recorded by the group consistent with the sharer's understanding of his or her communication?
2. As others related their interpretations of significant words or phrases, did you change your mind about the nature of the underlying theme?
3. Were the interpretations of pertinent information relatively similar or significantly different?
4. If they were different, what implications do you think such differences have for nurse-client relationships in nursing practice?
5. What did you learn from doing this exercise?

COMMUNICATION PATTERNS

Communication patterns provide a different type of information. Some clients exaggerate information; others characteristically leave out highly relevant details. Some talk a lot, using dramatic language and multiple examples; others say very little and have to be encouraged to provide details. Evaluation of the client's present overall pattern of interaction with others includes strengths and limitations, family communication dynamics, and developmental and educational levels. Culture, role, ways of handling conflict, and ways of dealing with emotions reflect and influence communication patterns. Being respectful of the client's communication pattern involves accepting the client's communication style as a part of who the person is, and not expecting the person to be different. For example, AJ is a client with chronic mental illness. She frequently interrupts and presents with a loud, ebullient opinion on most things. This is AJ's communication pattern. To engage successfully with her, you would need to listen, while accepting her way of communicating as a part of who she is, without getting lost in detail.

USING INTUITIVE FEELINGS

Intuitive feelings can emerge as a personal listening response from within the nurse during the course of a conversation with a client or family. Personal ways of knowing represent a body-centered way of listening to feelings about underlying issues and concerns (Klagsbrun, 2001). For example, if a nurse has no particular personal reason for reacting to the client with anger, fear, or sadness, this inner response may reflect a client's unexpressed feeling. Behavioral reactions that the nurse feels are out of proportion to the situation (e.g., complete calm before surgery, excessive anger, noncompliance or passive compliance with no questions asked, guarded verbalizations, incongruent facial expressions or body language, or social withdrawal) can be danger signals that need further exploration.

ACTIVE LISTENING RESPONSES

Active listening responses show the client that the nurse is fully present as a professional partner in helping the client understand a change in health status and the best ways to cope with it (Keller & Baker, 2000). Minimal verbal cues, clarification, restatement, paraphrasing, reflection, summarization, silence, and touch are examples of skilled listening responses nurses can use to guide therapeutic interventions (Table 10-1).

MINIMAL CUES AND LEADS

Simple, encouraging leads communicate interest. **Minimal cues** transmitted through body actions (e.g., smiling, nodding, and leaning forward) encourage clients to continue with their story. By not detracting from the client's message and by giving permission to tell the story as the client sees it, minimal cues promote client comfort in sharing intimate information. Short

TABLE 10-1	Listening Responses
Listening Response	**Example**
Minimal cues and leads	Body actions: smiling, nodding, leaning forward
	Words: "mm," "uh-huh," "oh really," "go on"
Clarification	"Could you describe what happened in sequence?" "I'm not sure I understand what you mean. Can you give me an example?"
Restatement	"Are you saying that... (repeat client's words)?" "You mean... (repeat client's words)?"
Paraphrasing	Client: "I can't take this anymore. The chemo is worse than the cancer. I just want to die."
	Nurse: "It sounds as though you are saying you have had enough."
Reflection	"It sounds as though you feel guilty because you weren't home at the time of the accident." "You sound really frustrated because the treatment is taking longer than you thought it would."
Summarization	"Before moving on, I would like to go over with you what I think we've accomplished thus far."
Silence	Briefly disconnecting but continuing to use attending behaviors after an important idea, thought, or feeling
Touch	Gently rubbing a person's arm during a painful procedure

phrases such as "Go on" or "And then?" or "Can you say more about...?" are useful prompts. Exercise 10-6 provides an opportunity to see the influence of minimal cues and leads on communication.

CLARIFICATION

Clarification seeks to understand the message of the client by asking for more information or for elaboration on a point. The strategy is most useful when parts of a client's communication are ambiguous or not easily understood. Failure to ask for clarification when part of the communication is poorly understood means that the nurse will act on incomplete or inaccurate information.

Clarification listening responses are expressed as a question or statement followed by a restatement or paraphrasing of part of the communicated message; for example, "You stated earlier that you were concerned about your blood pressure. Tell me more about what

EXERCISE 10-6	Minimal Cues and Leads

Purpose: To practice and evaluate the efficacy of minimal cues and leads.

Procedure:
1. Initiate a conversation with someone outside of class and attempt to tell the person about something with which you are familiar for 5 to 10 minutes.
2. Make note of all the cues that the person puts forth that either promote or inhibit conversation.
3. Now try this with another person and write down the different cues and leads you observe as you are speaking and your emotional response to them (e.g., what most encouraged you to continue speaking).

Discussion:
As a class, share your experience and observations. Different cues and responses will be compiled on the board. Discuss the impact of different cues and leads on your comfort and willingness to share about yourself. What cues and leads promoted communication? What cues and leads inhibited sharing?

Variation:
This exercise can be practiced with a clinical problem simulation in which one student takes the role of the professional helper and the other takes the role of client. Perform the same scenario with and without the use of minimum encouragers. What were the differences when encouragers were not used? Was the communication as lively? How did it feel to you when telling your story when this strategy was used by the helping person?

EXERCISE 10-7	Using Clarification

Purpose: To develop skill in the use of clarification.

Procedure:
1. Write a paragraph related to an experience you have had.
2. Place all the student paragraphs together and then pick one (not your own).
3. Develop clarification questions you might ask about the selected paragraph.

Discussion:
Share with the class your chosen paragraph and the clarification questions you developed. Discuss how effective the questions are in clarifying information. Other students can suggest additional clarification questions.

concerns you." The tone of voice used with a clarification response should be neutral, not accusatory or demanding. Practice this response in Exercise 10-7.

RESTATEMENT

Restatement is an active listening strategy used to broaden a client's perspective or when the nurse needs to provide a sharper focus on a specific part of the communication. Restatement is particularly effective when the client overgeneralizes or seems stuck in a repetitive line of thinking. To challenge the validity of the client's statement directly could be counterproductive, whereas repeating parts of the message in the form of a query serves a similar purpose without raising defenses; for example, "Let me see if I have this right..." (Coulehan et al., 2001). Restating a self-critical or irrational part of the message in a questioning manner focuses the client's attention on the possibility of an inaccurate or global assertion.

PARAPHRASING

Paraphrasing is a response strategy used to check whether the nurse's translation of the client's words is an accurate interpretation of the message. The strategy involves the nurse taking the client's original message and transforming it into his or her own words, without losing the meaning. The paraphrase is shorter and more specific than the client's initial statement so that the focus is on the core elements of the original statement.

Case Example

Client: "I don't know about taking this medicine the doctor is putting me on. I've never had to take medication before, and now I have to take it twice a day.

Nurse: It sounds like you don't know what to expect from taking the medication.

REFLECTION

Reflection as a listening response focuses on the emotional implications of a message. This listening response helps the client clarify important feelings and experience them with their appropriate intensity in relation to a particular situation or event. There are several ways to use reflection, for example:

- *Reflection on vocal tone:* "I can sense anger and frustration in your voice as you describe your accident."
- *Linking feelings with content:* "It sounds like you feel _____ because _____."
- *Linking current feelings with past experiences:* "It seems as if this experience reminds you of feelings you had with other health care providers where you didn't feel understood."

Reflection as a listening response gives clients permission to have feelings and helps them to identify feelings they may not be aware of in new and unfamiliar circumstances. Sometimes nursing students feel they are putting words into the client's mouth when they "choose" an emotion from their perception of the client's message. This would be true if you were choosing an emotion out of thin air, but not when the nurse empathetically considers the client's situation and presents the underlying feelings present in the client's narrative, without interpreting its meaning. Exercise 10-8 provides practice in using paraphrasing and reflection as listening responses.

SUMMARIZATION

Summarization is an active listening skill used to review content and process. Summarization pulls several ideas and feelings together, either from one interaction or a series of interactions, into a few succinct sentences. This would be followed by a comment seeking validation, such as "Tell me if my understanding of this

EXERCISE 10-8 | Role-Play Practice with Paraphrasing and Reflection

Purpose: To practice use of paraphrasing and reflection as listening responses.

Procedure:
1. The class forms into groups of three students each. One student takes the role of client, one the role of nurse, and one the role of observer.
2. The client shares with the nurse a recent health problem he or she encountered, and describes the details of the situation and the emotions experienced. The nurse responds, using paraphrasing and reflection in a dialogue that lasts at least 5 minutes. The observer records the statements made by the helper. At the end of the dialogue, the client writes his or her perception of how the helper's statements affected the conversation, including what comments were most helpful. The helper writes a short summary of the

listening responses he or she used, with comments on how successful they were.

Discussion:
1. Share your summary and discuss the differences in using the techniques from the helper, client, and observer perspectives.
2. Discuss how these differences related to influencing the flow of dialogue, helping the client feel heard, and the impact on the helper's understanding of the client from both the client and the helper positions.
3. Identify places in the dialogue where one form of questioning might be preferable to another.
4. How could you use this exercise to understand your client's concerns?
5. Were you surprised by any of the summaries?

---

agrees with yours." A summary statement is useful as a bridge to changing the topic or focus of the conversation. The summarization should be completed before the end of the conversation. A summary statement should not be delivered as the nurse leaves the room. Exercise 10-9 is designed to provide insight into the use of summarization as a listening response.

SILENCE

Silence, used deliberately and judiciously, is a powerful listening response. Intentional pauses can allow the client to think. A short pause also lets the nurse step back momentarily and process what he or she has heard before

responding. Too often a quick response addresses only a small part of the message or gives the client an insufficient opportunity to formulate an idea fully.

Silence can be used to emphasize important points that you want the client to reflect on. By pausing briefly after presenting a key idea and before proceeding to the next topic, you can encourage a client to notice vital elements. When a client falls silent, it can mean many things: something has touched the client, the client is angry or does not know how to respond, or the client is thinking. A verbal comment to validate meaning is helpful. Exercise 10-10 provides practice with the use of silences.

EXERCISE 10-9 | Practicing Summarization

Purpose: To provide practice in summarizing interactions.

Procedure:
1. Choose a partner for a pairs discussion.
2. For 10 minutes, discuss a medical ethics topic such as euthanasia, heroic life support for the terminally ill, or "Baby Doe" decisions to allow malformed babies to die if the parents desire.
3. After 10 minutes, both partners must stop talking until Participant A has summarized what Participant B has just said to Participant B's satisfaction, and vice versa.

Discussion:
After both partners have completed their summarizations, discuss the process of summarization, answering the following questions:
1. Did knowing you had to summarize the other person's point of view encourage you to listen more closely?
2. Did the act of summarizing help clarify any discussion points? Were any points of agreement found? What points of disagreement were found?
3. Did the exercise help you to understand the other person's point of view?
4. What should an effective summary contain? Is it hard to summarize a long conversation?
5. How did you determine which points to focus on in your summarization?

EXERCISE 10-10	Therapeutic Use of Silence

Purpose: To experience the effect of the use of silence as a listening response.

Procedure:
1. Two people act as Participants A and B.
2. Participant A plays the role of the nurse. Participant B is a healthy, ambulatory, 80-year-old female client in an extended-care facility who was placed there against her will by her family, who are moving to another state.
3. Participant B's role is to describe feelings (shock) at being institutionalized and to discuss the slow

adjustment to new surroundings and new companions, describing both the positive and the negative aspects.
4. Participant A's objective is to make at least three deliberate efforts to use silence during the conversation (as a therapeutic device to encourage Participant B's consideration of life and problems).

Discussion:
After 10 minutes of role-playing, have a general discussion to share feelings about the effective use of silence.

Not all listening responses are helpful. Nurses need to recognize when their responses are interfering with objectivity or inviting premature closure. Table 10-2 provides definitions of negative listening responses that block communication. Exercise 10-11 provides practice with using active listening responses.

VERBAL RESPONSES

Active listening and verbal responses are inseparable from each other. Each informs and reinforces the other.

Table 10-3 presents a summary of the therapeutic interviewing skills presented in this chapter as they apply to the phases of the nurse-client relationship. With shorter time frames for client contact, nurses need to verbally connect with clients, beginning with the first encounter.

As the relationship develops, the quality of verbal and listening responses ensure that care remains client centered. Most clients are not looking for brilliant answers from the nurse, but rather seek feedback and support that suggests a compassionate understanding of their particular dilemma. No matter what level of

TABLE 10-2	Negative Listening Responses	
Category of Response	**Explanation of Category**	**Examples**
False reassurance	Using pseudocomforting phrases in an attempt to offer reassurance	"It will be okay." "Everything will work out."
Giving advice	Making a decision for a client; offering personal opinions; telling a client what to do (using phrases such as "ought to," "should")	"If I were you, I would..." "I feel you should..."
False inferences	Making an unsubstantiated assumption about what a client means; interpreting the client's behavior without asking for validation; jumping to conclusions	"What you really mean is you don't like your physician." "Subconsciously, you are blaming your husband for the accident."
Moralizing	Expressing your own values about what is right and wrong, especially on a topic that concerns the client	"Abortion is wrong." "It is wrong to refuse to have the operation."
Value judgments	Conveying your approval or disapproval about the client's behavior or about what the client has said using words such as "good," "bad," or "nice"	"I'm glad you decided to..." "That really wasn't a nice way to behave." "She's a good patient."
Social responses	Polite, superficial comments that do not focus on what the client is feeling or trying to say; use of clichés	"Isn't that nice?" "Hospital rules, you know?" "Just do what the doctor says." "It's a beautiful day."

EXERCISE 10-11   Active Listening

Purpose: To develop skill in active listening and an awareness of the elements involved.

Procedure:
1. Students break up into pairs. Each will take a turn reflecting on and describing an important experience they have had in their lives. The person who shares should describe the details, emotions, and outcomes of his or her experience. During the interaction, the listening partner should use listening responses such as clarification, paraphrasing, reflection, and focusing, as well as attending cues, eye contact, and alert body posture to carry the conversation forward.

2. After the sharing partner finishes his or her story, the listening partner indicates understanding by: (a) stating in his or her own words what the sharing partner said; and (b) summarizing perceptions of the sharing partner's feelings associated with the story and asking for validation. If the sharing partner agrees, then the listening partner can be sure he or she correctly utilized active listening skills.

Discussion:
In the large group, have pairs of students share their discoveries about active listening. As a class, discuss aspects of nursing behavior that will foster active listening in client interactions.

TABLE 10-3	Interviewing and Relationship Skills		
Phase	**Stage**	**Purpose**	**Skills**
Orientation Phase	Rapport and structuring with the client	To build a working alliance	Basic listening and attending; information giving
Intervention Phase Assessment, engagement, and beginning active	Gathering information, defining the problem, identifying strengths	To determine how the client views problems; to identify values, beliefs, strengths to resolve problems and promote health/well-being	Basic listening and attending; open-ended questions, verbal cues, and leads
Planning, active	Determining outcomes: What needs to happen to reduce the self-care demand? Where does the client want to go?	To find out how the client would like to be: How would things be if the problems were solved?	Attending and basic listening; influencing; feedback
Implementation, active	Explaining alternatives and options	To work toward resolution of the client's self-care needs	Influencing; feedback balanced with attending and listening behaviors
Termination Phase Evaluation	Generalization and transfer of learning	To enable changes in thoughts, feelings, and behaviors; to evaluate the effectiveness of the changes in modifying the self-care need	Influencing; feedback; validation

communication exists in the relationship, the same needs—"hear me," "touch me," "respond to me," "feel my pain and experience my joys with me"—are fundamental themes. These are the themes addressed by client-centered communication.

Nurses use verbal responses to teach, encourage, support, provide and gather information, in guiding a client toward goal achievement. Words help clients assess the healthy elements of their personality (their strengths) and enables them to use these elements in coping with their current health problems. Accurate, appropriate language is critical for informed consent.

Verbal response strategies include mirroring, focusing, metaphors, humor, reframing, feedback, and validation, all of which are designed to strengthen the coping abilities of the client, alone or in relationship with others. Nurses use observation, validation, and patterns of knowing to gauge the effectiveness of verbal interventions. On the basis of the client's reaction, the nurse may decide to use simpler language or to try a different strategy in collaboratively working with a client.

When making verbal responses or providing information, do not overload the client with too many ideas or details. If you find you are doing most of the talking, you need to back up and use listening responses to elicit the client's perspective. People can absorb only so much information at one time, particularly if they are tired, fearful, or discouraged. Introducing new ideas one at a time allows the client to process data more efficiently. Repeating key ideas and reinforcing information with concrete examples facilitates understanding and provides an additional opportunity for the client to ask questions. Paying attention to nonverbal response cues from the client that support understanding or that reflect a need for further attention is an important dimension of successful communication.

MATCHING RESPONSES

Regardless of content, the nurse's verbal responses should match the client's message in level of depth, meaning, and language (Johnson, 1980). The client needs to lead the way to any exploration of deeper feeling. If the client makes a serious statement, the nurse should not respond with a flip remark. Likewise, a superficial statement does not warrant an intense response. Responses that encourage a client to explore feelings about limitations or strengths at a slightly deeper but related level of conversation are likely to meet with more success.

Verbal response should neither expand nor diminish the meaning of the client's remarks. Notice the differences in the nature of the following responses to a client.

Case Example

Client: I feel so discouraged. No matter how hard I try, I still can't walk without pain on the two parallel bars.

Nurse: You want to give up because you don't think you will be able to walk again.

At this point, it is unclear that the client wants to give up, so the nurse's comment expands on the client's meaning without having sufficient data to support it.

Although it is possible that this is what the client means, it is not the only possibility. The more important dilemma for the client may be whether his or her efforts have any purpose. The next response focuses only on the negative aspects of the client's communication and ignores the client's comment about his or her efforts.

Nurse: So you think you won't be able to walk independently again.

In the final response example below, the nurse addresses both parts of the client's message and makes the appropriate connection. The nurse's statement invites the client to validate the nurse's perception.

Nurse: It sounds to me as if you don't feel your efforts are helping you regain control over your walking.

USING UNDERSTANDABLE LANGUAGE

Using simple, clear-cut words, keeping the client's developmental and educational level in mind, and speaking with a general spirit of inquiry and concern for the client stimulates trust. Verbal messages should address core issues in a comprehensible, concise manner, taking into account the guidelines for effective verbal expressions, listed in Box 10-3.

Avoid using jargon or clinical language that clients may have trouble understanding. Unless clients can associate new ideas with familiar words and ideas that have meaning to him or her, the nurse might as well be talking in a different language. Clients may not tell the nurse that they do not understand for fear of offending the nurse or revealing personal deficits. Giving information that fails to take into account a client's previous experiences, or assumes that clients have knowledge they do not possess, tends to fall on deaf

BOX 10-3	What the Nurse Listens For

- Content themes
- Communication patterns
- Discrepancies in content, body language, and vocalization
- Feelings, revealed in a person's voice, body movements, and facial expressions
- What is not being said, as well as what is being said
- The client's preferred representational system (auditory, visual, tactile)
- The nurse's own inner responses
- The effect communication produces in others involved with the client

ears. Frequent validation with the client related to content helps reduce this problem.

FOCUSING

In the past, nurses had more time to talk with clients. In today's health care delivery system, nurses must make every second count. It is important for nurses and clients to select the most pressing health care topics for discussion. For example, the nurse can redirect the conversation to immediate nursing needs.

Case Example

"Mr. Solan, you have given me a lot to think about here, but I would like to hear more about how you are handling the surgery tomorrow. You mentioned that you were feeling afraid, and this is normal. I wonder if we could talk more about this."

Sensitivity to client need and preferences, and client readiness are factors to take into consideration. You should not force a client to focus on an issue that he or she is not yet willing to discuss unless it is an emergency situation. You can always go back to a topic when the client is more receptive. For example, you might say, "I can understand that this is a difficult topic for you, but I am here for you if you would like to discuss [identified topic] later."

PRESENTING REALITY

Presenting reality to a client who is misinterpreting it can be helpful as long as the client does not perceive that the nurse is criticizing the client's perception of reality. A simple statement such as "I know that you feel very strongly about _____, but I don't see it that way" is an effective way for the nurse to express a different interpretation of the situation. Another strategy is to put into words the underlying feeling implied but not directly stated.

Case Example

Client: I can't talk to anyone around here. All you people seem to care about is the money, not the patient.
   Nurse: It sounds like you are really feeling all alone right now.

GIVING FEEDBACK

Feedback is a message given by the nurse to the client in response to a message or observed behavior. Feedback can focus on the content, the relationship between people and events, the feelings generated by the message, or parts of the communication that are not clear. Feedback should be specific and directed to the behavior. It should not be an analysis of the client's motivations.

Feedback responses reassure the client that the nurse is directing full attention to what the client is communicating through words or nonverbal behavior. Verbal feedback provides the receiver's understanding of the sender's message and personal reaction to it. Effective feedback offers a neutral mirror, which allows a client to view a problem or behavior from a different perspective. Feedback is most relevant when it only addresses the topics under discussion and does not go beyond the data presented by the client.

Effective feedback is specific rather than general. Telling a client he or she is shy or easily intimidated is less helpful than saying, "I noticed when the anesthesiologist was in here that you didn't ask her any of the questions you had about your anesthesia tomorrow. Let's look at what you might want to know and how you can get the information you need." With this response, the nurse provides precise information about an observed behavior and offers a solution. The client is more likely to respond with validation or correction, and the nurse can provide specific guidance.

Feedback can be about the nurse's observations of nonverbal behaviors; for example, "You seem (angry, upset, confused, pleased, sad, etc.)." It can be framed as a question, requiring the client to elaborate; for example, "I want to be sure that we have the same understanding of what we have talked about. Can you summarize for me what we have discussed?"

Not all feedback is equally relevant, nor is it always uniformly accepted. The benchmark for deciding whether feedback is appropriate is to ask, "Does the feedback advance the goals of the relationship?" and "Does it consider the individualized needs of the client?" If the answer to either question is "no," then the feedback may be accurate but inappropriate for the moment.

Timing of feedback is important. Feedback given as soon as possible after a behavior is observed is most effective. Other factors (e.g., a client's readiness to hear feedback, privacy, and the availability of support from others) contribute to effectiveness. Providing feedback about behaviors over which the client has little control only increases the client's feelings of low self-esteem and leads to frustration. Feedback should be to the point and empathetic.

Case Example

An obese mother in the hospital was feeding her new-born infant 4 ounces of formula every 4 hours. She was concerned that her child vomited a considerable amount of the undigested formula after each feeding. Initially, the nursing student gave the mother instructions about feeding the infant no more than 2 ounces at each feeding in the first few days of life, but the mother's behavior persisted, and so did that of her infant. The nursing student began to ask questions and discovered that the client's mother had fed her 4 ounces right from birth with no problem, and she considered this the norm. This additional information helped the nurse work with the client in seeing the uniqueness of her child and understanding what the infant was telling her through his behavior. The client began to feel comfortable and confident in feeding her infant a smaller amount of formula consistent with his needs.

Effective feedback is clear, honest, and reflective. Feedback supported with realistic examples is believable, whereas feedback without documentation to support it can lack credibility. To illustrate from your nursing school experience, if you were told that you would have no trouble passing any of the exams in nursing school, you would wonder whether the statement was true. However, if your instructor said, "On the basis of past performance and the fact that your score on the entrance exams was high, I think you should have little problem with our tests as long as you study," you would have more confidence in the statement.

Nonverbal feedback registers the other's reaction to the sender's message through facial expressions such as surprise, boredom, or hostility. When you receive nonverbal messages suggesting uncertainty, concern, or inattention, use a listening response to fully inquire about what the client is having trouble understanding. Feedback can have a surprise twist leading to an unexpected conclusion, as shown in the following example.

Case Example

It was Jovan's third birthday. There was a party of adults (his mother and father; his grandparents; his great-uncle and great-aunt; and me, his aunt), because Jovan was the only child in the family. While we were sitting and chatting, Jovan was running around and playing. At a moment of complete silence, Jovan's great-uncle asked him solemnly: "Jovan, who do you love the best?" Jovan replied, "Nobody!" Then Jovan ran to me and whispered in my ear: "You are Nobody!" (Majanovic-Shane, 1996, p. 11).

ASKING FOR VALIDATION

Meanings are in people, not in the words themselves. Validation is a special form of feedback, used to ensure that both participants have the same basic understanding of messages. Simply asking clients whether they understand what was said is not an adequate method of validating message content. Instead, you might ask, "How do you feel about what I just said?" or "I'm curious what your thoughts are about what I just told you." If the client does not have any response, you can suggest that the client can respond later, "Many people do find they have reactions or questions about [the issue] after they have had a chance to think about it. I would be glad to discuss this further." Validation can provide new information that helps the nurse frame comments that match the client's need.

Case Example

Mr. Brown (to nurse taking his blood pressure): I can't stand that medicine. It doesn't sit well. (He grimaces and holds his stomach.)

Nurse: Are you saying that your medication for lowering your blood pressure upsets your stomach?

Mr. Brown: No, I just don't like the taste of it.

Sometimes validation is observational rather than expressed through words.

Case Example

Jane Smith has been coming to the clinic to lose weight. At first she was quite successful, losing 2 pounds per week. This week she has gained 3 pounds. The nurse validates the weight change with the client and asks for input.

Nurse: Jane, over the past 6 weeks you have lost 2 pounds per week, but this week you gained 3 pounds. There seems to be a problem here. Let's discuss what might have happened and how you can get back on track with your goal of losing weight.

OTHER FORMS OF COMMUNICATION

TOUCH

Touch, the first of our senses to develop, and the last to leave, is a nurturing form of communication and validation. Intentional comforting touch benefits the nurse, as well as the client (Connor & Howett, 2009). Touch is a powerful listening response used when words would break a mood or when verbalization would fail to convey the empathy or depth of feeling between nurse and client (Straneva, 2000). A hand placed on a frightened mother's shoulder or a squeeze of the hand can speak far more eloquently than words in times of deep emotion. Touch stimulates comfort, security, and a sense of feeling valued (Sundin & Jansson, 2003). Clients in pain, those who feel repulsive to others because of altered appearance, lonely and dying clients, and those experiencing sensory deprivation or feeling confused respond positively to the nurse who is unafraid to enter their world and touch them. Children and the elderly are comforted by touch.

Case Example

"I found out that if I held Sam's hand he would lie perfectly still and even drift off to sleep. When I sat with him, holding his hand, his blood pressure and heart rate would go down to normal and his intracranial pressure would stay below 10. When I tried to calm him with words, there was no response—he [had] a blood pressure of 160/90!" (Chesla, 1996, p. 202).

How you touch a client in providing everyday nursing care is a form of communication. For example, gentle massage of a painful area helps clients relax. Holding the hand of a client with dementia can reduce agitation. Gently rubbing a client's forehead or stroking the head is comforting to very ill clients.

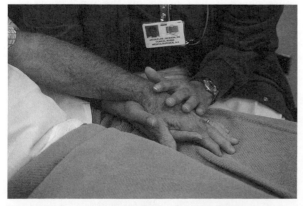

Touch can be an important form of communication.

People vary in their comfort with touch. Touch is used as a common form of communication in some cultures, whereas in others, it is reserved for religious purposes, or seldom used as a form of communication (Samovar, Porter, & McDaniel, 2009). Before touching a client, assess the client's receptiveness to touch. Observation of the client will provide some indication, but you may need to ask for validation. If the client is paranoid, out of touch with reality, verbally inappropriate, or mistrustful, touch is contraindicated as a listening response.

SPECIALIZED COMMUNICATION STRATEGIES

METAPHORS

Familiar images promote understanding. Metaphors can help clients and families process difficult new information by connecting it with familiar images from ordinary life experience. For example, Arroliga et al. (2002) describe chronic lung disease as "emphysema is like having lungs similar to 'swiss cheese,'" and the airways in asthma are "different sized drainpipes that can get clogged up and need to be unclogged" (p. 377). These are familiar images that the client can appreciate and connect with a disease that is harder to comprehend.

In health care situations, metaphors need to be used carefully. Periyakoil (2008) suggests that using war or sports metaphors with clients experiencing advanced metastatic cancer can result in an unintended impact when the client can no longer fight the valiant battle or win the game by playing according to prescribed moves.

HUMOR

Humor is a powerful therapeutic communication technique when used with deliberate intent for a specific therapeutic purpose. Humor recognizes the incongruities in a situation, or an absurdity present in human nature or conduct (Random House Dictionary, 2009). Humor allows taboo topics to be raised without creating hostility or discomfort.

Humor and laughter have healing purposes. Laughter generates energy and activates β-endorphins, a neurotransmitter that creates natural highs and reduces stress hormones (Hassed, 2001). Humorous remarks are best delivered as simple statements that contain positive kernels of truth and are conveyed with calmness. The surprise element in humor can cut through an overly intense situation and put it into perspective.

Case Example

Karen, the mother of 4-year-old Megan, had just returned from a long shopping trip in which she had purchased several packages of paper towels. While she was in another room, Megan took everything out of four kitchen drawers, put them on the floor, and put the paper towels in the drawers. Her mother expressed her anger to Megan in no uncertain terms. As she was leaving the kitchen, she heard Megan say to herself, "Well, I guess she didn't like that idea." Karen's anger was permanently interrupted by her daughter's innocent humorous remark.

Humor is most effective when rapport is well established and a level of trust exists between the nurse and client (McGhee, 1998). When humor is used, it should focus on the idea, event, or situation, or something other than the client's personal characteristics. Humor that ridicules is not funny. Some clients respond well to humor; others are insulted or perplexed by it. Humor is less effective when the client is tired or emotionally vulnerable. Instead, that client may need structure and calming support.

Humor should fit the situation, not dominate it. The following factors contribute to its successful use:

- Knowledge of the client's response pattern
- An overly intense situation
- Timing
- Situation that requires an imaginative or paradoxical solution
- Gearing the humor to the client's developmental level
- Focus on a situation or circumstance, rather than client characteristics

REFRAMING

Bandler and Grindler (1997) define **reframing** as "changing the frame in which a person perceives events in order to change the meaning" (p. 1). Reframing offers a different positive interpretation designed to broaden the client's perspective.

Reframing strategies should accentuate client strengths. The new frame must fit the current situation *and* be understandable to the client; otherwise, it will not work.

Reframing a situation is helpful when blame is a component of a family's response to the client's illness, for example, with alcoholism. Helping a family view the alcoholism as a disease rather than as a reaction to family members permits necessary detachment.

COGNITIVE BEHAVIORAL STRATEGIES

Reality often is not the problem; rather it lies with negative thinking that creates emotional responses and influences behavior. Cognitive behavioral communication strategies are helpful in helping clients challenge self-defeating thoughts that threaten productive engagement in recovery. Once the nurse helps clients identify negative thoughts, clients are taught to challenge the validity of those thoughts and/or to replace them with a positive thought. By interrupting negative thinking patterns and replacing them with positive thoughts, people can modify behavior.

Case Example

Jack Norris is receiving an antidepressant medication for depression symptoms associated with his cancer diagnosis. He tells the nurse he wants to stop the medication because it feels like a "crutch" to him, and he doesn't want to depend on medication "to make him feel better." When the nurse queries him about his other medications, he says, "That's different, those are medications I need. My antidepressant is just to make me feel better."

Applying the cognitive behavioral therapy model (Box 10-4), the activating event (A) is Jack's prescription for depressive symptoms associated with cancer. His belief (B) that using psychotropic medication is a sign of weakness and that he should be able to get along as well without it gets in the way of his being able to resolve his depressive symptoms. This belief affects his efforts to cope with his cancer. The consequence (C) of going off the medication is a return of his depressive symptoms. In this case example, how would you help the client receive the help he needs for his emotional well-being?

BOX 10-4	ABCs of a Cognitive Behavioral Approach

A refers to the Activating event, which creates an image in the person's mind.
B refers to the Beliefs surrounding the activating event. Beliefs can also include personal rules or demands a person makes on himself and fixed attitudes.
C refers to the Consequences, which include a person's decision and behaviors representing the person's beliefs.

USING TECHNOLOGY IN COMMUNICATION

Increasingly, nurses are using technology to communicate with clients and families. Although technology can never replace face-to-face time with clients, voice mail, e-mail, and telehealth virtual home visits help connect clients with care providers and provide critical information. Currently, technology is used as a form of communication to augment onsite communication. For example, routine laboratory results, appointment scheduling, and links to information on the Web can be transmitted through technology. Present-day technology allows people to use the Internet as a communication means to share common experiences with others who have a disease condition, to consult with experts about symptoms and treatment, and to learn up-to-date information about their condition.

The electronic nurse-client relationship begins when the nurse comes online or begins speaking to the client on the phone (Sharpe, 2001). From that point forward, the nurse needs to follow defined standards of nursing care, using communication principles identified in this chapter. At the end of each telehealth encounter, nurses need to provide their clients with clear directions and contact information should additional assistance be required. Confidentiality and protection of identifiable client information is an essential component of telehealth conversations.

Telephone communication is an essential communication link. Periodic informational telephone calls enhance family involvement in the long-term care of clients. Over time, some families lose interest or find it too painful to continue active commitment. Interest and support from the nurse reminds families that they are not simply nonessential, interchangeable parts in their loved one's life; their input is important.

SUMMARY

This chapter discusses basic therapeutic communication strategies nurses can use with clients across clinical settings. Nurses use active listening responses such as paraphrasing, reflection, **clarification**, silence, summarization, and touch to elicit complete information. Observation is a primary source of information, but all nonverbal behaviors need to be validated with clients for accuracy.

Open-ended questions give the nurse the most information because they allow clients to express ideas and feelings as they are experiencing them. Focused or closed-ended questions are appropriate in emergency clinical situations, when precise information is needed quickly.

Nurses use verbal communication strategies that fit the client's communication patterns in terms of level, meaning, and language to help clients meet treatment goals. Other strategies include use of metaphors, reframing, humor, confirming responses, feedback, and validation. Feedback provides a client with needed information.

ETHICAL DILEMMA   What Would You Do?

You have had a wonderful relationship with a client and the client's family. They have revealed issues they had never talked about before and raised questions that extended beyond the health care situation that they did not have the time to finish. You are about to end your rotation. What do you see as your ethical responsibility to this client and family?

REFERENCES

Arroliga AC, Newman S, Longworth DL, et al: Metaphorical medicine: using metaphors to enhance communication with patients who have pulmonary disease, *Ann Intern Med* 137(5 Part 1):376–379, 2002.

Bandler R, Cahill Grindler J: *Reframing*, Palo Alto, CA, 1997, Science and Behavior Books.

Bush K: Do you really listen to patients? *RN* 64(3):35–37, 2001.

Burgoon JK, Guerrero LK, Floyd K: *Nonverbal Communication*, Boston, MA, 2009, Allyn and Bacon.

Caughan G, Long A: Communication is the essence of nursing care: 2. Ethical foundations, *Br J Nurs* 9(15):979–984, 2000.

Chesla C: Reconciling technologic and family care in critical-care nursing, *Image J Nurs Sch* 28(3):199–203, 1996.

Connor A, Howett M: A conceptual model of intentional comfort touch, *J Holist Nurs* 27(2):127–135, 2009.

Coulehan JL, Platt FW, Egener B, et al: Let me see if I have this right...: words that help build empathy, *Ann Intern Med* 135: 221–227, 2001.

Definition of humor: *Random House Dictionary*, Available online at: dictionary.com. New York, 2009, Random House, Inc.

Epstein RM, Street RL Jr, : *Patient-centered communication in cancer care: promoting healing and reducing suffering* (NIH Publication No. 07-6225), Bethesda, MD, 2007, National Cancer Institute.

Hall E: *The silent language*, New York, 1959, Doubleday.

Hassed C: How humour keeps you well, *Aust Fam Physician* 30(1): 25–28, 2001.

Johnson M: Self-disclosure: a variable in the nurse-client relationship, *J Psychiatr Nurs* 18(1):17–20, 1980.

Kagan P: Feeling listened to: a lived experience of human becoming, *Nurs Sci Q* 21(1):59–67, 2008.

Keller V, Baker L: Communicate with care, *RN* 63(1):32–33, 2000.

Kettunen T, Poskiparta M, Liimatainen L: Empowering counseling—a case study: nurse-patient encounter in a hospital, *Health Educ Res* 16:227–238, 2001.

Klagsbrun J: Listening and focusing: holistic health care tools for nurses, *Nurs Clin North Am* 36(1):115–130, 2001.

Majanovic-Shane A: *Metaphor: a propositional comment and an invitation to intimacy, 1996,* Paper presented at the Second Conference for Sociocultural Research, Geneva, Switzerland September, 1996. Available online: www.speakeasy.org/~anamshane/intima.pdf.

McGhee P: Rx laughter, *RN* 61(7):50–53, 1998.

Moustakas C: *Finding yourself: finding others*, Englewood Cliffs, NJ, 1974, Prentice Hall.

Myers S: Empathetic listening: reports on the experience of being heard, *J Humanist Psychol* 40(2):148–174, 2000.

Nadzam D: Nurses' role in communication and patient safety, *J Nurs Care Qual* 24(3):184–188, 2009.

Peplau H: Talking with patients, *Am J Nurs* 60(7):964–966, 1960.

Periyakoil V: Using metaphors in medicine, *J Palliat Med* 11(6): 842–844, 2008.

Platt FW, Gaspar DL: Tell me about yourself"; the patient-centered interview, *Ann Intern Med* 134(11):1079–1085, 2001.

Ruesch J: *Therapeutic communication*, New York, 1961, Norton.

Samovar L, Porter R, McDaniel E: *Communication between Cultures*, Boston MA, 2009, Wadsworth Cengage Learning.

Sharpe C: *Telenursing: nursing practice in cyberspace*, Westport, CT, 2001, Auburn House.

Straka DA: Are you listening—have you heard? *Adv Pract Nurs Q* 3(2): 80–81, 1997.

Straneva JA: Therapeutic touch: coming of age, *Holist Nurs Pract* 14(3): 1–13, 2000.

Sundin K, Jansson L: Understanding and being understood" as a creative caring phenomenon: in care of patients with stroke and aphasia, *J Clin Nurs* 12:107–116, 2003.

Van Servellen G: Talking the talk to improve your skills, *Nursing* 39(12):22–23, 2009.

Weiten W, Lloyd M, Dun S, et al: *Psychology applied to modern life: adjustment in the 21st centtury*, Belmont CA, 2009, Wadsworth Cengage Learning.

CHAPTER 11

Intercultural Communication

Elizabeth C. Arnold

OBJECTIVES

At the end of the chapter, the reader will be able to:

1. Define culture and related terms.
2. Discuss the concept of intercultural communication.
3. Describe the concept of cultural competence.
4. Apply the nursing process to the care of culturally diverse clients.
5. Discuss characteristics of selected cultures as they relate to the nurse-client relationship.

This chapter is designed to equip nurses with the knowledge and skills needed to interact with clients from varied cultural backgrounds. The chapter describes communication principles and applications from a multicultural perspective. Included are social and cultural factors associated with the United States' four major cultural groups.

BASIC CONCEPTS

CULTURE

Culture is a complex social concept that encompasses the entirety of socially transmitted communication styles, family customs, political systems, and ethnic identity held by a particular group of people. "Culture is primarily learned and transmitted through family and other social institutions" (p. 213), for example schools and church. (Giger, Davidhizar, Purnell, Harden, Phillips, & Strickland, 2007(a)). Exercise 11-1 offers an opportunity to reflect on how culture is learned within the family.

Culture develops from the customs, beliefs, and social institutions associated with different ethnic, racial, religious, and social groups. Cultural patterns shape health-related beliefs, attitudes, values, and behaviors (Kleinman & Benson, 2006). Culture differences relate to some or all of the life issues identified in Box 11-1. Culture is a strong determinant of social behavior. The meaning of the word culture extends beyond country of origin and ethnic background to include professional, organizational, and religious cultures (Betancourt, 2004).

Multiculturalism describes a heterogeneous society in which diverse cultural worldviews can coexist with some general (-etic) characteristics shared by all cultural groups and some (-emic) perspectives that are unique to a particular population.

Worldview is defined as "the way people tend to look out upon their world or their universe to form a picture or value stance about life or the world around them" (Leininger & McFarland, 2006, p. 15). It is closely linked to cultural and spiritual beliefs, but it is not the same. Culture describes the social characteristics of a society. Worldview describes an individual's perceptions of his or her reality within that society. A teenager and an older adult can have similar beliefs about their culture, but their worldviews would be dissimilar because of the age difference.

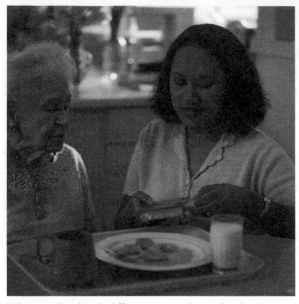

Ethnic and cultural differences need not be barriers to relationships

The existence of cultural patterns as part of personal identity and client preferences is fundamental to understanding nurse and client behavior in therapeutic relationships. Delivering safe, effective, client-centered care requires sensitivity to cultural differences, with specialized skill development in multicultural interpersonal communication skills.

RELATED CONCEPTS
Subculture

Subculture refers to a smaller group of people living within the dominant culture who have adopted a cultural lifestyle distinct from that of the mainstream population. The Amish are an important subculture. Dress, loyalty to a leader or cause, language, social patterns, philosophies, and behavior distinguish members of a subculture. The differences between subculture orientations and mainstream cultural expectations can create conflict (Drench, Noonan, Sharby, & Ventura, 2009).

EXERCISE 11-1 | Family Culture Experiences

Purpose: To help students appreciate how people learn about their culture within their family in the course of everyday living.

Procedure:
1. Identify and describe one family custom or tradition. It can relate to special family foods, a holiday custom, a child-rearing practice, or any other special tradition.
2. Describe the custom or tradition in detail.
3. Talk with a family member about how this family tradition originated in your family.
4. Discuss how this custom or tradition has changed over time.
5. Describe how this family tradition has affected your family functioning.

Discussion:
1. Share your family tradition with your classmates.
2. As a class, discuss how differences in family culture can influence health.
3. Discuss how knowledge of family customs can influence communication and health care promotion.

BOX 11-1 | Points of Cultural Diversity in Health Care

- People's feelings, attitudes, and behavioral standards
- Ways of living, language, and habits
- How people relate to others, including attitudes about health professionals
- Nutrition and diet
- Personal views of what is right and wrong
- Perspectives on health, illness, and death, including appropriate rituals

- Hearing about and discussing negative health information
- Decisional authority, role relationships, and truth-telling practices
- Child-rearing practices
- Use of advance directives, informed consent, and client autonomy (Calloway, 2009; Carrese & Rhodes, 2000; Karim, 2003; Searight & Gafford, 2005)

Ethnicity

Ethnicity is used to describe "groups in which members share a cultural heritage from one generation to another" (Day-Vines et al., 2007, p. 403). Personal awareness of a common racial, geographic, religious, or historical history binds people together, with a strong commitment to ethnic values and practices. Research indicates that ethnicity is an important aspect of a person's social identity (Malhi, Boon, & Rogers, 2009).

Ethnicity describes a sociopolitical construct, different from race and physical characteristics (Ford & Kelly, 2005). People with similar skin color and features can have a vastly different ethnic heritage: Jamaican versus African American. Ethnicity can reflect spiritually based membership, for example, Amish (Donnermeyer & Friedrich, 2006).

Ethnocentrism

Ethnocentrism refers to a belief that one's own culture should be the norm because it is considered better or more enlightened than others. Other cultures are judged as inferior (Lewis, 2000). Taking pride in one's culture is appropriate, but when a person fails to respect the value of other cultures, it is easy to develop stereotypes and prejudice. Ethnocentrism fosters the belief that one culture has the right to impose its standards of "correct" behavior and values on another. Prejudice can be felt or expressed, and directed to either a group as a whole or toward an individual associated with the group (Allport, 1979). The deadly consequences of prejudice were evidenced in the persecution of innocent people during Hitler's regime, and continue today with terrorist attacks and violence embedded in ethnocentric views and sectarian differences.

A variation of ethnocentrism labels people who are different from the mainstream as being inferior (Canales & Howers, 2001). Examples include physical or mental disability, sexual orientation, ageism, morbid obesity, and unusual physical or personal characteristics.

Case Example

"I knew a man who had lost the use of both eyes. He was called a 'blind man.' He could also be called an expert typist, a conscientious worker, a good student, a careful listener, and a man who wanted a job. But he couldn't get a job in the department store order room where employees sat and typed orders, which came over the phone. The personnel man was impatient to get the interview over.

'But you are a blind man,' he kept saying, and one could almost feel his silent assumption that somehow the incapability in one aspect made the man incapable in every other. So blinded by the label was the interviewer that he could not be persuaded to look beyond it" (Allport, 1979, p. 178). Exercise 11-2 explores the prevalence of cultural stereotypes.

Cultural Relativism

Cultural relativism holds that each culture is unique and should be judged only on the basis of its own values and standards. Behaviors viewed as unusual from outside a culture make perfect sense when they are evaluated within a cultural context (Aroian & Faville, 2005).

Case Example

Benjamin Franklin's Comments on Native Americans
"Savages we call them, because their Manners differ from ours, which we think the Perfection of Civility; they think the same of theirs. Perhaps if we could examine the Manners of Different Nations with Impartiality, we should find no people so rude, as to be without any Rules of Politeness; nor any so polite, as not to have some Remains of Rudeness" (Benjamin Franklin, quoted in Jandt, 2003, p. 76).

Exercise 11-3 examines how culture shapes values and perceptions.

Cultural Diversity

Cultural diversity refers to variations among cultural groups. People notice differences related to language, mannerisms, and behaviors in people of different cultures, in ways that do not happen with people from their own culture (Spence, 2001). Lack of exposure to and understanding of people from other cultures reinforces stereotypes and creates prejudice.

Diversity exists *within* a culture too. The Institute of Medicine (2002) identifies economic status and social class as components of diversity related to health risk and treatment outcomes. More differences can exist among individuals within a culture than between cultural groups related to educational and socioeconomic background, age, gender, and life experiences. This is true of providers and clients

EXERCISE 11-2	Exploring Cultural Stereotypes

Purpose: To help students examine stereotypes and their impact on communication and relationships.

Procedure:
The first part of this exercise should be written outside of class, anonymously, to encourage honest answers. The following list represents some of the groups in our society that carry familiar value-laden stereotypes:

African Americans	Alcoholics	Hispanics
AIDS victims	Immigrants	People on welfare
Asian Americans	Mentally ill persons	Homeless people
Native American	Elderly adults	Homosexuals
Teenage mothers	Hearing deficit	Migrant workers

1. Write down the first three words or phrases that come into your mind regarding each of these groups.
2. Make a grid with headings representative of positive, negative, and neutral connotations.
3. As a class group, take the collected words and phrases and place each word or phrase under the appropriate column for each group. Use an X to indicate repetitive words or phrases.

Discussion:
For each cultural group, consider the following:
1. Why do you think people believe that this cultural group possesses these characteristics? Are the characteristics good, bad, or evil as an abstract concept?
2. What were the common themes of these groups? Did certain groups have more negative than positive responses? If so, how would you account for this?
3. In what ways did this exercise help you to think about your own cultural socialization process?
4. Did this exercise cause you to question any of your own assumptions about culturally different values?
5. From your view, what implications do these stereotypes hold for providing appropriate nursing care?
6. How can you use this exercise in your future care of culturally different populations?

Modified from Eliason M, Macy N: A classroom activity to introduce cultural diversity, *Nurse Educ* 17(3):32–35, 1992.

EXERCISE 11-3	Values and Perceptions Associated with Different Cultures

Purpose: To help students appreciate values and generalized perceptions associated with different cultures.

Procedure:
1. Select a specific ethnic culture
2. Interview someone from that culture and ask them to tell you about their culture related to family values, religion, what is important in social interaction health care beliefs, and end-of-life rituals.
3. Write a short report on your findings.
4. Share your written report with your classmates.

Discussion:
1. What important values did you uncover?
2. In what ways did the person's answers agree or disagree with the generalized cultural characteristics of the culture?
3. What did you learn from doing this exercise that you could use in your clinical practice with culturally diverse clients?

even when they share the same spoken language. Exercise 11-4 examines cultural diversity in the nursing profession.

Acculturation

Acculturation describes how a person from a different culture initially learns the behavior norms and values of the dominant culture, and begins to adopt its behaviors and language patterns. Physical acculturation takes place before emotional acculturation. Higher socioeconomic status, social support, and education facilitate the process of acculturation. The client's level of acculturation is a factor in client assessment and nursing care.

Assimilation

Assimilation refers to a person's full adoption of the behaviors, customs, values, and language of the

---

EXERCISE 11-4 | Diversity in the Nursing Profession

Purpose: To help students learn about the experience of nurses from a different ethnic group.

Procedure:
1. Each student will interview a registered nurse from an ethnic minority group different from their own ethnic origin.
2. The following questions should be asked:
   a. In what ways was your educational experience more difficult or easier as a minority student?
   b. What do you see as the barriers for minority nurses in our profession?
   c. What do you see as the opportunities for minority nurses in our profession?
   d. What do you view as the value of increasing diversity in the nursing profession for health care?

   e. What do you think we can do as a profession and personally to increase diversity in nursing?
3. Write a one- to two-page narrative report about your findings to be presented in a follow-up class.

Discussion:
1. What were the common themes that seemed to be present across narratives?
2. How do professional nurses view diversity, and how did doing this exercise influence your thinking about diversity?
3. Did you find any of the answers to the interview questions disturbing or surprising?
4. How could you use this exercise in becoming culturally competent?

---

mainstream culture. By the third generation, people may have little knowledge of their traditional culture and language, or allegiance to their original heritage. Even so, people carry unconscious vestiges of cultural traditions with them throughout life (Bacallao & Smokowski, 2005).

INTERCULTURAL COMMUNICATION

Intercultural communication refers to conversations between people from different cultures. The concept embraces differences in perceptions, language, and non-verbal behaviors, and recognition of dissimilar contexts for interpretations (Samovar, Porter, & McDaniel, 2008). It is a primary means of sharing meaning and developing relationships between people of different cultures. Successful outcomes emphasize a common understanding and inclusion of issues and values that facilitate treatment (Purnell, Purnell, Paulanka, et al. 2008).

With intercultural communication, the perception of relationship between care provider and client is just as important as the words used to communicate. Interactions take place within "transcultural caring relationships" (Pergert, Ekblad, Enskar, & Bjork, 2007, p. 18). Relationships are carefully designed to provide a respectful, encouraging environment in which the client's cultural values and beliefs can be freely expressed and responded to with empathy (Pergert et al., 2007).

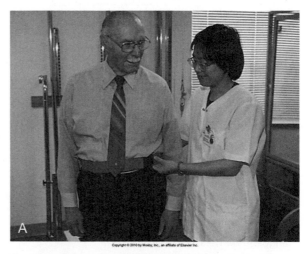

A

The goal of intercultural communication is to find a common ground through which people from different cultures can connect on many different levels with each other.

Case Example

A Chinese first-time mother, tense and afraid as she entered the transition phase of labor, spoke no English. Her husband spoke very little, and saw birthing as women's work. Callister (2001) relates, "The nurse could feel palpable tension that filled the room. The nurse could not speak Chinese either, but she tried to convey a sense of caring, touching the woman, speaking softly, modeling supportive behavior for her husband and

Continued

Case Example—cont'd

helping her to relax as much as possible. The atmosphere in the room changed considerably with the calm competence and quiet demeanor of the nurse. Following the birth ... the father conveyed to her how grateful he was that she spoke Chinese. She tactfully said, 'Thank you, but I don't speak Chinese.' He looked at her in amazement and said with conviction, 'You spoke Chinese.' The language of the heart transcends verbal communication" (p. 212).

LIMITED LANGUAGE PROFICIENCY

Limited language proficiency is a fundamental barrier to effective health care delivery. Different languages create and express different cultural and personal realities. Understanding vocabulary and grammar is not enough. Language competence requires "knowing what to say, and how, when, where, and why to say it" (Hofstede, Pedersen, & Hofsted, 2002, p. 18).

Linguistic rules, language structures, and meanings vary among cultures. Different dialects even within the same culture create language difficulties. Within the same language, words can have more than one meaning. For example, the words *hot, warm,* and *cold* can refer to temperature, or to impressions of strong personal characteristics, or responses to new ideas (Sokol & Strout, 2006). Idioms are particularly problematic because they represent a nonliteral expression of an idea.

Case Example

A nursing student from the Philippines said she was thoroughly confused by her instructor's slang expression, "I want to touch base with you." The student did not know how to respond because her literal translation of the instructor's sentence did not express its meaning to her. Had the instructor said, "I would like to talk with you," the student would have known how to respond.

Nonverbal behaviors, designed to clarify messages and demonstrate relations, are not the same in different cultures. Most people are reasonably comfortable about the meanings of common nonverbal symbols in their own culture—and even then, they have to clarify that the nonverbal has the same meaning for both parties. But consider going to a different culture, where the same gesture or nonverbal symbol has the opposite meaning or is meaningless (Anderson & Wang, 2008). Understanding cultural differences in nonverbal behavior is a dimension of intercultural communication. Exercise 11-5 provides an opportunity to consider the implications of language barriers.

CULTURAL COMPETENCE

Cultural competence is defined as "a set of cultural behaviors and attitudes integrated into the practice methods of a system, agency, or its professionals, that

EXERCISE 11-5	Understanding Language Barriers Role-Play

Purpose: To help students understand the role of language barriers.

Procedure:
Situation 1
Lee Singh is a 24-year-old Korean patient who speaks no English. She was admitted to the maternity unit and has just delivered her first child, a 9-pound infant. It was a difficult labor because the infant was so big. The initial objectives of the health care providers are to help the client understand what is happening to her and to help her become comfortable with her baby.
Situation 2
Jose Perot is a 30-year-old Hispanic man who was admitted to the emergency department with multiple injuries after a car accident. His family has been notified, but the nurse is not sure they understand what has happened. They have just arrived in the emergency department.

1. Break up into groups of four or five students. Each group acts as a unit. The groups role-play Situation 1 and reverse roles for Situation 2.
2. The client group should completely substitute made-up words that only they understand for the words they would normally use to communicate in this situation. The made-up words should have the same meaning to all members of the client group.
3. The health provider group must figure out creative ways to understand and communicate with the client group.

Discussion:
1. In what ways was it different being the client and being the health provider group?
2. What was the hardest part of this exercise?
3. In what ways did this exercise help you understand the frustrations of being unable to communicate?

enables them to work effectively in cross cultural situations" (Sutton, 2000, p. 58). The Institute of Medicine (2003) and the American Association of Colleges of Nursing (AACN, 2008) identify cultural competence as an essential skill set required for health care providers.

Self-awareness of unintentional bias in health care is essential. Value judgments are hard to eliminate, particularly those outside of awareness. Developing competence begins with self-awareness of your own cultural values, attitudes, and perspectives, followed by developing knowledge and acceptance of cultural differences in others (Gravely, 2001; Leonard & Plotnikoff, 2000). This allows you to own your own biases and not project them onto clients. Exercise 11-6 provides an opportunity for you to reflect on personal cultural beliefs, values, and behaviors.

Cultural competence is expressed through cultural sensitivity. The Office of Minority Health (U.S. Department of Health and Human Services [DHHS], 2001) describes **cultural sensitivity** in health care as "the ability to be appropriately responsive to the attitudes, feelings, or circumstances of groups of people that share a common and distinctive racial, national, religious, linguistic, or cultural heritage" (p. 131). Used with clients, cultural sensitivity is expressed through the use of neutral words, categorizations, and behaviors that respect the culture of the client, and avoidance of those that could be interpreted as offensive (AACN, 2008). Practiced by health care providers, cultural sensitivity refers to an understanding of one's own cultural beliefs, and how these beliefs and values affect their practice with minority clients. The goal of culturally sensitive communication is to find common ground.

Case Example

"There weren't many Filipino nurses [in that hospital] and a lot of them were Caucasian and I remember this Black nurse ... who was very, very nice. I think it was because she is not a Caucasian and she is able to feel with me. She probably sympathized with me who like her is from a different culture and had to move to Canada" (Pasco, Morse, & Olson, 2004, p. 243).

A valuable way to learn about another person's culture is to spend time with them and to ask questions about what is important to them about their culture (Jandt, 2003).

HEALTH DISPARITIES

Health disparities is defined as "a chain of events signified by a difference in the environment, access to, utilization of, and quality of care, health status, or a particular health outcome that deserves scrutiny" (Villarruel, 2004, p. 8). In 2002, the Institute of

---

EXERCISE 11-6 | Self-awareness Cultural Assessment

Purpose: To help students develop awareness of their own culture.

Procedure:
Think about your own culture and answer the following questions. Be as honest as you can; this will help you to be open and honest toward clients from culturally diverse backgrounds. There are no right or wrong answers.
1. Where did my family originate?
2. What do I attach importance to that could be considered a cultural value?
3. What do I believe about the gender roles of men and women? Are my beliefs different or consistent with those of my parents?
4. How much physical distance do I need in social interactions?
5. Who are the decision makers in my family, and whom do I look to for guidance in important matters?
6. What are my definitions of health and well-being?

7. If I needed health care, how would I respond to this need and what would be my expectations?
8. In a health care situation, what would be the role of my family?
9. In a health care situation, how important would religion be, and what would I need for spiritual comfort?

Discussion:
1. Share your observations with your classmates.
2. How difficult was it for you to really identify some of the behaviors and expectations that are part of your cultural self?
3. Were you surprised with any of your answers? If so, in what ways?
4. What did you learn about culture from hearing stories of other students? In what ways were their stories the same or different from your cultural story?
5. How can you use this exercise in communicating with clients from culturally diverse backgrounds?

Medicine reported that people of color and ethnic minorities receive a lower quality of care even when insurance and income are considered. This phenomena has been confirmed in a number of research studies (Giger, Davidhizar, Purnell, Harden, Phillips, Strickland, 2007(b)). *Healthy People 2010* identifies "eliminating health disparities" and "improving the quality of life" for U.S. citizens as overarching goals. The *National Healthcare Disparities Report* (2007) confirms that minority status accounts for significant differences and inequality in the quality of health care related to access, screenings, and level of care.

The National Center for Health Statistics (2007) indicates that ethnic and racial minorities, which make up 30% of the adult population, and almost 40% of the U.S. population younger than 18 have greater mortality and morbidity rates (Edwards, 2009; National Center for Health Statistics, 2007). These demographics, coupled with a sharp increase in the number of immigrants entering the United States and Canada, require a special focus on the role of culture in nurse-client relationships. By 2050, ethnic minorities are expected to become a numerical majority (Sue & Sue, 2003).

Developing an Evidence-Based Practice

McElmurry B, Park C, Buseh A: The nurse-community health advocate team for urban immigrant primary health care, *J Nurs Sch* 35(3):275–280, 2003.

This descriptive study was designed to describe an urban outreach health program for Latino immigrants, using a professional nurse and community advocate teamed together in providing health care delivery. Convenience samples of participants, staff, and other sources were used to describe the program and its effects in the Latino community.

Results: Findings indicated that pairing nurses with community health advocates greatly enhanced the project team's ability to provide preventive care in the Latino community. The combined resources provided culturally sensitive care to Latino immigrants, and enabled them to seek and obtain appropriate health care.

Application to Your Clinical Practice: As professionals working in an increasingly multicultural society, nurses need to develop innovative ways to reach out to immigrants with limited knowledge and limited ways to access the health care system. What steps would you need to take as an individual nurse to encourage a stronger connection between culturally sensitive nursing care and the needs of immigrant populations?

APPLICATIONS

Minorities are less likely to participate in screening or to seek early treatment for recognizable symptoms. They have misgivings about the health care system and feel uncomfortable about using it (Johnstone & Kanitsaki, 2009). Fundamental cultural differences in health beliefs, unfamiliarity with the health care system, language or literacy, and fear of discrimination contribute to gaps in assessment and treatment. Healthy People 2010 (DHHS, 2000) identifies eliminating health disparities among different population groups as one of its overarching goals.

Accessing health care for minority clients can be frustrating. Minority populations, especially new immigrants, often are marginalized economically, occupationally, and socially in ways that adversely affect their access to mainstream health care. Seeking treatment and compliance with treatment is complicated by an inability to effectively describe health problems in terms health providers understand. Undocumented immigrants have an added burden of fearing deportation if their legal status is revealed (Chung, Bernak, Otiz, & Sandoval-Perez, 2008).

CARE OF THE CULTURALLY DIVERSE CLIENT

This section describes the integration of cultural sensitivity into the assessment, diagnosis and treatment planning, implementation, and evaluation of client-centered professional nursing care. When health recommendations conflict with a client's worldview, it is unlikely they will be followed. Having knowledge and constructive attitudes about health traditions associated with different cultures increases client comfort and engagement with caregivers. Hulme (2010) distinguishes between the folk domain and alternative health care remedies. She emphasizes the need to understand the client's health care traditions which are "specific to—and fundamentally a part of—an individual's culture" (p. 276).

BUILDING RAPPORT

Minority clients often have limited firsthand experience with the complexity of the U.S. health care system that could help them negotiate it successfully. They respond better to providers who orient them to the setting and set the stage for a comfortable encounter. Ideally, when meeting a client for the first time, you should perform the following tasks:

- Pronounce the client's name correctly. Calling the client by title and last name shows respect. If the name presents a challenge, ask the client how to pronounce it correctly.
- Speak clearly and spend time with the client before asking assessment questions to make the client or family comfortable.
- Avoid assumptions or interpretations about what you are hearing without validating the information.
- Allot more time to conduct a health assessment, to accommodate language needs and cultural interpretations.
- Have as your goal the client's feelings of satisfaction and success in communicating health concerns and expectations.
- Take the position of interested co-learner when inquiring about cultural values and standards of behavior.
- Inquire about individual perceptions, as well as cultural explanatory models associated with the illness, and preferences for treatment.
- Explain treatment procedures at every opportunity and alert clients ahead of time of potential discomfort.
- Ask permission for and explain the necessity for any physical examination and use of assessment tools.

GUIDES TO CULTURAL ASSESSMENT

Cultural competence is described as "the adaptation of care in a manner that is congruent with the client's culture" (Giger, Davidhizar, Purnell, Harden, Phillips, & Strickland, 2007(b), p. 98). Madeleine Leininger's Theory of Culture Care (2006) is recognized as a major contribution to nursing's understanding of culture in health care. Leininger believes that nurses must have knowledge about diverse cultures to provide care that fits the client. Her sunrise model is composed of "enablers," which help explain each person's cultural environmental context, language, and ethnohistory. Enabling factors reflect the person's worldview and a person's social and culture structures. Each influences verbal and nonverbal expressions, patterns, and understandings of health and health practices.

Larry Purnell's model (see Table 11-1) examines cultural competence from both its macro aspects (global society, community, family, and the person), and its micro aspects consisting of 12 interconnected domains at the person level. Using Purnell's domains as a framework for understanding individual differences dictated by national cultural standards and practices allows for a comprehensive cultural assessment and a culturally congruent, individualized, patient-centered approach to client care.

ASSESSMENT THROUGH A CULTURAL LENS

Assessment should start with the client's reality. Although actual symptoms may be similar, clients will express symptoms consistent with their ethnic beliefs (DHHS, 2001). How clients answer questions about symptoms can reveal which aspects of their complaints are culturally acceptable, and how the client's culture permits their expression. Asking questions like "Can you tell me about your illness and how it developed?" provides information about cultural explanatory models of illness. The information you need would include the client's

- Identified cultural affiliation
- Health beliefs, and values
- Customary health practices
- Spiritual beliefs and practices
- Culturally specific social structures related to health care

Although clients from a different culture may not spontaneously volunteer information about their cultural practices, they often are willing to share this information when asked by an empathetic, interested health care provider. Table 11-2 provides sample questions to assess client preferences when the client is from a different culture.

DIAGNOSIS

Cultural beliefs and values play a role in the interpretation and response to a clinical diagnosis, especially if the culture relates the development of illness to personal weakness or the will of God. For example, it is not uncommon for Asian and Arab Israeli women to believe that breast cancer is God's will or fate (Kim & Flaskerud, 2008; Baron-Epel, Friedman & Lernau, 2009). Such cultural beliefs can affect use of early detection mammograms. Nurses need to be

TABLE 11-1 Purnell's Domains of Cultural Assessment

Domains of Cultural Assessment	Sample Areas for Inquiry
Personal Heritage	Country of origin, reasons for migration, politics, class distinctions, education, social and economic status
Communication	Dominant language and dialects, personal space, body language and touch, time relationships, greetings, eye contact
Family Roles and Organization	Gender roles; roles of extended family, elders, head of household; family goals, priorities, and expectations; lifestyle differences
Workforce Issues	Acculturation and assimilation, gender roles, temporality, current and previous jobs, variance in salary and status associated with job changes
Bioecology	Genetics, hereditary factors, ethnic physical characteristics, drug metabolism
High Risk Health Behaviors	Drugs, nicotine and alcohol use, sexual behaviors
Nutrition	Meaning of food, availability and food preferences, taboos associated with food, use of food in illness
Pregnancy and Childbearing	Rituals and constraints during pregnancy, labor and delivery practices, newborn and postpartum care
Death Rituals	How death is viewed, death rituals, preparation of the body, care after death, use of advance directives, bereavement practices
Spirituality	Religious practices, spiritual meanings, use of prayer
Health Care Practices	Traditional practices, magicoreligious health care beliefs, individual versus collective responsibility for health, how pain is expressed, transplantation, mental health barriers
Health Care Practitioners	Use of traditional and/or folk practitioners, gender role preferences in health care

Adapted from Purnell, J.D., and Paulanka, B.J. (2008). *Transcultural health care: A culturally competent approach* (3rd Ed.), FA Davis; and Purnell, J.D. (2009). *Guide to culturally competent health care* (2nd Ed.), F.A. Davis.

TABLE 11-2 Assessing Client Preferences When the Client Is from a Different Culture

Areas to Assess	Sample Assessment Approaches
Explanatory models of illness	"What do you think caused your health problem? Can you tell me a little about how your illness developed?"
Traditional healing processes	"Can you tell me something about how this problem is handled in your country? Are there any special cultural beliefs about your illness that might help me give you better care? Are you currently using any medications or herbs to treat your illness?"
Lifestyle	"What are some of the foods you like? How they are prepared? What do people do in your culture to stay healthy?"
Type of family support	"Can you tell me who in your family should be involved with your care? Who is the decision maker for health care decisions?"
Spiritual healing practices and rituals	"I am not really familiar with your spiritual practices, but I wonder if you could tell me what would be important to you so we can try to incorporate it into your care plan."
Cultural norms about cleanliness	"A number of our patients have special needs related to cleanliness and modesty of which we are not always aware. I am wondering if this is true for you and if you could help me understand what you need to be comfortable."
Truth-telling and level of disclosure	Ask the family about cultural ways of talking about serious illness. In some cultures, the family knows the diagnosis/prognosis, which is not told to the ill person (e.g., Hispanic, Asian).
Ritual and religious ceremonies at time of death	Ask the family about special rituals and religious ceremonies at time of death.

aware that the clinical diagnosis of a disease is embedded in cultural understandings about its etiology and its meaning. This is particularly true for the diagnosis and treatment of mental disorders. Cross and Bloomer (2010) caution that culturally specific expressions of mental illness vary and can lead to misdiagnosis.

Client-centered care in the United States advocates for a shared understanding of illness, diagnosis, and prognosis. Some cultures have strong beliefs about providing full disclosure of diagnosis and prognosis to clients. Cultural preference may dictate that the family be notified first. The family then decides when and if the disclosure should be made to the client. Before discussing important health matters, ask the client who should be involved. Careful, unhurried discussion and inclusion of family members in decision-making processes can be helpful. Asian and Hispanic cultures traditionally prefer family centered decision-making about care for a family member with a terminal diagnosis (Kwak & Haley, 2005). Although informed consent forms require full disclosure, the cultural acceptability of autonomous informed consent can be an ethical issue when interacting with clients who hold different cultural values (Calloway, 2009). When the family is authorized by the client to discuss diagnosis and make treatment decisions, the client's preference should be honored. Exploration of each client's preferences about disclosure should take place early in the clinical relationship.

Case Example

Wilma Martinez is a 67-year-old immigrant from El Salvador who moved to the United States to live with her daughter. Mrs. Martinez speaks only Spanish. Through her daughter's translations, the patient appears to comprehend details of her illness and treatment. When asked if she understands what the doctor is saying, she invariably nods affirmatively. During a clinic visit, when Mrs. Martinez's daughter is not present, the physician arranges for a trained medical interpreter to be present. Later, the interpreter explains that Mrs. Martinez could not understand why the staff was insistent that she, rather than her daughter, make decisions. Mrs. Martinez stated, "In my country, the family decides." Assuming that her daughter would make the decisions for her, she saw no reason to sign the forms. She worried that signing forms would cause legal problems because of her immigration status (Crawley, Marshall, Lo, & Koenig, 2002, p. 675).

COMMUNICATION ISSUES IN PLANNING AND INTERVENTION

Clients from different cultures often identify language barriers as the most frustrating aspect of communicating in health care situations. Following are communication principles to keep in mind when planning and implementing care.

- Limitations in English proficiency should not be construed as a limitation of intellectual functioning.
- People can be highly literate in their language of origin, but functionally illiterate in English.
- Internal interpretation of a message is often accompanied by visual imagery reflecting the person's cultural beliefs and experiences. (This can change the meaning of the original message, with neither party having awareness of the differences in interpretation.)

People tend to think and process information in their native language, translating back and forth from English. This results in delayed responses that need to be taken into account, particularly in health teaching. Sometimes the nurse is aware only that the client seems to be taking more time than usual. With clients demonstrating limited English proficiency, speak slowly and clearly; use simple words; and avoid slang, technical jargon, and complex sentences. All written information should be provided in the person's native language whenever possible, to avoid misinterpretation. It is important that the translator of information be as well versed in medical interpretations as in relevant terms used in both languages.

ROLE RELATIONS

Understanding that role interactions between health providers and clients are embedded in cultural influences helps nurses structure meaningful interactions. In many minority cultures, there is an unspoken tendency to view health professionals as authority figures, treating them with deference and respect. This value can be so strong that a client will not question the nurse or in any way indicate mistrust of professional recommendations. They just do not follow the professional advice.

Asian clients typically respond better to a formal relationship and an indirect communication style characterized by polite phrases and marked deference. They work better with well-defined boundaries and clear expectations (Galanti, 2008). The client waits for the information to be offered by the nurse as the authority figure. Sometimes this gets interpreted as timidity. A better interpretation is that the client is deferring to the health professional's expertise.

LEVEL OF FAMILY INVOLVEMENT

Level of family involvement can be an issue for people from collectivistic cultures. Distinctions between male and female roles are well defined in these cultures, and this can affect decision making in health care. In Hispanic and Asian cultures, male family members are likely to be the identified decision makers. Age and position in the family are relevant. Decisions may be deferred to elders, and there may be distinct role expectations of the eldest man, of women, and of children within the family. Identifying and including from the outset all those who will be taking an active part in the care of the client recognizes the communal nature of family involvement in health care. For the Native American client, this may include members of an immediate tribe or its spokesperson.

TIME ORIENTATION

Galanti (2008) distinguishes between present and future time. American culture is a future-oriented culture in which people are accustomed to meeting exact time frames for appointments and taking medications. Present time cultures do not consider the commitment to a future appointment as important as attending to what is happening in the moment. They deal with things as they come up, and not before. Giger and Davidhizar (1991) note, "A common belief shared by some African Americans and Mexican Americans is that time is flexible and events will begin when they arrive" (p. 105). Usually it is necessary to explain not once but many times why a precise schedule is required, and to extend some flexibility when possible.

Clock time versus activity time also reflects culture (Galanti, 2008). Contrast the difference in time orientation of a clock-conscious German person with that of his Italian counterpart.

Case Example

Germans and Swiss love clock-regulated time, for it appears to them as a remarkably efficient, impartial, and very precise way of organizing life—especially in business. For Italians, on the other hand, time considerations will usually be subjected to human feelings. "Why are you so angry because I came at 9:30?" an Italian asks his German colleague. "Because it says 9 a.m. in my diary," says the German. "Then why don't you write 9:30 and then we'll both be happy?" is a logical Italian response. The business we have to do and our close relations are so important that it is irrelevant at what time we meet. The meeting is what counts (Lewis, 2000, p. 55).

COMMUNICATION PRINCIPLES

Clients from minority backgrounds respond better to health care providers who ask about and take into account their social circumstances, values, and cultural experiences. Framing interventions within a culturally sensitive format that the client recognizes as familiar and valid, and openly discussing differences in backgrounds, norms, and health practices increases client understanding and compliance.

Interventions for culturally diverse clients use the same communication strategies discussed in other chapters, with special accommodation for cultural differences. Client-centered principles include:

- Respect for the client's belief in folk and natural traditional remedies
- Combining cultural folk treatments with standard medical practices to whatever extent is possible
- Familiarity with formal and informal sources of health care in the cultural community, including churches, Shamans, medicine men/women, curanderos, and other faith healers
- Respect for family position and gender distinctions when relating to family members about health care concerns
- Continuous use of active listening strategies, with frequent validation to ensure the cultural appropriateness of provider assumptions
- Remembering that the client is a person first and a cultural person second

Informed Consent and Client Autonomy

Issues such as client autonomy and informed consent need to be reframed within a cultural context (Calloway, 2009). Without full disclosure, consent forms are not valid.

Philosophical differences about end-of-life care exist between Western values and those of the four major minority groups. Many minority clients believe in prolonging life and are reluctant to use advance

| EXERCISE 11-7 | Applying Cultural Sensitivity to Care Planning |

Purpose: To practice cultural sensitivity in care planning.

Procedure:
This can be done in small, even-numbered groups rather than as an individual exercise.
1. Out of class, create a written clinical scenario based on a client from a cultural group. Be creative and write a situation in which ethnicity or cultural factors are present in the client's nursing needs.
2. Trade scenarios with another student.
3. Write what should be included in a culturally sensitive care plan.

4. Discuss each of the care plans and make any revisions.

Discussion:
1. What were the areas of agreement and disagreement about the care plan?
2. What questions would you need to ask to clarify needs?
3. In developing the plan, did you find any additional needs?
4. How could you use this exercise to improve your clinical practice?

directives (Thomas, 2001). Exercise 11-7 provides an opportunity to explore the role of cultural sensitivity in care planning.

HEALTH TEACHING PRINCIPLES

Health teaching strategies for culturally diverse populations is a challenge. Specific approaches include the following:

- Be patient when teaching; extra time is always needed.
- Look for facial expressions indicating bewilderment, frustration, or being overwhelmed. If the client seems confused, stop and ask the client to explain how it works in his or her culture.
- Use an English-as-a-second-language style of phrasing; that is, speak words slowly, with distinct separation of words and accentuation of important terms.
- Explain information in greater depth. Repeat explanations of important information in another way if the client does not seem to understand the original explanation.
- Use gestures, pantomime, body language, and visual cues to enhance words.
- Acknowledge effort and express belief in the client's ability to grasp the material (Tong, Huang, & McIntyre, 2006).

Cultural differences affect a nurse's coaching functions. A useful teaching sequence for clients from culturally diverse backgrounds is to use the mnemonic LEARN: Listen, Explain, Acknowledge, Recommend, and Negotiate (Campinha-Bacote, 1992). With this process, you *listen* carefully to the client's

perspective on his or her health problem, including cause, expectations for treatment, and information about family and others who traditionally are involved in the client's care.

Once you have a clear understanding of the client's perception of the problem, you can *explain* your understanding, using simple, concrete terminology, and then ask for validation that your perspective is accurate. Acknowledge the differences and similarities between perceptions. Specific *recommendations* to the client flow from shared understanding of the issues.

The final step is *negotiating* a mutually acceptable treatment approach. This may take longer because of language and cultural expectations. The client's right to hold different cultural views and to make decisions reflective of those views must be respected. If family members traditionally are involved in decision making (with the client's consent), they should be actively involved in decision making. Box 11-2 provides general guidelines for teaching clients from culturally diverse backgrounds.

USE OF INTERPRETERS

Federal law (Title VI of the Civil Rights Act) mandates the use of a trained interpreter for any client experiencing communication difficulties in health care settings because of language. Interpreters should have a thorough knowledge of the culture, as well as the language. They should be carefully chosen, keeping in mind variations in dialects, as well as differences in the sex and social status of the interpreter and the client if these are likely to be an issue. In general, family members, particularly children, should not be used

BOX 11-2	Communication Guidelines for Teaching Clients

- Use the same sequence and repeat phrases, expanding on the same basic questions.
- Speak slowly and clearly, and use concrete language the client can understand. Make the sentence structure as simple as possible.
- Encourage the client by smiling and by listening. Provide cues such as pictures and gestures.
- Avoid the use of technical language, and choose words that incorporate cultural terms whenever possible.
- Allow enough time, and do not assume that simply because the client nods or smiles that the communication is understood.
- Identify barriers to compliance, such as social values, environment, and language.
- Help the client develop realistic, culturally relevant goals.
- Incorporate culturally specific teaching formats (e.g., use an oral or storytelling format with clients who have oral teaching traditions).
- Close with cultural sensitivity: "I've really learned a lot today about [restate highlights]. Thanks for sharing with me."

BOX 11-3	Guidelines for Using Interpreters in Health Care

- Whenever possible, the translator should not be a family member.
- Orient the translator to the goals of the clinical interview and expected confidentiality.
- Look directly at the client when either you or the client is speaking.
- Ask the translator to clarify anything that is not understood by either the nurse or the client.
- After each completed statement, pause for translation.

as interpreters. Box 11-3 provides guidelines for the use of interpreters in health care interviews.

Cultural Brokering

Cultural brokering refers to advocacy actions of mediating between persons or groups from different cultural backgrounds for the purpose of increasing understanding, reducing conflict, or generating change. The cultural broker acts as a go-between and/or advocate for a specified person or group.

FEATURES OF KEY CULTURAL GROUPS

Having basic knowledge of the common cultural features of the four major cultures in the United States enhances service delivery and the nurse's capacity to respond with sensitivity to client needs and preferences (Eiser & Ellis, 2007). It provides a social context for understanding cultural differences.

As you review characteristics of each culture group, it is important to avoid overgeneralizing or viewing them as applicable to all members of a culture or **ethnic group**. Each client is a unique individual. Galanti (2008) distinguishes between generalizations, which can be helpful, and stereotypes. The generalization serves as a cue to ask further questions about social factors impacting health care. Stereotypes make an invalid assumption about an individual, based on general data.

Case Example

An example is the assumption that Mexicans have large families. If I meet Rosa, a Mexican woman, and I say to myself, "Rosa is Mexican; she must have a large family," I am stereotyping her. But if I think Mexicans often have large families and wonder whether Rosa does, I am making a generalization (Galanti, 2008, p. 7).

Education, income, individual characteristics, and level of acculturation are modifiers to be considered in cultural assessment and treatment planning (Kline & Huff, 2008).

Each minority culture discussed in the following sections is a collectivistic society, compared with the United States, which is an individualistic society. Collectivism views people as being fundamentally connected with each other as an integral part of a larger society. Duty to others is considered before duty to self. Individualism views people as being independent parts of the universe and society. Western health care approaches need to respect this difference in communication.

HISPANIC/LATINO CULTURE

Hispanic Americans account for 15% of the population (Office of Minority Health & Health Disparities [OMHD], 2010), making them the largest minority group in the United States. Identifying themselves as Hispanics, or Latinos, they are more racially diverse, and represent a wider range of cultures than other minority groups. Mexican Americans may refer to themselves as Chicanos.

Current growth in the Hispanic population of the United States consists mainly of first-generation and younger immigrants with lower socioeconomic status and undocumented legal status. Many do not speak English or do not speak it well enough to negotiate the U.S. health care system. Implementation of bilingual education in schools acknowledges the significance of the growth in the Hispanic population and social repositioning of diversity as a fact of life in the United States (Cavazos-Rehg & DeLucia-Waack, 2009).

Family

Familismo is a strong value in the Hispanic community (Juarez, Ferrell, & Boreman, 1998). The family is the center of Hispanic life and serves as a primary source of emotional support. Hispanic clients are "family members first, and individuals second" (Pagani-Tousignant, 1992, p. 10). Family units tend to live in close proximity with each other and close friends are considered a part of the family unit. Latino families have strong cultural values and beliefs about the sanctity of life. Families show their love and concern in health care situations by pampering the client.

Gender roles are rigid, with the father viewed as head of the household. Latino women are socialized to serve their husbands and children without question (*la sufrida,* or the long-suffering woman; Pagani-Tousignant, 1992). The nurse needs to be sensitive to gender-specific cultural values in treatment situations. Family inclusion in health care planning serves as a focus of care and as a resource to the client.

Religion

Hispanic clients take religion seriously. The predominant religion is Catholicism. Receiving the sacraments is important to Hispanics, and call for family celebration. The final sacrament in the Catholic Church, anointing of the sick, offers comfort for clients and families.

Hispanic clients view health as a gift from God, related to physical, emotional, and social balance (Kemp, 2004). Many believe that illness is the result of a great fright *(susto),* or falling out of favor with God.

Faith in God is closely linked with the Hispanic population's understanding of health care problems (Zapata & Shippee-Rice, 1999). Their relationship with God is an intimate one, which may include personal visions of God or saints. This should not be interpreted as a hallucination.

Health Beliefs and Practices

They identify a "hot-cold balance," referring to a cultural classification of illness resulting from an imbalance of body humors, as essential for health. When a person loses balance, illness follows (Juckett, 2005). "Cold" health conditions are treated with hot remedies, and vice versa. Mental illness is not addressed as such. Instead, a Hispanic client will talk of being sad *(triste).*

Modesty is important to Hispanic women. They may be reluctant to discuss matters of sexuality. Women may be reluctant to express their private concerns in front of their children, even adult children.

Hispanics use the formal health care system only as a short-term problem-solving strategy for health problems. The value of *familisimo* discourages revealing problems outside the family. Hispanic men may view asking for help as a weakness, incompatible with being machismo (Ramos-Sánchez & Atkinson, 2009). Many are illegal immigrants and/or have low incomes, limited education, and no health insurance. A source of health care outside the family is the use of *curanderos* (local folk healers and herb doctors) for initial care. The *curandera* uses a combination of prayers, healing practices, medicines, and herbs to cure illness (Amerson, 2008).

It is not uncommon for clients to share medications with other family members. Aponte (2009) suggests that nurses should ask Hispanic clients about the use of folk medicine and explain, if needed, the reason and importance of sharing this information with the nurse. A proactive prevention approach tailored to the health care needs of this minority population is essential.

Social Interaction Patterns

Spanish is the primary language spoken in all Latin American countries except Brazil (Portuguese) and Haiti (French). Hispanics are an extroverted people who value interpersonal relationships. They appreciate recognition that their speech comes from the heart. Hispanic clients trust feelings more than facts. Strict rules govern social relationships *(respeto),* with higher status being given to older individuals and to male over female individuals. Nurses are viewed as authority figures, to be treated with respect. Clients hesitate to ask questions, so it is important to ask enough questions to ensure that they understand their diagnosis and treatment plan (Aponte, 2009).

Hispanic clients look for warmth, respect, and friendliness *(personalismo)* from their health care providers. It is important to ask about their well-being and to take extra time with finding out what they need. They value smooth social relations, and avoid confrontation and criticism *(simpatia).* Hispanic people are sensitive and easily hurt.

Hispanic clients need to develop trust *(confianza)* in the health care provider. They do this by making small talk before getting down to the business of discussing their health problems. Knowing the importance of *confianza* to the Hispanic client allows nurses to spend initial time engaging in general topics before moving into assessment or care (Knoerl, 2007).

AFRICAN AMERICAN CULTURE

African Americans account for 13.5% of the population of the United States (OMHD, 2010), making them the second largest minority group in the nation A smaller group (referred to as African American or Black) emigrated voluntarily from countries such as Haiti and Jamaica.

Purnell and Paulanka (2008) note, "Black or African American refers to people having origins in any of the black racial groups of Africa, and includes Nigerians and Haitians or any person who self-designates this category regardless of origin" (p. 2). Although African Americans are represented in every socioeconomic group, approximately one-third of them live in poverty (Spector, 2004). For many, their cultural heritage traces back to slavery and deprivation. This unfortunate legacy colors the expectations of African Americans with health care issues, and explains the distrust many African Americans have about the American health care system (Eiser & Ellis, 2007). African Americans need to experience feeling respected by their caregivers to counteract the sense of powerlessness and lack of confidence they sometimes feel in health care settings.

The African American worldview consists of four fundamental characteristics:

- *Interdependence:* feeling interconnected and as concerned about the welfare of others as of themselves
- *Emotional vitality:* expressed with intensity and animation in lifestyle dance, language, and music
- *Harmonious blending:* "going with the flow" or natural rhythm of life
- *Collective survival:* sharing and cooperation is essential to everyone surviving and succeeding (Parham, White, & Ajamu, 2000)

Family

The family is considered the "primary and most important tradition in the African American community" (Hecht et al., 2003, p. 2). Women are often considered the head of the family, consistent with vestiges of a matriarchal tradition in many African villages. Many low-income African American children grow up in extended families. Grandparents assume caregiving responsibilities for working parents. Including grandparents, particularly grandmothers, is useful when caring for African American clients in the community (Purnell & Paulanka, 2005).

African Americans depend on kinship networks for support. Loyalty to the extended family is a dominant value, and family members rely on each other for emotional and financial support (Sterritt & Pokorny, 1998). The combination of strong kinship bonds and the value of "caring for one's own" are important aspects of the African American culture. Caring for less fortunate family members is viewed as a resource strength of African American families (Littlejohn-Blake & Darling, 1993). When planning interventions, taking advantage of kinship bonds and incorporating family as supportive networks can greatly enhance the quality of care.

Religion and Spiritual Practices

The church serves the dual purpose of providing a structure for meeting spiritual needs and functioning as a primary social, economic, and community life center. Chambers (1997) explains, "Since its inception, the black church has been more than a place of worship for African-Americans. It is where the community has gathered to lobby for freedom and equal rights" (p. 42). African American political leaders (e.g., Jesse Jackson and Dr. Martin Luther King, Jr.) are revered as influential church leaders.

Major religions include Christianity (predominantly Protestant), Islam, and to a lesser extent, Pentecostal. Although fairly rare, beliefs associated with ancient religious practices (voodoo) provide explanatory models for illness and emotional disturbance.

Case Example

Ms. Jones is a 56-year-old African American who was brought by her family to the psychiatric emergency service of a large city hospital. She claimed that her husband's lover had poisoned her. After a psychiatric examination, Ms. Jones was given the diagnosis of delusional disorder, jealous type. She was admitted to the inpatient psychiatric unit and started on a neuroleptic medication. However, the diagnostician failed to conduct a cultural assessment, which would have revealed that Ms. Jones felt she was experiencing voodoo illness. A more culturally relevant treatment would have included consultation with a folk healer (Campinha-Bacote, 1992).

Christianity is often associated with evangelical expression. Prayer and the "laying on of hands" may be very important to the African-American client (Purnell & Paulanka, 2005). Because of the central meaning of the church in African-American life, incorporating appropriate clergy as a resource in treatment is a useful strategy. Readings from the Bible and gospel hymns are sources of support during hospitalization.

African Americans account for approximately 30% of the U.S. Muslim population. Islam influences all aspects of life. Muslim clients are expected to follow the Hallal (lawful) diet, which calls for dietary restrictions on eating pork or pork products, and drinking alcohol (Rashidi & Rajaram, 2001).

Health Beliefs and Practices

Lower income African-American clients statistically are less likely to use regular preventive health services. They frequently delay seeking treatment for serious diseases, which results in a poorer prognosis and fewer, more expensive treatment options. Because of cost, many African Americans use emergency departments as a major health care resource (Lynch & Hanson, 2004).

African Americans tend to rely on informal helping networks in the community, particularly those associated with their churches, until a problem becomes a crisis. Purnell and Paulanka (2005) advise engagement of the extended family system, particularly grandmothers, in providing support and health teaching when working with African American clients in the community.

Social Interaction

Establishing trust is essential for successful communication with African American clients. They are more willing to participate in treatment when they feel respected and are treated as treatment partners in their health care. Allowing clients to have as much control over their health care as possible reinforces self-efficacy and promotes self-esteem.

Recognizing and respecting African American values of interdependence, emotional vitality, and collective survival helps facilitate confidence in health care. Awareness of community resources in the African American community and incorporation of informal care networks such as the church, neighbors, and extended family can help provide culturally congruent continuity of care.

African Americans suffer more health disparities than any other minority population. They have a greater rate of HIV infection and are less likely to be on appropriate treatment. African Americans have greater rates of hypertension, adolescent pregnancy, diabetes, heart disease, and stroke, and male African Americans have a significantly greater chance of developing cancer and of dying of it (Spector, 2004).

ASIAN AMERICAN

The third most common minority group in the United States is Asian Americans. Currently, they make up 5% of the population (OHMD, 2010) and represent the fastest growing of all major ethnic groups. Pagani-Tousignant (1992) notes that the cultural community of Asians and Pacific Islanders comprises more than 32 ethnic groups, with the best known being Chinese, Japanese, Indian, Korean, and Vietnamese.

Even within the same geographic grouping, significant cultural differences exist. For example, in India, there are more than 350 "major languages," with 18 being acknowledged as "official languages," and a complex caste system defines distinctive behavioral expectations for gender roles within the broader culture (Chaudhary, 2004).

Asian culture values hard work, education, and going with the flow of events. In most Asian countries, there is an emphasis on politeness and correct behavior. The correct cultural behavior is to put others first and not to create problems. This can lead to vagueness in communication that is not always understandable to cultures that use a more direct communication style. Traditionally, the Asian client exercises significant emotional restraint in communication. Interpersonal conflicts are not directly addressed, and challenging an expert is not allowed (Chen, 2001). Jokes and humor are usually not appreciated because "the Confucian and Buddhist preoccupation with truth, sincerity, kindliness and politeness automatically eliminates humour techniques such as sarcasm, satire, exaggeration and parody" (Lewis, 2000, pp. 20–21).

Family

Asian families traditionally live in multigenerational households, with extended family providing important social support. Individual privacy is uncommon. The Asian culture places family before individual welfare. The centrality of the family unit means that individuals will sacrifice their individuality if needed for the good of the family. The need to avoid "loss of face" by acting in a manner that brings shame to the individual is paramount, because loss of face brings shame to the whole family, including ancestors.

The family may consist of father, mother, and children; nuclear family, grandparents, and other relatives living together; or a broken family in which some family members are in the United States and other nuclear family members are still living in their country of origin (Gelles, 1995). There is family pressure on younger members to do well academically, and the behavior of individual members is always considered within the context of its impact on the family as a whole. Family members are obligated to assume a great deal of responsibility for each other, including ongoing financial assistance. Older children are responsible for the well-being of younger children.

Family communication takes place through prescribed roles and obligations, taking into account family roles, age, and position in the family. The husband (father) is the primary authority and decision maker. He acts as the family spokesperson in crisis situations. Elders in the Asian community are highly respected and well taken care of by younger members of the family (Pagani-Tousignant, 1992). The wisdom of the elders helps guide younger family members on many life issues, including major health decisions (Davis, 2000).

The family is a powerful force in maintaining the religious and social values in Asian cultures. "Good health" is described as having harmonious family relationships and a balanced life (Harrison et al., 2005). Tradition strongly regulates individual behavior. Traditional Chinese culture does not allow clients to discuss the full severity of an illness; this creates challenges for mutual decision making based on full disclosure that is characteristic of Western health care. Family members take an active role in deciding whether a diagnosis should be disclosed to a client. They frequently are the recipients of this information before the client is told of the diagnosis, prognosis, and treatment options.

Religion and Spiritual Practices

Religion plays an important role in Asian society, with religious beliefs tightly interwoven into virtually every aspect of daily life. Referred to as "Eastern religions," major groups include Hindus, Buddhists, and Muslims.

Hinduism is not a homogeneous religion, but rather a living faith and philosophical way of life with diverse doctrines, religious symbols, and moral and social norms (Michaels, 2003). Being a Hindu provides membership in a communal society. Hinduism represents a pragmatic philosophy of life that articulates harmony with the natural rhythms of life, and "right" or "correct" principles of social interaction and behavior. The *veda* refers to knowledge passed through many generations from ancient sages, which combined with Sanskrit literature provides the "codes of ritual, social and ethical behavior, called dharma, which that literature reveals" (Flood, 1996, p. 11).

Hindus are vegetarians: It is against their religion to kill living creatures. Sikhism is a reformed variation of Hinduism in which women have more rights in domestic and community life.

Buddhism represents a philosophical approach to life that identifies fate, Inn and Ko, as the primary factors impacting health and illness. Buddhists believe that In (cause) and Ko (effect) are variables that interact with fate and can influence people to be righteous and experience less stress and guilt, thereby promoting better health (Chen, 2001). Referred to as the four noble truths, Buddhists believe:

- All life is suffering.
- Suffering is caused by desire or attachment to the world.

- Suffering can be extinguished by eliminating desire
- The way to eliminate desire is to live a virtuous life (Lynch & Hanson, 2004).

Buddhists follow the path to enlightenment by leading a moral life, being mindful of personal thoughts and actions, and by developing wisdom and understanding. Buddhists pray and meditate frequently. They eat a vegetarian diet, and alcohol, cigarettes, and drugs are not permitted.

The Muslim religion (Islam) is a way of life. Muslims adhere to the Quran/Koran, the holy teaching of Muhammad. Faith, prayer, giving alms, and making a yearly pilgrimage to Mecca are requirements of the religion.

Identified as an Eastern monotheistic religion, Islam is practiced throughout the world. Followers are called Muslims. Allah is identified as a higher power or God. Muhammad is his prophet. Muslims submit to Allah and follow Allah's basic rules about everything from personal relationships to business matters, including personal matters such as dress and hygiene. Islam has strong tenets that affect health care, an important one being that God is the ultimate healer.

Dietary restrictions center on consuming Halaal (lawful) food. Excluded from the diet are pork and pork products, and alcohol. In the hospital, Muslims can order Kosher food because it meets the requirements for Halaal (Davidson, Boyer, Casey, Matzel, & Walden, 2008). The Muslim client values physical modesty, and the family may request that only female staff care for female family members. Physical contact, eye contact, touch, and hugs between members of the opposite sex who are not family are avoided (McKennis, 1999).

Muslims believe death is a part of Allah's plan, so to fight the dying process with treatment is wrong. They believe that the dying person should not die alone. A close relative should be present, praying for God's blessing or reading the Quran/Koran. Once the person actually dies, it is important to perform the following: turn the body toward Mecca; close the person's mouth and eyes, and cover the face; straighten the legs and arms; announce the death to relatives and friends; bathe the body (with men bathing men and women bathing women); and cover the body with white cotton (Servodido & Morse, 2001).

Health Care Beliefs and Practices

Ayurveda represents an ancient system of medicine endogenous to Asian culture, particularly India. The term describes a "way of living with awareness and promoting longevity" (Lic & Ayur, 2006, p. xix). Mind, body, and spirit are considered an integrated whole, and Ayurveda differentiates between substances, qualities, and actions that are life enhancing and those that are not. It is considered a form of complementary alternative treatment consisting of herbs, yoga, and massage, and is designed to reestablish harmony between the mind, body, and spirit.

Health, based on the ayurvedic principle, requires harmony and balance between yin and yang, the two energy forces required for health (Louie, 2001). A blockage of qi, defined as the energy circulating in a person's body, creates an imbalance between yin (negative energy force) and yang (positive energy force), resulting in illness (Chen, 2001). Yin represents the female force, containing all the elements that represent darkness, cold, and weakness. Yang symbolizes the male elements of strength, brightness, and warmth. Ayurveda emphasizes health promotion and disease prevention.

The influence of Eastern health practices and alternative medicine is increasingly incorporated into the health care of all Americans. Many complementary and alternative medical practices in the United States (acupuncture, botanicals, and massage and therapeutic touch) trace their roots to Eastern holistic health practices. Acupressure and herbal medicines are among the traditional medical practices used by Asian clients to reestablish the balance between yin and yang. In some Asian countries, healers use a process of "coining," in which a coin is heated and vigorously rubbed on the body to draw illness out of the body. The resulting welts can mistakenly be attributed to child abuse if this practice is not understood. Traditional healers, such as Buddhist monks, acupuncturists, and herbalists, also may be consulted when someone is ill.

Social Interaction Patterns

Health care providers are considered health experts, so they are expected to provide specific advice and recommendations (Lynch & Hanson, 2004). Asian clients prefer a polite, friendly, but formal approach in communication. They appreciate clinicians willing to provide advice in a matter-of-fact, concise manner.

Asian clients favor harmonious relationships. Confrontation is avoided; clients will nod and smile in agreement, even when they strongly disagree (Xu, Davidhizar, & Giger, 2004; Cross & Bloomer, 2010). Nurses need to ask open-ended questions and clarify issues throughout an interaction. If you use questions that require a yes or no answer, the answer may reflect the client's polite deference rather than an honest response. Explain treatment as problem solving, ask the client how things are done in his or her culture, and work with the Asian client to develop culturally congruent solutions (McLaughlin & Braun, 1998).

Asian clients are stoic. They may not request pain medication until their pain is quite severe (Im, 2008). Asking the client about pain and offering medication as normal management is helpful. Sometimes it is difficult to tell what Asian clients are experiencing. Facial expressions are not as flexible, and words are not as revealing as those of people in the dominant culture.

Health care concerns specifically relevant to this population include a higher-than-normal incidence of tuberculosis, hepatitis B, and liver cancer (OMHD, 2010). People with mental health issues do not seek early treatment because of shame and the lack of culturally appropriate mental health services (Louie, 2001).

Asian men may have a difficult time disclosing personal information to a female nurse unless the nurse explains why the data are necessary for care, because in serious matters, women are not considered as knowledgeable as men. Asian clients may be reluctant to be examined by a person of the opposite sex, particularly if the examination or treatment involves the genital area.

NATIVE AMERICAN CLIENTS

Native Americans account for 1.6% of the U.S. population (OMHD, 2010). They represent the smallest of the major ethnic groups in the United States. There are more than 500 federally recognized tribes, and another 100 tribes or bands that are state-recognized but are not recognized by the federal government. Native Americans include First or Original Americans, American Indians, Alaskan Natives, Aleuts, Eskimos, Metis (mixed blood), or Amerindians. Most will identify themselves as members of a specific tribe (Garrett & Herring, 2001). Tribal identity is maintained through regular powwows and other ceremonial events. Like other minority groups with an oppressed heritage, the majority of Native Americans are poor and

undereducated, with attendant higher rates of social and health problems (Hodge & Fredericks, 1999).

Family

The family is highly valued by the Native American. Multigenerational families live together in close proximity. When two individuals marry, the marriage contract implicitly includes attachment and obligation to a larger kinship system (Red Horse, 1997). Both men and women feel a responsibility to promote tribal values and traditions through their crafts and traditional ceremonies. However, women are identified as their culture's standard bearers. A Cheyenne proverb graphically states, "A nation is not conquered until the hearts of its women are on the ground. Then it is done, no matter how brave its warriors nor how strong their weapons" (Crow Dog & Erdoes, 1990, p. 3), and Cheshire (2001) notes, "It is the women—the mothers, grandmothers and aunties—that keep Indian nations alive" (p. 1534).

Gender roles are egalitarian, and women are valued. Being a mother and auntie gives a social standing as a life giver related to the survival of the tribe (Barrios & Egan, 2002). Because the family matriarch is a primary decision maker, her approval and support may be required for compliance with a treatment plan (Cesario, 2001).

Spiritual and Religious Practices

The religious beliefs of Native Americans are strongly linked with nature and the earth. There is a sense of sacredness in everyday living between "grandmother earth" and "grandfather sky" that tends to render the outside world extraneous (Kavanagh et al., 1999, p. 25).

Health Beliefs and Practices

Illness is viewed as a punishment from God for some real or imagined imbalance with nature. Native Americans believe illness to be divine intervention to help the individual correct evil ways, and spiritual beliefs play a significant role in the maintenance and restoration of health (Cesario, 2001; Meisenhelder, Bell, & Chandler, 2000). Spiritual ceremonies and prayers form an important part of traditional healing activities, and healing practices are strongly embedded in religious beliefs. Recovery occurs after the person is cleansed of "evil spirits."

Medical help is sought from tribal elders and Shamans (highly respected spiritual medicine men and women) who use spiritual healing practices and herbs to cure the ill member of the tribe (Pagani-Tousignant, 1992). For example, spiritual and herbal tokens or medicine bags placed at the bedside or in an infant's crib are essential to the healing process and should not be disturbed (Cesario, 2001). Native Americans view death as a natural process, but they fear the power of dead spirits and use numerous tribal rituals to ward them off.

Social Interaction Patterns

Building a trusting relationship with the health care provider is important to the Native American client. Native American clients respond best to health professionals who stick to the point and don't engage in small talk. On the other hand, they love story telling and appreciate humor.

Nurses need to understand the value of nonverbal communication and taking time in conversations with Native American clients. Direct eye contact is considered disrespectful. Listening is considered a sign of respect and essential to learning about the other (Kalbfleisch, 2009). The client is likely to speak in a low tone. Native Americans are private people who respect the privacy of others and prefer to talk about the facts rather than emotions about them.

Native Americans live in "present" time. They have little appreciation of scheduled time commitments, which in their mind do not necessarily relate to what needs to be achieved. For Native Americans, being on time or taking medication with meals (when three meals are taken on one day and two meals are eaten on another day) has little relevance (Kavanagh et al., 1999). Understanding time from a Native American perspective decreases frustration. Calling the client before making a home visit or to remind the client of an appointment is a useful strategy.

Native Americans are experiential learners.

Case Example

When the nurse is performing a newborn bath demonstration, the Native American mother is likely to watch from a distance, avoid eye contact with the demonstrator, ask few or no questions, and decline a return demonstration. This learning style should not be seen as indifference or lack of understanding. Being an experiential learner, the Native American woman is likely to assimilate the information provided and simply give the newborn a bath when it is needed (Cesario, 2001, p. 17).

Their learning style is observational and oral, so the use of charts, written instructions, and pamphlets is usually not well received. Verbal instructions delivered in a story-telling format is more familiar to Native Americans (Hodge et al., 2002).

Native Americans suffer from greater rates of mortality from chronic diseases such as tuberculosis, alcoholism, diabetes, and pneumonia. Domestic violence, often associated with alcoholism, is a significant health concern. Pain assessment is important, because the Native American client tends to display a stoic response to pain (Cesario, 2001). Homicide and suicide rates are significantly greater for Native Americans (Meisenhelder et al., 2000). Health concerns of particular relevance to the Native American population are unintentional injuries (of which 75% are alcohol related), cirrhosis, alcoholism, and obesity.

CULTURE OF POVERTY

The worldview of those who fall below the poverty line is significant enough to warrant special consideration of their needs in the nurse-client relationship. Raphael (2009) notes, "Poverty is not only the primary determinant of children's intellectual, emotional, and social development but also an excellent predictor of virtually every adult disease known to medicine" (p. 10).

Health disparities are as clearly tied to economy and social disparities in education as they are to other cultural factors. The uncertainty of today's economy is further likely to decrease the distribution of resources that influence health in ways we have not seen before.

People without money or insurance, or both, do not have the same access to the health care system that others have. The type of health insurance a person has determines the level of care that a person will receive and what treatments are allowable. Poor people have to think carefully about seeking medical attention for anything other than an emergency situation. Medications are expensive and may not be taken. The emergency department becomes a primary health care resource, and health-seeking behaviors tend to be crisis oriented. Things that most of us take for granted, such as food, housing, clothing, the chance for a decent job, and the opportunity for education, are not available, or are insufficient to meet needs. People at the poverty level have to worry on a daily basis about how to provide for basic human needs.

Poverty is a difficult but important sociocultural concept because it has an adverse effect on a large segment of the population, limiting their options in health care. Lack of essential resources is associated with political and personal powerlessness (Reutter et al., 2009). The idea that the poor can exercise choice or make a difference in their lives is not part of their worldview. People living in poverty may overlook opportunities simply because life experience tells them that they cannot trust their own efforts to produce change. Poor people often look to but do not expect others to work with them in making things better. This mindset prompts the poor to avoid and distrust the health care system for anything other than emergencies. Care strategies require a proactive, persistent, client-oriented approach to helping clients and families self-manage health problems (Minick et al., 1998). Communication strategies that acknowledge, support, and empower the poor to take small steps to independence are most effective.

Respect for the human dignity of the poor client is a major component of care. This means that the nurse pays strict attention to personal biases and stereotypes so as not to distort assessment or implementation of nursing interventions. It means treating each client as "culturally unique," with a set of assumptions and values regarding the disease process and its treatment, and acting in a nonjudgmental manner that respects the client's cultural integrity (Haddad, 2001). Ethics become particularly important in client situations requiring informed consent, health care decision making, involvement of family and significant others, treatment choices, and birth and death.

SUMMARY

This chapter explores the intercultural communication that takes place when the nurse and client are from different cultures. Culture is defined as a common collectivity of beliefs, values, shared understandings, and patterns of behavior of a designated group of people. Culture needs to be viewed as a human structure with many variations in meaning.

Related terms include cultural diversity, cultural relativism, subculture, ethnicity, ethnocentrism, and ethnography. Each of these concepts broadens the definition of culture. Intercultural communication is defined as a communication in which the sender of a message is a member of one culture and the receiver of the message is from a different culture. Different languages create and express different personal realities.

A cultural assessment is defined as a systematic appraisal of beliefs, values, and practices conducted to determine the context of client needs and to tailor nursing interventions. It is composed of three progressive, interconnecting elements: a general assessment, a problem-specific assessment, and the cultural details needed for successful implementation.

Knowledge and acceptance of the client's right to seek and support alternative health care practices dictated by culture can make a major difference in compliance and successful outcome. Health care professionals sometimes mistakenly assume that illness is a single concept, but illness is a personal experience, strongly colored by cultural norms, values, social roles, and religious beliefs. Interventions that take into consideration the specialized needs of the client from a culturally diverse background follow the mnemonic LEARN: Listen, Explain, Acknowledge, Recommend, and Negotiate.

Some basic thoughts about the traditional characteristics of the largest minority groups (African American, Hispanic, Asian, Native American) living in the United States relating to communication preferences, perceptions about illness, family, health, and religious values are included in the chapter. The culture of poverty is discussed.

ETHICAL DILEMMA   What Would You Do?

Antonia Martinez is admitted to the hospital and needs immediate surgery. She speaks limited English, and her family is not with her. She is frightened by the prospect of surgery and wants to wait until her family can be with her to help her make the decision about surgery. As a nurse, you feel there is no decision to be made: She must have the surgery, and you need to get her consent form signed now. What would you do?

REFERENCES

Allport G: *The nature of prejudice*, Reading, MA, 1979, Addison-Wesley Publishers.

American Association of Colleges of Nursing (AACN): *The essentials of baccalaureate education for professional nursing practice*, Washington, DC, 2008, AACN.

Amerson R: Reflections on a conversation with a curandera, *J Transcult Nurs* 19(4):384–387, 2008.

Anderson P, Wang H: Beyond language: nonverbal communication across cultures. In Samovar L, Porter R, McDaniel E, editors: *Intercultural communication: a reader*, ed 12, Belmont, CA, 2008, Wadsworth.

Aponte J: Addressing cultural heterogeneity among Hispanic subgroups by using Campinha-Bacote's model of cultural competency, *Holist Nurs Pract* 23(1):3–12, 2009; quiz 13–14.

Aroian K, Faville K: Reconciling cultural relativism for a clinical paradigm: what's a nurse to do? *J Prof Nurs* 21(6):330, 2005.

Bacallao M, Smokowski P: "Entre dos mundos" (between two worlds): bicultural skills with Latino immigrant families, *J Prim Prev* 26(6): 485–509, 2005.

Baron-Epel O, Friedman N, Lernau O, et al: Fatalism and mammography in a multicultural population, *Oncol Nurs Forum* 36(3):353–361, 2009.

Barrios PG, Egan M: Living in a bicultural world and finding the way home: native women's stories, *Affilia* 17:206–228, 2002.

Betancourt J: Cultural competence—marginal or mainstream movement, *N Engl J Med* 35(10):953–955, 2004.

Callister L: Culturally competent care of women and newborns: knowledge, attitude, and skills, *J Obstet Gynecol Neonatal Nurs* 30(2):209–215, 2001.

Calloway S: The effect of culture on beliefs related to autonomy and informed consent, *J Cult Divers* 16(2):68–70, 2009.

Campinha-Bacote J: Voodoo illness, *Perspect Psychiatr Care* 28(1): 11–16, 1992.

Canales M, Howers H: Expanding conceptualizations of culturally competent care, *J Adv Nurs* 36(1):102–111, 2001.

Carrese JA, Rhodes LA: Bridging cultural differences in medical practice, *J Gen Intern Med* 15:92–96, 2000.

Cavazos-Rehg P, Delucia-Waack J: Education, ethnic identity, and acculturation as predictors of self-esteem in Latino adolescents, *J Couns Dev* 87(1):47–54, 2009.

Cesario S: Care of the Native American woman: strategies for practice, education and research, *J Obstet Gynecol Neonatal Nurs* 30(1):13–19, 2001.

Chambers V: Say amen, indeed, *American Way* 30(4):38–43, 102–105, 1997.

Chaudhary N: *Listening to culture: constructing reality from every day talk*, Thousand Oaks CA, 2004, Sage Publications, Inc.

Chen YC: Chinese values, health and nursing, *J Adv Nurs* 36(2): 270–273, 2001.

Cheshire T: Cultural transmission in urban American Indian families, *Am Behav Sci* 44(9):1528–1535, 2001.

Chung RC, Bernak F, Otiz D, et al: Promoting the mental health of immigrants: a multicultural/social justice perspective, *J Couns Dev* 86:310–317, 2008.

Crawley L, Marshall P, Lo B, et al: Strategies for culturally effective end-of-life care, *Ann Intern Med* 136(9):673–679, 2002.

Cross W, Bloomer M: Extending boundaries: clinical communication with culturally and linguistically diverse mental health clients and carers, *Int J Ment Health Nurs* 19:268–277, 2010.

Crow Dog M, Erdoes R: *Lakota woman*, New York, 1990, Grove Weidenfeld.

Davidson J, Boyer M, Casey D, et al: Gap analysis of cultural and religious needs of hospitalized patients, *Crit Care Nurs Q* 31(2):119–126, 2008.

Davis R: The convergence of health and family in the Vietnamese culture, *J Fam Nurs* 6(2):136–156, 2000.

Day-Vines N, Wood S, Grothaus T, et al: Broaching the subjects of race, ethnicity and culture during the counseling process, *J Couns Dev* 85:401–409, 2007.

Donnermeyer J, Friedrich L: Amish society: an overview reconsidered, *J Multicult Nurs* 12(3):36–43, 2006.

Drench M, Noonan A, Sharby N, et al: *Psychosocial aspects of health care*, ed 2, Upper Saddle River, NJ, 2009, Pearson Prentice Hall.

Edwards K: Disease prevention strategies to decrease health disparities, *J Cult Divers* 16(1):3–4, 2009.

Eiser A, Ellis G: Cultural competence and the African American experience with health care: the case for specific content in cross-cultural education, *Acad Med* 82:176–183, 2007.

Flood G: *An introduction to Hinduism*, Cambridge, 1996, Cambridge University Press.

Ford M, Kelly P: Conceptualizing and categorizing race and ethnicity in health services research, *Health Serv Res* 40(5 pt 2):1658–1675, 2005.

Galanti GA: *Caring for patients from different cultures*, ed 4, Philadelphia, 2008, University of Pennsylvania Press.

Garrett M, Herring R: Honoring the power of relations: counseling Native adults, *J Humanist Couns Educ Dev* 40(20):139–140, 2001.

Gelles R: *Contemporary families*, Thousand Oaks, CA, 1995, Sage.

Giger J, Davidhizar R: *Transcultural nursing: assessment and intervention*, St Louis, 1991, Mosby.

Giger J, Davidhizar R, Purnell L, et al: Understanding cultural language to enhance cultural competence, *Nurs Outlook* 55(4):212–214, 2007(a).

Giger J, Davidhizar R, Purnell L, et al: American Academy of Nursing Expert panel Report: developing competence to eliminate health disparities in ethnic minorities and other vulnerable populations, *J Transcult Nurs* 18(2):95–102, 2007(b).

Gravely S: When your patient speaks Spanish—and you don't, *RN* 64(5):64–67, 2001.

Haddad A: Ethics in action, *RN* 64(3):21–22, 24, 2001.

Harrison G, Kagawa-Singer M, Foerster S, et al: Seizing the moment, *Cancer* 15(104–112 Suppl.):2962–2968, 2005.

Hecht M, Ronald L, Jackson L, et al: *African American communication: identity and cultural interpretation*, Mahwah, NJ, 2003, Lawrence Erlbaum Associates.

Hodge F, Fredericks L: American Indian and Alaska Native population in the United States: an overview. In Huff R, Kline M, editors: *Promoting health in multicultural populations*, Thousand Oaks, CA, 1999, Sage Publications.

Hodge FS, Pasqua A, Marquez C, et al: Utilizing traditional storytelling to promote wellness in American Indian communities, *J Transcult Nurs* 13(1):6–11, 2002.

Hofstede GJ, Pedersen P, Hofsted GH, et al: *Exploring culture: exercises, stories, and synthetic cultures*, Yarmouth, ME, 2002, Intercultural Press, Inc.

Hulme P: Cultural considerations in evidence-based practice, *J Transcult Nurs* 21(3):271–280, 2010.

Im E: The situation specific theory of pain experience for Asian American cancer patients, *Adv Nurs Sci* 31(4O):319–331, 2008.

Institute of Medicine: *Unequal treatment: confronting racial and ethnic disparities in health care*, Washington, DC, 2003, National Academies Press.

Institute of Medicine: *Speaking of health: assessing health communication strategies for diverse populations*, Washington DC, 2002, National Academies Press.

Jandt F: *An introduction to intercultural communication: identities in a global community*, Thousand Oaks, CA, 2003, Sage Publications.

Johnstone M, Kanitsaki O: Ethics and advance care planning in a culturally diverse society, *J Transcult Nurs* 20(4):405–416, 2009.

Juarez G, Ferrell B, Borneman T: Influence of culture on cancer pain management in Hispanic patients, *Cancer Pract.* 6(5):262–269, 1998.

Juckett G: Cross cultural medicine, *Am Fam Physician* 1(72):2189–2190, 2005.

Kalbfleisch P: Effective health communication in native populations in North America, *J Lang Soc Psychol* 28(2):158–173, 2009.

Karim K: Informing cancer patients: truth telling and culture, *Cancer Nurs Pract* 2:23–31, 2003.

Kavanagh K, Absalom K, Beil W, et al: Connecting and becoming culturally competent: a Lakota example, *Adv Nurs Sci* 21(3):9–31, 1999.

Kemp C: *Mexican & Mexican-Americans: health beliefs & practices*, Cambridge, 2004, Cambridge University Press.

Kim S, Flaskerud J: Does culture frame adjustment to the sick role? *Issues Ment Health Nurs* 29:315–318, 2008.

Kleinman A, Benson P: Antropology in the clinic: the problem of cultural competency and how to fix it, *PLOS Med* 3:1672–1675, 2006.

Kline M, Huff R, editors: *Health promotion in multicultural populations*, ed 2, Thousand Oaks, CA, 2008, Sage Publications.

Knoerl AM: Cultural considerations and the Hispanic cardiac client, *Home Health Care Nurse* 25(2):82–86, 2007.

Kwak J, Haley W: Current research findings on end-of-life decision making among racially or ethnically diverse groups, *Gerontologist* 45(5):634–641, 2005.

Leininger M, McFarland MR, editors: *Culture care diversity and universality: a worldwide nursing theory*, Sudbury, MA, 2006, Jones and Bartlett.

Leonard B, Plotnikoff G: Awareness: the heart of cultural competence, *AACN Clin Issues* 11(1):51–59, 2000.

Lewis R: *When cultures collide: managing successfully across cultures*, London, 2000, Nicholas Brealey Publishing.

Lic OHM, Ayur HCS: *Ayurvedic medicine: the principles of traditional practice*, Philadelphia, 2006, Elsevier.

Littlejohn-Blake SM, Darling CA: Understanding the strengths of African-American families, *J Black Stud* 23(4):460–471, 1993.

Louie K: White paper on the health status of Asian-Americans and Pacific Islanders and recommendations for research, *Nurs Outlook* 49:173–178, 2001.

Lynch E, Hanson M: *Developing cross-cultural competence: a guide for working with children and families*, ed 3, Baltimore, MD, 2004, Paul H. Brookes Publishing Co.

Malhi R, Boon S, Rogers T, et al: "Being Canadian" and "being Indian": subject positions and discourses used in South Asian-Canadian women's talk about ethnic identity, *Culture Psychol* 15(2):255–283, 2009.

McKennis A: Caring for the Islamic patient, *AORN J* 69(6):1185–1206, 1999.

McLaughlin L, Braun K: Asian and Pacific Islander cultural values: considerations for health care decision-making, *Health Soc Work* 23(2):116–126, 1998.

Meisenhelder M, Bell J, Chandler E, et al: Faith, prayer, and health outcomes in elderly Native Americans, *Clin Nurs Res* 9(2):191–204, 2000.

Michaels A: *Hinduism: past and present*, Princeton, NJ, 2003, Princeton University Press.

Minick P, Kee C, Borkat L, et al: Nurses' perceptions of people who are homeless, *West J Nurs Res* 20(3):356–369, 1998.

National Center for Health Statistics: *Health, United States, 2007 with Chartbook on trends in the health of Americans*, Hyattsville, MD, 2007, Author. Available online: http://www.cdc.gov/nchs/data/hus/hus07.pdf#027. Accessed February 2, 2009.

Office of Minority Health, U.S. Department of Health and Human Services (DHHS): *National standards for culturally and linguistically appropriate services in health care*, Washington, DC, 2001, Author. Available online: www.omhrc.gov/assets/pdf/checked/finalreport.pdf.

Office of Minority Health: *Populations*, Available at http://www.cdc.gov/omhd/Populations/populations.htm. Accessed July 20, 2010.

Pagani-Tousignant C: *Breaking the rules: counseling ethnic minorities*, Minneapolis, MN, 1992, The Johnson Institute.

Parham TA, White JL, Ajamu A, et al: *The psychology of Blacks: an African centered perspective*, Upper Saddle River, NJ, 2000, Prentice Hall.

Pasco A, Morse J, Olson J, et al: The cross-cultural relationships between nurses and Filipino Canadian patients, *J Nurs Sch* 36(3):239–246, 2004.

Pergert P, Ekblad S, Enskar K, et al: Obstacles to transcultural caring relationships: experiences of health care staff in pediatric oncology, *J Pediatr Oncol Nurs* 24(6):314–328, 2007.

Purnell L, Purnell JD, Paulanka BJ, et al: *Transcultural health care: A culturally competent approach*, ed 3, Philadelphia, PA, 2008, F.A. Davis.

Purnell JD: *Guide to culturally competent health care*, ed 2, Philadelphia PA, 2009, F.A. Davis.

Raphael D: Poverty, human development, and health in Canada: research, practice, and advocacy dilemmas, *Can J Nurs Res* 41(2):7–18, 2009.

Ramos-Sánchez L, Atkinson D: The relationships between Mexican American acculturation, cultural values, gender, and help seeking intentions, *J Couns Dev* 87:62–71, 2009.

Rashidi A, Rajaram S: Culture care conflicts among Asian-Islamic immigrant women in US hospitals, *Holist Nurs Pract* 16(1):55–64, 2001.

Red Horse J: Traditional American Indian family systems, *Fam Syst Health* 15(3):243–250, 1997.

Reutter L, Stewart M, Veenstra G, et al: Who do they think we are anyway? Perceptions and responses to poverty stigma, *Qual Health Res* 19(3):297–311, 2009.

Samovar L, Porter R, McDaniel E, et al: *Intercultural communication: a reader*, ed 12, Belmont, CA, 2008, Wadsworth.

Searight H, Gafford J: Cultural diversity at the end of life: issues and guidelines for family physicians, *Am Fam Physician* 71:3, 2005.

Servodido C, Morse E: End of life issues, *Nurs Spectr* 11(8DC):20–23, 2001.

Sokol R, Strout S: A complete theory of human emotion: the synthesis of language, body, culture and evolution in human feeling, *Culture Psychol* 12(1O):115–123, 2006.

Spector R: *Cultural diversity in health and illness*, ed 6, Upper Saddle River, NJ, 2004, Pearson Prentice Hall.

Spence D: Prejudice, paradox, and possibility: nursing people from cultures other than one's own, *J Transcult Nurs* 12(2):100–106, 2001.

Sterritt P, Pokorny M: African American caregiving for a relative with Alzheimer's disease, *Geriatr Nurs* 19(3):127–128, 133–134, 1998.

Sue DW, Sue D: *Counseling the culturally diverse: theory and practice*, ed 4, New York, 2003, Wiley.

Sutton M: Cultural competence, *Fam Pract Manag* 7(9):58–62, 2000.

Thomas N: The importance of culture throughout all of life and beyond, *Holist Nurs Pract* 15(2):40–46, 2001.

Tong V, Huang C, McIntyre T, et al: Promoting a positive cross-cultural identity: reaching immigrant students, *Reclaiming Children and Youth* 14(4):203–208, 2006.

U.S. Department of Health and Human Services (DHHS): *Healthy People 2010: national health promotion and disease prevention objectives*, Washington, DC, 2000, Author.

U.S. Department of Health and Human Services: *National standards for cultural and linguistically appropriate services in health care: final report*, Washington, DC, 2001, Author.

U.S. Department of Health and Human Services (DHHS), Agency for Healthcare Research and Quality: *2006 national healthcare disparities report*, Rockville, MD, 2007, Author.

Villarruel: A Health disparities research: issues, strategies, and innovations, *The Journal of Multicultural Nursing and Health* 10(2):7–12, 2004.

Xu Y, Davidhizar R, Giger J, et al: What if your nursing student is from an Asian culture, *J Cult Divers* 12(1):5–12, 2004.

Zapata J, Shippee-Rice R: The use of folk healing and healers by six Latinos living in New England, *J Transcult Nurs* 10(2):136–142, 1999.

Communicating in Groups

Elizabeth C. Arnold

OBJECTIVES

At the end of the chapter, the reader will be able to:

1. Define group communication.
2. Identify the stages of group development.
3. Discuss theory-based concepts of group dynamics.
4. Apply group concepts in therapeutic groups.
5. Compare and contrast different types of therapeutic groups.
6. Apply concepts of group dynamics to work groups.

This chapter describes concepts related to group dynamics in therapeutic and organizational settings. Theoretical frameworks related to the stages of group development and role functioning provide a background. Different types of group formats and the stages of group relationships are identified. Applications of group concepts in therapeutic and in work groups complete chapter content.

BASIC CONCEPTS

DEFINITIONS OF GROUP

A *group* is more than a random number of individuals occupying the same space. Forsyth (2009) defines group as "two or more individuals who are connected by and within social relationships" (p. 3). Relationships among members are interdependent; each member's behavior affects the behavior of other group members. Group cultures develop through shared images, values, and meanings that over time become the stories, myths, and metaphors about the group and how it functions.

PRIMARY AND SECONDARY GROUPS

Groups are categorized as primary or secondary groups. *Primary* groups are characterized by an informal structure and social process. Group membership is automatic (e.g., in a family) or is voluntarily chosen because of a common interest (e.g., in scouting, religious, or civic groups). Primary groups are an important part of a person's self-concept, revealed in self-descriptions such as "I am Jamie's mother."

Secondary groups differ from primary groups in structure and purpose; they have a planned, time-limited association; a prescribed structure; a designated leader; and a specific, identified purpose. When groups achieve their goals, the group disbands. Examples include focus groups, therapy and health-related groups, discipline-specific work groups, interdisciplinary health care teams, and educational groups. People join secondary groups for one of three reasons: to meet personally established goals, to develop more effective coping skills, or because it is required by the larger community system to which the individual belongs. Exercise 12-1 identifies the role that group communication plays in a person's life.

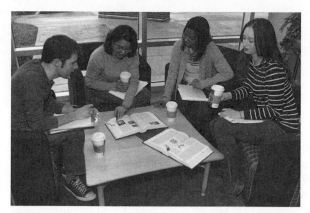

Groups offer a special forum for learning and emotional support.

THERAPEUTIC GROUPS

The value of group communication as a therapeutic tool was first introduced by Joseph Pratt, who found that he was able to expand positive outcomes with people treated for tuberculosis (TB), through group classes. Group therapy for psychological issues became apparent during World War II when it was used as a primary treatment modality to treat soldiers for war-related stress (Corey & Corey, 2008). The outcomes were so successful that mental health professionals continued to use group therapy to treat people with psychological problems. Jacob Moreno later developed psychodrama as an experiential form of group therapy, and introduced sociometry as a way to diagram group participation. In the 1930s, Samuel Slavson introduced the idea of using therapeutic activity groups for disturbed children (Rutan, Stone, & Shay, 2007).

Many others contributed to the development of group communication as a treatment modality for psychological problems and general medical issues. Some health related groups are one session; most meet on a regular basis to share common concerns and experiences, and to learn new skills. With the exception of self-help groups, and some support groups, a trained group facilitator guides groups in health care.

Irvin Yalom's classic work (2005) on interactional group process is recognized as the gold standard for describing group communication processes and dynamics in therapeutic settings. Curative changes occur in therapy groups as a result of 11 therapeutic process factors. Yalom and Leszcz (2005) identify these as follows:

1. Instillation of hope
2. Universality
3. Imparting information
4. Altruism
5. The corrective recapitulation of the primary family group
6. Development of socializing techniques
7. Imitative behavior
8. Interpersonal learning
9. Group cohesiveness
10. Catharsis
11. Existential factors (pp. 1–2).

GROUP DYNAMICS

Group dynamics is a term used to describe the communication processes and behaviors occurring during the life of the group. They represent a complex blend of individual and group characteristics that interact

---

EXERCISE 12-1	Groups in Everyday Life

Purpose: To help students gain an appreciation of the role group communication plays in their lives.

Procedure:

1. Write down all the groups in which you have been a participant (e.g., family; scouts; sports teams; community, religious, work, and social groups).
2. Describe the influence membership in each of these groups had on the development of your self-concept.
3. Identify the ways in which membership in different groups was of value in your life.
4. Identify the primary reason you joined each group. If you have discontinued membership, specify the reason.

Discussion:

1. How similar or dissimilar were your answers from those of your classmates?
2. What factors account for differences in the quantity and quality of your group memberships?
3. How similar were the ways in which membership enhanced your self-esteem?
4. If your answers were dissimilar, what makes membership in groups such a complex experience?
5. Could different people get different things out of very similar group experiences?
6. What implications does this exercise have for your nursing practice?

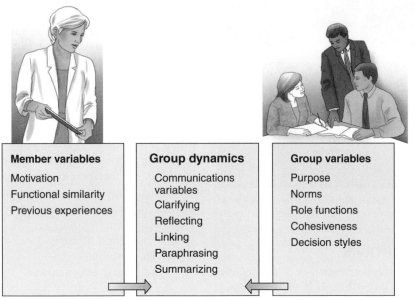

Member variables	Group dynamics	Group variables
Motivation	Communications variables	Purpose
Functional similarity	Clarifying	Norms
Previous experiences	Reflecting	Role functions
	Linking	Cohesiveness
	Paraphrasing	Decision styles
	Summarizing	

Figure 12-1   Factors that affect group dynamics.

with each other to achieve a group purpose. Factors that influence dynamics are illustrated in Figure 12-1.

Functional Similarity

Careful selection of group members, based on the person's capacity to derive benefit from the group and to contribute to group goals, is a critical variable in successful groups. One variable is **functional similarity**, defined as choosing group members who have enough in common intellectually, emotionally, and experientially to interact with each other in a meaningful way. Exercise 12-2 shows the value of finding things in common. An older, highly educated adult placed in a group of young adults with limited verbal and educational skills can be a group casualty or scapegoat simply because there is not enough in common to be viewed as a peer. Placed in a different group, with clients of a similar intellectual, emotional, and experiential level, the outcome might be quite different.

Whereas it is important that group members have enough in common to understand each other, differences in interpersonal styles help clients learn a broader range of behavioral responses.

EXERCISE 12-2   Group Self-Disclosure: The Impact of Universality

Purpose: To provide students with the experience of universality and insight.

Procedure:
1. Break into groups of four to six people.
2. One person should act as a scribe.
3. Identify three things all members of your group have in common other than that you are in the same class and you are human (e.g., have siblings, have parents in the military, like sports or art).
4. Identify two things that are unique to each person in your group (e.g., only child, never moved from the area, born in another country, collects stamps).

5. Each person should elaborate on both the common and different experiences.

Discussion:
1. What was the effect of finding common ground with other group members?
2. In what ways did finding out about the uniqueness of each person's experience add to the discussion?
3. Did anything in either the discussion of commonalities or differences in experience stimulate further group discussion?
4. How could you use what you have learned in this exercise in your clinical practice?

Group Purpose

Group purpose supplies the rationale for each group's existence (Powles, 2007). It provides direction for decisions, encourages the development of relevant group norms, and determines the type of communication and activities required to meet group goals. For example, if a group's purpose relates to medication compliance, the interventions would be educational. The purpose of a therapy group would be to improve interpersonal functioning and insight into behavior. Purposes of different group types are presented in Table 12-1.

Norms

Group norms refer to the behavioral rules of conduct expected of group members. Norms provide needed predictability for effective group functioning and make the group safe for its members. There are two types of group norms: universal and group specific. *Universal norms* are stated behavioral standards that must be present in all groups for effective outcomes. Examples include confidentiality, regular attendance, and not socializing with members outside of group (Burlingame et al., 2006). Unless group members can trust that personal information will not be shared outside the group setting (confidentiality), trust will not develop. Regular attendance at group meetings is critical to group stability and goal achievement. Personal relationships between group members outside of the group threaten the integrity of the group as the therapeutic arena for the group's work.

Group-specific norms evolve from the group itself in the storming phase. They represent the shared beliefs, values, and unspoken operational rules governing group function. Examples include tolerance for latecomers, use of humor or confrontation, and talking directly to other group members rather than about them. Exercise 12-3 will help you develop a deeper understanding of group norms.

TABLE 12-1	Group Type and Purpose

Group	Purpose
Therapy	Reality testing, encouraging personal growth, inspiring hope, strengthening personal resources, developing interpersonal skills
Support	Giving and receiving practical information and advice, supporting coping skills, promoting self-esteem, enhancing problem-solving skills, encouraging client autonomy, strengthening hope and resiliency
Activity	Getting people in touch with their bodies, releasing energy, enhancing self-esteem, encouraging cooperation, stimulating spontaneous interaction, supporting creativity
Education	Learning new knowledge, promoting skill development, providing support and feedback, supporting development of competency, promoting discussion of important health-related issues

EXERCISE 12-3	Identifying Norms

Purpose: To help identify norms operating in groups.

Procedure:
1. Divide a piece of paper into three columns.
2. In the first column, write the norms you think exist in your class or work group. In the second column, write the norms you think exist in your family. Examples of norms might be as follows: no one gets angry, decisions are made by consensus, assertive behaviors are valued, and missed sessions and lateness are not tolerated.
3. Share your norms with the group, first related to the school or work group and then to the family. Place this information in the third column.

Discussion:
1. Were there many similarities between the norms you think exist in your school or work group and those that others in the same group had on their list?
2. Were there any "universal" norms on either of your lists?
3. Were you surprised either by some of the norms you wrote down when you thought about it or by those of your classmates?
4. Did you or other members in the group feel a need to refine or discuss the meaning of the norms on your list?
5. How difficult was it to determine implicit norms operating in the group?

Group Role Positions

People in groups assume and/or are ascribed roles that influence their communication and the responses of others. A person's role position in the group corresponds with the status, power, and internal image that other members in the group have of the member. Group members usually have trouble breaking away from roles they have been cast in despite their best efforts. For example, people will look to the "helper" group member for advice, even when that person lacks expertise or personally needs the group's help. Other times, group members "project" a role position onto a particular group member that represents a hidden agenda or unresolved issue for the group as a whole (Gans & Alonso, 1998). If the group as a whole seems to scapegoat, ignore, defer to, or consistently idealize one of its members, this group phenomenon can signify a group projection (Moreno, 2007). Exercise 12-4 considers group role position expectations.

GROUP DYNAMICS

PHASES OF THE GROUP LIFE CYCLE

Group process refers to the structural development of the group, and describes the phases of its life cycle. Tuckman's (1965, 1977) model of small-group development provides a framework for examining group process at different stages in the life of the group. He describes five stages: forming, storming, norming, performing, and adjourning (see Figure 12-2). Stages of group development are applicable to work groups, as well as therapeutic groups. Each sequential phase has its own set of tasks that build and expand on the work of previous phases. The concept of stage development is operationalized in the application section of the chapter.

Forming Phase

The forming phase begins when members come together to form a group. Members enter group relationships as strangers to each other. There is high dependence on the leader for direction, and orientation

---

EXERCISE 12-4	Headbands: Group Role Expectations

Purpose: To experience the pressures of role expectations on group performance.

Procedure:
1. Break the group up into a smaller unit of six to eight members. In a large group, a small group performs while the remaining members observe.
2. Make up mailing labels or headbands that can be attached to or tied around the heads of the participants. Each headband is lettered with directions on how the other members should respond to the role. Examples include:
   - Comedian: laugh at me
   - Expert: ask my advice
   - Important person: defer to me
   - Stupid: sneer at me
   - Insignificant: ignore me
   - Loser: pity me
   - Boss: obey me
   - Helpless: support me
3. Place a headband on each member in such a way that the member cannot read his or her own label, but the other members can see it easily.
4. Provide a topic for discussion (e.g., why the members chose nursing, the women's movement) and instruct each member to interact with the

others in a way that is natural for him or her. Do not role-play, but be yourself. React to each member who speaks by following the instructions on the speaker's headband. You are not to tell each other what the headbands say, but simply to react to them.
5. After about 20 minutes, the facilitator halts the activity and directs each member to guess what his or her headband says and then to take it off and read it.

Discussion:
Initiate a discussion, including any members who observed the activity. Possible questions include:
1. What were some of the problems of trying to "be yourself" under conditions of group role pressure?
2. How did it feel to be consistently misinterpreted by the group—to have them laugh when you were trying to be serious or ignore you when you were trying to make a point?
3. Did you find yourself changing your behavior in reaction to the group treatment of you—withdrawing when they ignored you, acting confident when they treated you with respect, giving orders when they deferred to you?

Modified from Pfeiffer J, Jones J: *A handbook of structured experiences for human relations training, Vol. VI,* La Jolla, CA, 1977, University Associate Publishers.

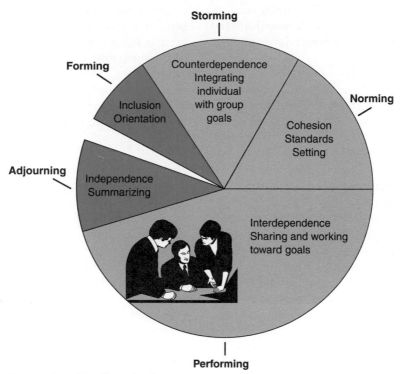

Figure 12-2   The life cycle of groups.

of members to purpose and expectations for behavior is a fundamental leadership responsibility. Getting to know each other, finding common threads in personal experience, and learning about group goals and tasks are emphasized. Members have a basic need for acceptance. Minimal work on the task is accomplished, but this phase cannot be shortchanged without having a serious impact on the evolving effectiveness of the group (Yalom & Leszcz, 2005).

Storming Phase

When a group moves into the storming phase, the gloves come off. This phase is characterized by conflict around interpersonal issues. Members focus on power and control issues. They use testing behaviors around boundaries, communication styles, and personal reactions with other members and the leader. Characteristic behaviors include disagreement with the group format, topics for discussion, the best ways to achieve group goals, and comparisons of member contributions. Although the storming phase is uncomfortable, successful resolution leads to the development of group-specific norms.

Norming Phase

In the norming phase, cohesiveness develops as standards evolved by members are accepted as operational norms. Individual goals become aligned with group goals. The group holds members accountable and challenges individual members who fail to adhere to expected behaviors. Group norms make the group safe, and members begin to experience the cohesiveness of the group as "their group."

Performing Stage

The group's "work" is accomplished in the performing phase, which is characterized by interdependence and cohesion. People feel loyal to the group and to individual members. Members are comfortable taking risks, and are invested enough in each other and the group process to offer constructive comments.

Adjourning Phase

Tuckman introduced the adjourning phase as a final phase of group development at a later date (Tuckman & Jensen, 1977). This phase is characterized by reviewing what has been accomplished, reflecting on the meaning of the group's work together, and making plans to move on in different directions.

FUNCTIONAL GROUP ROLES

Functional roles differ from positional roles group members assume in that they are related to the type of member contributions needed to achieve group goals. Benne and Sheats (1948) described constructive role functions as the behaviors members use to move toward goal achievement (**task functions**) and behaviors designed to ensure personal satisfaction (**maintenance functions**).

Balance between task and maintenance functions increases group productivity. When task functions predominate, member satisfaction decreases and a collaborative atmosphere is diminished. When maintenance functions override task functions, members have trouble reaching goals. Members do not confront controversial issues, so the creative tension needed for successful group growth does not occur. Task and maintenance role functions found in successful small groups are listed in Box 12-1. Exercise 12-5 provides practice in identifying task and maintenance functions.

Benne and Sheats (1948) also identified nonfunctional role functions. *Self-roles* are roles a person uses to meet self-needs at the expense of other members' needs, group values, and goal achievement. Self-roles, identified in Table 12-2, detract from the group's work and compromise goal achievement by taking time away from group issues and creating discomfort among group members.

GROUP LEADERSHIP

Two basic assumptions support the function of group leadership: (1) Group leaders have a significant influence on group process; and (2) most problems in groups can be avoided or reworked productively if the leader is aware of and responsive to the needs of individual group members, including the needs of the leader (Corey & Corey, 2008).

Effective leadership behaviors require adequate preparation, professional leadership attitudes and behavior, responsible selection of members, and use of a responsible scientific rationale for determining a specific group approach. Personal characteristics demonstrated by effective group leaders include commitment to the group purpose, self-awareness of personal biases and

---

| BOX 12-1 | Task and Maintenance Functions in Group Dynamics |

Task Functions: Behaviors Relevant to the Attainment of Group Goals

- *Initiating*: identifies tasks or goals; defines group problem; suggests relevant strategies for problem solving
- *Seeking information or opinion*: requests facts from other members; asks other members for opinions; seeks suggestions or ideas for task accomplishment
- *Giving information or opinion*: offers facts to other members; provides useful information about group concerns
- *Clarifying, elaborating*: interprets ideas or suggestions placed before group; paraphrases key ideas; defines terms; adds information
- *Summarizing*: pulls related ideas together; restates key ideas; offers a group solution or suggestion for other members to accept or reject
- *Consensus taking*: checks to see whether group has reached a conclusion; asks group to test a possible decision

Maintenance Functions: Behaviors That Help the Group Maintain Harmonious Working Relationships

- Harmonizing: attempts to reconcile disagreements; helps members reduce conflict and explore differences in a constructive manner
- Gatekeeping: helps keep communication channels open; points out commonalties in remarks; suggests approaches that permit greater sharing
- Encouraging: indicates by words and body language unconditional acceptance of others; agrees with contributions of other group members; is warm, friendly, and responsive to other group members
- Compromising: admits mistakes; offers a concession when appropriate; modifies position in the interest of group cohesion
- Setting standards: calls for the group to reassess or confirm implicit and explicit group norms when appropriate

Note: Every group needs both types of functions and needs to work out a satisfactory balance of task and maintenance activity.

Modified from Rogers C: The process of the basic encounter group. In Diedrich R, Dye HA, editors: *Group procedures: purposes, processes and outcomes*, Boston, 1972, Houghton Mifflin.

EXERCISE 12-5 Task Functions versus Maintenance Functions

Purpose: To help students identify task functions versus maintenance functions.

Procedure:
1. Break up into groups of eight students each.
2. Choose a topic to discuss (e.g., how you would restructure the nursing program; nursing and the women's movement; the value of a group experience; nursing as a profession).
3. Two students should volunteer to be the observers.
4. The students discuss the topics for 30 minutes; observers use the initial of each student and the grid below to mark with a tick (/) the number of times each student uses a task or maintenance function.
5. After completion of the group interaction, each observer shares his or her observations with the other group members.

Task Functions
Initiating _____.
Information seeking _____.
Clarifying _____.

Consensus taking _____.
Testing _____.
Summarizing _____.
Maintenance Functions
Encouraging _____.
Expressing _____.
Group feeling _____.
Harmonizing _____.
Compromising _____.
Gatekeeping _____.
Setting standards _____.

Discussion:
1. Was there an adequate balance between task and maintenance activity?
2. What roles did different members assume?
3. Were the two observers in agreement as to members' assumptions of task versus maintenance functions? If there were discrepancies, what do you think contributed to their occurrence?
4. What did you learn from this exercise?

TABLE 12-2	Nonfunctional Self-Roles
Role	**Characteristics**
Aggressor	Criticizes or blames others, personally attacks other members, uses sarcasm and hostility in interactions
Blocker	Instantly rejects ideas or argues an idea to death, cites tangential ideas and opinions, obstructs decision making
Joker	Disrupts work of the group by constantly joking and refusing to take group task seriously
Avoider	Whispers to others, daydreams, doodles, acts indifferent and passive
Self-confessor	Uses the group to express personal views and feelings unrelated to group task
Recognition	Seeks attention by excessive talking, seeker trying to gain leader's favor, expressing extreme ideas, or demonstrating peculiar behavior

Modified from Benne KD, Sheats P: Functional roles of group members, *J Soc Issues* 4(2):41–49, 1948.

interpersonal limitations, careful preparation for the group and with the group, and an open attitude toward group members. Knowledge of group dynamics, training, and supervision are additional requirements for leaders of psychotherapy groups. Educational group leaders need to have expertise on the topic for discussion.

Throughout the group's life, the leader models attitudes of caring, objectivity, and integrity. Effective leaders are good listeners, and are able to adapt their leadership style to fit the changing needs of the group. They respectfully support the integrity of group members as equal partners in meeting group goals. Successful leaders trust the group process enough to know that group members can work through conflict and difficult situations. They know that even mistakes can be used to promote group member growth (Rubel & Kline, 2008).

Some individuals, because of the force of their personalities, knowledge, or experience, will emerge as informal leaders within the group. Power is given to members who best clarify the needs of the other group members, or who move the group toward goal achievement. They are not always the group members making the most statements.

Case Example

Al is a powerful informal leader in a job search support group. Although he makes few comments, he has an excellent understanding of and sensitivity to the needs of individual members. When these are violated, Al speaks up and the group listens. Al's observations reflect that the group themes are trustworthy.

Emergent informal leaders such as Al are recognized by other group members as being powerful, and their comments are equated with those of the designated leader. Ideally, group leadership is a shared function of all group members, with many opportunities to divide up responsibility for achieving group goals. Exercise 12-6 is designed to help you develop an appreciation of leadership role preferences.

Co-Leadership

Yalom and Leszcz (2005) suggest that co-leadership has advantages and disadvantages. The advantages are that co-leaders can complement and support each other. Co-leaders provide a wider variety of responses, dual points of view that can be helpful to group members, and feedback to each other. When one leader is under fire, it can increase the other's confidence, knowing that in-group support and an opportunity to process the session afterward is available.

Problems arise when co-leaders have different theoretical orientations or are competitive. Needing to pursue solo interpretations rather than explore or support the meaning of co-leader's interventions is distracting to the group. Yalom and Leszcz (2005) state, "You are far better off leading a solo group with good supervision than being locked into an incompatible co-therapy relationship" (p. 447).

If you decide to co-lead a group, you need to spend sufficient prep time together before meeting with a therapy group to ensure personal compatibility, and that you have the same understanding of the group purpose. Depending on time availability, it is sometimes advantageous for both group co-leaders to hold pregroup interviews with clients. You will also need to process the group dynamics together, preferably after each meeting.

It is important for co-leaders to work together harmoniously. This requires developing respect for each other's skills, maintaining authenticity for yourself, and sensitivity to your co-leaders style of communicating (Corey & Corey, 2008).

Developing an Evidence-Based Practice

Erwin P, Purves D, Johannes K: Involvement and outcomes in short-term interpersonal cognitive problem solving groups, *Couns Psychol Q* 18(1):41–46, 2005.

This quantitative study was designed to explore the extent to which involvement in a short-term, interpersonal, cognitive problem-solving group could predict improvement in interpersonal cognitive problem-solving skills. A convenience sample of 31 children were assigned to either an experimental ($N = 16$) or control ($N = 15$) group. All study participants were given a pre-test and post-test for interpersonal cognitive problem-solving skills.

Results: Findings indicated significantly greater improvement in these skills with study participants in the experimental group compared with the control group ($N = 761$) regarding barriers and facilitators to their utilizing research in clinical practice. Reported barriers included time constraints, lack of awareness about availability of research literature, insufficient authority and/or lack of support to make changes based on research findings, and lack of knowledge

---

EXERCISE 12-6   Clarifying Leadership Role Preferences

Purpose: To help students focus on how they personally experience the leadership role.

Procedure:
Answer the following questions briefly:
1. What do you enjoy most about the leadership role?
2. What do you like least about the leadership role?
3. What skills do you bring to the leadership role?
4. What are the differences in your functioning as a group member and as a group leader?

Discussion:
1. What types of transferable skills did you find you bring to the leadership role? For example, are you an oldest child? Did you organize a play group? Did you teach swimming to mentally handicapped children in high school? Are you a member of a large family?
2. Were some of the uncomfortable feelings "universal" for a majority of the group?
3. What skills would you need to develop to feel comfortable as a group leader?
4. What did you learn about yourself from doing this exercise?

needed for critique of research studies. Facilitators included availability of time, access and support for review and implementation of research findings, and support of colleagues.

Application to Your Clinical Practice: Study findings suggest a significant relationship between group learning and positive outcomes for problem-solving skills. What kinds of problems do you see in your clinical experience that might lend themselves to short-term group intervention?

APPLICATIONS
APPLYING GROUP CONCEPTS TO THERAPEUTIC GROUPS

DIFFERENCES BETWEEN INDIVIDUAL AND GROUP COMMUNICATION

Group communication encompasses characteristics of individual communication. Acceptance, respect, understanding, and listening responses found in individual relationships are essential components of effective group communication. Similar therapeutic strategies of using open-ended questions, listening responses, and minimal cues are important in group communication.

There also are key differences. Group communication is more complex than individual communication because each member brings to the group a different set of perspectives, perception of reality, communication style, and personal agenda. Counselman (2008) suggests, "Group demonstrates that there truly are multiple realities" (p. 270). Group themes, rather than individual feelings with situations, form the basis for conversation.

Case Example

Martha: I was upset with last week's meeting because I didn't feel we made any progress. Everyone complained, but no one had a solution.

Leader: I wonder if other people feel as Martha does?

In therapeutic groups, clients are sources of help, as well as recipients. Groups offer a simulated forum for learning. Members not only talk about interpersonal issues; they can practice interpersonal skills with other group members. Disclosures from other group members help individuals recognize the universality of their problems at a personal level (Forsyth, 2009; Yalom & Leszcz, 2005). The leader relates to the group as a whole, instead of with only one person.

Case Example

Carrie: I feel like giving up. I've tried to do everything right, and I still can't seem to get good grades in my classes.

Leader: I wonder if the discouragement you are feeling is similar to Mary's disenchantment with her job, and Bill's desire to throw in the towel on his marriage.

GROUP STRUCTURE AND FORMAT

Group purpose and goals dictate group structure, membership, and format. For example, a medication group would have an educational purpose. A group for parents with critically ill children would have a supportive design, whereas a therapy group would have restorative functions. Exploration of personal feelings would be limited and related to the topic under discussion in an education group. In a therapy group, such probing would be encouraged.

GROUP SIZE

The size of the group depends on its purpose. In general, therapy and personal growth groups consist of six to eight members. Generally, therapy groups should not have fewer than five members. With less than this number, interaction tends to be limited, and if one or more members are absent, the group interaction can become intense and uncomfortable for the remaining members. Powles (2007) argues, "The threesome rarely leads to solid group formation or a productive group work" (p. 107). Support, education, and skills training groups can have from 10 to 30 members.

Group Membership Issues

Groups are categorized as closed or open groups, and as having homogeneous or heterogeneous membership (Corey, 2007). *Closed* groups have a predefined selected membership with an expectation of regular attendance for an extended time period, usually at least 12 sessions. Group members may be added, but their inclusion depends on a match with group-defined criteria. Most psychotherapy groups fall into this category. *Open* groups do not have a defined membership. Individuals come and go depending on their needs. One week the group might consist of 2 or 3 members and the next week 15 members. Most community support groups are open groups. Some groups, such as Alcoholics Anonymous, have "open" meetings, which anyone can attend, and "closed" meetings, which only alcoholic members can attend.

Therapeutic groups are composed of a homogeneous or heterogeneous membership. **Homogeneous** groups share common characteristics, for example, diagnosis (e.g., breast cancer support group) or a personal attribute (e.g., gender or age). Twelve-step programs for alcohol or drug addiction, eating disorder groups, and gender-specific consciousness-raising groups are familiar examples of homogeneous groups.

Heterogeneous groups represent a wider diversity of human experience and problems. Members vary in age, gender, and psychodynamics. Most psychotherapy and insight-oriented personal growth groups have a heterogeneous membership. Educational groups held on inpatient units (e.g., medication groups) may have a homogeneous membership related to diagnosis or specific learning needs.

Group Goals

Group goals define the therapeutic outcome that a group hopes to achieve. Group goals need to be achievable, measurable, and within the capabilities of group membership. Identifying a group goal helps the leader determine the time frame and type of membership needed to achieve the goal. Evidence of goal achievement justifies the existence of the group and increases client satisfaction.

Matching group goals with client needs and characteristics is essential. The leader needs to ask, "How will being in this group enhance a client's health and well-being?" When there is a good match and the mix of clients has the capacity to contribute to the group (functional similarity), members develop commitment and perceive the group as having value.

CREATING A SAFE GROUP ENVIRONMENT

Privacy and freedom from interruptions are key considerations in selecting an appropriate location. A sign on the door indicating the group is in session promotes privacy. Seating should be comfortable and arranged in a circle so that each member has face-to-face contact with all other group members. Being able to see facial expressions and to respond to several individuals at one time is essential to effective group communication.

The number of sessions, times, and frequency of meetings depend on the type of group and group goals. Therapy groups usually meet weekly. Support groups meet at regular intervals, ranging from weekly

to monthly. Educational groups meet for a predetermined number of sessions and then disband. Once established, agreed-on times and days should be maintained, except for emergency situations. Meetings should start and end on time.

Most groups, other than educational groups, meet for 60 to 90 minutes on a regular basis with established, agreed-on meeting times. A regular time that does not conflict with a member's other obligations should be established. Groups that begin and end on time foster trust and predictability. Characteristics of effective and ineffective groups are presented in Table 12-3.

LEADER TASKS APPLIED TO GROUP STAGE DEVELOPMENT

PREGROUP INTERVIEW

Pregroup interview has several purposes. This individual interview is used to explain group goals and commitment, and affirm the client's suitability for the group.

Adequate preparation of group members in pregroup interviews and the early stages of the group life cycle enhances the effectiveness of therapeutic groups (Corey, 2007; Yalom & Leszcz, 2005). Leaders should keep the description of the group and its members short and simple. Ask clients about previous group experiences and concerns. Allow ample time for questions and comments.

FORMING STAGE

The forming stage is an orientation phase. Communication is tentative and structured to allow members to learn about each other and develop trust. The leader takes an active role in helping group members feel accepted during the forming stage. Members are asked to introduce themselves and share a little of their background or their reason for coming to the group. Corey and Corey (2008) state that how well leaders prepare themselves and group members has a direct impact on building the trust needed within the group.

In the first session, the leader identifies the purpose and goals of the group and allows ample time for questions. Although members may know the purpose ahead of time, taking the time to verbalize the purpose allows group members to hear it in the same way. The leader clarifies how the group will be conducted and what the group can expect from the leader and other members in achieving group goals. It is helpful to

TABLE 12-3	Characteristics of Effective and Ineffective Groups

Effective Groups	Ineffective Groups
Goals are clearly identified and collaboratively developed.	Goals are vague or imposed on the group without discussion.
Open, goal-directed communication of feelings and ideas is encouraged.	Communication is guarded; feelings are not always given attention.
Power is equally shared and rotates among members, depending on ability and group needs.	Power resides in the leader or is delegated with little regard to member needs. It is not shared.
Decision making is flexible and adapted to group needs.	Decision making occurs with little or no consultation. Consensus is expected rather than negotiated based on data.
Controversy is viewed as healthy because it builds member involvement and creates stronger solutions.	Controversy and open conflict are not tolerated.
There is a healthy balance between task and maintenance role functioning.	There is a one-sided focus on task or maintenance role functions to the exclusion of the complementary function.
Individual contributions are acknowledged and respected. Diversity is encouraged.	Individual resources are not used. Conformity, the "company man," is rewarded. Diversity is not respected.
Interpersonal effectiveness, innovation, and problem-solving adequacy are evident.	Problem-solving abilities, morale, and interpersonal effectiveness are low and undervalued.

ask clients in round robin fashion about their personal expectations.

Clients need to be educated about the nature of the group process and the behaviors required to achieve group goals. Successful short-term groups focus on "here and now" interactions, giving practical feedback, sharing personal thoughts and feelings, and listening to each other (Corey & Corey, 2008). Orienting statements may need to be restated in subsequent early sessions if there is a lot of anxiety in the group.

The leader introduces universal behavioral norms such as confidentiality, attendance, and mutual respect (Corey & Corey, 2008). Confidentiality is harder to implement in group formats because members are not held to professional legal standards. However, for the integrity of the group, all members need to commit to confidentiality as a group norm (Lasky & Riva, 2006). Limits to confidentiality related to treatment disclosures to other providers for therapeutic purposes need to be clearly stated and agreed to by all members early in the group.

STORMING PHASE

The storming phase helps group members move to a deeper level. In the storming phase, the gloves come off and communication can become controversial. The leader plays an important facilitative role in the

storming phase by accepting differences in member perceptions as being normal and growth producing. By affirming genuine strengths in individual members, leaders model handling conflict with productive outcomes. Linking constructive themes while stating the nature of the disagreement is an effective modeling strategy.

Members who test boundaries through sexually provocative, flattering, or insulting remarks should have limits set promptly. Refer to the work of the group as being of the highest priority, and tactfully ask the person to align remarks with the group purpose. Resolution of the storming stage is evidenced in the willingness of members to take stands on their personal preferences without being defensive, and to compromise.

NORMING PHASE

Once initial conflict is resolved in the storming phase, the group moves into the norming phase. Group-specific norms have developed from discussions in the previous phase. The leader encourages member contributions and emphasizes cooperation in recognizing each person's talents related to group goals.

During the norming phase, cohesion begins to develop and is carried forward into the remaining stages of group development as a critical variable related to success. Similar to the concept of therapeutic alliance in individual relationships, cohesion is considered the most central therapeutic factor, influencing all others (Bernard et al., 2008). The group itself now becomes the agent of change.

Group Cohesion

Cohesion refers to the value a group holds for its members and their investment in being a part of the group. It describes the emotional bonds among members for each other and underscores their commitment to the group (Yalom & Leszcz, 2005). Evidence of group cohesion occurs when the group demonstrates a sense of common purpose, caring, collaboration in problem solving, a sense of feeling personally valued, and a team spirit (Powles, 2007). Research suggests that cohesive groups experience more personal satisfaction with goal achievement, and that members of such groups are more likely to join other group relationships. See Box 12-2 for communication principles that facilitate cohesiveness. Exercise 12-7 provides experience with understanding the relationship between individual involvement and group cohesion.

FACILITATING THE PERFORMING PHASE

In the performing stage of group development, members focus on problem solving. Working together and participating in another person's personal growth allows members to experience one another's personal strengths and the collective caring of the group. Of all the possibilities that can happen in a group, feeling affirmed and respected is most highly valued by group members (Table 12-4).

Dissent is expected, but because members function interdependently and respect each other, they are able to work through issues in ways that are acceptable to the individual and the group. Effective group leaders trust group members to develop their own solutions, but call attention to important group dynamics when needed. This can be done with a simple statement such as "I wonder what is going on with her right now" (Rubel & Kline, 2008).

Monopolizing

Despite clear operational roles, the performance stage can get bogged down when one person monopolizes

---

BOX 12-2	Communication Principles to Facilitate Cohesiveness

- Group tasks are within the membership's range of ability and expertise.
- Comments and responses are nonevaluative; they are focused on behaviors rather than on personal characteristics.

- The leader points out group accomplishments and acknowledges member contributions.
- The leader is empathetic and teaches members how to give feedback.
- The leader sanctions creative tension as necessary for goal achievement.

EXERCISE 12-7	Cohesion and Member Commitment

Purpose: To help students understand the concept of cohesion.

Procedure:
1. In small groups of three to five students, think of a group to which you belonged that you would characterize as being successful.
2. What did you do in this group that contributed to its success?
3. What made this group easier to commit to than other groups to which you belonged? Be as specific as you can be about the factors that enhanced your commitment.
4. Have one student act as scribe and write down the factors that increased commitment to share with the rest of the class.

Discussion:
1. What are the common individual themes that emerged from the discussion?
2. Discuss the relationship of commitment to success.
3. Did commitment emerge as a major factor related to goal achievement?
4. Did commitment emerge as a major factor related to personal satisfaction?
5. What factors emerged as important variables in personal commitment?
6. How could you use what you learned in this exercise in client groups?

TABLE 12-4	Leader Strategies in the Performing (Working) Stage	
Strategic Action	**Sample Leader Statement**
Maintain focus on main themes related to group goals	"I think that maybe we're straying a little away from our discussion of the triggers that make people feel like drinking. I wonder what people are feeling right now."
Emphasize the here and now	
Between members	"I wonder if we could look at what happened between Barbara and Bill just now."
Between a group member and the group as a whole	"Would you be willing to let the members of the group give you some feedback about how they experienced your story tonight?"
Leader self-disclosure	"May I share some of my personal reactions about what I experienced when you told your story?" This can be followed by a statement such as "I wonder how other group members experienced what you were saying."
Summarize at critical points and at the end of each session (this helps the group members to feel heard, allows correction of distortions, and provides transitions to future topics)	"I think we did a lot of good work tonight. My sense is that the group is saying that..." Alternatively, the group leader can ask group members if anyone would like to summarize what they think happened in the group.

conversation. *Monopolizing* is a negative form of power communication used to advance a personal agenda without considering the needs of others. When one person monopolizes the conversation, the leader should address the behavior, not an individual's motivation. For example, the leader might affirm the monopolizer's contribution and ask for group input: "Has anyone else had a similar experience?" Looking in the direction of positive group members as the statements are made also encourages member response. If a member continues to monopolize, the leader can respectfully acknowledge the person's comment and refocus the issue within the group directly: "I appreciate your thoughts, but I think it would be important to hear from other people as well. What do you think about this, Jane?"

COMPLETING THE ADJOURNING PHASE

The final phase of group development, termination or adjournment, ideally occurs when the group members have achieved desired outcomes. This phase is about task completion and disengagement. The leader encourages the group members to express their feelings about one another with the stipulation that any concerns the group may have about an individual member or suggestions for future growth should be stated in a constructive way. The leader closes the group with a summary of goal achievement. By being the last person to share closing comments, the leader has an opportunity to soften or clarify previous comments, and to connect cognitive with feeling elements that need to be addressed. The leader needs to remind members that the norm of confidentiality continues after the completion of the group (Mangione, Forti, & Iacuzzi, 2007). Referrals are handled on an individual basis. Exercise 12-8 considers group closure issues.

TYPES OF THERAPEUTIC GROUPS

Individuals tend to act in groups as they do in real life. The group provides a mirror with which clients can learn how others perceive them so that they can learn more adaptive responses.

The term *therapeutic*, as it applies to group relationships, refers to more than treatment of emotional and behavioral disorders. In today's health care arena, short-term groups are being designed for a wide range of different client populations as a first-line intervention to either remediate problems or prevent them (Corey & Corey, 2008). Therapeutic groups offer a structured format that encourages a person to experience his or her natural healing potential (instillation of hope), and other group members reinforce individual group member's resolve.

Therapeutic groups provide reality testing. People under stress lose perspective. Other group members can gently challenge cognitive distortions. They rarely

EXERCISE 12-8	Group Closure Activities

Purpose: To experience summarizing feelings about group members.

Procedure:

1. Focus your attention on the group member next to you and think about what you like about the person, how you see him or her in the group, and what you might wish for that person as a member of the group.
2. After 5 minutes, your instructor will ask you to tell the person next to you to use the three themes in making a statement about the person. For example, "The thing I most like about you in the group is..."; "To me you represent the _____ in the group"; and so on.

3. When all of the group members have had a turn, discussion may start.

Discussion:

1. How difficult was it to capture the person's meaning in one statement?
2. How did you experience telling someone about your response to him or her in the group?
3. How did you feel being the group member receiving the message?
4. What did you learn about yourself from doing this exercise?
5. What implications does this exercise have for future interactions in group relationships?

accept unsubstantiated comments at face value and can say things to the client that friends and relatives are afraid to say. It is difficult to turn aside the energy and caring of five or six people when member comments are delivered in a caring, but reality-based way.

THERAPY GROUPS

Therapy groups are designed to remediate or correct behavioral disorders and issues that limit a person's potential in personal and work relationships.

Group psychotherapy is a primary form of treatment for inpatient stabilization of mental disorders. In a number of studies, clients ranked group psychotherapy as one of the most valuable components of their treatment (Hoge & McLoughlin, 1991). Psychotherapy groups focus on "here and now group interaction" as the primary vehicle of treatment (Beiling, McCabe, & Antony, 2009). Treatment goals relate to modification of maladaptive interpersonal behaviors and development of constructive coping strategies. Clients are expected to share personal feelings, develop insights about personal behaviors, and practice new and more productive interpersonal responses. When situations cannot be changed, psychotherapy groups help clients accept that reality and move on with their lives by empowering and supporting their efforts to make constructive behavioral changes. A hidden benefit of group therapy is the opportunity to experience giving, as well as receiving help from others. Helping others enhances self-esteem (altruism), especially for people who feel they have little to offer others.

Therapy groups in inpatient settings are designed to stabilize the client's behavior enough for them to

functionally transition back into the community. Therapeutic groups in the community are particularly effective for adolescents as a preventive strategy because peer group interaction is such an intrinsic part of the adolescent's life (Aronson, 2004).

Leading Groups for Psychotic Clients

Staff nurses are sometimes called on to lead or co-lead unit-based group psychotherapy on inpatient units for chronically ill clients (Clarke, Adamoski, & Joyce, 1998). Other times, staff nurses participate in community group meetings composed mostly of psychotic clients. Although acutely psychotic clients usually cannot participate until they are stabilized, community groups and small, structured therapy groups can be useful.

A directive, but flexible leadership approach is needed. Because the demands of leadership are so intense with psychotic clients, co-leadership is recommended. Co-therapists can share the group process interventions, model healthy behaviors, offset negative transference from group members, and provide useful feedback to each other. Every group session should be processed immediately after its completion.

If a group topic is not forthcoming from members, the leader can introduce a relevant, concrete, problem-centered topic of potential interest to the group. For example, the group might discuss how to handle a simple behavior in a more productive way. Other members can provide feedback, and the group can choose the best solution.

A primary goal in working with psychotic clients is to understand each person as a unique human being.

Although their needs are disguised as symptoms, you can help clients "decode" a psychotic message by uncovering the underlying theme and translating it into understandable language. Sometimes other members will translate the message if called on by the nurse leader. The leader might say to the group, "I wonder if anyone in the group can help us understand better what John is trying to say." Keep in mind how difficult it is for the psychotic client to tolerate close interaction, and how necessary it is interact with others, if the client is to succeed in the outside environment.

THERAPEUTIC GROUPS IN LONG-TERM SETTINGS

Therapeutic groups in long-term settings offer opportunities for socially isolated individuals to engage with others. Common types of groups include reminiscence, reality orientation, resocialization, remotivation, and activity groups.

Reminiscence Groups

Reminiscence groups focus on life review and/or pleasurable memories (Stinson, 2009). They are not designed as insight groups, but rather to provide a supportive, ego-enhancing experience. Each group member is expected to share a few memories about a specific weekly group focus (holiday, first day of school, family photos, songs, favorite foods, pets, etc.). The leader encourages discussion. Depending on the cognitive abilities of members, the leader will need to be more or less directive. Sessions are held on a weekly basis and meet for an hour.

Reality Orientation Groups

Used with confused clients, reality orientation groups help clients maintain contact with the environment and reduce confusion about time, place, and person. Reality orientation groups are usually held each day for 30 minutes. Nurses can use everyday props such as a calendar, a clock, and pictures of the seasons to stimulate interest. The group should not be seen as an isolated activity; what occurs in the group should be reinforced throughout the 24-hour period. For example, on one unit, nurses placed pictures of the residents in earlier times on the doors to their bedrooms.

Resocialization Groups

Resocialization groups are used with confused clients who are too limited to benefit from a remotivation group but still need companionship and involvement with others. Resocialization groups focus on providing a simple social setting for clients to experience basic social skills again, for example, eating a small meal together. Although the senses and cognitive abilities may diminish in the elderly, basic needs for companionship, interpersonal relationships, and a place where one is accepted and understood remain the same throughout the life span. Improvement of social skills contributes to an improved sense of self-esteem.

Remotivation Groups

Remotivation groups are designed to stimulate self-esteem and socialization in a small group environment of acceptance and appreciation. Originally developed by Dorothy Hoskins Smith for use with patients with chronic mental illness, remotivation groups represent an effort to reach the unwounded healthy areas of the patient's personality. It differs from other forms of therapy because of its exclusive focus on client strengths and abilities rather than on his or her disabilities (Dyer & Stotts, 2005).

Remotivation groups are composed of 10 to 15 members who sit in a circle. They focus on everyday topics, such as the way plants or trees grow, or they might consist of poetry reading or art appreciation. Visual props engage the participant and stimulate more responses. Steps for conducting remotivation groups are presented in Box 12-3.

THERAPEUTIC ACTIVITY GROUPS

Activity groups offer clients a variety of self-expressive opportunities through creative activity rather than through words. The nurse may function as group leader or as a support to other disciplines in encouraging client participation. Activity groups include the following:

BOX 12-3 | **Steps for Conducting Remotivation Groups**

1. Provide an accepting environment and greet each member by name.
2. Offer a bridge to reality by discussing topics of interest, such as news items and historical items.
3. Develop topic with group members through the use of questions, props, or visual aids.
4. Encourage members to discuss the topic in relation to themselves.
5. Express verbal appreciation to members for their contributions and plan the following session.

- *Occupational therapy groups* allow clients to work on individual projects or to participate with others in learning life skills. Examples are cooking, making ceramics, or activities of daily living groups. Tasks are selected for their therapeutic value, as well as for client interest. Life skills groups use a problem-solving approach to interpersonal situations.
- *Recreational therapy groups* offer opportunities to engage in leisure activities that release energy and provide a social format for learning interpersonal skills. Some people never learned how to build needed leisure activities into their lives.
- *Exercise groups* allow clients to engage in structured exercise. The nurse models the exercise behaviors, either with or without accompanying music, and encourages clients to participate. This type of group works well with chronically mentally ill clients.
- *Art therapy groups* encourage clients to reveal feelings through drawing or painting. It is used in different ways. The art can be the focus of discussion. Children and adolescents may engage in a combined group effort to make a mural. Clients are able to reveal feelings through expression of color and abstract forms that they have trouble putting into words.
- *Poetry and bibliotherapy groups* select readings of interest and invite clients to respond to literary works. Sluder (1990) describes an expressive therapy group for the elderly in which the nurse leader first read free verse poems and then invited the clients to compose group poems around feelings such as love or hate. Clients then wrote free verse poems and read them in the group. In the process of developing their poetry, clients got in touch with their personal creativity.

SELF-HELP AND SUPPORT GROUPS

Self-help and support groups provide emotional and practical support to clients and/or families experiencing chronic illness, crises, or the ill health of a family member. Held in the community, most support groups are led informally by group members rather than professionals, although often a health professional acts as an adviser. A suggested format for leading a support group is presented in Table 12-5.

TABLE 12-5	Sample Introductory Format for Support Group Leaders
Steps	**Examples**
Introduce self.	"I am Christy Atkins, a staff nurse on the unit, and I am going to be your group facilitator tonight."
Explain purpose of the group.	"Our goal in having the group is to provide a place for family members to get support from each other and to provide practical information to families caring for victims of Alzheimer's disease."
Identify norms.	"We have three basic rules in this group: (1) We respect one another's feelings; (2) we don't preach or tell you how to do something; and (3) the meetings are confidential, meaning that everything of a personal nature stays in this room."
Ask members to identify themselves and have each one tell something about his or her situation.	"I'd like to go around the room and ask each of you to tell us your name and something about your situation."
Link common themes.	"It seems as if feeling powerless and out of control is a common theme tonight. What strategies have you found help you to feel more in control?"
Allow time for informal networking (optional).	Providing a 10-minute break with or without refreshments allows members to talk informally with each other.
Provide closure.	"Now I'd like to go around the group and ask each of you to identify one thing you will do in the next week for yourself to help you feel more in control."

Self-help groups are voluntary groups, led by consumers and designed to provide peer support for individuals and their families struggling with mental health issues (Solomon, 2004). Examples include 12-step groups, On our own for chronic mentally ill clients, bipolar support alliance, and National Alliance on Mental Illness. Self-help groups are often associated with hospitals, clinics, and national health organizations.

Support groups, for example, for Alzheimer's and related dementias, compassionate friends, and cancer support groups foster creative problem solving and provide community-based opportunities for people with serious health care problems to interact with others experiencing the same kinds of problems. Support groups have an informational function in addition to social support (Percy, Gibbs, Potter, & Boardman, 2009).

Nurses are encouraged to learn about support group networks in their community. Exercise 12-9 offers an opportunity to learn about them.

EDUCATIONAL GROUPS

Community health agencies provide education groups to impart important knowledge about lifestyle changes needed to promote health and well-being and to prevent illness. Family education groups provide families of clients with the knowledge and skills they need to care for their loved ones.

Educational groups are reality-based and related to client needs. They are time-limited group applications (e.g., the group might be held as four 1-hour sessions over a 2-week period or as an 8-week, 2-hour seminar). Examples of primary prevention groups are childbirth education, parenting, stress reduction, and professional support groups for nurses working in critical care settings. Suitable adolescent groups include those that deal with values clarification, health education, and sex education, as well as groups to increase coping skills (e.g., avoiding peer pressure to use drugs).

Medication groups are an excellent example of educational group formats used in hospitals and community clinics. Clients are taught effective ways to carry out a therapeutic medication regimen while learning about their disorder. A typical sequence would be to provide clients with the following information:

- Details about their disorder and how the medication works to reduce symptoms
- Medications, including purpose, dosage, timing, and side effects; what to do when they do not take the medication as prescribed; what to avoid while on the medication (e.g., some medications cause sun sensitivity); and tests needed to monitor the medication

Giving homework, written instructions, and materials to be read between sessions can be helpful if the medication group is to last more than one session. You should allow sufficient time for questions and, by encouraging an open, informal discussion of the topic, engage individual members in the group activity.

FOCUS GROUPS

Clark et al. (2003) describe a focus group as "a group of people who have personal experience of a topic of interest and who meet to discus their perceptions and perspectives on that topic" (p. 457). Focus groups

---

EXERCISE 12-9 | **Learning about Support Groups**

Purpose: To provide direct information about support groups in the community.

Procedure:
1. Contact a support group in your community. (Ideally, students will choose different support groups so that a variety of groups are shared.)
2. Identify yourself as a nursing student and ask for information about the support group (e.g., the time and frequency of meetings, purpose and focus of the group, how a client joins the group, types of services provided, who sponsors the group, issues the group might discuss, and fee schedules).

3. Write a two-paragraph report including the information you have gathered, and describe your experience in asking for the support group information.

Discussion:
1. How easy was it for you to obtain information?
2. Were you surprised by any of the informants' answers?
3. If you were a client, would the support group you chose to investigate meet your needs?
4. What did you learn from doing this exercise that might be useful in your nursing practice?

are used to elicit feedback about important social and health issues as a basis for health policy recommendations. Focus groups allow qualitative researchers to "see the world from the participants' perspectives" (Heary & Hennessy, 2002, p. 47). It is a very powerful and respected tool. In the process of participating in a focus group, clients learn more about health care issues affecting them, and have the opportunity to reflect on their own perceptions (Laube & Wieland, 1998).

DISCUSSION GROUPS

Functional elements appropriate to discussion groups are found in Table 12-6. Careful preparation, formulation of relevant questions, and use of feedback ensure that personal learning needs are met. Group participation on an equal basis should be a group expectation. Although the level of participation is never quite equal, discussion groups in which only a few members actively participate are disheartening to group members and limited in learning potential. Because the primary purpose of a discussion group is to promote the learning of all group members, other members are charged with the responsibility of encouraging the participation of more silent members. Sometimes, when more verbal participants keep quiet, the more reticent group member begins to speak. Cooperation, not competition, needs to be developed as a conscious group norm in all discussion groups. Discussion group topics often include prepared data and group-generated material, which then is discussed in the group. Before the end of each meeting, the leader or a group member should summarize the major themes developed from the content material.

GROUP PRINCIPLES APPLIED TO PROFESSIONAL WORK GROUPS

PROFESSIONAL WORK GROUPS

Multiple group membership is a fact of life in most organizations. Groups found in organizational settings (e.g., standing committees, ad hoc task forces, and quality circles) accomplish a wide range of tasks related to organizational goals.

In work groups, there are two main elements: content and process. Task group content is predetermined by an assignment or charge given to the group. Group process relates to the ways in which group members interact with each other to achieve goals.

APPLYING GROUP CONCEPTS TO WORK GROUPS

LEADERSHIP STYLES

Flexibility of leadership style is an essential characteristic of successful work groups. Effective leadership develops from leader characteristics, situational features, and member needs in combination with each other. Different groups require different leadership behaviors. Leadership is contingent on a proper match between a group situation and the leadership style.

Three types of **leadership** styles found in groups are authoritarian, democratic, and laissez-faire. Leaders demonstrating an **authoritarian leadership** style take full responsibility for group direction and control group interaction. Authoritarian leadership styles work best when the group needs structure and there is limited time to reach a decision. **Democratic leadership** involves members in active discussion and

TABLE 12-6	Elements of Successful Discussion Groups
Element	**Rationale**
Careful preparation	Thoughtful agenda and assignments establish a direction for the discussion and the expected contribution of each member.
Informed participants	Each member should come prepared so that all members are communicating with relatively the same level of information and each is able to contribute equally.
Shared leadership	Each member is responsible for contributing to the discussion.
Good listening skills	Members concentrate on the material and listen to content; challenge, anticipate, and weigh the evidence; they listen between the lines to emotions about the topic.
Relevant questions	Focused questions keep the discussion moving toward the group objectives.
Useful feedback	Thoughtful feedback maintains the momentum of the discussion by reflecting different perspectives of topics raised and confirming or questioning others' views.

decision making. Democratic leaders are goal-directed but flexible. They offer members a functional structure, whereas preserving individual member autonomy, and members feel ownership of solutions. Members of a group with a **laissez-faire** leader function without significant leader input or structure. They are likely to be less productive or satisfying to group members.

Another way to look at leadership styles in professional group life is by using a situational leadership framework, originally developed by Hershey and Blanchard (Hershey, Fowler, Hawkins, et al., 2005). This format requires group leaders to match their leadership style to the situation and the maturity of the group members. The situational leader varies the amount of direction and support a group needs based on the complexity of the task and the follower's experience and confidence with achieving task or group goals.

Group maturity involves two forms of maturity: *job maturity* and *psychological maturity* related to the work. Job maturity refers to the level of work abilities, skills, and knowledge. Psychological job maturity refers to the followers' accurate knowledge of personal assets and limitations, feelings of confidence, willingness, and motivation. The capacity and readiness of situational maturity plays a role in the type of preferred leadership style to accomplish goals. A basic assumption is that leadership should be flexible and adapted to group needs. The situational leadership framework describe four leadership styles, matched to employee's maturity level in a particular work situation and dependent on their need for structure and direction.

- Telling: high structure, low consideration
- Selling: high structure, high consideration
- Participating: high consideration, low structure
- Delegating: low consideration, low structure

The leader must consistently monitor group member readiness level and must be willing to adapt to changes in the group's maturity in working together. As the group matures, leaders turn more of the responsibility for the group to its members. Decision making is collaborative. The leader seeks member input, acts as discussion facilitator, and seeks consensus.

Leader and Member Responsibilities

Box 12-4 summarizes guidelines for groups charged with making organizational changes. The group leader takes the following responsibilities:

- Forms the committee structure and establishes the agenda
- Clarifies the group's tasks and goals (providing background data and material if needed)

BOX 12-4	Guidelines for Organizational Planning Groups

1. Clarify plans.
   - Make one person responsible for implementation plans.
   - Formulate clear, simple, time-bound goals.
   - Make specific plans with milestones and outcomes.
   - Make plans public.
   - Give and solicit frequent face-to-face feedback.
2. Integrate new practices.
   - Limit the amount of change introduced at any one time.
   - Slow the change process.
   - Introduce the change to receptive users first.
   - Ensure that the rationale and procedure for change are well-known.
3. Provide education.
   - Involve the end users and incorporate their experience.
   - Provide "hands-on" training whenever possible.
   - Design training from the end-user's perspective.
   - Train motivated or key end-users first.

- Evaluate the effects of training or work practices and end-users' attitudes.
4. Foster ownership.
   - Ensure that the change improves end-users' ability to accomplish work.
   - Provide incentives for end-users applying the change.
   - Specify milestones for obtaining end-user feedback.
   - Incorporate end-user suggestions in the implementation plans.
   - Publicize end-user suggestions.
5. Give feedback.
   - Document and communicate the expected outcomes of the change.
   - Ensure frequent face-to-face feedback.
   - Identify clear milestones.
   - Make sure feedback includes the large organization.
   - Acknowledge key successes.

From Schoonover S, Dalziel M: Developing leadership for change. In Cathcart R, Samovar L, editors: *Small group communication: a reader*, ed 5, Dubuque, IA, 1988, WC Brown.

- Notifies each member of meeting dates, times, and place
- Keeps group members focused on tasks
- Adheres to time limits
- Concludes each meeting with a summarization of progress

Group members take responsibility for coming prepared to meetings, demonstrating respect for other members' ideas, and taking an active participatory role in the development of viable solutions. Each member should take responsibility for the overall functioning of the group and the achievement of group goals.

STAGE DEVELOPMENT LEADER TASKS APPLIED TO WORK GROUPS

PREGROUP TASKS

Before the group starts, participants should have a clear idea of what the group task commitment will entail in terms of time, effort, and knowledge. Group members should have enough in common to engage in meaningful communication, relevant knowledge of the issues and/or expertise needed for resolution, a willingness to make a contribution to the group solution, and the ability to complete the task.

FORMING

Even if members are known to each other, it is useful to have each person give a brief introduction that includes his or her reason for being part of the work group. The leader should explain the group's purpose and structural components (e.g., time, place, and commitment). Member responsibilities should be outlined clearly with time for questions. A task group with vague or poorly understood goals or structure can breed boredom or frustration, and lead to power struggles and inadequate task resolution.

NORMING

To be successful, group norms should support accomplishment of stated goals. In general, all data developed within the group context should be kept confidential until officially ready for publication. Otherwise, the "grapevine" can distort information and sabotage group efforts. Members should be accountable for regular attendance. If administrative staff is part of the group membership, they should attend all or designated meetings. Few

circumstances are more threatening to a work-related group than having a supervisor enter and exit the task group at will.

PERFORMING

In the performing phase, leader interventions should be consistent and well defined as the group works to fulfill its charge. Most of the group's work is accomplished, including development of recommendations and preparation of final reports. Suggestions for leader feedback in work groups are presented in Box 12-5. Brainstorming is a commonly used strategy to generate solutions. Exercise 12-10 provides practice in the use of brainstorming. Guidelines for brainstorming include:

- Entertaining all ideas without censure
- Testing the more promising ideas for relevance
- Exploring consequences of each potential solution
- Identifying human and instrumental resources, including availability
- Achieving agreement about best possible solutions

Group formats are particularly useful for facilitating changes in organizational life.

Group Think

Although cohesiveness is an essential characteristic of effective work groups, carried to an extreme, it results in **group think**, defined by Janis (1971, 1982) as a

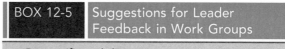

BOX 12-5	Suggestions for Leader Feedback in Work Groups

- Be specific and direct.
- Support comments with evidence.
- Separate the issue from the person.
- "Sandwich" negative messages between positive ones.
- Pose the situation as a mutual problem.
- Mitigate or soften negative messages to avoid overload.
- Deliver feedback close to occurrence.
- Manner of delivery:
  - Assertive, dynamic
  - Trustworthy, fair, and credible
  - Relaxed and responsive
  - Preserve public image of recipient

EXERCISE 12-10	Brainstorming: A Family Dilemma

Purpose: To increase self-awareness and provide practical experience with the use of brainstorming as a group activity.

Procedure:

1. Using the format on brainstorming identified in this chapter, consider the following clinical problem:
   Mrs. Joan Smith is an 80-year-old woman living in Florida. Her husband recently suffered a stroke, which has affected his speech. All he is able to say to his wife is that he loves her, although he seems to understand her words to him. He is paralyzed on one side. When he tried to get out of bed, he fell and broke his hip, so he is confined to a wheelchair. No longer able to care for him, Mrs. Smith moved to Virginia to be close to her daughter, and Mr. Smith is being cared for in a nearby nursing home. Mrs. Smith is living temporarily in her daughter's home, sleeping on the couch because her daughter has a 15-year-old boy and a 3-year-old girl occupying the bedrooms.
   Mrs. Smith visits her husband every day and entertains the idea that he will get well enough that they will be able to return to Florida. She tries to be there at mealtime because she thinks no one will feed him if she doesn't, and he can't eat by himself. Now that the evenings are getting darker, her daughter fears her driving after dark. She hesitates to bring up the idea of selling the house in Florida for fear it will distress her mother. Mrs. Smith is not sleeping at night and seems driven to be with her husband. Her daughter worries that her mother will collapse if she keeps up her current pace. Meanwhile, the house in Florida remains empty, her mother has taken no steps to secure legal advice, and the current living situation is becoming more permanent by default.

2. Divide the class into groups of three to six students, depending on class size.
3. Each group should identify a spokesperson to the larger group. Use a flip chart or board to record ideas.
4. Brainstorm to generate ideas for a practical solution to the Smith family's problem. Allow 15 minutes for the first part of the exercise and 20 minutes for the brainstorming section.
5. Describe your group's solution, and give the rationale for your selection.

Discussion:

In the larger group, each spokesperson presents the smaller group's solution to the Smith family's problem.

1. How did your group's answers compare with those of other groups?
2. What did you learn about the brainstorming process as a problem-solving format?
3. What was the most difficult part of the process for your group?
4. As you listen to how other groups implemented the process, what ideas came to mind?
5. How might you use this format in your nursing practice?

phenomenon that occurs when loyalty and approval by other group members become so important that members are afraid to express conflicting ideas and opinions for fear of being excluded from the group. The group exerts pressure on members to act as one voice in decision making, so that realistic appraisal of issues gets lost. The warning signs of group think are listed in Box 12-6. Group think can create irrational decisions and dissatisfaction with goal achievement. Figure 12-3 displays the characteristics.

Ways to reduce the potential for group think in work groups include developing norms that make it acceptable to disagree with other group members, and to seek fresh information and outside opinions. Individual members who act as "devil's advocate" about important issues should be respected and their ideas explored.

BOX 12-6	Warning Signs of Group Think

1. Illusion of invulnerability
2. Collective rationalization that disregards warnings
3. Belief in inherent morality of the decision
4. Stereotyped or negative views of people outside of group
5. Direct pressure on dissenters to not express their concerns
6. Self-censorship: individual members with doubts do not express them
7. Illusion of unanimity in which majority view is held to be unanimous
8. Self-appointed "mindguards" within the group who withhold problematic or contradictory data

Adapted from Janis I: *Groupthink: psychological studies of policy decisions and fiascoes,* ed 2, New York, 1982, Houghton Mifflin.

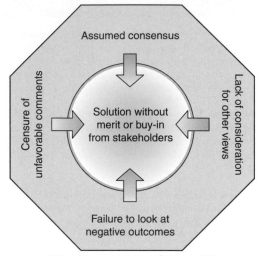

Figure 12-3   Characteristics of Group Think.

ETHICAL DILEMMA What Would You Do?

Mrs. Murphy is 39 years old and has had multiple admissions to the psychiatric unit for bipolar disorder. She wants to participate in group therapy but is disruptive when she is in the group. The group gets angry with her monopolization of their time, but she says it is her right as a patient to attend if she chooses. Mrs. Murphy's symptoms could be controlled with medication, but she refuses to take it when she is "high" because it makes her feel less energized. How do you balance Mrs. Murphy's rights with those of the group? Should she be required to take her medication? How would you handle this situation from an ethical perspective?

ADJOURNING PHASE

Termination in work groups takes place when the group task is accomplished. The leader should summarize the work of the group, allow time for processing level of goal achievement, and identify any follow-up. Work groups need to disband once the initial charge is satisfied. They should not simply move on into a never-ending commitment without negotiation and the agreement of participants to continue with another assignment.

SUMMARY

This chapter outlines key concepts associated with group communication and explores how it is used to help clients cope with their health or personal issues more effectively. Differences between individual and group communication are described. Group dynamics include individual member commitment, functional similarity, and leadership style. Group concepts related to group dynamics consist of purpose, norms, cohesiveness, roles, and role functions.

Group processes refer to the structural phases of group development as described by Tuckman (1965, 1977): forming, storming, norming, performing, and adjourning. In the forming phase of group relationships, the basic need is for acceptance. The storming phase focuses on issues of power and control in groups. Behavioral standards are formed in the norming phase that will guide the group toward goal accomplishment, and the group becomes a safe

environment in which to work and express feelings. Once this occurs, most of the group's task is accomplished during the performing phase. Feelings of warmth, caring, and intimacy follow; members feel affirmed and valued. Finally, when the group task is completed to the satisfaction of the individual members, or of the group as a whole, the group enters an adjourning (termination) phase. Different types of groups found in health care include therapeutic, support, educational, and discussion focus groups. Group communication principles can be applied to task groups in work settings and strategies for conducting successful work groups are addressed.

REFERENCES

Aronson S: Where the wild things are: the power and challenge of adolescent group work, *Mt Sinai J Med* 71(3):174–180, 2004.

Beiling P, McCabe R, Antony M, et al: *Cognitive-behavioral therapy in groups*, New York, 2009, Guilford Press.

Benne KD, Sheats P: Functional roles of group members, *J Soc Issues* 4(2):41–49, 1948.

Bernard H, Birlingame G, Flores P, et al: Clinical practice guidelines for group psychotherapy, *Int J Group Psychother* 58(4):455–542, 2008.

Burlingame G, Strauss B, Joyce A, et al: *Core battery—revised*, New York, 2006, American Group Psychotherapy Association.

Clark M, Cary S, Diemert G, et al: Involving communities in community assessment, *Public Health Nurs* 20(6):456–463, 2003.

Clarke D, Adamoski E, Joyce B, et al: In-patient group psychotherapy: the role of the staff nurse, *J Psychosoc Nurs Ment Health Serv* 36(5): 22–26, 1998.

Corey G: *Theory and practice of group counseling*, ed 7, Pacific Grove, CA, 2007, Brooks Cole.

Corey M, Corey G: *Groups: process and practice*, ed 8, Pacific Grove, CA, 2008, Brooks/Cole.

Counselman E: Reader's forum: why study group therapy? *Int J Group Psychother* 58(2):265–272, 2008.

Dyer J, Stotts M, editors: *Handbook of Remotivation Therapy*, Binghamton NY, 2005, The Haworth Press, Inc.

Forsyth D: *Group dynamics*, ed 5, Belmont, CA, 2009, Wadsworth Cengage Learning.

Gans J, Alonso A: Difficult patients: their construction in group therapy, *Int J Group Psychother* 48(3):311–326, 1998.

Heary C, Hennessy E: The use of focus group interviews in pediatric health care research, *J Pediatr Psychol* 27(1):47–57, 2002.

Hershey K, Fowler S, Hawkins L, et al: *Self Leadership and the One Minute Manager*, New York, 2005, Harper Collins Publishers.

Hoge M, McLoughlin K: Group psychotherapy in acute treatment settings: theory and technique, *Hosp Commun Psychiatry* 42(2):153–157, 1991.

Janis I: Groupthink, *Psychol Today* 5:43–46, 74–76, 1971.

Janis I: *Groupthink: Psychological studies of policy decisions and fiascos*, ed 2, Boston, 1982, Houghton Mifflin.

Lasky G, Riva M: Confidentiality and privileged communication in group psychotherapy, *Int J Group Psychother* 56(4):455–476, 2006.

Laube J, Wieland V: Nourishing the body through use of process prescriptions in group therapy, *Int J Eat Disord* 24(1):1–11, 1998.

Mangione L, Forti R, Iacuzzi C, et al: Ethics and endings in group psychotherapy: saying good-bye and saying it well, *Int J Group Psychother* 57(1):25–40, 2007.

Moreno KJ: Scapegoating in group psychotherapy, *Int J Group Psychother* 57(1):93–104, 2007.

Percy C, Gibbs T, Potter L, et al: Nurse-led peer support group: experiences of women with polycystic ovary syndrome, *J Adv Nurs* 65(10):2046–2055, 2009.

Powles W: Reader's forum: reflections on "what is a group?" *Int J Group Psychother* 57(1):105–113, 2007.

Rogers C: The process of the basic encounter group. In Diedrich R, Dye HA, editors: *Group procedures: purposes, processes and outcomes*, Boston, 1972, Houghton Mifflin.

Rubel D, Kline W: An exploratory study of expert group leadership, *J Specialists Group Work* 3(2):138–160, 2008.

Rutan JS, Stone W, Shay J, et al: *Psychodynamic group psychotherapy*, New York, 2007, The Guilford Press.

Sluder H: The write way: using poetry for self-disclosure, *J Psychosoc Nurs Ment Health Serv* 28(7):26–28, 1990.

Solomon P: Peer support/peer provided services underlying processes, benefits, and critical ingredients, *Psychiatr Rehab J* 27(4):392–401, 2004.

Stinson C: Structured group reminiscence: an intervention for older adults, *J Contin Educ Nurs* 40(11):521–528, 2009.

Tuckman B: Developmental sequence in small groups, *Psychol Bull* 63:384, 1965.

Tuckman B, Jensen M: Stages of small-group development revisited, *Group Organ Manag* 2(4):419–427, 1977.

Yalom I, Leszcz M: *The theory and practice of group psychotherapy*, ed 5, New York, 2005, Basic Books.

CHAPTER 13

Communicating with Families

Elizabeth C. Arnold

OBJECTIVES

At the end of the chapter, the reader will be able to:
1. Define family and identify its components.
2. Compare and contrast theoretical frameworks used to study family relationships.
3. Apply family-centered concepts to the care of the family in clinical settings, using standardized family assessment tools.
4. Apply the nursing process to the care of families in clinical settings.
5. Identify nursing interventions for families in the intensive care unit (ICU).
6. Identify nursing interventions for families in the community.

The purpose of this chapter is to describe family-centered relationships and communication strategies that nurses can use to support family integrity in health care settings. The chapter identifies family theory frameworks, which provide a common language for describing family relationships. Practical assessment and intervention strategies address family issues that affect a client's recovery, and support self-management of chronic health conditions, or peaceful death in clinical practice.

BASIC CONCEPTS

DEFINITION OF FAMILY

Wright and Leahey (2009) state, "A **family** is who they say they are" (p. 70). Identified family members may or may not be blood related. Strong emotional ties and durability of membership characterize family relationships regardless of how uniquely they are defined. Even when family members are alienated, or distanced geographically, they "can never truly relinquish family membership" (Goldenberg & Goldenberg, 2008, p. 3).

Some people identify their family as those with whom they have close relationships and who care for them (Kristjanson & Aoun, 2004). Each family member relates to the other and to crisis affecting the family in unique ways. Communication, even when reactive, is designed to maintain the integrity of the family. Understanding the family as a system is relevant in today's health care environment, as the family is an essential part of the health care team.

The family represents the primary sociocultural system, in which children learn values and behavior patterns (Novilla, Barnes, De La Cruz, & Williams, 2006). Family health beliefs, past family experience with illness or injury, family loyalties and conflicts are important pieces of information that help explain client and family responses to health disruptions.

Families have a profound influence on sick clients as advisors, caretakers, supporters, and sometimes irritants. Clients who are very young, very old, and those requiring assistance with self-management of chronic illness are particularly dependent on their families.

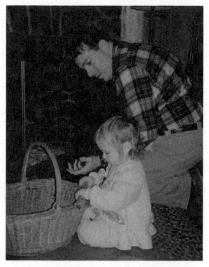

Young children learn family rules for communication from their parents.

Learning about the family's dynamics provides:

- Awareness of family relationships that can be rallied for support, or that may need special attention because of a negative impact on the client's situation
- Awareness of who else in the family has had a similar illness or medical problem and family coping strategies
- Awareness of cultural and family factors that influence a client's attitudes, beliefs, and willingness to take action related to health care (Cole-Kelly & Seaburn, 1999).

FAMILY COMPOSITION

There is significant diversity in the composition of families, family beliefs and values, how they communicate with each other, ethnic heritage, life experiences, commitment to individual family members, and connections with the community (Schor, 2003). Box 13-1 identifies different types of family composition.

Families today are much more complex than in past generations. Modern definitions of family include "declared commitment" family households without marriage (Levine, 2004). Single-parent families must accomplish the same developmental tasks as two-parent families, but in many cases, they do it without the support of the other partner or sufficient financial resources.

Blended families have a different life experience than those in an intact family because their family structure is more complex. Children may be members of more than one family unit, linked biologically, physically, and emotionally to people who may or may not be part of their daily lives. Their "family" may include two or more sets of grandparents, step- or half-brothers and sisters, and multiple aunts and uncles (Byng-Hall, 2000). The child may spend extended periods in separate households, each with a full set of family expectations that may or may not be similar. Blended families can offer a rich experience for everyone concerned, but they are more complex because of multiple connections. Table 13-1 displays

---

| BOX 13-1 | Types of Family Composition |

- **Nuclear family**: a father and mother, with one or more children, living together as a single family unit
- **Extended family**: nuclear family unit's combination of second- and third-generation members related by blood or marriage but not living together
- **Three-generational family**: any combination of first-, second-, and third-generation members living within a household
- **Dyad family**: husband and wife or other couple living alone without children
- **Single-parent family**: divorced, never married, separated, or widowed male or female and at least one child; most single-parent families are headed by women
- **Stepfamily**: family in which one or both spouses are divorced or widowed with one or more children from a previous marriage who may not live with the newly reconstituted family

- **Blended or reconstituted family**: a combination of two families with children from one or both families and sometimes children of the newly married couple
- **Common law family**: an unmarried couple living together with or without children
- **No kin**: a group of at least two people sharing a nonsexual relationship and exchanging support who have no legal, blood, or strong emotional tie to each other
- **Polygamous family**: one man (or woman) with several spouses
- **Same-sex family**: a homosexual or lesbian couple living together with or without children
- **Commune**: more than one couple living together and sharing resources
- **Group marriage**: all individuals are "married" to one another and are considered parents of all the children

TABLE 13-1	Comparing Differences Between Biological and Blended Families
Biological Families	**Blended Families**
Family is created without loss.	Family is born of loss.
There are shared family traditions.	There are two sets of family traditions.
One set of family rules evolves.	Family rules are varied and complicated.
Children arrive one at a time.	Instant parenthood of children at different ages occurs.
Biological parents live together.	Biological parents live apart.

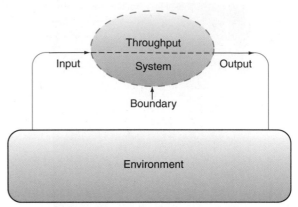

Figure 13-1 Systems model: Interaction with the Environment.

some of the differences between biological and blended families. Issues for blended families include discipline, money, use of time, birth of an infant, death of a stepparent, inclusion at graduation, and marriage and health care decisions.

THEORETICAL FRAMEWORKS

GENERAL SYSTEMS THEORY

Kurt von Bertalanffy's (1968) general systems theory provides a conceptual foundation for family system models (Barker, 1998). A systems perspective examines the interdependence among all parts of the system and how they support the system as a functional whole. Systems' thinking maintains that the whole is greater than the sum of its parts with each part reciprocally influencing its function. If one part of the system changes or fails, it affects the functioning of the whole. A clock is a useful metaphor. It displays time correctly, but only if all parts work together. If any part of the clock breaks down, the clock no longer tells accurate time.

A system interacts with other systems in the environment. An interactional process occurs when "*inputs*" are introduced into the system in the form of information, energy, and resources. Within each system, the information is processed internally as the system actively processes and interprets its meaning. The transformation process of raw data into desired outputs is referred to as *throughput*. The *output* refers to the result or product that leaves the system. Each system is separated from its environment by boundaries that control the exchange of information, energy,

and resources into and out of the system. Evaluation of the output and feedback loops from the environment inform the system of changes needed to achieve effective outputs. Figure 13-1 identifies the relational components of a human system's interaction with the environment, using von Bertalanffy's model.

Applied to the human system, individuals take in food, liquids, and oxygen to nourish the body (inputs). Within the body, a transformational process occurs through enzymes and other metabolic processes (throughputs). so that the body can use them. This interactional process results in the human organism's growth, health, and capacity to interact with the external environment (outputs). Nonusable outputs excreted from the body include urine, feces, sweat, and carbon dioxide. A person's skin represents an important boundary between the environment and the human system.

Family systems have boundaries that regulate information coming into and leaving the family system. Family systems theory helps explain how families strive for harmony and balance *(homeostasis),* how the family is able to maintain its continuity despite challenges, *(morphostasis),* and how the family is able to change and grow over time in response to challenges *(morphogenesis). Feedback loops* describe the patterns of interaction that facilitate movement toward morphogenesis, or morphostasis. They impact goal setting in behavior systems. The systems principle of *equifinality* describes how the same outcome or end state can be reached through different pathways. This principle helps explain why some individuals at high risk for poor outcomes do not develop maladaptive behaviors

(Cicchetti & Blender, 2006). Hierarchy is the term used to describe the complex layers of smaller systems that exist within a system. *Subsystems* refer to the smaller parts within the system, and *suprasystems* help describe the larger economic, social, and political systems in which the family system exists.

BOWEN'S SYSTEMS THEORY

Murray Bowen (1978) family systems theory conceptualizes the family as an interactive emotional unit. He believed that family members assume reciprocal family roles, develop automatic communication patterns, and react to each other in predictable connected ways, particularly when family anxiety is high. Once anxiety heightens within the system, an emotional process gets activated (Nichols & Schwartz, 2009) and dysfunctional communication patterns can emerge. For example, if one person is overly responsible, another family member is less likely to assume normal responsibility. Until one family member is willing to challenge the dysfunction of an emotional system by refusing to play his or her reactive part, the negative emotional energy fueling a family's dysfunctional communication pattern persists.

Bowen developed eight interlocking concepts to explain his theoretical construct of the family system (Bowen Center, 2004; Gilbert, 2006). He viewed self-differentiation as the fundamental means of reducing chronic anxiety within the family system and enhancing effective problem solving. Self-differentiation emphasizes thinking rather than feeling in communication.

- **Self-differentiation** refers to a person's capacity to define himself/herself within the family system as an individual having legitimate needs and wants. It requires making "I" statements based on rational thinking rather than emotional reactivity. Self-differentiation takes into consideration the views of others but is not dominated by them. Poorly differentiated people are so dependent on the approval of others that they discount their own needs.
- **Multigenerational transmission** refers to the emotional transmission of behavioral patterns, roles, and communication response styles from generation to generation. It explains why family patterns tend to repeat behaviors in marriages, child rearing, choice of occupation, and emotional responses across generations without understanding why it happens.

- **Nuclear family emotional system** refers to the way family members relate to one another within their immediate family when stressed. Family anxiety shows up in one of four patterns: (1) dysfunction in one spouse, (2) marital conflict, (3) dysfunctional symptoms in one or more of the children, or (4) emotional distancing.
- **Triangles** refer to a defensive way of reducing, neutralizing, or defusing heightened anxiety between two family members by drawing a third person or object into the relationship (Glasscock & Hales, 1998). If the original triangle fails to contain or stabilize the anxiety, it can expand into a series of "interlocking" triangles, for example, into school issues or an affair.
- **Family projection process** refers to an unconscious casting of unresolved anxiety in the family on a particular family member, usually a child. The projection can be positive or negative, and it can become a self-fulfilling prophecy as the child incorporates the anxiety of the parent as part of his or her self-identity.
- **Sibling position**, a concept originally developed by Walter Toman (1992), refers to a belief that sibling positions shape relationships and influence a person's expression of behavioral characteristics. Each sibling position has its own strengths and weaknesses. This concept helps explain why siblings in the same family can exhibit very different characteristics. For example:
  - Oldest or only children are more serious, assume leadership roles, and like to be in control. They may experience more trouble with staying connected with others, or depending on them.
  - Youngest siblings are characterized as being followers, spontaneous and fun loving, with a stronger sense of humor. They are more likely to be interested in quality of life and relationships.
  - Middle child positions embrace characteristics of oldest and youngest; they are likely to be adventuresome and independent, but not leaders. The child in the middle position may feel neglected or take on the role of peacemaker.
  - An age differential of 6 years or more, illness, life circumstances, gender, and personality can modify typical sibling position characteristics. Children in well-differentiated families are less likely to be affected by sibling position characteristics than those in fused family systems.

Complementary matches, for example, oldest/youngest work best in marriage and work situations. When two people occupy the same sibling position, issues can arise. For example, competitiveness in two oldest or only child marital partners, or difficulty making decisions with two youngest pairings is not uncommon.

- Although sibling position is a factor in explaining different relational behaviors, it is not useful as a descriptor of life functioning as a person occupying any sibling position can be successful or unsuccessful (Gilbert, 2006).
- **Emotional cutoff** refers to a person's withdrawal from other family members as a means of avoiding family issues that create anxiety. Emotional cutoffs range from total avoidance to remaining in physical contact, but in a superficial manner. Emotional cutoffs contain a negative anxiety that drains personal energy. The problems creating the emotional cutoff persist.
- **Societal emotional process** refers to parallels that Bowen found between the family system and the emotional system operating at the institutional level in society. As anxiety grows within a society, many of the same polarizations, lack of self-differentiation, and emotion-based thinking dominate behavior and system outcomes.

Family legacies have a powerful influence on family relationships and in shaping parenting practices. Knowledge of family relationships helps explain behaviors that would not be clear without having a family context. Helping families gain clarity about how their family heritage can be used as an asset in health care and/or what areas need work strengthens the potential for effective family-centered care.

MINUCHIN'S STRUCTURAL MODEL

Family structure models, pioneered by Salvador Minuchin (1974), emphasize the structure (subsystems, hierarchies, and boundaries) of the family unit as the basis for understanding family function. Family structure refers to how the family is constructed legally and emotionally. The concept of *hierarchy* describes how families organize themselves into various smaller units, referred to as the subsystems that comprise the larger family system.

Subsystems are organized by position, gender, generation, interest, or function to accomplish the goals of the family through related tasks. Common subsystems include spousal, parental, and sibling units. Family members typically belong to several subsystems simultaneously (Goldenberg & Goldenberg, 2008). Their behaviors in each subsystem reflect the nature of the relationship, for example, an adult feeling like a child when visiting parents. Being in multiple subsystems can generate conflict when the expectations of one subsystem interfere with those of another, for example, being a parent while having caregiving responsibility as a daughter for a frail elder and finding time for the spousal subsystem.

Boundaries, defined as invisible limits surrounding the family unit, protect the integrity of the family system. Boundaries draw a line in the sand by identifying what belongs within the family system and what is external to it. They define the level of participation between family members (Nichols & Schwartz, 2009). Clear generational boundaries provide security for family members, for example, setting legitimate limits with children and balancing individual needs with caring for the needs of chronically ill family members.

Boundaries regulate the flow of information into and out of the family. Permeable boundaries welcome interactions with others and allow information to flow freely. Families with clear, permeable boundaries are better able to balance the demands of the illness with other family needs and can communicate more effectively with care providers (Dalton & Kitzmann, 2008). Diffuse boundaries lead to family overinvolvement, whereas rigid boundaries are operative in families with little interaction between members and family secrets. Rigid boundaries restrict flow of information. Interaction with outsiders is discouraged or heavily regulated. Diffuse boundaries are found in enmeshed families.

Exercise 13-1 provides an opportunity to look at the communication process of family from a structural functional perspective. Structural and functional aspects of families determine the nature of interactions between family members. Family interactions offer protective and health-promoting support for members in crisis when they function well, and are an area of concern when they function ineffectively.

The family performs its functions through subsystem alliances and coalitions to maintain the system as a whole (homeostasis). Wright and Leahey (2009) describe two ways of examining family functioning: instrumental

EXERCISE 13-1	Family Structures and Processes

Purpose: To develop an awareness of the different structures and processes within families.

Procedure:
Each student will attempt to spend time with a family other than his or her own family of origin. (Family can be any two or more persons of relation.) Students should observe the communication patterns, roles, and norms of the family and write a descriptive summary of their experience. How do you think this family

would cope with one of the members becoming ill? Think about how this family differs from your own regarding structure and process.

Discussion:
Each student will share experiences with the group. Identify how families are different and similar. What are some of the coping strategies that you predicted based on observations? Discuss how the nurse can interface with families and assist them with coping.

and expressive. Both are important descriptors of family functioning.

- *Instrumental* functioning refers to task activities of daily living (e.g., eating, sleeping, or caring for a sick member).
- *Expressive* functioning looks at the communication, problem-solving skills, roles, beliefs, spheres of influence, and power that govern how individual members interact with one another.

Assessment of a family's structure and function for strengths and weaknesses, and comparing current functionality with previous functioning helps focus nursing interventions and supports.

DUVALL'S DEVELOPMENTAL FRAMEWORK

Evelyn Duvall (1958) proposed a family life stage framework for understanding issues that normal families experience based on expected family development through the life span, each with its own set of tasks. Her model describes the life cycle of a family, using the age of the oldest child in the family as the benchmark for determining the family's developmental stage. Developmental tasks represent the challenges and growth responsibilities each family experiences at different life stages (Table 13-2).

Duvall's stages of family development are helpful in guiding nurses about possible concerns families may have at different stages of family development. It helps nurses appreciate a family's current developmental needs that may coincide with their family member's illness or injury. Nurses can provide information about natural family development as a basis for discussion of the limitations imposed by the health deviation.

Duvall (1958) identified nine family characteristics indicative of successful family development:

1. An independent home
2. Satisfactory ways of earning and spending money
3. Mutually acceptable patterns in the division of labor
4. Continuity of mutually satisfying sexual relationships
5. An open system of communication
6. Workable relationships with relatives
7. Ways of interacting with the larger social community
8. Competency in childbearing and child-rearing
9. A workable philosophy of life

Developmental family theory helps nurses appreciate the family's current developmental needs that may coincide with their family member's illness or injury. This knowledge helps nurses craft a developmentally appropriate level of involvement for each family system (Leon, 2008). Families benefit from information about normal developmental patterns and typical limitations imposed by a health deviation. For example, hair loss for the adolescent having chemotherapy can be devastating because of the heightened attention to appearance during this developmental stage. Anticipatory guidance about natural developmental milestones and associated behaviors is helpful.

MCCUBBIN'S RESILIENCY MODEL OF FAMILY COPING

McCubbin's Resiliency Model of Family Stress, Adjustment, and Adaptation is considered the most extensively studied model of family coping with traumatic and chronic illness (McCubbin, McCubbin, Thompson, et al, 1993; Clark, 1999). In this model, A (an event) interacts with B (resources) and with C (family's perception of the event) to produce X (the crisis). An expansion of this model adds the concepts of *"pileup of demands, family system resources,* and

TABLE 13-2	Duvall's Family Life Cycle and Related Developmental Tasks
State Family Life Cycle Stage	**Family Development Tasks**
I. Beginning families (married couples without children)	Establishing a mutually satisfying marriage; adjusting to pregnancy and the promise of parenthood; fitting into the kin network
II. Child-bearing families (oldest child birth through 30 months)	Having, adjusting to, and encouraging the development of infants; establishing a satisfying home for both parents and infants
III. Families with preschool-age children (oldest child 2.5–6 years of age)	Adapting to the critical needs and interests of preschool-age children in stimulating, growth-promoting ways; coping with energy depletion and lack of privacy as parents
IV. Families with school-age children (oldest child 6–13 years of age)	Fitting into the community of school-age families in constructive ways; encouraging children's educational achievement
V. Families with teenagers (oldest child 13–20 years of age)	Balancing freedom with responsibility as teenagers mature and emancipate themselves; establishing postparental interests and careers as growing parents
VI. Families launching young adults (first child leaving home through last child leaving home)	Releasing young adults into work, college, marriage with appropriate rituals and assistance; maintaining supportive home base
VII. Middle-age parents (empty nest to retirement)	Rebuilding the marriage relationship; maintaining kin ties with older and younger generations
VIII. Family during retirement and aging (retirement)	Adjusting to retirement; closing the family home or adapting it to aging; coping with bereavement and living alone

From Duvall EM, Miller BC: *Marriage and family development*, ed 6, Boston, 1985, Allyn and Bacon. Copyright © 1985 by Pearson Education. Adapted by permission of the publisher.

postcrisis behavior" (McCubbin, McCubbin, & Thompson et al., 1998, p. 49). With any serious illness, most people experience a roller coaster emotional response that parallels the course of the illness—optimism and hope when things are going well, disappointment and anger when they are not.

Protective factors related to stress adaptation include good problem-solving skills and flexibility to try different constructive actions. Successful coping built on family capabilities, strengths, and resources leads to positive adaptation. Unsuccessful coping strategies result in maladaptive behaviors (Greeff & Human, 2004). Exercise 13-2 provides an opportunity to look at the differences between positive and negative family interactions.

Pile-up demands (McCubbin et al., 1998) from the environment such as job loss, unexpected expenses, overcrowded housing conditions, and limited caregiving skills can place children and vulnerable adults at risk for significant stress. Family violence, substance abuse, neglect, and dysfunction are on the rise as families become more and more stressed while trying to cope with the demands of chronically ill clients. Nurses must be able to recognize families who are providing unsafe environments for individual family members or who have reached dangerous stress levels themselves.

Recognizing Families at Risk

Medalie and Cole-Kelly (2002) describe the course of chronic illness as being a series of health crises with relatively stable times in between. Knowledge of risk factors for family coping is an important dimension of providing family-centered care for the person with chronic illness and the family caring for the family member. Equally essential is knowledge and an assessment of family assets. Assets can include support from other family members, shared family activities, connections with supportive people in the community, and parental involvement in child care and school activities.

An atmosphere of openness to family concerns helps families feel comfortable in sharing painful

EXERCISE 13-2	Positive and Negative Family Interactions

Purpose: To examine the effects of functional versus dysfunctional communication.

Procedure:
Answer the following questions in a brief essay:
1. Recall a situation in dealing with a client's family that you felt was a positive experience? What characteristics of that interaction made you feel this way?
2. Recall a situation in dealing with a client's family that you felt was a negative experience? What

characteristics of that interaction made you feel this way?

Discussion:
Compare experiences, both positive and negative. What did you see as the most striking differences? In what ways were your responses similar or dissimilar from those of your peers? What do you see as the implications of this exercise for enhancing family communication in your nursing practice?

feelings of anger or guilt. Psychosocial screening for risk factors should include asking relevant questions about family relationships, domestic violence, maternal depression, substance abuse, and suicidal ideation. There are brief written screening tools for depression and stress that nurses can also use. Individuals found to be at risk through screening can be referred to appropriate resources.

Just talking about the impact of a significant illness on family roles and function is helpful for families. Relevant questions should focus on how each family member is coping with the situation, what types of changes are needed in family functioning to cope with the illness over time, and the degree to which the family is able to meet the requirements of the crisis situation. Exercise 13-3 examines coping strategies that families use in crisis situations.

The McCubbin model is helpful in assessing and responding to a family's psychosocial needs around the serious illness of a family member, particularly a

child. Families of seriously ill children face many competing demands—care for the ill child, attention to other children, balancing work responsibilities, and having any kind of a normal life for themselves. Using this model, the nurse might inquire about how the family is able to work together in dealing with the challenges of the current illness.

Providing timely information and promoting connections with community supports and parent-to-parent networks is helpful. When significant problems exist, referring families to professionals able to deal with these complex problems and notifying protective service authorities become essential roles. Nurses are considered reporting agents in most states and, therefore, are required by law to report suspicion of child physical or sexual abuse to child protection agencies.

Family Resilience

Resilience refers to the ability to cope positively with adversity. It is recognized as a protective factor in

EXERCISE 13-3	Family Coping Strategies

Purpose: To broaden awareness of coping strategies among families.

Procedure:
Each student is to recall a time when his or her family experienced a significant health crisis and how they coped. (Alternative strategy: Pick a health crisis you observed with a family in clinical practice.) Respond to the following questions:
1. Did the crisis cause a readjustment in roles?
2. Did it create tension and conflict, or did it catalyze members, turning to one another

for support? Look at individual members' behavior.
3. What would have helped your family in this crisis? Write a descriptive summary about this experience.

Discussion:
Each student shares his or her experience. Coping strategies and helpful interventions will be compiled on the board. Discuss the differences in how families respond to crisis. Discuss the nurse's role in support to the family.

times of family stress. Family resilience is associated with a healthy family atmosphere of positive support, warmth, and affection. Walsh (1996) identifies four characteristics found in resilient families:

- Capacity to derive meaning from adversity
- A positive outlook
- The capacity to affirm strengths and consider alternative possibilities
- Transcendent and spiritual beliefs that allow families to connect with a larger purpose and commitment to help others

Serious illness or injury creates many challenges to family integrity, all occurring within a short period. In addition to fear and anxiety about the illness itself, the internal image of what the family is and the meaning it holds for each person within it is challenged. In some cases, the experience strengthens the family unit. In others, it leads to disruption of family functioning. Normal life routines are suspended. Families automatically become involved in the client's care as participant, critic, support, or advocate with health care providers.

Nurses can support family resilience by providing emotional support for individual family members and vital updated information about the client's condition. Psychosocial support makes a difference. Families need attention, repeated information, and assurances (Van Horn & Kautz, 2007). Other strategies include encouraging collaboration among family members, reinforcing a sense of teamwork. Referrals to support groups for peer support of shared experiences and verbalizing observations of personal and family strengths are helpful.

Developing an Evidence-Based Practice

Wigert H, Berg M, Hellstrom AL: Parental presence when their child is in neonatal intensive care, *Scand J Caring Sci* 23:139–146, 2010.

This article describes a study of parents with children hospitalized in a neonatal intensive care unit (NICU) in a university-based hospital and a rural hospital in a smaller city. The goal of the study was to identify parent-identified factors that facilitated or obstructed family presence with their child in the NICU. These data can help inform nurses about the types of optimal conditions needed to encourage parental presence with their children in the NICU. The study used a quantitative descriptive design to assess the amount of time parents spent with their hospitalized child, combined with an interview guide. The interview guide asked parents to answer questions about the reasons for their presence at the NICU, and factors that facilitated or obstructed their presence. The use of the interview allowed parents to expand their answers and ask for clarification. Data were collected over a 2-week period on each unit with the parents of 43 infants hospitalized at one of the NICUs (N = 67; 36 mothers, 31 fathers). Descriptive data analysis was conducted with a one-way analysis of variance designed to describe variance with the type of accommodation and time of presence within and between groups. Choice of accommodation was limited to availability at the time and the condition of the infant (maternity ward, parent rooms at the ICU, a family hotel, and the family home).

Results: Study findings indicated that parents having the availability of a parent room at the NICU resulted in parents spending more time with their children ($P < 0.001$) in the NICU. Reasons given by parents for wanting to be present with their child centered around wanting to have more control over what was happening with their infant and wanting to assume as much parental responsibility as possible. The most important factors facilitating parental presence were good treatment by the staff and a family-friendly environment. Availability of staff and being given attention and support were other important factors. Parents appreciated being invited to participate, being given permission to choose visiting times, and getting regular information. Obstacles to being present, as identified by parents, included a non–family-friendly environment and poor treatment by staff. Responsibilities for children and care of the home were other obstacles. Lack of information and not knowing whom to turn to with questions was viewed as an obstruction. Other reasons for limited presence, as identified by parents, consisted of distance and economic situations that precluded spending significant amounts of time with the child in the NICU. Findings from this study point out that parental presence can be facilitated with a family-friendly environment, and a supportive nursing staff dedicated to providing tangible supports and optimal conditions for parents to be with their child in an NICU.

Application to Your Clinical Practice: Family presence is an important dimension of family-centered care for infants in the NICU. Presence promotes bonding between parent and child, helps parents develop the skills they need to care for their infant, and reduces the parent's psychological stress. Understanding the factors that encourage parental presence and involvement with critically ill infants in the NICU can help nurses develop carefully targeted interventions.

APPLICATIONS

FAMILY-CENTERED CARE

Family-centered care allows health care providers to have a more uniform understanding of the client and family's knowledge, preferences, and values in health care as the basis for shared decision making. This information allows them to provide consistent information to all those involved in the client's care, and to identify any barriers that might arise with the care plan.

The health events of one family member affect the whole family. Trotter and Martin (2007) note, "Families share genetic susceptibilities, environments, and behaviors, all of which interact to cause different levels of health and disease" (p. 561). Families bear a bulk of the care and/or support of client self-management of chronic health conditions. They are instrumental in helping clients appreciate the need for diagnosis and treatment, and in encouraging the patient to seek treatment. Family members are involved in a client's health care decisions ranging from treatment options to critical decisions about end of life care. Families play a pivotal advocacy role in treatment by monitoring and insisting on quality care actions for an individual family member.

The challenges for the nurse in family-centered care are:

- To understand the impact of the medical crisis on family functioning and dynamics
- To appreciate and respond empathetically to the emotional intensity of the experience for the family
- To determine the appropriate level of family involvement in holistic care of the client, based on an understanding of fundamental family system concepts (Leon & Knapp, 2008)

ASSESSMENT

For immediate health care purposes, family is defined as the significant people in the client's environment who are capable and willing to provide family-type support. This definition of family includes members who may not be related by blood, marriage, or adoption (Medalie & Cole-Kelly, 2002). Regardless of how it occurs, any health disruption becomes a family event. Even when the family is not directly involved in the client's care, they will have feelings about it—individually or collectively—that support or sabotage

BOX 13-2	Indicators for Family Assessment

- Initial diagnosis of a serious physical or psychiatric illness/injury in a family member
- Family involvement and understanding needed to support recovery of client
- Deterioration in a family member's condition
- Illness in a child, adolescent, or cognitively impaired adult
- A child, adolescent, or adult child having an adverse response to a parent's illness
- Discharge from a health care facility to the home or an extended care facility
- Death of a family member
- Health problem defined by family as a family issue
- Indication of threat to relationship (abuse), neglect, or anticipated loss of family member

the effectiveness of treatment and the client's quality of life (Bell, 2000). Box 13-2 lists sample indicators that could warrant family assessment and nursing intervention.

ASSESSMENT TOOLS

Wright and Leahey's (2009) 15-minute interview, consisting of the genogram, ecomap, therapeutic questions, and commendations provide a comprehensive look at family relationships. Assessment tools such as the genogram, ecomap, and family time lines are used to track family patterns. The structured format of these tools focuses on getting relational data quickly and can sensitize clinicians to systemic family issues that affect patterns of health and illness (Gerson, McGoldrick, & Petry, 2008).

Genograms

Most family members enjoy constructing a genogram and learn about themselves in the process (Cole-Kelly & Seaburn, 1999). A **genogram** uses a standardized set of connections to graphically record basic information about family members and their relationships over three generations. Genograms are updated and/or revised as new information emerges.

There are three parts to genogram construction: mapping the family structure, recording family information, and describing the nature of family relationships. Figure 13-2 identifies the symbols used to map family structure, with different symbols representing pregnancies, miscarriages, marriages, deaths, and other nodal family events. Male family members

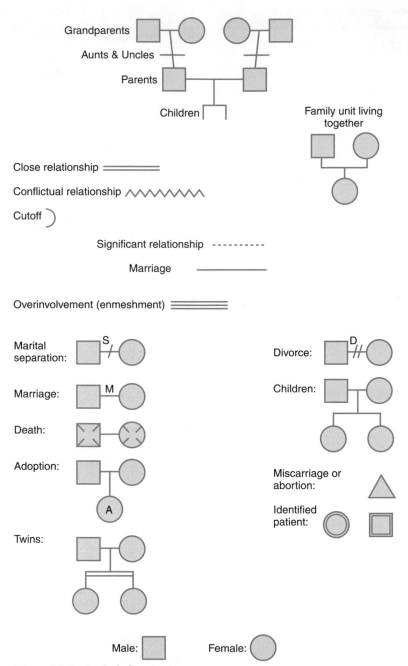

Figure 13-2   Symbols for a genogram.

are drawn on the left of the horizontal line as a square and female members on the right as a circle. The oldest sibling is placed on the left, with younger siblings following from left to right, in order of birth. In the case of multiple marriages, the earliest is placed on the left and the most recent on the right. Lines drawn between significant family members identify the strength of relational patterns that are overly close, close, distant, cut off, or conflicted. An example of a family genogram is presented in Figure 13-3. Exercise 13-4 provides practice with developing a family genogram.

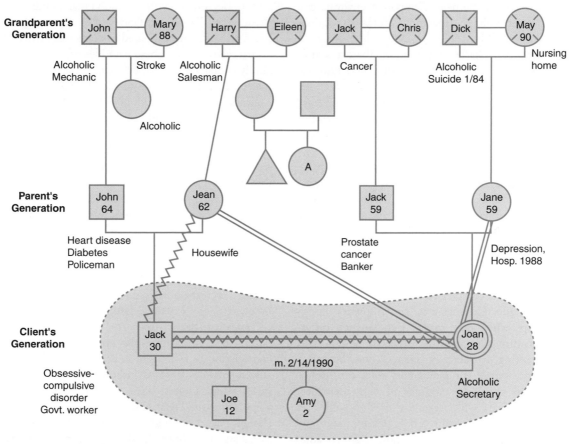

Grandparent's Generation

John   Mary 88   Harry   Eileen   Jack   Chris   Dick   May 90

Alcoholic Mechanic   Stroke   Alcoholic Salesman   Cancer   Alcoholic Suicide 1/84   Nursing home

Alcoholic

A

Parent's Generation

John 64   Jean 62   Jack 59   Jane 59

Heart disease Diabetes Policeman   Housewife   Prostate cancer Banker   Depression, Hosp. 1988

Client's Generation

Jack 30   Joan 28

Obsessive-compulsive disorder Govt. worker   m. 2/14/1990   Alcoholic Secretary

Joe 12   Amy 2

Figure 13-3   Basic family genogram.

EXERCISE 13-4 | Family Genograms

Purpose: To learn to create a family genogram.

Procedure:
Students will break into pairs and interview one another to gain information to develop a family genogram. The genogram should include demographic information, occurrence of illness or death, and relationship patterns for three generations. Use the symbols for diagramming in Figure 13-2 to create a visual

picture of the family information. Ask the author for validation of accuracy as you develop the genogram.

Discussion:
Each person will display their genogram and discuss the process of obtaining information. Discuss strategies for obtaining information expediently yet sensitively and tactfully. Discuss how genograms can be used in a helpful way with families.

The genogram explores the basic dynamics of a multigenerational family. Its multigenerational format, which traces family structure and relationships through three generations is based on the assumption that family relationship patterns are systemic, repetitive, and adaptive. Data about ages, birth and death dates, miscarriages, relevant illnesses, immigration, geographical

location of current members, occupations and employment status, educational levels, patterns of family members entering or leaving the family unit, religious affiliation or change, and military service are written near the symbols for each person. The recorded information about family members allows families and health professionals to simultaneously analyze complex family interaction patterns in a supportive environment. The impact of multiple generations on family relationships is more readily visible.

The genogram offers much more than a simple diagram of family relationship. Formal and informal learning about appropriate social behaviors and roles takes place within the family of origin. People learn role behaviors and responsibilities expected in different life stages experientially, by way of role modeling, and through direct instruction.

As you help a client construct a family genogram, you can ask questions regarding family thoughts about the role of gender, spiritual beliefs, or cultural values in shaping personal identity, managing conflict, and handling life issues (McCormick & Hardy, 2008). For example, girls are exposed to different role behaviors and social expectations than their male siblings. Although they are less rigid than in previous generations, the differences persist. Both men and women carry these understandings into "contemporary" family relationships when they marry. Fundamental differences in family rules and role expectations especially about parenting, handling of finances, and the nature of male and female complementary roles can lead to conflict and misunderstandings if not identified, shared, and dealt with. Exercise 13-5 provides an opportunity to trace gender role development and socialization within a family and how it affects adult communication and behaviors.

Ecomaps

An **ecomap** is essentially a sociogram, illustrating the shared relationships between family members and the external environment (Rempel, Neufeld, & Kushner,

2007). Beginning with an individual family unit or client, the diagram extends to include significant social and community-based systems with whom they have a relationship. These data identify at a glance the family's interaction with environmental supports, and their use of resources available through friends and community systems. Adding the ecomap is an important dimension of family assessment, providing awareness of community supports that could be or are not being used to assist families. Ecomaps can point out resource deficiencies and conflicts in support services that can be corrected.

An ecomap starts with an inner circle representing the family unit, labeled with relevant family names. Smaller circles outside the family circle represent significant people, agencies, and social institutions with whom the family interacts on a regular basis. Examples include school, work, church, neighborhood friends, recreation activities, health care facilities or home care, and extended family.

Lines are drawn from the inner family circle to outer circles indicating the strength of the contact and relationship. Straight lines indicate relation, with additional lines used to indicate the strength of the relationship. Dotted lines suggest tenuous relationships. Stressful relationships are represented with slashes placed through the relationship line. Directional arrows indicate the flow of the relational energy. Figure 13-4 shows an example of an ecomap. Exercise 13-6 provides an opportunity to construct an ecomap.

Family Time Lines

A family systems framework acknowledges that each family is unique with its own set of expertise,

---

EXERCISE 13-5	Using a Gendergram to Understand Gender Role Development in Families and Its Influence on Current Role Enactments

Purpose: To assist students in developing an understanding of family contributions to gender role development.

Procedure:
Each student should ask older family members of the same sex (e.g., mother, aunt, grandmother or father, uncle, grandfather) to talk about their experience growing up as a girl or a boy. Dialogue about what they see as different about gender roles today and how their gender has influenced who they are today.

Compare their impressions with your own gender role development in a short essay.

Discussion:
Each student will share his or her findings with the larger group. Discussion can focus on how gender role expectations are different and similar to those held in the past. Discuss differences and similarities in the gender role development of men and women. Discuss implications of this exercise for health care delivery.

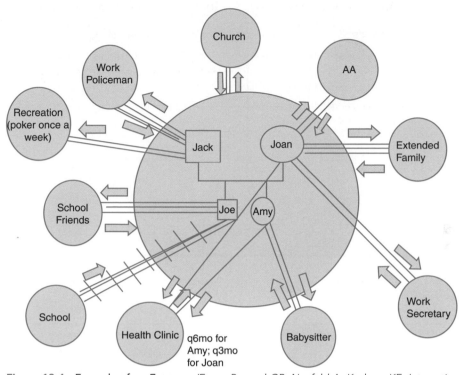

Figure 13-4 **Example of an Ecomap.** *(From: Rempel GR, Neufeld A, Kushner KE: Interactive use of genograms and ecomaps in family caregiving research, J Fam Nurs 13(4):403-419, 2007.)*

EXERCISE 13-6	Family Ecomaps

Purpose: To learn to create a family ecomap.

Procedure:
Using the interview process, students will break into pairs and interview one another to gain information to develop a family ecomap. The ecomap should include information about resources and stressors in the larger community system, such as school, church, health agencies, and interaction with extended family and friends for each student's family.

Discussion:
Each person will display his or her ecomap and discuss the process of obtaining information. Discuss strategies for obtaining information expediently yet sensitively and tactfully. Discuss how ecomaps broaden the structural information about a family and can be used in a helpful way with families.

---

knowledge, and skills. Vertical and horizontal stressors affect the family systems level of functioning in both positive and negative ways. Medical crises tend to exacerbate unresolved issues, which can create additional challenges for nurses (Leon & Knapp, 2008).

Time lines offer a visual diagram that captures significant family stressors, life events, health, and developmental patterns through the life cycle. Family history and patterns developed through multigenerational transmission are represented as vertical lines. Horizontal lines indicate timing of life events occurring over the current life span. These include such milestones as marriages, graduations, and unexpected life events such as disasters, war, illness, death of person or pet, moves, births, and so forth (Figure 13-5). Time lines are useful in looking at how the family history, developmental stage, and concurrent life events might interact with the current health concern.

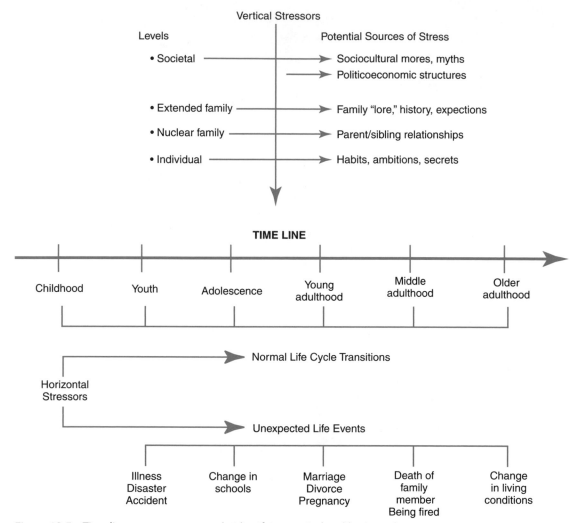

Figure 13-5   Time line assessment example identifying vertical and horizontal stressors.

APPLYING THE NURSING PROCESS

ORIENTING THE FAMILY

The nurse-family relationship in client care depends on a reciprocal relationship between the nurses and family in which both are equal partners and sources of information. Nurses should begin offering information to the family as soon as the client is admitted to the hospital or service agency. Orientation to the unit, location of the cafeteria and restrooms, parking options, nearby lodging, and access to the hospitalist or physician are important data points.

The initial encounter sets the tone for the relationship. How nurses interact with each family member may be as important as what they choose

to say. Begin with formal introductions and explain the purpose of gathering assessment data. Even this early in the relationship, you should listen carefully for family expectations and general anxiety that may be revealed more through behavior than through words.

GATHERING ASSESSMENT DATA

Inquiring about the relationship the family member has with the identified client is an initial step nurses can take in establishing a relationship with the family. For example, you can initially say, "I would like to understand more about the effect of your husband's heart attack on the family." This simple statement frames the information needed. It also serves as a reminder that each family member plays a role in the health care scenario and has associated support needs that the nurse needs to consider (Vandall-Walker, Jensen, & Oberle, 2007). Box 13-3 illustrates a framework for a family assessment with a client entering cardiac rehabilitation.

Family participation in the data assessment process enhances the therapeutic relationship and completeness of the data. It is important to inquire about the family's cultural identity, rituals, values, level of family involvement, decision making, and traditional behaviors as it relates to the health care of the client (Leon & Knapp, 2008).

| BOX 13-3 | Family Assessment for Client Entering Cardiac Rehabilitation |

Coping/Stress
- Who lives with you?

  _____
- How do you handle stress?

  _____
- Have you had any recent changes in your life (e.g., job change, move, change in marital status, loss)?

  _____
- On whom do you rely for emotional support?

  _____
- Who relies on you for emotional support?

  _____
- How does your illness affect your family members/ significant other? _____
- Are there any health concerns of other family members? _____
- If so, how does this affect you?

  _____

Communication/Decision Making
- How would you describe the communication pattern in your family?

  _____
- How does your family address issues/concerns?

  _____
- Can you identify strengths/weaknesses within the family? _____
- Are family members supportive of each other?

  _____
- How are decisions that affect the entire family made? _____
- How are decisions implemented?

  _____

Role
- What is your role in the family?

  _____
- Can you describe the roles of other family members? _____

Value Beliefs
- What is your ethnic/cultural background?

  _____

- What is your religious background?

  _____
- Are there any particular cultural/religious healing practices in which you participate?

  _____

Leisure Activities
- Do you participate in any organized social activities? _____
- In what leisure activities do you participate?

  _____
- Do you anticipate any difficulty with continuing these activities? _____
- If so, how will you make the appropriate adjustments? _____
- Do you have a regular exercise regimen?

  _____

Environmental Characteristics
- Do you live in a rural, suburban, or urban area?

  _____
- What type of dwelling do you live in?

  _____
- Are there stairs in your home?

  _____
- Where is the bathroom?

  _____
- Are the facilities adequate to meet your needs?

  _____
- If not, what adjustments will be needed?

  _____
- How do you plan to make those adjustments?

  _____
- Are there any community services provided to you at home? (explain) _____
- Are there community resources available in your area? _____
- Do you have any other concerns at this time?

  _____
- Is there anything that we have omitted?

  _____
- Signature _____ (must be completed by RN) Date/Time

Developed by Conrad J, University of Maryland School of Nursing, 1993.

Knowledge of a family's past medical experiences, particularly whether they were positive or negative, the family's medical beliefs, major family events a family is struggling with concurrently, plus family expectations for treatment and care are essential pieces of family assessment data. Suggested questions include:

- How does the family view the current health crisis?
- What is each family member's most immediate concern?
- Has anyone else in the family experienced a similar problem?
- What do family members believe would be most helpful to the client at this time?
- How does the family explain the reasons for the illness or injury?
- Are there any other recent changes or sources of stress in the family that make the current situation worse (pile up of demands?)
- How has the family handled the problem to date?
- What would the family like to achieve with the nurse's help in resolving issues related to the client's health and well-being (McBride, 2004)?
- As you close the session, ask, "Is there anything else I should know about your family and this experience?"

PLANNING

INTERVENTIVE QUESTIONING

Wright and Leahey (2009) identify therapeutic questioning as a nursing intervention that nurses can use with their client families to identify family strengths; help family members sort out their personal fears, concerns, and challenges in health care situations; and provide a vehicle for exploring alternative options. Interventive questioning can be either linear or circular.

Circular questions focus on family interrelationships and the impact a serious health alteration has on individual family members and the equilibrium of the family system. Examples of therapeutic questions are found in Box 13-4. The nurse uses information the family provides as the basis for additional questions.

The following case example demonstrates its use when the nurse asks a family, "What has been your biggest challenge in caring for your mother at home?"

BOX 13-4	Examples of Therapeutic Questions

- What is the greatest challenge facing your family now?
- On whom in the family do you think the illness has the most impact?
- Who is suffering the most?
- What has been most and least helpful to you in similar situations?
- If there were one question you could have answered now, what would it be?
- How can we best help you and your family?
- What are your needs/wishes for assistance now?

From Leahey M, Svaavarsdottir E: Implementing family nursing: how do we translate knowledge into clinical practice. *J Fam Nurs* 15 (4):445–460, 2009.

Case Example

Daughter: My biggest challenge has been finding a balance between caring for my mother and also caring for my children and husband. I have also had to learn a lot about the professional and support resources that are available in the community.

Son-in-law: For me, the biggest challenge has been convincing my wife that I can take over for a while, in order for her to get some rest. I worry that she will become exhausted.

Mother: I have appreciated all the help that they give me. My biggest challenge is to continue to do as much as possible for myself so that I do not become too much of a burden on them. Sometimes I wonder about moving to a palliative care setting or a hospice (Leahey & Harper-Jaques, 1996, p. 135).

In this example, each family member's concern is related but different. The therapeutic circular question opens a discussion about each person's anxiety. As family members hear the concerns of other family members, and as they hear themselves respond, their perspective broadens. The resulting conversation forms the basis for developing strategies that are mutually acceptable to all family members.

Selekman (1997) identifies four elements to consider when designing therapeutic interventions within a family context:

- The family's definition of the problem
- Key family characteristics (e.g., language, beliefs, and strengths)
- Unique cooperative response patterns of family members
- Family treatment goals

Meaningful involvement in the client's care not only differs from family to family, it differs among individual family members (Sydnor-Greenberg, Dokken, & Ahmann, 2000). Individual family members have different perspectives. Hearing each family member's perspective helps the family and nurse develop a unified understanding of significant treatment goals and implications for family involvement.

Although treatment plans should be tailored around personal client goals, acknowledging family needs, values, and priorities enhances compliance, especially if they are different. Shared decision making

and development of realistic achievable goals makes it easier for everyone concerned to accomplish them with a sense of ownership and self-efficacy about the process. Taking little achievable steps is preferred to attempting giant steps that misjudge what the family can realistically do.

Exercise 13-7 provides practice with developing a family nursing care plan.

IMPLEMENTATION

Nurses can only *offer* interventions; it is up to the family to accept them (Wright & Leahey, 2009).

EXERCISE 13-7	Developing a Family Nursing Care Plan

Purpose: To practice skills needed with difficult family patterns.

Procedure:
Read the case study and think of how you could interact appropriately with this family.

Mr. Monroe, age 43 years, was chairing a board meeting of his large, successful manufacturing corporation when he developed shortness of breath, dizziness, and a crushing, viselike pain in his chest. An ambulance was called, and he was taken to the medical center. Subsequently, he was admitted to the coronary unit with a diagnosis of an impending myocardial infarction (MI).

Mr. Monroe is married, with three children: Steve, age 14; Sean, age 12; and Lisa, age 10. He is the president and majority stockholder of his company. He has no history of cardiovascular problems, although his father died at the age of 38 of a massive coronary occlusion. His oldest brother died at the age of 42 from the same condition, and his other brother, still living, became a semi-invalid after suffering two heart attacks, one at the age of 44 and the other at 47.

Mr. Monroe is tall, slim, suntanned, and very athletic. He swims daily; jogs every morning for 30 minutes; plays golf regularly; and is an avid sailor, having participated in every yacht regatta and usually winning. He is very health-conscious and has had annual physical checkups. He watches his diet and quit smoking to avoid possible damage to his heart. He has been determined to avoid dying young or becoming an invalid like his brother.

When he was admitted to the coronary care unit, he was conscious. Although in a great deal of pain, he seemed determined to control his own fate. While in the unit, he was an exceedingly difficult patient, a trial to the nursing staff and his physician. He constantly watched and listened to everything going on

around him and demanded complete explanations about any procedure, equipment, or medication he received. He would sleep in brief naps and only when he was totally exhausted. Despite his obvious tension and anxiety, his condition stabilized. The damage to his heart was considered minimal, and his prognosis was good. As the pain diminished, he began asking when he could go home and when he could go back to work. He was impatient to be moved to a private room so that he could conduct some of his business by telephone.

When Mrs. Monroe visited, she approached the nursing staff with questions regarding Mr. Monroe's condition, usually asking the same question several times in different ways. She also asked why she was not being "told everything."

Interactions between Mr. Monroe and Mrs. Monroe were noted by the staff as Mr. Monroe telling Mrs. Monroe all of the things she needed to do. Little intimate contact was noted.

Mr. Monroe denied having any anxiety or concerns about his condition, although his behavior contradicted his denial. Mrs. Monroe would agree with her husband's assessment when questioned in his company.

Discussion:
1. What questions would you ask the client and family to obtain data regarding their adaptation to crisis?
2. What family nursing diagnosis would apply with this case study?
3. What nursing interventions are appropriate to interact with this client and his family?
4. How would you plan to transmit the information to the family?
5. What outcomes and measures would you use to determine success or failure of the nursing care plan?

Developed by Conrad J: University of Maryland School of Nursing, Baltimore, MD, 1993.

Suggested nursing actions to promote positive change in family functioning include

- Encouraging the telling of illness narratives
- Commending family and individual strengths
- Offering information and opinions
- Validating or normalizing emotional responses
- Encouraging family support
- Supporting family members as caregivers
- Encouraging respite

Encouraging Family Narratives

Families need to tell their story about the experience of their loved one's illness or injury; it may be quite different from how the client is experiencing it. The differences can lead to a more complete understanding.

Case Example

Frances is a client with a diagnosis of breast cancer. When she sees her oncologist, Frances reports that she is feeling fine, eating and able to function in much the same way as before receiving chemotherapy. Her husband's perception differs. He reports that her appetite has declined such that she only eats a few spoonfuls of food and she spends much of the day in bed. What Frances is reporting is true. When she is up, she enjoys doing what she did previously, although at a slower pace, and she does eat at every meal. Frances is communicating her need to feel normal, which is important to support. What her husband adds is also true. Her husband's input allows Frances to receive the treatment she needs to stimulate her appetite and give her more energy.

Nurses play an important role in helping families understand, negotiate, and reconcile differences in perceptions without losing face.

Incorporating Family Strengths

Otto (1963) introduced the concept of family strengths as potential and actual resources families can use to make their life more satisfying and fulfilling to its members. When health care changes are required, and they usually are with clients suffering from serious illness or injury, working through family strengths rather than focusing on deficits is useful. Viewing the family as having strengths to cope with a problem rather than *being* a problem is a healing strategy, giving the family hope that a problem is not the end point but rather only a circumstance in need of a solution.

Feeley and Gottlieb (2000) identify four different types of strengths nurses can help the family use to achieve important health outcomes:

- Traits that reside within an individual or a family (e.g., optimism, resilience)
- Assets that reside within or are associated with an individual or a family (e.g., finances, social, spiritual, or work relationships)
- Capabilities, skills, or competencies that an individual or a family has developed (e.g., problem-solving skills)
- A quality that is more transient in nature than a trait or asset (e.g., motivation)

Questions nurses can use specifically to elicit family strengths include:

- What has the family been doing so far that has been helpful?
- What is going well for this family?
- How have they (family) been able to do as well as they have done?
- What beliefs or previous experiences or relationships are sustaining them and preventing the problem from being worse?
- What advice would they give to other people in the same situation? (Tapp & Moules, 1997)

Giving Commendations

Limacher and Wright (2003) define **commendations** as "the practice of noticing, drawing forth, and highlighting previously unobserved, forgotten, or unspoken family strengths, competencies or resources" (p. 132). Commendations are particularly effective when the family seems dispirited or confused about a tragic illness or accident. More than a simple compliment, commendations should reflect *patterns* of behavior existing in the family unit over time. Wright and Leahey (2009) differentiate between a commendation ("Your family is showing much courage in living with your wife's cancer for 5 years.") and a compliment ("Your son is so gentle despite feeling so ill.") (p. 270). They suggest giving at least one commendation per interview.

Ryan and Steinmiller (2004) recommend naming family strengths in front of the family. For example, nurses can verbally reflect on the strength of the family in coping with multiple problems, the capacity to stay involved when client anger threatens the relationship, or the ability of the family to thoroughly research a health problem. Exercise 13-8 provides practice with giving commendations.

EXERCISE 13-8	Offering Commendations

Purpose: To provide practice with using commendation skills with families.

Procedure:
Students will work in groups of three students. Each student will develop a commendation about the two other students in the group. The commendation should reflect a personal strength that the reflecting student has observed over a period time. Examples might include kindness, integrity, commitment, persistence, goal-directedness, tolerance, or patience. Write a simple paragraph about the trait or behavior you observe in this person. If you can, give some examples of why you have associated this particular characteristic with the person. Each student, in turn, should read his or her reflections about the other two participants, starting the conversation with good eye contact, the name of the receiving student, and a simple orienting statement (e.g., "Kelly, this is what I have observed in knowing you...").

Discussion:
Class discussion should focus on the thought process of the students in developing particular commendations, the values they focused on, and any consideration they gave to the impact of the commendation on the other students. The students can also discuss the effect of hearing the commendations about themselves and what it stimulated in them. Other areas of focus might be how commendations can be used with families and how they can be used to counteract family resistance to working together.

Informational Support

Helping a family become aware of information from the environment and how to access it empowers families. By showing interest in the coping strategies that have and have not worked, the nurse can help the family see progress in their ability to cope with a difficult situation.

You can offer family members informational support related to talking with extended family, children, and others about the client's illness. You can help family members prepare questions for meeting with physicians. Finally, you can engage with families in discussions about the cultural, ethical, and physical implications of using or discontinuing life support systems. This is nursing's special niche, as these conversations are rarely one-time events, and nurses can provide informal opportunities for discussing them during care provision.

Meeting the Needs of Families with Critically Ill Clients

Having a family member in an ICU represents a serious crisis for most families. Eggenberger and Nelms (2007) suggest, "Patients enter a critical care unit in physiological crisis, while their families enter the hospital in psychological crisis" (p. 1619). Box 13-5 identifies care needs of families of critically ill clients. Family-centered relationships are key dimensions of quality care in the ICU.

BOX 13-5	Caring for Family Needs in the Intensive Care Unit

Families of critically ill clients need to:
- Feel there is hope
- Feel that hospital personnel care about the patient
- Have a waiting room near the patient
- Be called at home about changes in the patient's condition
- Know the prognosis
- Have questions answered honestly
- Know specific facts about the patient's prognosis
- Receive information about the patient at least once a day
- Have explanations given in understandable terms
- Be allowed to see the patient frequently

Perrin K: *Understanding the essentials of critical care nursing* (pp. 40–41), Upper Saddle River, NJ, 2009, Pearson Prentice Hall.

PROXIMITY TO THE CLIENT

The need to remain near the client is a priority for many family members of clients in the ICU (Perrin, 2009; Verhaeghe et al., 2005). Although the family may appear to hover too closely, it is usually an attempt to rally around the client in critical trouble (Leon, 2008). Viewed in this way, nurses can be more empathetic. As the family develops more confidence in the genuine interest and competence of staff, the hovering tends to lessen. Liberal visitation policies can result in "increased family involvement with patient care, increased family communication with nurses, and greatly decreased number of complaints from families" (Van Horn & Kautz, 2007, p. 102).

Families can be a primary support to clients, but they usually need encouragement and concrete suggestions for maximum effect and satisfaction. Family members feel helpless to reverse the course of the client's condition and appreciate opportunities to help their loved one. Suggesting actions that family members can take at the bedside include doing range-of-motion exercises, holding the client's hand, positioning pillows, providing mouth care or ice chips. Talking with the client, even if the person is unresponsive, can be meaningful.

Helping families balance the need to be present with the client's needs to conserve energy and have some alone time to rest or regroup is important. Family members also need time apart from their loved one for the same reasons. Tactfully explaining the need of critically ill clients to have family presence without feeling pressure to interact can be supportive. Encouraging families to take respites is equally important.

At the same time, nurses need to be sensitive to and respect a family member's apprehension or emotional state about their critically ill family member. Individual family members may need the nurse's support in talking about difficult feelings.

Nurses can role model communication with clients, using simple caring words and touch. Families are quick to discern the difference between nurses who are able to connect with a critically ill client in this way, as evidenced in a family member's comment that "some seem to have a way with him and they talk to him like he is awake" (Eggenberger & Nelms, 2007, p. 1623).

Caring for Families in the Pediatric Intensive Care Unit

Parents of children in the pediatric intensive care unit (PICU) want to be with their children as often as possible, but particularly when the child is having a procedure or is uncomfortable (Aldridge, 2005). Parents of children in the PICU need frequent reassurance from the nurse about why things are being done for their child and about treatment-related tubes and equipment. They want to actively participate in their child's care and have their questions honestly answered (Aldrich).

Families often act as the child's advocate during hospitalization, either informally by insisting on high-quality care or formally as the legal surrogate decision maker designated to make health care decisions on behalf of the client. The nurse is a primary health care provider agent in working with families facing these issues. A critical intervention for the family as a whole and its individual members is to help them recognize their limitations and hidden strengths, and to maintain a balance of health for all members.

PROVIDING INFORMATION

Families with clients in the ICU have a fundamental need for information, particularly if the patient is unresponsive—"Not knowing is the worst part." This cannot be stressed enough. Providing updated information as a clinical situation changes is critical. Even if there is no change in the client's condition, most families will need to have information repeated because of anxiety that may limit processing of complex or emotionally difficult information (Van Horn & Kautz, 2007). They need to know exactly what is being done for their loved one in simple understandable terms, and to have their questions answered honestly (Miracle, 2006). This information is particularly critical when family members must act as decision makers for clients who cannot make them on their own (Perrin, 2009).

How health care providers deliver information is important. Even if the patient's condition or prognosis leaves little room for optimism, the family needs to feel some hope and that the staff genuinely cares about what is happening with the client and family (Perrin, 2009; Verhaeghe, Defloor, Van Zuuren, et al., 2005).

Daily contact with the nurse assigned to the client in the ICU is a critical nursing action (Miracle, 2006) that the family needs. Identifying one family member to act as the primary contact helps ensure continuity between staff and family. A short daily phone call when family members cannot be present keeps the family connection and reduces family stress (Leon, 2008). Families need ongoing information on the client's progress, modifications in care requirements, and any changes in expected outcomes, with opportunities to ask questions and clarify information. Nurses in the ICU often serve as mediators between client, family, and other health providers to ensure that data streams remain open, coordinated, and relevant.

FAMILY-CENTERED RELATIONSHIPS IN THE COMMUNITY

The Centers for Disease Control and Prevention (CDC) estimates that approximately 70% of deaths in the United States are the result of chronic disease. Although many of these individuals are able to self-manage their disease, an increasing number will require family support with coping, self-management, and palliative care. Increasingly, nurses are called on to help families effectively manage the care of people with chronic illness who can no longer take care of themselves or who require additional support to maintain their independence (McKenry & Price, 2005).

The concept of the family caregiver as a key member of the health care team has become increasingly important as more people live with chronic illness on a daily basis in the community or subacute care facility. Medalie and Cole-Kelly (2002) define the functional family as the group coping with the everyday affairs of the client. Caregiving responsibilities can include providing personal care, performing medical procedures, managing a client's affairs, and facilitating or coordinating medical care and social services for the client (Levine, 2004).

Healthy family members have concurrent demands on their time from their own nuclear families, work, church, and community responsibilities. This is particularly true when spouses have to become caregivers in younger families (Gordon & Perrone, 2004). A significant change in health status can cause previous unresolved relationship issues, which may need advanced intervention in addition to the specific health care issues. When individual family members are experiencing a transition, for example, ending or entering a relationship, or job change, they may not be as available as support and can experience unnecessary guilt about it. Nurses need to consider the broader family responsibilities people have as an important part of the context of health care in providing holistic care to a particular family.

MEETING FAMILY INFORMATIONAL NEEDS

Sharing information is a mutual process. Nurses need to welcome and respect family input and engage the family in mutual decision making (Levine, 2004).

Helping client families anticipate what will happen as a chronic disease progresses and how the day-to-day needs will change helps eliminate the stress of the unknown. Nurses can offer suggestions about how to respond to these changes, and offer support to the family caregiver as they emerge. Helping family members access services, support groups, and natural support networks at each stage of their loved one's illness empowers family members because they feel they are helping in a tangible way.

SUPPORTING THE CAREGIVER

Providing emotional support is crucial to helping families cope. Remaining aware of one's own values and staying calm and thoughtful can be very helpful to a family in crisis. Remember that your words can either strengthen or weaken a family's confidence in their ability to care for an ill family member.

Focus initially on issues that are manageable within the context of home caregiving. This provides a sense of mastery and satisfaction. The nurse can encourage the family to develop new ways of coping or can list alternatives and allow the family to choose coping styles that might be useful to them. Focus on what goes well, and ask the family to share with you their ideas about how to best care for the client.

Many families will need information about additional home care services, community resources and options needed to meet the practical, and financial and emotional demands of caring for a chronically ill family member.

Encouraging families to use natural helping systems increases the network of emotional and economic support available to the family in time of crisis. Examples include contact with other relatives, neighbors, friends, and churches. Spiritual beliefs and support from extended family and friends enhance family resilience in times of trauma and loss (Greeff & Human, 2004).

VALIDATING AND NORMALIZING EMOTIONS

Families can experience many conflicting emotions when placed in the position of providing protracted care for a loved one. Compassion, protectiveness, and caring can be intermingled with feelings of helplessness and being trapped. Major role reversals can stimulate anger and resentment for both client and family caregiver.

Sibling or family position or geographic proximity may put pressure on certain family members to provide a greater share of the care. Criticism or advice from less involved family members can be disconcerting and conflicts about care decisions can create rifts in family relationships. Some caregivers find themselves mourning for their loved one, even though the person is still alive, wishing it could all end and feeling guilty about having such thoughts.

These emotions are normal responses to abnormal circumstances. Listening to the family caregiver's feelings and struggles without judgment can be the most healing intervention you can provide. Nurses can normalize negative feelings by offering insights about common feelings associated with chronic illness. Family members may need guidance and permission to get respite and recharge their commitment by attending to their own needs. Support groups can provide families with emotional and practical support, and a critical expressive outlet.

Psychosocial issues for parents with chronically ill children can cover many relationship issues, for example, how to respond and discipline children with chronic illness. Siblings sometimes get short-changed emotionally, if not physically, when the focus necessarily is on the child with a serious illness or disability (Drench, Noonan, Sharby, & Ventura, 2007). Well siblings may experience feelings of resentment, worry that they might contract a similar illness, or have unrealistic expectations of their part in the treatment process. Siblings need clear information about the sick child's diagnosis and care plan. They need to be treated as children with needs of their own and should not be expected to assume adult caretaker responsibility for younger siblings while parents focus on the ill child (Fleitas, 2000). Exercise 13-9 provides practice with using intervention skills with families.

EVALUATION

Referrals, continuing the contact with another health professional, or family education about when to contact the health system may be needed (Wright & Leahey, 2004). The referral should include a summary of the information gained to date and should be communicated by the health team member most knowledgeable about the client's condition. Discuss with the client what will be shared with the referral resource.

SUMMARY

This chapter provides an overview of family communication and the complex dynamics inherent in family relationships. Families have a structure, defined as the way in which members are organized. Family function refers to the roles people take in their families, and family process describes the communication that takes place within the family. Theoretical frameworks, developed by Bowen, Minuchin, Duvall, and McCubbin, are particularly relevant for nurses in understanding family dynamics in health care settings.

EXERCISE 13-9	Using Intervention Skills with Families

Purpose: To provide practice with using intervention skills with families.

Procedure:
Each student will work with a family related to a specific problem. This can be a current or previous situation for the family. Talk with the family about the problem and learn how they have dealt with the problem, their perception of the problem, and its impact on their family. Use some of the approaches identified in the text to help them explore the problem in more depth and begin to develop viable options.

Write a descriptive summary of your experiences, including a self-evaluation. Evaluate the experience with the family as well, specifically for feedback regarding your approach. Did they feel you were too intrusive or not assertive enough? Did you validate all members' perceptions and perspectives? Did you clarify information and feelings? Did you remain nonjudgmental and objective? Did you respect the family's values and beliefs without imposing your own? Did you assist the family in clarifying and understanding the problem in a way that could lead to resolution?

Discussion:
Students share their experience and the feedback they received from the family. Discuss the obstacles encountered when communicating with families. Discuss strategies to facilitate goal-directed communication and resolution of problems. How can nurses best provide support to families? How could families learn to use honest communication most of the time? How does one influence this in one's own family?

Family-centered care is developed through a combination of strategies designed to gather information in a systematic, efficient manner starting with the genogram and ecomap. Therapeutic questions and giving family commendations are interventions nurses can use with families.

Families with critical illness need continuous updated information, and the freedom to be with their family member as often as possible. Involving the family in the care of the client is important. Parents want to participate in the care of their acutely ill client.

Nursing interventions are aimed at strengthening family functioning and supporting family coping during hospitalization and in the community.

ETHICAL DILEMMA   What Would You Do?

Terry Connors is a 90-year-old woman living alone in a two-story house. Her daughter Maggie lives in another state. So far, Terry has been able to live by herself, but within the past 2 weeks, she fell down a few stairs in her house and she has trouble hearing the telephone. Terry walks with a cane and relies on her neighbors for assistance when she cannot do things for herself. Maggie worries about her and would like to see her in a nursing home close to Maggie's home. Terry will not consider this option. As the nurse working with this family, how would you address your ethical responsibilities to Terry and Maggie?

REFERENCES

Aldridge M: Decreasing parental stress in the pediatric intensive care unit, *Crit Care Nurse* 25(6):40–51, 2005.

Barker P: Different approaches to family therapy, *Nurs Times* 94(14): 60–62, 1998.

Bell JM: Encouraging nurses and families to think interactionally: revisiting the usefulness of the circular pattern diagram, *J Fam Nurs* 6(3):203–209, 2000.

Bowen M: *Family therapy in clinical practice*, Northvale, NJ, 1978, Jason Aronson.

Byng-Hall J: Therapist reflections: diverse developmental pathways for the family, *J Fam Ther* 22:264–272, 2000.

Cicchetti D, Blender JA: A multiple levels of analysis perspective on resilience: implications for the developing brain, neural plasticity, and preventive interventions, *Ann N Y Acad Sci* 1094:248–258, 2006.

Clark S: The double ABCX model of family crisis as a representation of family functioning after rehabilitation from a stroke, *Health Med* 4(2):203–220, 1999.

Cole-Kelly K, Seaburn D: Five areas of questioning to promote a family oriented approach in primary care, *Fam Syst Health* 17(3):341–348, 1999.

Dalton W, Kitzmann K: Broadening parental involvement in family-based interventions for pediatric overweight: implications from family systems and child health, *Fam Commun Health* 31(4):259–268, 2008.

Drench M, Noonan AC, Sharby N, Ventura S: *Psychosocial aspects of health care*, ed 2, Upper Saddle River, NJ, 2007, Pearson Prentice Hall.

Duvall E: *Marriage and family development*, Philadelphia, 1958, JB Lippincott.

Eggenberger S, Nelms T: Being family: the family experience when an adult member is hospitalized with a critical illness, *Issues Clin Nurs* 16:1618–1628, 2007.

Feeley N, Gottlieb L: Nursing approaches for working with family strengths and resources, *J Fam Nurs* 6(1):9–24, 2000.

Fleitas J: When Jack fell down, Jill came tumbling after: siblings in the web of illness and disability, *Am J Matern Child Nurs* 25(5):267–273, 2000.

Gerson R, McGoldrick M, Petry S: *Genograms: assessment and intervention*, ed 3, New York, NY, 2008, WW Norton & Co.

Gilbert R: *The eight concepts of Bowen theory*, Falls Church, VA, 2006, Leading Systems Press.

Glasscock F, Hales A: Bowen's family systems theory: a useful approach for a nurse administrator's practice, *J Nurs Adm* 28(6):37–42, 1998.

Goldenberg H, Goldenberg I: *Family therapy: an overview*, Belmont, CA, 2008, Thomson Brooks/Cole.

Gordon P, Perrone K: When spouses become caregivers: counseling implications for younger couples, *J Rehabil* 70(2):27–32, 2004.

Greeff A, Human B: Resilience in families in which a parent has died, *Am J Fam Ther* 32:27–42, 2004.

Kristjanson L, Aoun S: Palliative care for families: remembering the hidden patients, *Can J Psychiatry* 49(6):359–365, 2004.

Leahey M, Harper-Jaques S: Family-nurse relationships: core assumptions and clinical implications, *J Fam Nurs* 2(2):133–152, 1996.

Leahey M, Svavarsdottir E: Implementing family nursing: how do we translate knowledge into clinical practice, *J Fam Nurs* 15(4):445–460, 2009.

Leon A: Involving family systems in critical care nursing: challenges and opportunities, *Dimens Crit Care Nurs* 27(6):255–262, 2008.

Leon A, Knapp S: Involving family systems in critical care nursing: challenges and opportunities, *Dimens Crit Care Nurs* 27(6):255–262, 2008.

Levine C: *Always on call: when illness turns families into caregivers*, Nashville, TN, 2004, Vanderbilt University Press.

Limacher L, Wright L: Commendations: listening to the silent side of a family intervention, *J Fam Nurs* 9(2):130–150, 2003.

McBride JL: Managing family dynamics, *Fam Pract Manag* 11(7):70, 2004.

McCormick M, Hardy K: *Re-visioning family therapy: race, culture and gender in clinical practice*, ed 2, New York, 2008, The Guilford Press.

McCubbin HI, McCubbin MA, Thompson A: Resiliency in families: the role of family schema and appraisal in family adaptation to crisis. In Brubaker TH, editor: *Family relations: challenges for the future*, Newbury Park, CA, 1993, Sage.

McCubbin HI, McCubbin MA, Thompson AI, et al: Resiliency in ethnic families: a conceptual model for predicting family adjustment and adaptation. In McCubbin HI, McCubbin MA, Thompson AI, et al, editors: *Resiliency in Native American and immigrant families*, Thousand Oaks, CA, 1998, Sage Publications.

McKenry P, Price S: *Families and change: coping with stressful events and transitions*, Thousand Oaks, CA, 2005, Sage.

Medalie J, Cole-Kelly K: The clinical importance of defining family, *Am Fam Physician* 65(7):1277–1279, 2002.

Minuchin S: *Families and family therapy*, Boston, 1974, Harvard University Press.

Miracle V: Strategies to meet the needs of families of critically ill patients, *Dimens Crit Care Nurs* 25(3):121–125, 2006.

Nichols M, Schwartz R: *Family therapy: concepts & methods*, ed 9, Prentice Hall, 2009, Upper Saddle River NJ.

Novilla M, Barnes N, De La Cruz N, Williams P: Public health perspectives on the family, *Fam Commun Health* 29(1):28–42, 2006.

Otto H: Criteria for assessing family strength, *Fam Process* 2:329–338, 1963.

Perrin K: *Understanding the essentials of critical care nursing*, Upper Saddle River, NJ, 2009, Pearson Prentice Hall.

Rempel G, Neufeld A, Kushner K: Interactive use of genograms and ecomaps in family caregiving research, *J Fam Nurs* 13(4):403–419, 2007.

Rivera-Andino J, Lopez L: When culture complicates, *RN* 63(7):47–49, 2000.

Ryan E, Steinmiller E: Modeling family-centered pediatric nursing care: strategies for shift report, *J Spec Pediatr Nurs* 9(4):123–129, 2004.

Schor EL: Family pediatrics: report of the Task /force on the Family, *Pediatrics* 111(6 Pt2):154–171, 2003.

Selekman M: *Solution focused therapy with children: harnessing family strengths for systemic change*, New York, 1997, Guilford Press.

Sydnor-Greenberg N, Dokken D, Ahmann E: Coping and caring in different ways: understanding and meaningful involvement, *Pediatr Nurs* 26(2):185–190, 2000.

Tapp D, Moules N: Family skills labs: facilitating the development of family nursing skills in the undergraduate, *J Fam Nurs* 3(3):247–267, 1997.

The Bowen Center: *Bowen theory: societal emotional process*, Washington, DC, 2004. Available online http://www.thebowencenter.org/pages/conceptsep.html. Accessed May 25, 2009.

Toman W: *Family therapy and sibling position*, New York, 1992, Jason Aronson Publishers.

Trotter T, Martin H: Family history in pediatric primary care, *Pediatrics* 120:S60–S65, 2007.

Vandall-Walker V, Jensen L, Oberle K: Nursing support for family members of critically ill adults, *Qual Health Res* 17(9):1207–1218, 2007.

Van Horn E, Kautz D: Promotion of family integrity in the acute care setting: a review of the literature, *Dimens Crit Care Nurs* 26 (3):101–107, 2007.

Verhaeghe S, Defloor T, Van Zuuren F, et al: The needs and experiences of family members of adult patients in an intensive care unit: a review of the literature, *J Adv Nurs* 14:501–509, 2005.

von Bertalanffy L: *General systems theory*, New York, 1968, George Braziller.

Walsh F: The concept of family resilience: crisis and challenge, *Fam Process* 35(3):261–279, 1996.

Wigert H, Berg M, Hellstrom AL: Parental presence when their child is in neonatal intensive care, *Scand J Caring Sci* 23:139–146, 2010.

Wright L, Leahey M: How to conclude or terminate with families, *J Fam Nurs* 10(3):379–401, 2004.

Wright LM, Leahey M: *Nurses and families: a guide to family assessment and intervention*, ed 5, Philadelphia, 2009, FA Davis.

CHAPTER 14

Resolving Conflict Between Nurse and Client

Kathleen Underman Boggs

OBJECTIVES

At the end of the chapter, the reader will be able to:

1. Define conflict and contrast the functional with the dysfunctional role of conflict in a therapeutic relationship.
2. Recognize and describe personal style of response to conflict situations.
3. Discriminate among passive, assertive, and aggressive responses to conflict situations.
4. Specify the characteristics of assertive communication.
5. Identify four components of an assertive response and formulate sample assertive responses.
6. Identify appropriate assertive responses and specific nursing strategies to promote conflict resolution in relationships.
7. Discuss how findings from research studies can be applied to clinical practice.

Conflict is a natural part of human relationships. We all have times when we experience negative feelings about a situation or person. When this occurs in a nurse-client relationship, clear, direct communication is needed. This chapter emphasizes the dynamics of conflict and the skills needed for successful resolution.

Effective nurse-client communication is critical to efficient care provision and to receiving quality care (Finke, Light, & Kitko, 2008). Knowing how to respond in emotional situations allows you to use feelings as a positive force. Nurses often find themselves in dramatic situations in which a calm response is required. Some clients approach their initial encounter with a nurse with hostility or embarrassment, such as the intoxicated client admitted to an emergency department (Baillie, 2005). To listen and to respond creatively to intense emotion when your first impulse is to withdraw or to retaliate demands a high level of skill. It requires self-control and empathy for what your client may be experiencing. It is difficult to remain cool under attack, and yet your willingness to stay with the angry client may mean more than any other response.

Assertive skills, described in this chapter, can help you deal constructively with conflict. As nurses, our goal is to prevent or reduce levels of conflict (Bowers et al., 2008). We know that resolving some long-standing conflicts is a gradual process in which we may have to revisit the issue several times to fully resolve the conflict. Workplace conflict between nurse and colleagues will be discussed in Chapter 23. The focus of this chapter is conflict between nurse and client.

BASIC CONCEPTS

Conflict has been defined as tension arising from incompatible goals or needs, in which the actions of one frustrate the ability of the other to achieve their goal, resulting in stress or tension (Wikipedia). Conflicts in any relationship are inevitable: They serve as warning that something in the relationship needs closer attention. Conflict can lead to improved relationships.

NATURE OF CONFLICT

All conflicts have certain things in common: (a) a concrete *content problem issue*; and (b) relationship or *process issues,* which involve our emotional response to the situation. It is immaterial whether the issue makes realistic sense to you. They feel real to your client and need to be dealt with. Unresolved, they will interfere with success in meeting goals. Most people experience conflict as discomfort. Previous experiences with conflict situations, the importance of the issue, and possible consequences all play a role in the intensity of our reaction. For example, a client may have great difficulty asking appropriate questions of the physician regarding treatment or prognosis, but experience no problem asking similar questions of the nurse or family. The reasons for the discrepancy in comfort level may relate to previous experiences. Alternatively, it may have little to do with the actual persons involved. Rather, the client may be responding to anticipated fears about the type of information the physician might give.

CAUSES OF CONFLICT

Lack of communication is a main cause of misunderstanding and conflict (Jasmine, 2009). Other psychological causes of conflict include poor communication, differences in values, personality clashes, and stress. Clashes occur between nurse and client or even between two clients. If your nursing care does not fit in with your client's cultural belief system, conflict can result (Chang & Kelle, 2007).

Case Example

Two women who gave birth this morning are moved to a semiprivate room on the postpartum floor. Ms. Patton is 19 years old, likes loud music, and is feeling fine. Her roommate, Mrs. DiSauro, is 36 years old, has four children at home, and wants to rest (*latent*). The music and visitors to Ms. Patton repeatedly wake up Mrs. DiSauro (*perceived*), who yells at them (*overt*). The nurse arranges to transfer Mrs. DiSauro to an unoccupied room (*resolution*).

WHY WORK FOR CONFLICT RESOLUTION?

Unresolved conflicts impede quality of client care. Conflicts, even those between two clients, poison the working environment. Nurse-client conflict undermines your therapeutic relationship with your client. Energy is transferred to conflict issues instead of being used to build the relationship. Once you identify a conflict, take action immediately and work to resolve it.

UNDERSTANDING OWN PERSONAL RESPONSES TO CONFLICT

Conflicts between nurse and client are not uncommon. The first step is to gain a clear understanding of your own personal response. No one is equally effective in all situations. Completing Exercise 14-1 may help you identify your personal responses.

The second step is to understand the context of the situation. Most interpersonal conflicts involve some threat to one's sense of control or self-esteem. Nurses have been shown to respond to the stress of not having enough time to complete their work by imposing more controls on the client, who then often reacts by becoming more difficult (Macdonald, 2007). Other situations that may lead to conflict between you and your client include:

- Having your statements discounted
- Being asked to give more information than you feel comfortable sharing
- Encountering sexual harassment
- Being the target of a personal attack
- Having the client's family make demands
- Wanting to do things the old way instead of trying something new

Clients who feel listened to and respected are generally receptive. Be careful what you say and how you say it. Avoid acting in ways which create anger or conflict with your client; examples are listed in Box 14-1.

FOUR STYLES OF PERSONAL CONFLICT MANAGEMENT

There are distinct styles of response to conflict. Although not specifically addressing nurse-client conflict, the literature shows that, in the past, corporate managers felt that any conflict was destructive and needed to be suppressed. Current thinking holds that

---

EXERCISE 14-1 | Personal Responses to Conflict

Purpose: To increase awareness of how students respond in conflict situations and the elements in situations (e.g., people, status, age, previous experience, lack of experience, or place) that contribute to their sense of discomfort.

Procedure:
Break up into small groups of two. You may do this as homework or create an Internet discussion room. Think of a conflict situation that could be handled in different ways.

The following feelings are common correlates of interpersonal conflict situations that many people say they experienced in conflict situations that they have not handled well:

Anger	Competitiveness	Humiliation
Annoyance	Defensiveness	Inferiority
Antagonism	Devaluation	Intimidation
Anxiousness	Embarrassment	Manipulation
Bitterness	Frustration	Resentment

Although these feelings generally are not ones we are especially proud of, they are a part of the human experience. By acknowledging their existence within ourselves, we usually have more choice about how we will handle them.

Using words from the list, describe the following as concretely as possible:
1. The details of the situation: How did it develop? What were the content issues? Was the conflict expressed verbally or nonverbally? Who were the persons involved, and where did the interaction take place?
2. What feelings were experienced before, during, and after the conflict?
3. Why was the situation particularly uncomfortable?

Discussion:
Suggest different ways to respond. Might these lead to differences in outcome?

BOX 14-1 | Behaviors That Create Anger in Others

- Providing unsolicited advice
- Conveying ideas that try to create guilt
- Offering reassurances that are not realistic
- Communicating using "gloss it over" positive comments
- Speaking in a way that shows you do not understand your client's point of view
- Exerting too much pressure to make a person change their unhealthy behavior
- Placing blame, speaking in an accusing tone
- Portraying self as an infallible expert
- Using excessively histrionic language or sarcastic retorts
- Using an authoritarian tone
- Using "hot button" words that have heavy emotional connotations

conflict can be healthy and can lead to growth. These concepts can be applied to nursing.

A common response to conflict by nurses is to distance themselves from their client or to provide them less support (Macdonald, 2007); this is known as **avoidance**. Sometimes an experience makes you so uncomfortable that you want to avoid the situation or person at all costs, so you withdraw. This style is appropriate when the cost of addressing the conflict is higher than the benefit of resolution. Sometimes you just have to "pick your battles," focusing your energy on the most important issues. However, use of avoidance postpones the conflict, leads to future problems, and damages your relationship with your client, making it a *lose-lose* situation.

Accommodation is another common response. We surrender our own needs in a desire to smooth over the conflict. This response is cooperative but nonassertive. Sometimes this involves a quick compromise or giving false reassurance. By giving into others, we maintain peace but do not actually deal with the issue, so it will likely resurface in the future. It is appropriate when the issue is more important to the other person. This is a *lose-win situation*. Harmony results and credits may be accumulated that can be used at some future time (McElhaney, 1996).

Competition is a response style characterized by domination. In this contradictory style, one party exercises power to gain his own goals at the expense of the other person. It is characterized by aggression and lack of compromise. Authority may be used to suppress the conflict in a dictatorial manner. This leads to increased stress. It is an effective style when there is a need for a quick decision, but it leads to problems in the long term, making it a *lose-lose situation*.

Collaboration is a solution-oriented response in which we work together cooperatively to problem solve. To manage the conflict, we commit to finding a mutually satisfying solution. This involves directly confronting the issue, acknowledging feelings, and using open communication to solve the problem. Steps for productive confrontation include identifying concerns of each party; clarifying assumptions; communicating honestly to identify the real issue; and working collaboratively to find a solution that satisfies everyone. This is considered to be the most effective style for genuine resolution. This is a *win-win situation*.

FACTORS THAT INFLUENCE RESPONSES TO CONFLICT
Gender

Expression of emotion may differ according to gender. A traditional female socialized response was to "smooth over" conflicts. Women still tend to use more accommodative conflict management styles such as compromise and avoidance, whereas men tend to use collaboration more often and prefer competitive or aggressive methods. However, the literature is inconclusive regarding the effects of gender and style on the outcome of conflict resolution.

Culture

Many of a nurse's responses are determined by cultural socialization, which prescribes proper modes for behaviors. Personal style and past experiences influence the typical responses to conflict situations. Individuals from societies that emphasize group cooperation tend to use more avoidance and less confrontation in their conflict resolution styles. People from cultures that value

individualism more tend to more often use competing/dominating styles. Nurses are individuals with different attitudes toward the existence of conflict and different ways of responding. The underlying feelings generated by conflict situations may be quite similar. Common emotional responses to conflict include anger, embarrassment, and anxiety. Awareness of how we cope with conflict is the first step in learning assertiveness strategies. Fortunately, assertiveness and other skills essential to conflict resolution are learned behaviors that any nurse can master.

TYPES OF CONFLICT: INTRAPERSONAL VERSUS INTERPERSONAL

A conflict can be internal (intrapersonal); that is, it can represent opposing feelings within an individual. Intrapersonal conflict arises when nurses are faced with two different choices, each supported by a different ethical principle. For example, nurses traditionally were socialized to follow orders. Studies have shown that up to 75% of the ethical dilemmas reported in nurse surveys involve their perceptions about inadequate client care (Redman & Fry, 1996). Conflict more often occurs between two or more people (interpersonal).

FUNCTIONAL USES OF CONFLICT

Traditionally, conflict was viewed as a destructive force to be eliminated. Actually, conflicts that are successfully resolved lead to stronger relationships. The critical factor is the willingness to explore and resolve it mutually. Appropriately handled, conflict can provide an important opportunity for growth. Box 14-2 gives helpful guidelines regarding your responsibilities when involved in a conflict.

BOX 14-2 Personal Rights and Responsibilities in Conflict Situations

I have the right to:
- respect from other people as a unique human being
- make my own decisions
- have feelings
- make mistakes
- decide how I will act
- my own opinions

I have the responsibility to:
- respect the human rights of others
- allow others to make their own decisions
- express my feelings in ways that do not violate the rights of others
- accept full accountability for my mistakes
- act in ways that will not be harmful to myself or to others
- respect the rights of others to hold opinions different from mine

NATURE OF ASSERTIVE BEHAVIOR

Assertive behavior is defined as setting goals, acting on those goals in a clear, consistent manner, and taking responsibility for the consequences of those actions. The assertive nurse is able to stand up for the rights of others, as well as for her own rights. Box 14-3 lists characteristics of assertive behaviors.

Components of assertion include the following four abilities: (1) to say no; (2) to ask for what you want; (3) to appropriately express both positive and negative thoughts and feelings; and (4) to initiate, continue, and terminate the interaction. This honest expression of yourself does not violate the needs of others but does demonstrate self-respect rather than deference to the demands of others.

The goal of assertiveness is to communicate directly, standing up for your personal rights while respecting the rights of others (Stuart, 2009). Conflict creates anxiety that may prevent us from behaving assertively. Assertive behaviors range from making a direct, honest statement about your beliefs to taking a very strong, confrontational stand about what will and will not be tolerated in the relationship. Assertive responses contain "I" statements that take responsibility. This behavior is in contrast with **aggressive behavior**, which has a goal of dominating while suppressing the other person's rights. Aggressive responses often consist of "you" statements that fix blame on the other person.

Assertiveness is a learned behavior. Some nurses were socialized to act passively. Passive behavior is defined as a response that denies our own rights to avoid conflict. An example is remaining silent and not responding to a client's demands for narcotics every 4 hours when he displays no signs of pain out of fear that he might report you to your superior.

Assertiveness needs to be practiced to be learned (Exercises 14-2 and 14-3). Effective nursing encompasses mastery of assertive behavior (see Box 14-3). Nonassertive behavior in a professional nurse is related to lower levels of autonomy. Continued patterns of nonassertive responses have a negative influence on you and on the standard of care you provide. Evaluate your own assertiveness with Exercise 14-4.

DYSFUNCTIONAL CONFLICT

Several elements may occur in **dysfunctional conflict**. The dysfunction occurs when emotions distort the content issue (e.g., when some information is withheld so that you must guess at what is truly going on in the mind of the other person). Sometimes the conflict is obscured by hidden messages, denied feelings, or feelings projected onto others. Nonproductive conflicts are characterized by feelings that are misperceived or stated too intensely. In other dysfunctional conflicts, the feelings are stated accurately, but they are expressed so strongly that the listener feels attacked. The listener then tends to respond in a defensive manner.

PRINCIPLES OF CONFLICT RESOLUTION

Figure 14-1 describes the principles of conflict resolution. Recognize your own "trigger" or "hot buttons." What words or client actions trigger an immediate emotional response from you? These could include having someone yelling at you or speaking to you in an angry tone of voice. Once you recognize the triggers, you can better control your own response. It is imperative that you focus on the current issue. Put aside past history. Listing prior problems will raise emotions and prevent both of you from reaching a solution. Identify *available options*. Rather than immediately trying to solve the problem, look at the range of possible options. Create a list of these options and work with the other party to evaluate the feasibility of each option. By working together, the expectation shifts from adversarial conflict to an

BOX 14-3	Characteristics Associated with the Development of Assertive Behavior

- Express your own position, using "I" statements.
- Make clear statements.
- Speak in a firm tone, using moderate pitch.
- Assume responsibility for personal feelings and wants.
- Make sure verbal and nonverbal messages are congruent.
- Address only issues related to the present conflict.
- Structure responses so as to be tactful and show awareness of the client's frame of reference.
- Understand that undesired behaviors, not feelings, attitudes, and motivations, are the focus for change.

EXERCISE 14-2   Pitching the Assertive Message

Purpose: To increase awareness of how the meaning of a verbal message can be significantly altered by changing one's tone of voice.

Procedure:
Place individual slips of paper in a hat so that every student in class can draw one. On each slip of paper should be written one of the five vocal pitches commonly used in conversation: whisper, soft tone with hesitant delivery, moderate tone and firm delivery, loud tone with agitated delivery, and screaming. Divide into groups, and have each student take a turn drawing and demonstrating the tone while the others in the group try to identify correctly which person is giving the assertive message.

Discussion:
How does tone affect perceptions of a message's content?

EXERCISE 14-3   Assertive Responses

Purpose: To increase awareness of assertiveness.

Procedure:
Have three students volunteer to read each answer to the following scenario:

You are working full time, raising a family, and taking 12 credits of nursing classes. The teacher asks you to be a student representative on a faculty committee. You say the following:

1. "I don't think I'm the best one. Why don't you ask Karen? If she can't, I guess I can."
2. "Gee, I'd like to, but I don't know. I probably could if it doesn't take too much time."
3. "I do want students to have some input to this committee, but I am not sure I have enough time. Let me think about it and let you know in class tomorrow."

Discussion:
Ask students to choose the most assertive answer and comment about how other options could be altered.

EXERCISE 14-4   Assertiveness Self-Assessment Quiz

Purpose: To help students gain insight into their own responses.

Procedure:
Read and answer "yes" (2 points), "sometimes" (1 point), or "no" (0 points). A score of more than 10 points suggests the need to practice assertiveness. Do you:

1. Feel self-conscious if someone watches you work with a client?
2. Not feel confident in your nursing judgment?
3. Hesitate to express your feelings?
4. Avoid questioning people in authority?
5. Feel uncomfortable speaking up in class?
6. Ever say, "I hate to bother you..."?
7. Feel people take advantage of you at work?
8. Ever feel reluctant to turn down a classmate who asks you to do his or her work?
9. Avoid protesting an unfair grade or evaluation?
10. Have trouble starting a conversation?

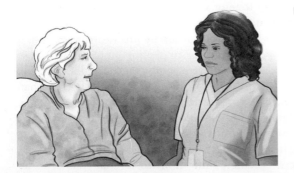

Figure 14-1   Principles of conflict resolution.
- Identify conflict issue
- Know own response
- Stay focused on issue
- Identify options
- User standards/criteria
- Seperate issue from people involved

expectation of a win-win outcome. After discussing possible solutions, select the best one to resolve the conflict. Evaluate the outcome based on fair, objective criteria.

Developing an Evidence-Based Practice

Kelly J, Ahern K: Preparing nurses for practice: a phenomenological study of the new graduate in Australia, *J Clin Nurs* 18:910–918, 2008.

This exploratory descriptive study examined the views of 13 graduating baccalaureate student nurses before employment, after 1 month, and again after 6 months of employment. Semistructured interviews were conducted using a phenomenologic "lived experience" approach. Findings were analyzed for themes.

Results: The major theme that emerged was workplace bullying/"eating your young," All these new graduate professional nurses struggled with socialization in their employment roles, experiencing "reality shock." They were unprepared for the culture of "cliques" that existed on their units and the lack of support they received. More experienced nurses gave them limited assistance with unfamiliar tasks; were perceived to act in a "bitchy" manner; used silence to communicate lack of acceptance; and seemed to subscribe to a philosophy that new nurses should learn by being "thrown into the deep end."

Application to Your Clinical Practice: As new graduates, you are a valuable resource. Seek positions with agencies that want to promote retention and thus provide extensive orientation programs with experienced staff nurse mentors.

APPLICATIONS

PREVENTING CONFLICT

In addition to managing your own responses to client provocations by adopting a professional, "calm" demeanor and low tone of voice, other conflict prevention strategies may be useful. Signal your readiness to listen with attending behaviors such as good body position, eye contact, and receptive facial expression (Jasmine, 2009). Give your undivided extra attention to a client or a visitor whom you identify as potentially becoming aggressive. Finke et al.'s (2008) review of 12 nurse-client communication studies showed that nurses' anti-communication attitudes were cited in

half the studies as a barrier to communication. Increasing your positive appreciation of your client does facilitate communication. As nurses, we hold the belief that all clients have worth as human beings. Remind yourself of this basic belief whenever you are in a conflict situation with your client. Remember we "choose" to enter into each relationship in a therapeutic manner (Milton, 2008). These strategies may be effective in preventing conflict or in preventing escalation of the conflict. Remember your primary goal is to prevent conflict or defuse escalating aggressive behavior (Phillips, 2007).

ASSESSING THE PRESENCE OF CONFLICT IN THE NURSE-CLIENT RELATIONSHIP

To get resolution, you need to acknowledge the presence of conflict. Often the awareness of our own feelings of discomfort is an initial clue. Evidence of the presence of conflict may be *overt*, that is, observable in the client's behavior and expressed verbally. For example, the client may criticize you. No one likes to be criticized, and a natural response might be anger, rationalization, or blaming others. But as a professional nurse, you recognize your response, recognize the conflict, and work toward resolution so that constructive changes may take place.

More often, conflict is *covert* and not so clear-cut. The conflict issues are hidden. Your client talks about one issue, but talking does not seem to help and the issue does not get resolved. He continues to be angry or anxious. Subtle behavioral manifestations of covert conflict might include a reduced effort by your client to engage in self-care; frequent misinterpretation of your words; behaviors that are out of character for him such as excessive anger. For example, when your client seems unusually demanding, has a seemingly insatiable need for your attention, or is unable to tolerate reasonable delays in having needs met, the problem may be anxiety stemming from conflictive feelings. Client behaviors are often negatively affected by feelings of pain, loss, frustration, or fear. As nurses, we affect the behavior of our clients through our actions. This can lead to positive or negative outcomes. See Exercise 14-5 for practice in defining conflict issues.

Sometimes the feelings themselves become the major issue, so that valid parts of the original conflict issue are hidden; consequently, conflict escalates. Consider the following situation.

EXERCISE 14-5 | **Defining Conflict Issues**

Purpose: To help students begin to organize information and define the problem in interpersonal conflict situations.

Procedure:
In every conflict situation, it is important to look for specific behaviors (including words, tone, posture, and facial expression); feeling impressions (including words, tone, intensity, and facial expression); and need (expressed verbally or through actions).

Identify the behaviors, your impressions of the behaviors, and needs that the client is expressing in the following situations. Then suggest an appropriate nursing action. Situation 1 is completed as a guide.

Situation 1
Mrs. Patel, an Indian client, does not speak much English. Her baby was just delivered by cesarean section, and it is expected that Mrs. Patel will remain in the hospital for at least 4 days. Her husband tells the nurse that Mrs. Patel wants to breast-feed, but she has decided to wait until she goes home to begin because she will be more comfortable there and wants privacy. The nurse knows that breast-feeding will be more successful if it is initiated soon after birth.

Behaviors: The client's husband states that his wife wants to breast-feed but does not wish to start before going home. Mrs. Patel is not initiating breast-feeding in the hospital.

Your impression of behaviors: Indirectly, the client is expressing physical discomfort, possible insecurity, and awkwardness about breast-feeding. She may also be acting in accordance with cultural norms of her country or family.

Underlying needs: Safety and security. Mrs. Patel probably will not be motivated to attempt breast-feeding until she feels safe and secure in her home environment.

Suggested nursing action: Provide family support and guarantee total privacy for feeding.

Situation 2
Mrs. Moore is returned to the unit from surgery after a radical mastectomy. The doctor's orders call for her to ambulate, cough, and deep breathe, and to use her arm as much as possible in self-care activities. Mrs. Moore asks the nurse in a very annoyed tone, "Why do I have to do this? You can see that it is difficult for me. Why can't you help me?"

Case Example

Ms. Denton is scheduled for surgery at 8 a.m. tomorrow. As the student nurse assigned to care for her, you have been told that she was admitted to the hospital 3 hours ago, and that she has been examined by the house resident. The anesthesia department has been notified of the client's arrival. Her blood work and urine have been sent to the laboratory. As you enter her room and introduce yourself, you notice that Ms. Denton is sitting on the edge of the bed and appears tense and angry.

Client: I wish people would just leave me alone. Nobody has come in and told me about my surgery tomorrow. I don't know what I'm supposed to do—just lay around here and rot, I guess.

At this point, you probably can sense the presence of conflictive feelings, but it is unclear whether the emotions being expressed relate to anxiety over the surgery or to anger over some real or imagined invasion of privacy because of the necessary laboratory tests and physical examination. Your client might also be annoyed by you or by a lack of information from her surgeon. She may feel the need to know that hospital personnel see her as a person and care about her

feelings. Before you can respond empathetically to the client's feelings, they will have to be decoded.

> *Nurse* (in a concerned tone of voice): You seem really upset. It's rough being in the hospital, isn't it?

Notice that the reply is nonevaluative and tentative, and does not suggest specific feelings beyond those the client has shared. There is an implicit request for her to validate your perception of her feelings and to link the feelings with a concrete issue. You process verbal as well as nonverbal cues. Concern is expressed through your tone of voice and words. The content focus relates to the client's predominant feeling tone, because this is the part of the conflict that she has chosen to share with you. It is important to maintain a nonanxious presence.

NURSING STRATEGIES TO ENHANCE CONFLICT RESOLUTION

One goal is to *de-escalate* the conflict (Pryor, 2006). Use the strategies for conflict resolution described in this section. Mastery takes practice. Although this

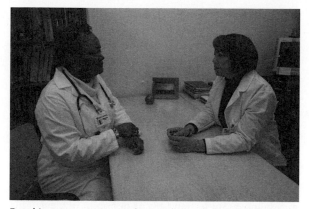

Reaching a common understanding of the problem in a direct, tactful manner is the first step in conflict resolution.

seems like a lot of information, Susanne Gaddis, the "Communications Doctor," calls these a "4-second rule" to improve communications.

PREPARE FOR THE ENCOUNTER

Careful preparation often makes the difference between being successful or failing to assert yourself when necessary. Clearly identify the issue in conflict. In discussing assertive communication, For communication to be effective, it must be carefully thought out in terms of certain basic questions:

- *Purpose.* What is the purpose or objective of this information? What is the central idea, the one most important statement to be made?
- *Organization.* What are the major points to be shared, and in what order?
- *Content.* Is the information to be shared complete? Does it convey who, what, where, when, why, and how?
- *Word choice.* Has careful consideration been given to the choice of words?

If you wish to be successful, you must consider not only what is important to you in the discussion but what is important to the other person. Bear in mind the other person's frame of reference when acting assertively. The following clinical example illustrates this idea.

Case Example

Mr. Pyle is an 80-year-old bachelor who lives alone. He has always been considered a proud and stately gentleman. He has a sister, 84 years old, who lives in Florida. His only other living relatives, a nephew and his wife, also live in another state. He recently changed his will so that it excludes his relatives, and he refuses to eat.

When his neighbor brings in food, he eats it, but he won't fix anything for himself. He tells his neighbor that he wants to die and that he read in the paper about a man who was able to die in 60 days by not eating. As the visiting nurse assigned to his area, you have been asked to make a home visit and assess the situation.

The issue in this case example is not one of food intake alone. Any attempt to talk about why it is important for him to eat or expressing your point of view in this conflict immediately on arriving is not likely to be successful. Mr. Pyle's behavior suggests that he feels there is little to be gained by living any longer. His actions suggest further that he feels lonely and may be angry with his relatives. Once you correctly ascertain his needs and identify the specific issues, you may be able to help Mr. Pyle resolve his intrapersonal conflict. His wish to die may not be absolute or final, because he eats when food is prepared by his neighbor and he has not yet taken a deliberate, aggressive move to end his life. Each of these factors needs to be assessed and validated with him before an accurate nursing diagnosis can be made.

ORGANIZE INFORMATION

Organizing your information and validating the appropriateness of your intervention with another knowledgeable person who is not directly involved in the process is useful. Sometimes it is wise to rehearse out loud what you are going to say. Remember to adhere to the principle of focusing on the conflict issue. Avoid bringing up the past.

MANAGE YOUR OWN ANXIETY OR ANGER

Recognizing and controlling your own natural emotional response to your client's upsetting behavior may be one key factor in managing conflict. Conflict produces anxiety, but anxiety increases your perception of conflict, creating feelings of helplessness (Stuart, 2009). This discomfort should signal you that you need to deal with the situation. Confronting the client's behavior now should keep you from losing control later as the problem escalates. Most people experience some variation of a physical response when taking interpersonal risks. A useful strategy for managing your own anger is to vent to a friend using "I" statements, as long as this does not become a complaining, whining session. Another strategy to manage your own anger is to "take a break." A cooling-off period, doing something else for a few minutes or hours until your anger subsides, is acceptable. Take care that you reengage, however, so that this does not become just an avoidance response style. Communicate with the correct person; do not take out your frustration on someone else. Focus on the one issue with the client involved. Try saying, "I would like to talk something over with you before the end of shift/ before I go." Before you actually enter the client's room, do the following:

- Cool off. Wait until you can speak in a calm, friendly tone.
- Take a few deep breaths. Inhale deeply and count "1-2-3" to yourself. Hold your breath for a count of 2 and exhale, counting again to 3 slowly.
- Fortify yourself with positive statements (e.g., "I have a right to respect."). Anticipation is usually far worse than the reality.
- Defuse your own anger before confronting the patient.
- Focus on one issue.

TIME THE ENCOUNTER

Timing is a determinant of success. Know specifically the behavior you wish to have the client change. Make sure that the client is capable physically and emotionally of changing the behavior. Select a time when you both can discuss the matter privately and use neutral ground, if possible. Select a time when the client is most likely to be receptive.

Timing is also important if an individual is very angry. The key to assertive behavior is choice. Sometimes it is better to allow your client to let off some "emotional steam" before engaging in conversation. In this case, the assertive thing to do is to choose silence accompanied by a calm, relaxed body posture. These nonverbal actions convey acceptance of feeling and a desire to understand. Validating the anger and reframing are useful. Comments such as "I'm sorry you are feeling so upset" recognize the significance of the emotion being expressed without getting into the cause.

PUT SITUATION INTO PERSPECTIVE

Don't play the blame game. Put the issue into perspective. Will the issue be significant in a year? In 10 years? Will there be a significant situational change with resolution? This is another way of saying to pick your battles. Not every situation is worth using up your time and energy. Remind yourself that anger may be caused by a problem communicating; the client who is frustrated may become angry when he cannot make staff understand.

USE THERAPEUTIC COMMUNICATION SKILLS

Refer to the discussion on therapeutic communication in Chapter 10. Particularly useful is *active listening*. Really trying to understand what the client is upset about requires more skill than just listening to his or her words. Listening closely to what the client is saying may help you understand his or her point of view. This understanding may decrease the stress. Repeat to assure the client you have heard what was said.

USE CLEAR, CONGRUENT COMMUNICATION

Riley (2008) adapted a CARE acronym to help nurses confront conflict situations. Refer to Box 14-4. The C is *clarify*. Choose direct, declarative sentences. Use

---

BOX 14-4 Potential Approaches for Dealing with Difficult Clients

1. **C**larify the behavior that is a problem:
   - Use active listening skills to identify issues of concern to the client.
   - Use a calm tone and avoid conveying irritation.
   - Use medical and nonmedical interventions to decrease anxiety (e.g., medicine, touch, relaxation, and guided imagery).
   - Factually state the problem.
2. **A**rticulate why the behavior is a problem:
   - Explain the institution policies.
   - Explain the limits of your role.
   - Set limits.
   - Give family permission (e.g., to rest or to leave).
3. **R**equest a change in the problem behavior:
   - Work with staff so all use the same uniform approach to the client's demands.
   - Develop a nursing care plan: involve patient in care and set goals; review and reevaluate whether nurse and client have same goals.
4. **E**ncourage change:
   - Evaluate progress.
   - Provide education; explain all options, with outcomes.
   - Use incentives and withdrawal of privileges to modify unacceptable behavior.
   - Promote trust by providing immediate feedback.

objective words, and directly state the behavior that is the problem. Then proceed to A and *articulate* why their behavior is a problem by stating facts.

Make sure verbal and nonverbal communication is congruent. Maintain an open stance and omit any gestures that might be interpreted as criticism, such as rolling your eyes or sighing heavily. Avoid mixed messages. One example of inappropriate communication might be found in the case of Larry, a staff nurse who works the 11-7 shift. Larry needs to get home to make sure his children get on the bus to school. A geriatric client routinely asks for a breathing treatment while Larry is reporting off. Instead of setting limits, Larry uses a soft voice and smiles as he tells her he can be late to begin the report. Another example is Mr. Carl, the 29-year-old client in Room 122 who constantly makes sexual comments to a young student nurse. She laughs as she tells him to cut it out.

TAKE ONE ISSUE AT A TIME

You may need to first focus on acknowledging the feelings associated with the conflict, because it is these that generally escalate conflict. It is always best to start with one issue at a time.

- Choose words that may lead to a positive outcome.
- Focus only on the present issue. The past cannot be changed.

Limiting your discussion to one topic issue at a time enhances the chance of success. Usually it is impossible to resolve a conflict that is multidimensional in nature with one solution. By breaking the problem down into simple steps, enough time is allowed for a clear understanding. In the case example just given, you might paraphrase the client's words, reflecting the meaning back to the client to validate accuracy. Once the issues have been delineated clearly, the steps needed for resolution may appear quite simple.

MUTUALLY GENERATE SOME OPTIONS FOR RESOLUTION

Focus on ways to resolve the problem by listing possible options. You are familiar with the "fight-or-flight" response to stress: Many people can respond to conflict only by either fighting or avoiding the problem. But brainstorming possible options and discussing pros and cons can turn the "fight" response into a more mutual "seeking a solution" mode of operations.

MAKE A REQUEST FOR A BEHAVIOR CHANGE

Avoid blaming. This would only make your client feel defensive or angry. As in Box 14-4, the R in the CARE acronym is your *request for a change* in his behavior. Clearly ask him or her for the needed behavior change. Take into consideration his developmental stage, values, and life experiences. His willingness to change needs to be considered. In addition, for an ill client, level of self-care, as well as outside support systems, are factors. To approach the task without this information is risky.

Rather than just stating your position, try to use some objective criteria to examine the situation. Saying, "I understand your need to_____, but the hospital has a policy intended to protect all our clients" might help you talk about the situation without escalating into anger. Psychiatric units have known rules against verbal abuse, violence such as throwing objects, violence against others, and so on. You can restate these "rules," together with their known violation outcomes (medication, seclusion, manual restraint), in a calm but firm voice.

There obviously will be situations in which such a thorough assessment is not possible, but each of these variables affects the success of the confrontation. For example, a client with dementia who makes a pass at a nurse may simply be expressing a need for affection in much the same way that a small child does; this behavior needs a caring response rather than a reprimand. A 30-year-old client with all his cognitive faculties who makes a similar pass needs a more confrontational response.

Client readiness is vital. The behavior may need to be confronted, but the manner in which the confrontation is approached and the amount of preparation or groundwork that has been done beforehand may affect the outcome.

UNDERSTAND CULTURAL IMPLICATIONS

Often what appears to be an inappropriate response in Western culture is a highly acceptable way of interacting in a different culture. For example, some clients experience conflict related to taking pain medication. In the cultures of these clients, pain is supposed to be endured with stoicism. It is often necessary to help such clients express their discomfort when it occurs and to give them guidelines, as well as explicit permission to develop a different behavior. It is easier for these clients to take such medication when they can assure their families that the nurse said it was necessary to take it. By focusing on the behavior required to meet the client's physical needs, the nurse bypasses placing a value on the rightness or wrongness of the behavior. Refer to chapter 11 for a more detailed discussion of cultural differences that can create conflict.

EVALUATE THE CONFLICT RESOLUTION

The E is the CARE acronym stands for encouraging the client to change by stating the outcomes, the positive consequences of changing or the negative implications for failing to change (Riley, 2008). The E could also stand for *evaluation of conflict resolution*. Evaluate the degree to which the interpersonal conflict has been resolved. This depends somewhat on the nature of the conflict. Sometimes a conflict cannot be resolved in a short time, but the willingness to persevere is a good indicator of a potentially successful outcome. Accepting small goals is useful when large goal attainment is not possible. Your goal is open communication with frequent feedback leading to successful problem solving.

For a client, perhaps the strongest indicator of conflict resolution is the degree to which he is actively engaged in activities aimed at accomplishing tasks associated with treatment goals. As the nurse, there are two questions you might want to address if modifications are necessary:

- What is the best way to establish an environment that is conducive to conflict resolution? What else needs to be considered?
- What self-care behaviors can be expected of the client if these changes are made? These need to be stated in ways that are measurable.

IDENTIFY CLIENT INTRAPERSONAL CONFLICT SITUATIONS

The initial interpersonal strategy used to help clients reduce strong emotion to a workable level is to provide a neutral, accepting, interpersonal environment. Within this context, you can acknowledge your client's emotion as a necessary component of adaptation to life. You convey acceptance of the individual's legitimate right to have feelings. Telling a client, "I'm not surprised that you are angry about..." or simply stating, "I'm sorry you are hurting so much," acknowledges the presence of an uncomfortable emotion in the client, conveys an attitude of acceptance, and encourages the client to express himself or herself.

Once a feeling can be put into words, it becomes manageable because it has concrete boundaries.

TALK ABOUT IT

The second step in defusing the strength of an emotion is to talk the emotion through with someone. For the client, this someone is often the nurse. For the nurse, this might be a nursing supervisor or a trusted colleague. Unlike complaining, the purpose of talking the emotion through is to help the person connect with all of his or her personal feelings surrounding the incident. If one client seems to produce certain negative emotional reactions on a nursing unit, the emotional responses may need the direct attention of all staff on the unit.

USE TENSION-REDUCING ACTIONS

The third phase is to take action. The specific needs expressed by the emotion suggest actions that might help the client come to terms with the consequences of the emotion. This responsibility might take the form of obtaining more information or of taking some concrete risks to change behaviors that sabotage the goals of the relationship. Convey mutual respect and avoid any "put-down" type of comment about yourself or the client.

Sometimes the most effective action is simply to listen. Active listening in a conflict situation involves concentrating on what the other person is upset about. Listening can be so powerful that it alone may reduce the client's feelings of anxiety and frustration.

Physical activity can reduce tension. For example, taking a walk can help your client control his anxiety behaviors and can defuse an emotionally tense situation. If your client is so upset that he constitutes a danger to himself or others, talk softly in a calm tone; face him but allow maximum space and an exit for yourself should it become necessary. Many hospitals and psychiatric units have a "code word " that is used to summon trained help.

Humor is frequently used by nurses to engage a client or to initiate an interaction. Humor can also be used as a means of reducing tension. To paraphrase a famous advice columnist, two of the most important words in a relationship are "I apologize." And she recommended making amends immediately when you've made a mistake, because it is easier to eat crow while it is still warm. Is this advice easier to take (we won't say swallow) since it comes with a chuckle? Humor serves as an immediate tension reliever.

DEFUSE INTRAPERSONAL CONFLICT

Intrapersonal conflicts develop when you hold opposing feelings within yourself. The client with a myocardial infarction who insists on conducting business from the bedside probably feels conflicted about the restraints placed on his or her activities, as does the diabetic client who sneaks off to the food vending machine for a candy bar.

There are times when the conflictive feelings begin intrapersonally within the nurse (e.g., in working with parents of an abused child or treating a foul-mouthed alcoholic client in the emergency department). Such situations often stir up strong feelings of anger or resentment in us. In this case, we may need to defuse destructive emotions before proceeding further. The following are interventions you can use to defuse intrapersonal conflicts:
- Identify the presence of an emotionally tense situation.
- Talk the situation through with someone.
- Provide a neutral, accepting environment.
- Take appropriate action to reduce tension.
- Evaluate the effectiveness of the strategies.
- Generalize behavioral approaches to other situations.

For the nurse, the first step in coping with difficult emotional responses is to recognize their presence and to assess the appropriateness of expressing emotion in the situation. If expressing the emotion does not fit the circumstances, one must deliberately remain unruffled when every natural instinct argues against it. Ambivalence, described as two opposing ideas or feelings related to any life situation or relationship coexisting within the same individual, is relatively common. It is not the responsibility of the nurse to help a client resolve all intrapersonal conflict. Long-standing conflicts require more expertise to resolve. In such cases, refer your client to the appropriate resource.

EVALUATE

The final step in the process is to evaluate the effectiveness of responses to emotions and to generalize the experience of confronting difficult emotions to other situations. Each step in the process may need to be taken more than once and refined or revised as circumstances dictate.

INTERPERSONAL CONFLICT INTERVENTIONS

DEVELOPING ASSERTIVE SKILLS

Demonstrate Respect

Responsible, assertive statements are made in ways that do not violate the rights of others or diminish their standing. They are conveyed by a relaxed, attentive posture and a calm, friendly tone of voice. Statements should be accompanied by the use of appropriate eye contact.

Use "I" Statements

Statements that begin with "You" sound accusatory and always represent an assumption because it is impossible to know exactly, without validation, why someone acts in a certain way. Because such statements usually point a finger and imply a judgment, most people respond defensively to them.

"We" statements should be used only when you actually mean to look at an issue collaboratively. Thus, the statement "Perhaps we both need to look at this issue a little closer" may be appropriate in certain situations. However, the statement "Perhaps we shouldn't get so angry when things don't work out the way we think they should" is a condescending statement thinly disguised as a collaborative statement. What is actually being expressed is the expectation that both parties should handle the conflict in one way—the nurse's way.

Use of "I" statements are one of the most effective conflict management strategies you can use. Assertive statements that begin with "I" suggest that the person making the statement accepts full personal responsibility for his or her own feelings and position in relation to the presence of conflict. It is not necessary to justify your position unless the added message clarifies or adds essential information. "I" statements seem a little clumsy at first and take some practice. The traditional format is this:

"I feel _____ (use a name to claim the emotion you feel) when _____ (describe the behavior nonjudgmentally) because _____ (describe the tangible effects of the behavior)."

Example:

"I feel uncomfortable when a client's personal problems are discussed in the cafeteria because someone might overhear confidential information."

Make Clear Statements

Statements, rather than questions, set the stage for assertive responses to conflict. When questions are used, "how" questions are best because they are neutral in nature, they seek more information, and they imply a collaborative effort. "Why" questions ask for an explanation or an evaluation of behavior and often put the other person on the defensive. It is always important to state the situation clearly; describe events or expectations objectively; and use a strong, firm, yet tactful manner. The following example shows how a nurse can use the three levels of assertive behaviors to meet the client's needs in a hospital situation without compromising the nurse's own needs for respect and dignity.

Case Example

Mr. Gow is a 35-year-old executive who has been hospitalized with a myocardial infarction. He has been acting seductively toward some of the young nurses, but he seems to be giving Miss O'Hara an especially hard time.

Client: Come on in, honey, I've been waiting for you.

Nurse (using appropriate facial expression and eye contact, and replying in a firm, clear voice): Mr. Gow, I would rather you called me Miss O'Hara.

Client: Aw, come on now, honey. I don't get to have much fun around here. What's the difference what I call you?

Nurse: I feel that it does make a difference, and I would like you to call me Miss O'Hara.

Client: Oh, you're no fun at all. Why do you have to be so serious?

Nurse: Mr. Gow, you're right. I am serious about some things, and being called by my name and title is one of them. I would prefer that you call me Miss O'Hara. I would like to work with you, however, and it might be important to explore the ways in which this hospitalization is hampering your natural desire to have fun.

In this interaction, the nurse's position is defined several times using successively stronger statements before the shift can be made to refocus on underlying client needs. Notice that even in the final encounter, however, the nurse labels the behavior, not the client, as unacceptable. Persistence is an essential feature when first attempts at assertiveness appear too limited. After careful analysis, if you find that a client's behavior is infringing on your rights, it is essential that the issues be addressed directly in a tactful manner. If they are not, it is quite likely that the undesirable behavior will continue until you are no longer willing to tolerate it.

Use Proper Pitch and Tone

The amount of force used in delivery of an assertive statement depends on the nature of the conflict situation, as well as on the amount of confrontation needed to resolve the conflict successfully. Starting with the least amount of assertiveness required to meet the demands of the situation conserves energy and does not place the nurse into the bind of overkill. It is not necessary to use all of one's resources at one time or to express ideas strongly when this type of response is not needed. You can sometimes lose your effectiveness by becoming long-winded in your explanation when only a simple statement of rights or intent is needed. Long explanations detract from the true impact of the spoken message. Getting to the main point quickly and saying what is necessary in the simplest, most concrete way cuts down on the possibility of misinterpretation. This approach increases the probability that the communication will be constructively received.

Pitch and tone of voice contribute to another person's interpretation of the meaning of your assertive message. A soft, hesitant, passive presentation can undermine an assertive message as much as vocalizing the message in a harsh, hostile, and aggressive tone. A firm but moderate presentation often is as effective as content in conveying the message (see Exercise 14-3).

Analyze Personal Feelings

As mentioned earlier, part of an initial assessment of an interpersonal conflict situation includes recognition of the nurse's intrapersonal contribution to the conflict, as well as that of the client. It is not wrong to have ambivalent feelings about taking care of clients with different lifestyles and values; however, this needs to be acknowledged to yourself.

Focus on the Present

The focus of assertive responses should always be on the present. Because it is impossible to do anything about the past except learn from it, and because the future is never completely predictable, the present is the only reality in which we have much decision-making power as to how we act. To be assertive in the face of an emotionally charged situation demands thought, energy, and commitment. Assertiveness also requires the use of common sense, self-awareness, knowledge, tact, humor, respect, and a sense of perspective. Although there is no guarantee that the use of assertive behaviors will produce desired interpersonal goals, the chances of a successful outcome are increased because the information flow is optimally honest, direct, and firm. Often the use of assertiveness brings about changes in ways that could not have been anticipated. Changes occur because the nurse offers a new resource in the form of objective feedback with no strings attached.

Structure Your Response

In mastering assertive responses, it may be helpful initially to use these steps in an assertive response.

1. Express empathy: "I understand that _____"; "I hear you saying _____."

Example:

"I understand that things are difficult at home."

2. Describe your feelings or the situation: "I feel that _____"; "This situation seems to me to _____."

Example:

"But your 8-year-old daughter has expressed a lot of anxiety, saying, 'I can't learn to give my own insulin shots.'"

3. State expectations: "I want _____"; "What is required by the situation is _____."

Example:

"It is necessary for you to be here tomorrow when the diabetic teaching nurse comes so you can learn how to give injections and your daughter can, too, with your support."

4. List consequences: "If you do this, then _____ will happen" (state positive outcome); "If you don't do this, then _____ will happen" (state negative outcome).

Example:

"If you get here on time, we can be finished and get her discharged in time for her birthday on Friday."

CLINICAL ENCOUNTERS WITH DEMANDING, DIFFICULT CLIENTS

Every nurse encounters clients who seem overly demanding of your limited time and resources. Although this may reflect a personality characteristic, most often it is sign of their anxiety. Box 14-1 describes behaviors that increase anger in others.

Nurses often respond to difficult clients, especially those who display inappropriate sexual aggression, by ignoring their verbal comments, physically avoiding the client, or by adopting a very "no-nonsense" professional behavior (Higgins, 2009). Try some of the more therapeutic approaches in Box 14-4. Usually we have labeled people as "difficult to deal with" when our normal way of dealing with them has failed. So remember, we cannot change other's personalities, but we can change the way we react to them (Salazar, 2004).

CLINICAL ENCOUNTERS WITH ANGRY CLIENTS

You can expect to encounter clients who express anger. This may take the form of refusal to comply with the treatment plan, exhibition of hostile behaviors toward staff, verbal or even physical actions, or perhaps withdrawal from any positive interaction with you. When dealing with a difficult client, ask yourself what the client is gaining from such behavior. Some people have not learned successful communication, so they revert to behavior that has gained them something in the past. For example, as children they may have only gotten needed attention when they acted out in a negative way or when they pouted or sulked. Ask yourself if the client behaving in a difficult way is getting rewarded by focusing a lot of staff attention on himself, for example. Does the client just need to learn a more effective way of communicating? Remind yourself that usually the client's feeling center on their disease or treatment and are not a reflection of their feeling about you. Nurses cited by Servodidio (2008) comment, "One of the hardest things to learn as a nurse is not to take a patient's frustration or anger personally" (p. 17).

Nonverbal clues to anger include grimacing, clenching jaws or fists, turning away, and refusing to maintain eye contact. Verbal cues by a client may, of course, include use of an angry tone of voice, but they may also be disguised as witty sarcasm or as condescending or insulting remarks. To become comfortable in dealing with client anger, the nurse must first become aware of his or her own reactions to anger so that the nurse does not threaten or reject the individual expressing anger, or respond in anger. Interventions include those listed in Box 14-5.

Help the client own the angry feelings by getting the client to verbalize things that make him or her

BOX 14-5	Strategies for Dealing with an Angry Client

- Call the client by name while making occasional eye contact.
- Use active listening while allowing client to ventilate some of his or her anger and discuss his problem.
- Use body language that is confident but nonthreatening: neutral position, hands down by your side, one foot in front of the other in a relaxed posture; do not "crowd" the client, maintain space (a safe distance).
- Take a deep breath and respond in a low, calm, gentle tone of voice (avoid being defensive).
- Restate the issue briefly, be friendly.
- For some clients with brain damage or mental illness, it is appropriate to remove them from the source of their irritation to a calm environment, sort of a time-out.

- Help client identify his or her own anger, for example: "I notice you are clenching your fists and talking more loudly than usual. These are things people do when angry. Are you feeling angry right now?"
- Give permission to feel angry, but set limits on acting out/violent behavior: "It's okay to feel angry about...but not okay to act on it," or "It's natural to feel angry about...but throwing isn't okay..."
- Avoid arguing, saying no, hurrying, or touching.
- Offer to work with client to help him deal with the issue.
- Get help *immediately* or *leave* if you feel in danger of physical harm; always maintain a space for safety and plan an exit.

angry. Acknowledging a client's anger may prevent an expression of abusive ranting. It is essential that you use empathetic statements or active listening to acknowledge the client's anger and maintain a non-threatening demeanor *before* moving on to try to discuss the issue. Remember your goal is to maintain *safety* while helping your client.

Defuse Hostility

Avoid responding to a client's anger by getting angry yourself. Verbal attacks follow certain rules, in that the abusive person expects you to react in specific ways. Usually people will respond by becoming aggressive and attacking back or by becoming defensive and intimidated. Keep your cool using strategies discussed earlier. Take a deep breath! Remember, if you lose control, you lose! If you become defensive, you lose! Abusive people want to provoke confrontations as a means of controlling you.

- Use empathy in your communication. An angry client needs to have you acknowledge both the issue and their feelings about that issue. Only then can the client begin to interact in a meaningful way. Your empathy may help defuse the situation (Nau, Dassen, Halfewns, & Needham, 2007).
- Deliberately begin to lower your voice and speak more slowly. When we get upset, we tend to speak quickly and use a higher tone of voice. If you do the opposite, the client may begin to mimic you and thus calm down.

- Realistically analyze the current situation that is disturbing the client.
- Be assertive in setting limits. If the client persists, you need to assert limits, saying, for example, "Jim, I want to help you sort this out, but if you continue to raise your voice, I'm going to have to leave. Which do you want?" or, "Yelling at me isn't going to get this worked out. I will not argue with you. Come back when you can talk calmly and I will try to help you."
- Assist the client in developing a plan to deal with the situation (e.g., use techniques such as role-playing to help the client express anger appropriately, using "I" statements such as "I feel angry" rather than "You make me angry"). Bringing behavior up to a verbal level should help alleviate the need for other acting out of destructive behaviors.

Prevent Escalation of Conflict

Depending on the type of feedback received, an intrapersonal conflict can take on interpersonal dimensions. In the following example, the mother initially experiences an intrapersonal conflict. The wished-for perfect infant has not appeared, and her personal ambivalence related to coping with her infant's defect is expressed indirectly through her partial noncompliant behavior. If the nurse interprets the client's behavior incorrectly as poor mothering and acts in a manner that reflects this attitude, the basically intrapersonal conflict can become interpersonal.

Case Example

A mother with her first infant is informed soon after delivery that her child has a cleft palate (missing roof of mouth). The physician explains the infant's condition in detail and answers the mother's questions. The mother requests rooming in and seems genuinely interested in the infant. Each time the nurse enters the client's room, the mother complains that her child does not seem hungry and states how difficult it is to feed the baby. Although the nurse spends a great deal of time teaching the mother the special techniques necessary for feeding, and the mother seems interested at the time, she seems unable or unwilling to follow any of the nurse's suggestions when she is by herself. Later, the nurse finds out that the mother has been asking for guidance and appears to be resisting what is offered. Although she may simply need further instruction in technique, the presence of an underlying intrapersonal conflict is worth investigating. Before proceeding with teaching, the nurse needs to find out about the mother's perceptions. Does she feel competent in the mothering role? What does having a less than perfect child mean to her? What are her fears about caring for an infant with this particular type of defect? Until the underlying feelings are identified, client teaching is likely to have limited success.

This client appears to reframe the experience from her own perspective. In this situation, a client strength would be the mother's ability and willingness to express her uncomfortable feelings so that they can be addressed. Even though the mother may be unclear about the nature of her feelings, reframing the issues in this way builds on strengths instead of on personal deficits.

Prevent any escalation in interpersonal conflict. Hurt feelings or misunderstandings can quickly escalate a conflict. In talking to an angry client, as his voice rises, lower yours. If eye contact seems confrontational, then break eye contact. If the client is acting out by throwing or hitting, set limits: "No hitting (spitting, or other physical behavior) is allowed here." If you set limits, be sure to follow through. Ask the client to verbalize his or her anger (e.g., "Talk about how you feel, instead of throwing things"). Studies show that talking will dramatically reduce aggressive behavior. Use other strategies described in this book for defusing conflict situations. Active listening (i.e., really listening to your client's viewpoint), using attentive body language, and summarizing the client's viewpoint can defuse some of the tension of the conflict.

CLINICAL ENCOUNTERS WITH AGGRESSIVE/VIOLENT CLIENTS

Some clients have mental problems, are truly confused, intoxicated, or have cognitive deterioration. The U.S. Preventive Services Task Force (USPSTF, 2008) recommends clinicians assess the client's level of cognitive functioning when this is suspected, using the Mini-Mental Status Examination (MMSE). It helps you to respond more positively if you perceive that their behavior is not "evil" but a result of their illness. Be aware that escalating conflict can be a threat not only to your client, but to your own safety. In no case is violence acceptable. Limits must be set. Failing this, you need to remove yourself from a potentially harmful situation. Starcher (1999) describes the behavior of an emotionally disturbed client admitted to a geriatric unit. Sam's behavior ranged from bullying or pushing other clients to noncompliance with his treatment. Staff tried setting clear limits and identifying specific negative outcomes, including restraints and medication, without success. Eventual successful interventions included consistent response by all staff members and using written patient contracts for each of his unacceptable behaviors. Outcomes were specifically stated for both negative behaviors (restrictions) and positive acceptable behaviors (rewards with his favorite activities).

Box 14-5 lists some useful strategies for coping with angry clients. Deliberate use of "calming interventions" have been validated in Pyror's (2006) analysis of expert nurses' behaviors. An additional strategy for helping nurse-client problem interactions is the staff-focused consultation. Consider the following situation.

Case Example

Mr. Plotsky, age 29, has been employed for 6 years as a construction worker. About 4 weeks ago, while operating a forklift, he was struck by a train, leaving him paraplegic. After 2 weeks in intensive care, he was transferred to a neurologic unit. When staff members attempt to provide physical care, such as changing his position or getting him up in a chair, Mr. Plotsky throws things, curses angrily, and sometimes spits at the nurses. Staff members become very upset; several nurses have requested assignment changes. Some staff members try bribing him with food to encourage good behavior; others threaten to apply restraints. The manager schedules a behavioral consultation meeting with a psychiatric nurse or clinical specialist. The immediate goal of this staff conference is to bring staff feelings out into the open and to facilitate increased awareness of the staff's behavioral responses when confronted with this client's behavior. The outcome goal is to use a problem-solving approach to develop a behavioral care plan, so that all staff members respond to Mr. Plotsky in a consistent manner.

Students are particularly prone to feeling rebuffed when they first encounter negative feedback from a client. Support from staff, instructors, and peers, coupled with efforts to understand the underlying reasons for the client's feelings, help you resist the trap of avoiding the relationship. To develop these ideas further, practice Exercise 14-5.

DEFUSING POTENTIAL CONFLICTS WHEN PROVIDING HOME HEALTH CARE

Recognizing potential situations lending themselves to conflict is, of course, an important initial step. Caregivers have been shown to experience conflict through incompatible pressures suffered between caregiver demands and demands from their other roles, such as parenting their children or maintaining employment (Stephens et al., 2001). In addition to this inter-role conflict, caregivers suffer pressures when a nurse comes into their home to participate in the care of an ill relative. A Canadian study of home health nurses and family caregivers of elderly relatives identified four evolving stages in the nurse-caregiver relationship. The initial stage is "worker-helper," with the nurse providing care to the ill client and the family helping. Next comes "worker-worker," when the nurse begins teaching the needed care skills to family members. Third is "nurse as manager; family as worker," as the family members learn needed care skills. The final stage, "nurse as nurse for family caregiver," occurs as the family member becomes exhausted (Butt, 2000). A source of conflict for nurses was the dual expectation of the family that the nurse would provide care not only for the identified client but also provide relief for the exhausted primary caregiver. When the nurse operated as manager and treated the caregiver as worker, the discrepancy in expectations and values resulted in increased tension in the relationship. Discussion of role expectations is essential. Because of the high cost of providing direct care to chronically ill clients, home health nurses may be expected to quickly shift to teaching the necessary skills to the family members. You can clarify that this shift in responsibility results in a reduction of expensive professional time but not in your commitment to the family.

SUMMARY

Conflict represents a struggle between two opposing thoughts, feelings, or needs. It can be intrapersonal in nature, deriving from within a particular individual; or interpersonal, when it represents a clash between two or more people.

All conflicts have certain things in common: a concrete content problem issue and relationship issues arising from the process of expressing the conflict. Generally, intrapersonal conflicts stimulate feelings of emotional discomfort. Strategies to defuse strong emotion include talking the emotion through with someone and temporarily reducing stress through the use of distraction or additional information. Most interpersonal conflicts involve some threat, either to one's sense of power to control an interpersonal situation or to ways of thinking about the self. Giving up ineffective behavior patterns in conflict situations is difficult; such patterns are generally perceived to be safer because they are familiar.

Behavioral responses to conflict situations fall into four categories. Nurses most commonly choose avoidance. However, this chapter describes other strategies (e.g., assertion) that have been more successfully used by nurses to manage client-nurse conflicts. Assertive behaviors range from making a simple statement, directly and honestly, about one's beliefs, to taking a very strong, confrontational stand about what will and will not be tolerated.

The principles of conflict management are described. To apply conflict management principles, you need to identify your own conflictive feelings or reactions. For internal conflict, feelings usually have to be put into words and related to the issue at hand before the meaning of the conflict becomes understandable. In conflict between nurse and client, you need to think through the possible causes of the conflict, as well as your own feelings, before making a response. To resolve these kinds of conflict, you need to use "I" statements and respond assertively.

ETHICAL DILEMMA What Would You Do?

You are caring for Kim, born at the gestational age of 24 weeks in a rural hospital and transferred this morning to your neonatal intensive care unit. Today her father arrives on the unit. Seeing you taking a blood sample from one of the many intravenous lines attached to her body, he yells at you to "Stop poking at her! What are you trying to prove by keeping her alive? Turn off those machines." This is both a communication and an ethics problem. How do you respond to his anger?

REFERENCES

Baillie L: An exploration of nurse-patient relationships in accident and emergency, *Accid Emerg Nurs* 13(9):9–14, 2005.

Bowers L, Flood C, Brennan G, et al: A replication study of the city nurse intervention: reducing conflict and containment on three acute psychiatric wards, *J Psychiatr Ment Health Nurs* 15(9):739–742, 2008.

Butt G: Nurses and family caregivers of elderly relatives engaged in 4 evolving types of relationships, *Evid Based Nurs* 3:134, 2000.

Chang M, Kelle AE: Patient education: addressing cultural diversity and health literacy issues, *Urol Nurs* 27(5):411–417, 2007.

Finke EH, Light J, Kitko L, et al: A systematic review of the effectiveness of nurse communication with patients with complex communication needs with a focus on the use of argumentative and alternative communication, *J Clin Nurs* 17(16):2102–2115, 2008.

Higgins A, Barker P, Begley CM, et al: Clients with mental health problems who sexualize the nurse-client encounter: the nursing discourse, *J Adv Nurs* 65(3):616–624, 2009.

Jasmine TJX: The use of effective therapeutic communication skills in nursing practice, *Singapore Nurs J* 36(1):35–40, 2009.

Macdonald M: Origins of difficulty in the nurse-patient encounter, *Nurs Ethics* 14(4):510–521, 2007.

McElhaney R: Conflict management in nursing administration, *Nurs Manag* 27(3):49–50, 1996.

Milton C: Boundaries: ethical implications for what it means to be therapeutic in the nurse-person relationship, *Nurs Sci Q* 21(1):18–21, 2008.

Nau J, Dassen T, Halfewns R, et al: Nursing students' experiences in managing patient aggression, *Nurs Educ Today* 27(8):933–946, 2007.

Phillips S: Countering workplace aggression: an urban tertiary care institution exemplar, *Nurs Adm Q* 31(3):209–218, 2007.

Pryor J: What do nurses do in response to their predictors of aggression? *J Neurosci Nurs* 28(3):177–182, 2006.

Redman BK, Fry ST: Ethical conflicts reported by RN/certified diabetes educators, *Diabetes Educ* 22(3):219–224, 1996.

Riley JB: *Communication in nursing*, ed 6, St. Louis, MO, 2008, Mosby/Elsevier Inc.

Salazar J: *Dealing with difficult people, Michigan Nurses Association*, Available online: http://www.minurses.org. Accessed May 5, 2009.

Servodidio CA: Nurses discuss working with challenging patients, *ONS Connect* 23(3):17, 2008.

Starcher S: Sam was an emotional terrorist, *Nursing* 99(2):40–41, 1999.

Stephens MA, Townsend AL, Martire LM, et al: Balancing parent care with other roles: interrole conflict, *J Gerontol B Psychol Sci Soc Sci* 56 (1):24–34, 2001.

Stuart GW: *Principles and practice of psychiatric nursing*, St. Louis, 2009, Mosby/Elsevier.

USPSTF, U.S. Preventive Services Task Force: *The Guide to Clinical Preventive Services*, 2008. Available online: www.preventiveservices.ahrq.govhttp://en.wikipedia.org/wiki/Conflict.

CHAPTER 15

Health Promotion and Client Learning Needs

Elizabeth C. Arnold

OBJECTIVES

At the end of the chapter, the reader will be able to:

1. Define health promotion and disease prevention and related concepts.
2. Identify national agendas for health promotion and disease prevention.
3. Describe relevant theory frameworks for health promotion strategies.
4. Apply health promotion and disease prevention strategies for individuals.
5. Apply health promotion strategies at the community level.
6. Discuss the role of learner variables in client education.

This chapter focuses on health promotion and disease prevention concepts used in health care. Included in the chapter are theory-based frameworks for health promotion as the starting point for improving the health of our nation and reducing health disparities. The chapter describes communication strategies designed to support clients, families, and targeted populations in achieving a better health quality of life, through education and lifestyle changes. The chapter addresses health literacy, readiness, and ability to learn as important components of health promotion/disease prevention efforts. A framework for developing and implementing community-based health promotion programs completes the chapter.

BASIC CONCEPTS

DEFINITIONS

HEALTH AND HEALTH PROMOTION

The concept of health and its importance as an essential underpinning in nursing practice are explored from the perspective of the social determinants influencing health and well-being in this chapter. Quality of life is viewed as a constituent of health.

Contemporary thinking recognizes that many determinants of health and well-being are embedded in the economics, culture, and social community in which people live and work. Health communication is conceptualized as being more than simple information transfer. Clients are held accountable for their health care decisions and expected to actively participate in shared decision making with their health care providers. Client education is viewed as part of a larger context of health promotion and disease prevention strategies (Hoving, Visser, Mullen & Borne, 2010).

Health in 2010 is described as "being free from disease, being able to function normally, experiencing well-being, and having a healthy lifestyle" (Fagerlind et al., 2010, p. 104). Health is identified as a fundamental human right intimately tied to a nation's social and economic development (Jakarta Declaration; World Health Organization [WHO], 1997). Engaging in activities to promote a healthy lifestyle is viewed as a personal responsibility. Clients are expected to actively change lifestyle behaviors and make treatment choices to enhance personal health and well-being. Contemporary thinking is that the dialogue between providers and clients about health should be an equal exchange of information. The emotional impact of the health disruption, environmental factors, and client preferences are parts of clinical assessment. A focus on teaching self-management skills, with clients taking primary responsibility for implementation, directs content in client-centered care (Hoving et al., 2010).

Health promotion is an interactive education and support process. It enables and empowers people to reach their highest health potential by taking control of and improving the circumstances pertaining to their health and well-being (Green, 2008). Health promotion and disease prevention activities are essential elements of U.S. health, as "treatment alone is unlikely to have marked effects on health inequities or health status" (Frankish et al., 2006, p. 271).

Health promotion is more than disease prevention. The concept of health promotion embraces resources and actions to improve quality of life and well-being. For health promotion activities to fully succeed, they need to address environmental circumstances that can be detrimental to a healthy living style, and include advocacy for change through health policy initiatives and social action. Reliable access to resources and leadership training are part of an essential infrastructure needed to support health promotion approaches in the community.

Organized health promotion strategies can target individuals, families, high-risk groups, or communities. Health promotion interventions focus on helping people develop the self-management skills they need to achieve maximum functional health and personal well-being. Examples range from coaching new mothers (individual) to parenting groups (group or community). Health promotion activities related to exercise, nutrition, job stress, and a balanced lifestyle are increasingly incorporated as essential components into occupational settings.

Health Promotion as a Population Concept

Health promotion as a population concept recognizes the community as its principal voice in assuming control of and improving health and well-being. Strategies involve organized actions and educational programs to support and inform individuals, families, and communities about better ways to improve and maintain a healthy lifestyle.

In 1986, the WHO's *Ottawa Charter for Health Promotion* documented essential prerequisites and resources needed for health promotion as "peace, shelter, education, food, income, a stable ecosystem, sustainable resources, social justice, and equity" (WHO, 1986). Desired outcomes of health promotion activities are optimum health and well-being. The Jakarta Declaration on Health Promotion (1997) reaffirmed its relevance and called for the following actions:

- Building *healthy public* policy
- Creating *supportive environments* for health
- Strengthening *community action* for health
- Developing *personal skills*
- Reorienting *health services*

DISEASE PREVENTION

Health promotion and disease prevention are related concepts. **Disease prevention** is concerned with identifying modifiable risk and protective factors associated with diseases and disorders. Zubialde, Mold, and Eubank (2009) assert, "The goal of prevention is managing risk of future disease, disability, or premature death" (p. 194). Interventions are designed to help individuals at risk for chronic disease avoid the occurrence of a disease, disorder, or injury, to slow the progression of detectable disease and/or reduce its consequences (WHO, 1998).

The emphasis is always on averting health problems *before* they occur or decreasing their impact once the health problem occurs. Disease prevention activities involve proactive decision making at all levels of prevention (Edelman & Mandel, 1998). The three tiers of prevention—primary, secondary, and tertiary prevention—represent a continuum of health care delivery focus.

- *Primary prevention* strategies emphasize reduction of risk factors, including genetic susceptibility as a methodology for preventing the initial appearance of a disease or disorder. Strategies emphasize establishing and maintaining lifestyles favorable to health and well-being. Examples include prenatal clinics, parenting classes, and stress management programs. Nutrition, exercise, and environmental safety are other examples, easily incorporated into ordinary health teaching conversations.
- *Secondary prevention* involves interventions designed to promote early diagnosis of symptoms through health screening, or timely treatment after the onset of the disease, thus minimizing

their effects on a person's life. Examples include mammograms, diabetes, respiratory, and blood pressure screenings. Screening for mental health problems during the course of primary care visits can detect undiagnosed depression, anxiety, and substance abuse. Early diagnosis has a direct impact on the course and treatment of acute and chronic illness (WHO, 2008).

- *Tertiary prevention* describes rehabilitation strategies designed to minimize the handicapping effects of a disease or injury once it occurs. Examples include teaching a cancer victim to manage chemotherapy symptoms, helping a stroke victim with bladder retraining to avoid infection, and teaching a client to cope effectively with the necessary adjustments a serious physical, social, or emotional illness imposes.

Well-being

Health promotion activities incorporate the WHO concept of an inseparable construct of health and well-being (Figure 15-1). Wellness or **well-being** is defined as a person's subjective experience of satisfaction about his or her life related to six personal dimensions: intellectual, physical, emotional, social, occupational, and spiritual (Edlin & Golanty, 2009). People experience well-being as being at peace with themselves and others. People can experience well-being even with a serious health problem or terminal diagnosis (Saylor, 2004).

Lifestyle

Milio (1976) defines **lifestyle** as "patterns of choices made from the alternatives that are available to people according to their socioeconomic circumstances and the ease with which they are able to choose certain ones over others" (quoted in Cody, 2006, p. 186). The significance of this statement is that not everyone has the same options for having a healthy lifestyle.

Lifestyle factors are implicated as root factors in up to half of deaths in the United States (Edlin & Golanty, 2009). Deaths and chronic disease that compromise quality of life because of lifestyle factors can be prevented with changes in health habits. Chronic diseases and degenerative health conditions can be prevented or put off with changes in lifestyle. At the same time, it is important that lifestyle reflects socioeconomic and environmental circumstances such as diet, social isolation, lack of access, language barriers, and poverty. Action plans to help people take charge of their health and make a commitment to positive lifestyle changes must take into account the close relationship between individual factors and environmental supports in health promotion.

Ideally, building healthy lifestyles begins in childhood. As Frederick Douglass (Brainy Quotes, 2010) noted years ago, "It is easier to build strong children than to repair broken men." Pender, Murdaugh, and Parsons (2006) identified six principles for achieving a healthy lifestyle: eating well, staying active, getting adequate sleep, managing stress, building supportive

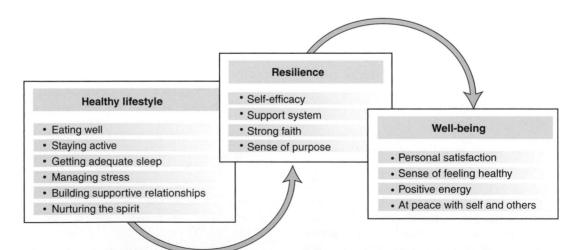

Figure 15-1 Critical elements for maintaining health and well-being.

relationships, and nurturing one's spirit. Comprehensive health promotion activities focused on individuals and their families, set within community, and larger ecosystem initiatives produce the best benefit, particularly when paired with social and resource support.

Resilience

Resilience is defined as "strength in the midst of change and stressful life events; the power of springing back or recovering readily from adversity" (Chapman, Lesch, & Aitken, 2005, p. 4). Resilience is a concept that helps explain why some people seem to weather adversity more easily than others and are able to grow from the experience. People can do this more easily when their stress is balanced with mechanisms to help them process it, and they acquire the skills they need to move forward with their lives (Schieveld, 2009). Psychosocial resilience is associated with self-efficacy, developing an organized way of coping with stressors, and the cultivation of a meaningful support system. A strong faith and sense of purpose also are factors (Freedman, 2008).

NATIONAL HEALTH PROMOTION AND DISEASE PREVENTION AGENDAS

The Committee on Assuring the Health of the Public in the 21st Century (2003) has cited three major trends influencing health care in the United States:

1. Demographic changes with the "population growing larger, older, and more racially and ethnically diverse, with a higher incidence of chronic disease"
2. Technical and scientific advances, which "create new channels for information and communication, as well as novel ways of preventing and treating disease"
3. "Globalization and health, to include the geopolitical and economic challenge of globalization, including international terrorism" (pp. 34–41)

HEALTHY PEOPLE: NATIONAL HEALTH PROMOTION AND DISEASE PREVENTION AGENDAS

Each decade, the U.S. Department of Health and Human Services (HHS) publishes an updated health promotion and disease prevention agenda for the nation with specific national goals and objectives. *Healthy People* 2010 (HHS, 2000) presents the health promotion and disease prevention agenda for the

nation. The third document of its kind, *Healthy People 2010* puts forth 28 focus areas with corresponding national health objectives designed to identify and reduce the most preventable threats to health. Federal agencies intimately involved with health care developed the document with input from more than 350 national membership organizations and 250 state health, mental health, substance abuse, and environmental agencies.

The overarching goals for Healthy People 2010 are to "achieve increased quality and years of healthy life and the elimination of health disparities" (U.S. Department of Health and Human Services, HHS, 2002). *Healthy People 2010* provides strong support for the nation's move from a predominantly medical model of health care to a public health model. It incorporates the most relevant scientific expertise on health care as the basis for evaluating leading health indicators against outcome benchmarks for preventive health care. Each leading health indicator listed in Box 15-1 has associated objectives.

Healthy People 2020 is conceptualized as continuing earlier Healthy People initiatives related to addressing environmental factors contributing to the health status of individuals and populations, with a stronger focus on action plans and strategies. The vision for *Healthy People 2020* is to have "a society in which all people live long, healthy lives" (U.S. Department of Health and Human Services, HHS, 2010). Proposed overarching goals to achieve this vision include the following:

- Eliminate preventable disease, disability, injury, and premature death.
- Achieve health equity, eliminate disparities, and improve the health of all groups.

BOX 15-1 | *Healthy People 2010:* Leading Health Indicators

- Physical activity
- Overweight and obesity
- Tobacco use
- Substance abuse
- Responsible sexual behavior
- Mental health
- Injury and violence
- Environmental quality
- Immunization
- Access to health care

From U.S. Department of Health and Human Services: What are the leading health indicators? *Healthy People 2010;* available online: http://www.healthypeople.gov/LHI/lhiwhat.htm. Accessed September 19, 2009.

- Create social and physical environments that promote good health for all.
- Promote healthy development and healthy behaviors across every stage of life.

Action models, proposed to achieve these goals, will provide clear priorities for what needs to be done, with focused strategies for addressing each goal. Objectives are projected to be organized in three categories— interventions, determinants, and outcomes—rather than in specific focus areas. More information about recommendations for the framework and format for *Healthy People 2020* is available online (www.healthypeople. gov/HP2020).

CENTERS FOR DISEASE CONTROL AND PREVENTION

Surveillance of health events is an important component of population-focused health promotion and disease prevention because it alerts health care providers to potential and actual health problems, and provides morbidity and mortality rates for evaluation purposes. The Centers for Disease Control and Prevention (CDC) is "the nation's premiere health promotion, prevention and preparedness agency and a global leader in public health" (CDC, 2006). It is the operational part of the HHS, which is directly responsible for protecting the health and safety of the nation's citizens and is committed to achieving improvement in people's health. As such, it is an important resource for health promotion activities.

The CDC collects data about the incidence and prevalence of diseases and chronic illnesses, and ranks illnesses that kill Americans. It tracks the development of new health problems and illnesses appearing in the United States and is recognized globally for its dedication to promoting people's health and well-being. This agency provides funding to states to implement health programs for Americans, and funding to developing countries related to prevention and treatment of AIDS. The CDC applies research findings to improve people's daily lives. State and municipal health departments receive support from the CDC to detect and reduce health threats from bioterrorism. The CDC has four health promotion impact goals:

- *Healthy people in every stage of life:* All people, and especially those at greater risk for health disparities, will achieve their optimal life span with the best quality of life in every stage of life.
- *Healthy people in healthy places:* The places where people live, work, learn, and play will protect and promote their health and safety, especially those at greater risk for health disparities.
- *People prepared for emerging health threats:* People in all communities will be protected from infectious, occupational, environmental, and terrorist threats.
- *Healthy people in a healthy world:* People around the world will live safer, healthier, and longer lives through health promotion, health security, and health diplomacy (CDC, n.d.).

In 2001, the Institute of Medicine (IOM) published a landmark report, *Crossing the Quality Chasm: A New Health System for the 21st Century,* which identified six areas of focus for improvement of health care. The areas identified for health care improvement (Table 15-1) have relevance for preventive interventions. A second report in 2006 outlined recommendations to improve the quality of health care for mental and substance-use conditions (IOM, 2006).

TABLE 15-1	Institute of Medicine's Six Aims for Improvement of Health Care
Aim	**Descriptor**
Safe	Avoiding injuries to patients from the care that is intended to help them
Effective	Providing services based on scientific knowledge to all who could benefit and refraining from providing services for those not likely to benefit
Patient centered	Providing care that is respectful of and responsive to individual patient preferences, needs, and values, and ensuring that patient values guide all clinical decisions
Timely	Reducing waits and sometimes harmful delays for both those who receive and those who give care
Efficient	Avoiding waste, including waste of equipment, supplies, ideas, and energy
Equitable	Providing care that does not vary in quality because of personal characteristics such as gender, ethnicity, geographic location, and socioeconomic status

Source: Institute of Medicine: *Crossing the quality chasm: a new health system for the 21st century* (p. 3), Washington, DC, 2001, Author.

THEORY FRAMEWORKS FOR HEALTH PROMOTION

Theory frameworks for health promotion focus on how people make choices and decisions about their health. Redman (2004) suggests that the health belief model, the transtheoretical model, and social learning theory are particularly relevant in health education for self-management of chronic diseases. This section presents three theoretical frameworks, each of which takes into consideration a person's beliefs about his or her ability to determine and influence health status and well-being.

PENDER'S HEALTH PROMOTION MODEL

Pender's (2006) revised health promotion model expands on an earlier health belief model developed by Rosenstock and his associates in the 1950s. The health belief model proposed that a person's willingness to engage in health promotion behaviors is best understood through examining a person's beliefs about the seriousness of a health condition and his or her capacity to influence its outcome.

Nola Pender's revised health promotion model continues to include perceived benefits, barriers, and ability to take action related to health and well-being as important components of people's health decision making. Added to these prior considerations is an emphasis on personal factors, including interpersonal influences and situational pressures, that can sway a person's commitment to plan of action and health-promoting behaviors (Figure 15-2). Taken together, these dynamics act as internal or external "cues to action" influencing a person's decision to seek health care or to engage in health-promoting activities. Examples include required school immunizations; interpersonal reminders, such as a family member's experience with the health care system; the mass

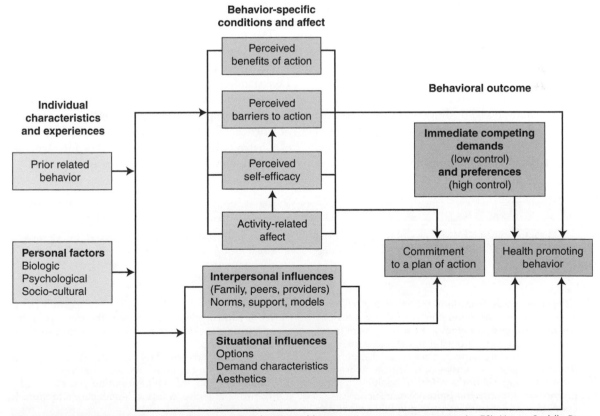

Figure 15-2 **Health promotion model.** *(From Pender N: Health promotion in nursing practice (p. 50), Upper Saddle River, NJ, 2006, Prentice Hall.)*

media; and ethnic approval. Using the health promotion model allows nurses to understand each person's combination of personal and behavioral variables as a consideration in choosing the best approach to engage a client in advancing health and well-being.

Case Example

Mary Nolan knows that walking will help diminish her risk for developing osteoporosis, but the threat of having this problem in her 60s is not sufficient to motivate her to take action in her 40s. Mary does not feel any signs or symptoms of the disorder, and it is easier to maintain a sedentary lifestyle. The nurse will have to understand the client's internal value system and other factors that influence readiness to learn to create the most appropriate learning conditions and types of teaching strategies Mary will need to effect positive change in health habits. The nurse might show Mary a video of the changes osteoporosis creates in spinal structure or ask an older adult with this disease to share her experience.

Exercise 15-1 provides practice with applying Pender's health promotion model to common health problems.

TRANSTHEORETICAL MODEL OF CHANGE

Prochaska's model provides a simple way to help identify the motivational readiness of people to engage in specific health-promoting behaviors (Daley, Fish, Frid, & Mitchell, 2009; Prochaska, DiClemente, & Norcross, 1992). The transtheoretical model of change recognizes the difficulty most people have with changing longstanding unhealthy lifestyle habits. Their model describes motivation to change as a state of readiness, which fluctuates and can be influenced by external encouragement (DiClemente, Schlundt, & Gemmell 2004). The model identifies five stages through which people make a decision to make an intentional behavioral change and carry through with implementation.

The transtheoretical model proposes that the client's intrinsic motivation is key to behavioral change and establishing preventive health behavior practices. Even people who are highly resistant to change can be motivated to change unhealthy behaviors. Assessment of the client's motivation, or lack thereof, is coupled with targeted interventions to match an individual's level of motivation or "readiness" to change the behavior. When motivational strategies match an individual's readiness, the likelihood that the client will follow a recommended course of action toward behavior change increases. The strategies challenge, support, and accept the client's readiness to change as the starting point for intervention.

The transtheoretical model is not a linear model. Clients can cycle through one or more of the stages several times before a permanent change takes place. Longstanding habits are hard to break. Setbacks and relapse with return to old behaviors can be expected, with an assumption that people will learn from the experience. Table 15-2 presents Prochaska's Model of Change with suggested approaches for each stage and corresponding sample statements.

EXERCISE 15-1	Pender's Health Promotion Model

Purpose: To help students understand the value of the health promotion model in assessing and promoting healthy lifestyles.

Procedure:
1. Using the health promotion model as a guide, interview a person in the community about his or her perception of a common health problem (e.g., heart disease, high cholesterol, osteoporosis, breast or prostate cancer, obesity, or diabetes).
2. Record the person's answers in written diagram form following Pender's model of health promotion. Identify the behavior-specific cognitions and affect action that would best fit the person's situation.

3. Share your findings with your classmates, either in a small group of four to six students with a scribe to share common themes with the larger class or in the general class.

Discussion:
1. Were you surprised by anything the client said, his or her perception of the problem, or interpretation of its meaning?
2. As you compare your findings with other classmates, do common themes emerge?
3. How could you use the information you obtained from this exercise in future health care situations?

TABLE 15-2	Prochaska's Stages of Change with Suggested Approaches and Sample Statements Applied to Alcoholism		
Stage	**Characteristic Behaviors**	**Suggested Approach**	**Sample Statement**
Precontemplation	Client does not think there is a problem; not considering the possibility of change.	Raise doubt; give informational feedback to raise awareness of a problem and health risks	"Your lab tests show liver damage. These tests can be predictive of serious health problems and premature death."
Contemplation	Client thinks there may be a problem; thinking about change; goes back and forth between concern and unconcern.	Tip the balance; allow open discussion of pros and cons of changing behavior; build motivation for change; help client justify a positive commitment	"It sounds as though you think you may have a drinking problem, but are not sure you are an alcoholic. What would your life be like without alcohol?"
Preparation	Client decides there is a problem and is willing to make a change: "I guess I do need to stop drinking."	Help the client choose the best course of action to take in resolving the problem	"What kinds of changes will you need to make to stop drinking? Most people find Alcoholics Anonymous (AA) helpful as a support. Have you heard of them?"
Action	Client engages in concrete actions to effect needed change.	Help the client take active steps to resolve health problem; review progress; give feedback	"I am impressed that you went to two AA meetings this week and have not had a drink either. What has this been like for you?"
Maintenance	Client perseveres with positive behavioral change.	Help client identify and use strategies to sustain progress; point out positive changes; accept temporary setbacks and use steps in preparation phase, if needed	"It's hard to let go of old habits, but you have been abstinent for three months now, and your liver tests are significantly improved."

Case Example

Client: "I'm ready to go home now. I know once I get home, that I'll be able to get along without help. I've lived there all my life and I know my way around."

Nurse: "I know that you think you can manage yourself at home. But most people need some rehabilitation after a stroke to help them regain their strength. If you go home now without the rehabilitation, you may be shortchanging yourself by not taking the time to develop the skills you need to be independent at home. Is that something important to you?" *(precontemplation approach to raise awareness of the problem)*

Exercise 15-2 provides an opportunity to work with the transtheoretical model in understanding learning readiness.

MOTIVATIONAL INTERVIEWING

Motivational interviewing (MI) is "theoretically congruent" with the transtheoretical model of behavior change (Goodwin, Bar, Reed & Ashford, 2009, p. 204). Originally conceptualized for use in the treatment of alcoholism, the MI framework is used with a growing range of chronic health conditions that are caused by or exacerbated by unhealthy lifestyle behaviors, for example, diabetes and obesity (Carels et al., 2007; Kirk, Mutrie, Macintyre, & Fisher, 2004).

MI is an evidenced-based treatment approach to helping clients address resistance or ambivalence about health-related lifestyle changes. Motivational learning represents an interactive process in which the clinician strives to learn about the client's goals,

| EXERCISE 15-2 | Assessing Readiness Using Prochaska's Model |

Purpose: To identify elements in teaching that can promote readiness using Prochaska's Model.

Procedure:

Identify as many specific answers as possible to the following questions:

1. Patrick drinks four to six beers every evening. Last year he lost his job. He has a troubled marriage and few friends. Patrick does not consider himself an alcoholic and blames his chaotic marriage for his need to drink. There is a strong family history of alcoholism.

    What kinds of information might help Patrick want to learn more about his condition?

2. Lily has just learned she has breast cancer. Although there is a good chance that surgery and chemotherapy will help her, she is scared to commit to the process and has even talked about taking her life.

    What kinds of health teaching strategies and information might help Lily become ready to learn about her condition?

3. Shawn has just been diagnosed as having epilepsy. He is ashamed to tell his friends and teachers about his condition. Shawn is considering breaking up with his girlfriend because of his newly diagnosed illness.

    How would you use health teaching to help Shawn cope more effectively with his illness?

values, and concerns as they relate to consideration of targeted health behavior changes. Developed by Miller and Rollnick (2002), MI is part of a cooperative partnership between client and clinician characterized by "an active collaborative conversation and joint decision making process" (Rollnick, Miller, & Butler, 2008, p. 6). Strategies include listening carefully to the client's description of the problem and the client's ideas about how the problem might be resolved. This step is followed by mutually exploring the pros and cons of each proposed solution. It is important for the nurse to express empathy for the challenges faced by the client and to affirm the client's opinions and progress (Levensky, Forcehimes, O'Donohue, & Bietz, 2007).

A motivational framework to change unhealthy behaviors is based on a person's values, beliefs, and preferences and fits well with the current emphasis on client-centered health care (Miller, 2004; Sandelowski, DeVellis, & Campbell, 2008). The client and clinician form a collaborative relationship in which they are equal partners, each contributing a knowledge and expertise to the situation. The clinician provides guidance, knowledge, and support. The final decision is always the client's responsibility. A critical component of MI is an acceptance of the client's right to make the final decision and the need for the clinician to honor each client's right to do so.

SOCIAL LEARNING THEORY

Bandura's (1997) contribution to the study of health promotion is his concept of self-efficacy. He believed that *self-efficacy*, described as a personal belief in one's ability to execute the actions required to achieve a goal, is a powerful mediator of behavior and behavioral change. Having self-confidence in one's ability to determine and implement actions has a direct influence on motivation and readiness to learn.

Self-efficacy and **motivation** are reciprocal processes; increased self-efficacy strengthens motivation, which, in turn, strengthens the client's capacity to complete the learning task. A person's perception of his her capability is a strong motivator even if it is not completely validated by the reality of the person's abilities. This is a critical concept because both clients and family caregivers may have reservations about their competence to carry out treatments in the home or make changes in lifestyle. Providing support at critical junctions can improve motivation and beliefs in one's ability to master essential tasks. Mastery is considered to be the strongest foundation of self-efficacy (Srof & Velsor-Friedrich, 2006).

Bandura considers learning to be a social process. He identified three sets of motivating factors that promote the learning necessary to achieve a predetermined goal: physical motivators, social incentives, and cognitive motivators. Physical motivators can be internal, such as memory of previous discomfort or a symptom that the client cannot ignore. Social incentives such as praise and encouragement increase self-esteem and give the client reason to continue learning.

Bandura refers to a third set of motivators as cognitive motivators, describing them as internal thought processes associated with change.

Case Example

Francis Edison agrees wholeheartedly with his nurse that smoking is bad and is likely to cause an earlier death from emphysema. However, in his mind, it is impossible for him even to contemplate giving up smoking. His mindset precludes learning until he can see the connection between giving up cigarettes and avoiding painful symptoms. A severe bronchitis creating air hunger and a hacking cough finally convinces Francis to give up cigarettes.

Below, the nurse combines the concept of a physical motivator with a social incentive related to something the client values (his grandson). The intervention is designed to help Francis recognize how changes in his health behavior can not only improve his health and well-being but give him a social outlet that could be important to him.

> *Nurse:* I'm worried that you are continuing to smoke, because it does affect your breathing. There is nothing you can do about the damage to your lungs that is already there, but if you stop smoking it can help preserve the healthy tissue you still have *(physical motivator)* and you won't have as much trouble breathing. I bet your grandson would appreciate it if you could breathe better and be able to play with him *(social incentive).* As Francis notices that he is coughing less when he gives up smoking, this new perceptual knowledge can act as an internal *cognitive motivator* to remain abstinent.

Developing an Evidence-Based Practice

Markle-Reid M, Weir R, Browne G, et al: Health promotion for frail older home care clients, *J Adv Nurs* 54(3):381–395, 2006.

This experimental study was designed to evaluate the comparative effects and costs of a proactive health promotion intervention provided to frail, elderly, home care clients. The sample, with an 84% completion rate, was randomly assigned to a control group (N = 120) or the experimental group (N = 120), who received health promotion nursing care in addition to their normal home care. This health promotion strategy consisted of a health assessment combined with their regular home visits or telephone contacts, education about the management of their illness, coordination of community services, and the use of empowerment strategies to enhance their independence.

Results: The frail elderly home care clients receiving the health promotion strategy in addition to their usual health care demonstrated significantly better mental health functioning, a reduction in depression, and enhanced perceptions of social support. Offering home-based health promotion activities can enhance the quality of life without increasing overall cost of services to homebound clients.

Application to Your Clinical Practice: As a profession, nurses are providing more and more community services reflective of a public health model. The frail elderly are a population that is growing exponentially. Finding creative, cost-effective ways to promote health and independence for this population needs to be a goal of professional nursing. What are some ways you can think of to promote health and quality of life for homebound clients with chronic illnesses?

APPLICATIONS

APPLYING HEALTH PROMOTION AND DISEASE PREVENTION STRATEGIES

The American Association of Colleges of Nursing (2008) identifies health promotion and disease prevention at individual and population levels as an essential component of professional nursing practice. It can be integrated informally into everyday nursing care, and formally in client education and screening programs. Nurses can play an important role in health promotion and disease prevention regardless of whether they work in primary or hospital care settings.

Nurses have unique opportunities to include primary and secondary prevention strategies with clients during routine health maintenance examinations and routine treatment. In the 21st century, health promotion strategies should be a part of everyday nursing care (Beckford-Ball, 2006). All nurses can participate in health screenings and client education. Examples of individualized health promotion strategies include encouraging regular medical checkups, providing client education, and offering health screenings to promote health and prevent disease (Maltby & Robinson, 1998).

Health promotion instruction can focus on condition-specific topics, or they can emphasize general education about healthy lifestyles. Condition-specific activities might include anticipatory guidance, and coaching for new mothers and caregivers of clients with chronic illness. Secondary prevention strategies focus on lifestyle/rehabilitative planning and interventions for clients with chronic conditions such as cardiac disorders or diabetes.

EXERCISE 15-3 | Developing a Health Profile

Purpose: To help students understand the relationship between lifestyle health assessment factors and related health goals from a personal perspective.

Procedure:
Out of class assignment:
1. Assess your own personal risk factors related to each of the following:
   a. Family risk factors (diabetes, cardiac, cancer, osteoporosis)
   b. Diet and nutrition
   c. Exercise habits
   d. Weight
   e. Alcohol and drug use
   f. Safe sex practices
   g. Perceived level of stress

   h. Health screening tests: cholesterol, blood pressure, blood sugar
2. Identify unhealthy behaviors or risk factors
3. Develop a personalized action plan, to identify strategies to address areas that need strengthening.
4. Identify any barriers that might prevent you from achieving your personal goals.

Discussion:
1. In small groups, discuss findings that you feel comfortable sharing with others.
2. Get input from others about ways to achieve health-related goals.
3. In the larger group, discuss how doing this exercise can inform your practice related to lifestyle changes and health promotion.

General education strategies related to positive lifestyle habits would emphasize diet, physical activity, regular sleep patterns, and stress reduction. Exercise 15-3 provides an opportunity to develop your own personal health portfolio.

A wide variety of topics lend themselves to health promotion focus. A sampling includes the following:

- Alcohol, nicotine, and other drug abuse prevention
- Anger management
- Prevention and early detection of common chronic diseases such as diabetes, cancer, heart disease, osteoporosis, co-occurring disorders
- Behaviors needed for a healthy lifestyle
- Family issues related to communication and parenting
- Job stress and burnout prevention for informal caregivers and at work sites
- Coping with grief and crisis

PROMOTING HEALTH FOR INDIVIDUALS

MI emphasizes a person's capacity to take charge of their health and to master the lifestyle factors that interfere with optimal health and well-being. The communication process starts with establishing a collaborative relationship with a client and family before beginning to assess their readiness for change. You can use the stages of change identified in Table 15-2 to determine where you should start. Focusing on the family's beliefs and values about health behaviors allows nurses to ease into a dialogue in which clients

explore the pros and cons of different behaviors. Open-ended questions that place health issues within the context of everyday life provide broader information about issues that otherwise might not be identified. For example, asking a client about exercise may yield a one-sentence answer. Asking the same client to describe his activity and exercise during a typical day, and what makes it easier or harder for him to exercise provides better data. Potential concerns about strategies that may not be consistent with values, preferences, or goals are more readily identified. Client-centered and family perspectives on disease and treatment are not necessarily the same as those of their health care providers.

Assessment of social and environmental supports is important. Because *perception* of self-efficacy and competence influences a person's willingness to participate in health-promoting behaviors, the assistance and support that others can provide to enable client success is critical. With this information, nurses are able to tailor their interventions to the client's capacity to change. Although initially an MI approach may take a little longer, it is likely to be more effective because the client chooses actions with personal meaning and will be more committed to it.

Nurturing the development of self-efficacy helps people to feel more confident. Opportunities for shared decision making and learning self-management skills empower clients to take an active role in treatment and health promotion activities (Hoving et al., 2010). Nurses empower clients and families through provision of accurate, timely information, coaching supports, and targeted links to health screening and community services. Educational and referral supports enable clients and families to learn the skills they need to effectively manage chronic conditions and to live a healthy lifestyle. Helping people use technology to find information and resources is another form of encouraging clients to take charge of their health and well-being.

Gance-Cleveland (2007) suggests setting an agenda with clients as a way of determining what is most important to clients and what they are willing to change. Effective health promotion activities perceived as being relevant are more likely to produce positive results. Tailoring instruction and coaching to the needs, abilities, and characteristics of the client and/or target population is important.

Timing is important for full effectiveness. For example, providing pregnant mothers with a tour of the obstetrics (OB) unit and providing information before admission is more effective than providing it after admission.

Working with Disparities

Although disparities refer to differences in health across ethnic groups, gender, education, or income, the term usually is associated with inequalities in access, service use, and health outcomes. Although major advances in health care have occurred since the beginning of the 21st century these developments have not benefited target health populations equally (Kline & Huff, 2008, p. 180).

People with the greatest health burdens often have the least access to information, communication technologies, health care, and supporting social services. For example, people living in extreme poverty may not have access to preventive care, adequate nutrition, or the opportunity to live in a healthy environment, because of finances. They may not even think about it because they are at the survival level. Noting environmental deficits in the client's environment that are beyond individual control can help you tailor meaningful health promotion supports.

Case Example

Michelle is a nurse practitioner in an inner city pediatric clinic. After examining a child with strep throat, she prescribed an antibiotic for her. She instructed the mother to give the child the medication four times a day, and to store it in the refrigerator between doses.

She asked the mother if she had any questions or concerns, and the mother indicated she did not have any. But as the mother and child were leaving the exam room, the mother turned to the nurse practitioner and said, "You know, we don't have a refrigerator. Will anything happen if I don't refrigerate the antibiotic?" If you were the nurse in this situation, how would you respond to this client? What supports would you suggest?

Health promotion and disease prevention strategies help people to recognize health problems and support them in choosing the most effective ways to self-manage their symptoms in the community. In many instances, clients presenting with physical complaints in primary care have an underlying mental disorder or substance abuse problem. Making it a practice to assess for mental problems and co-occurring disorders during intake with a few well-placed questions can help detect mental health issues or negative substance use.

Nurses use one-to-one counseling and community-based group education formats to meet educational health care objectives related to health promotion and maintenance of health, prevention of illness, restoration of health, coping with impaired functioning, and rehabilitation.

HEALTH PROMOTION STRATEGIES AT THE COMMUNITY LEVEL

At the community level, nurses help locate populations at risk for health problems. They can use case-finding strategies to recognize individuals and families with identified risk factors and to connect them with needed supports, resources, and services. Uncovering unhealthy physical and social environments or living circumstances can start within the formal health system during intake, or informally through liaisons with the justice system and schools.

Nurses can help design and provide health education, social marketing, and screening services to targeted populations with unrecognized health risk factors. They can instruct targeted populations about the nature of an illness, disability, or unhealthy environment, and the use of their medications. Nurses can identify what community supports are available, and/or how services can be obtained and how to access them. Examples include drug prevention and teenage pregnancy prevention programs, plus one-on-one coaching with step-by-step instructions on how to access critical supports.

COMMUNITY-BASED HEALTH PROMOTION STRATEGIES

Although health promotion strategies at the individual level are associated with improved health and well-being, health promotion is also a community concept. It is difficult to change attitudes and lifestyles to promote health when a client's social environment does not support these changes. Reducing generic environmental risks to maintaining health and well-being requires a community approach to health promotion.

Community is defined as "any group of citizens that have either a geographic, population-based, or self-defined relationship and whose health may be improved by a health promotion approach" (Frankish et al., 2006, p. 174). Equity and empowerment related to health care are the expected outcome of health promotion activities at the community level. Equity corresponds to the WHO directive that all people should have an equal opportunity to enjoy good health and well-being.

Empowerment at the community level recognizes the need for citizen participation in improving and promoting health. Community empowerment "seeks to enhance a community's ability to identify, mobilize, and address the issues that it faces to improve the overall health of the community (Yoo, Weed, & Lempa, 2004, p. 256).

Unless the community as a whole can collectively challenge and eradicate inequities in health care access and treatment provision, health promotion activities will fall short of their targeted goals (Messias, De Jong, & McLoughlin, 2005). Health promotion activities use a proactive approach to capture the attention of people who otherwise might not be predisposed to taking charge of their health and/or may not know that they are at risk.

Grass roots health promotion activities provided for "at-risk" populations are a community resource designed to influence personal lifestyle choices, coping skills, and health behaviors. They are designed to engage those people who are most involved with a common environmental concern related to health as active participants. Key health issues in economically disadvantaged communities often are those with social roots such as violence or abuse, substance abuse, teen pregnancies, and AIDS (Blumenthal, 2009). Socioenvironmental factors that affect health include income, education, health insurance, cultural health practices, social support, and accessibility of health services.

Successful health promotion programs require individuals, groups, and organizations to act as active agents in shaping health practices and policies that have meaning to the target population. Community-based health promotion activities must be grounded in a community analysis of health issues of concern, as identified by the community itself. They must begin with an engagement and buy-in of the community in which the activity is to take place. WHO notes that health promotion activities should be "carried out by and with people, not on, or to people" (Jakarta Declaration; WHO 1997). Active participation of individuals, communities, and systems means a stronger and more authentic commitment to the establishment of realistic regulatory, organizational, and sociopolitical supports needed to achieve targeted health outcomes (Kline & Huff, 2008).

USING THE PRECEDE-PROCEED MODEL IN COMMUNITY EDUCATION

Community education is an important component of health promotion and disease prevention. The precede-proceed community-based health education model that Green and Kreuter (2005) developed is based on two fundamental assumptions: (1) health and health risks are multidetermined, and (2) health teaching must be multidimensional and participatory to be effective.

The PRECEDE component of the health education model refers to the assessment and planning components of program planning. The acronym PRECEDE stands for Predisposing, Reinforcing, Enabling Causes in Educational Diagnosis and Evaluation factors associated with the targeted problem area. Examples of these diagnostic behavioral factors are presented in Table 15-3. Careful assessment of these factors provides direction for the type of program and content most likely to engage the interest of diverse learners in community-based settings. The PRECEDE assessment takes place as a part of the planning process before the educational program is offered. Nurses also determine population needs and establish evaluation methods before implementation. Evaluation is a continuous process that begins when the program is implemented, and is exercised throughout the educational experience.

The PROCEED component (Policy, Regulatory, Organizational Constructs in Educational and Environmental Development) was added to the model by

TABLE 15-3	PRECEDE-PROCEED Model: Examples of PRECEDE Diagnostic Behavioral Factors
Factors	**Examples**
Predisposing factors	Previous experience, knowledge, beliefs, and values that can affect the teaching process (e.g., culture and prior learning)
Enabling factors	Environmental factors that facilitate or present obstacles to change (e.g., transportation, scheduling, and availability of follow-up)
Reinforcing factors	Perceived positive or negative effects of adopting the new learned behaviors, including social support (e.g., family support, risk for recurrence, and avoidance of a health risk)

Green in the late 1980s. He realized that any viable educational model needed political, managerial, and administrative supports for full implementation of a community-based approach to health promotion and disease prevention. The utility of including the PRO-CEED component is that it explicitly considers critical environmental and cost variables such as budget, personnel, and critical organizational relationships as part of the planning process. Having the resources in place and assessing their sustainability is important in health promotion planning, though it is not always thought through in the planning phase. Bernard

(2006) also observes that, because health promotion and disease prevention activities do not generate the same level of revenue, they may not be as sustainable when resources become tight. Nurses can play an important role in advocating for public policies supporting sustainable access to appropriate health resources. The full PRECEDE-PROCEED model is presented in Table 15-4. Exercise 15-4 provides an opportunity to think about community health problems that could be addressed with the PRECEDE-PROCEED model in planning appropriate health promotion interventions.

TABLE 15-4	PRECEDE-PROCEED Model Definitions
Phase	**Definition**
PRECEDE Components	
1. Social diagnosis	People's perceptions of their own health needs, quality of life
2. Epidemiologic diagnosis	Determination of the extent, distribution, causes of health problem in target population
3. Behavioral and environmental diagnosis	Determination of specific health-related actions likely to affect problem (behavioral); systematic assessment of factors in the environment likely to influence health and quality-of-life outcomes (environmental)
4. Educational and organizational diagnosis	Assessment of all factors that must be changed to initiate or sustain desired behavioral changes and outcomes
5. Administrative and policy diagnosis	Analysis of organizational policies, resources, circumstances relevant to the development of the health program
PROCEED Components	
6. Implementation	Converting program objectives into actions taken at the organizational level
7. Process evaluation	Assessment of materials, personnel performance, quality of practice or services offered, and activity experiences
8. Impact evaluation	Assessment of program effects of intermediate objectives inclusive of all changes as a result of the training
9. Outcome evaluation	Assessment of the teaching program on the ultimate objectives related to changes in health, well-being, and quality of life

Adapted from Green L, Kreuter M: *Health program planning: an educational and ecological approach*, ed 4, New York, 2005, McGraw Hill.

| EXERCISE 15-4 | Analyzing Community Health Problems for Health Promotion Interventions |

Purpose: To develop an appreciation for the multidimensional elements of a community health problem.

Procedure:

In small groups of four to six students, brainstorm about health problems you believe exist in your community and develop a consensus about one public health problem that the group would prioritize as being most important.

Use the following questions to direct your thinking about developing health promotion activities for a health-related problem in your community.

What are the most pressing health problems in your community?

What are the underlying causes or contributing factors to this problem?

In what ways does the selected problem impact the health and well-being of the larger community?

What is the population of interest you would need to target for intervention?

What types of additional information would you need to have to propose a solution?

Who are the stakeholders, and how should they be involved?

What step would you recommend as an initial response to this health problem?

What is one step the nurse could take to increase awareness of this problem as a health promotion issue?

Discussion:

How hard was it for your group to arrive at a consensus about the most pressing problem? Were you surprised with any of the discussion that took place about this health problem? How could you use what you learned in doing this exercise in your nursing practice?

LEARNER VARIABLES IN EDUCATION FOR HEALTH PROMOTION

Pender's health promotion model serves as a guide for planning successful education with individuals and targeted high-risk groups. A person's capacity to absorb and use health promotion information depends to a large degree on what the person believes about his or her health, and the extent to which personal actions will influence their health. Nurses can use the health belief model to focus on behaviors that have the greatest potential to meet specific health needs. Examples of health promotion education topics can relate to sexual health; developing a healthy lifestyle through eating well, physical activity, and stress reduction; organizational wellness; parenting skills; and anger management.

Guidelines proposed by the U.S. Preventive Services Task Force for health-promoting education and counseling are presented in Box 15-2. As with all types of education and counseling, learners need to be actively engaged in goal setting and developing action plans that have meaning to them. Choosing the right strategies requires special attention to the learner's readiness, capabilities, and skills (see Chapter 16).

Ochieng (2006) contends that socioeconomic factors, level of education, age, and social networks are important contributors to understanding client preferences and working with clients to enable them to make the changes needed for a healthy lifestyle.

| BOX 15-2 | Strategies in Health Education and Counseling: Recommendations of the U.S. Preventive Services Task Force |

- Frame the teaching to match the client's perceptions.
- Fully inform clients of the purposes and expected outcomes of interventions, and when to expect these new effects.
- Suggest small changes and baby steps rather than large ones.
- Be specific.

- Add new behaviors rather than eliminating established behaviors whenever possible.
- Link new behaviors to old behaviors.
- Obtain explicit commitments from the client and client family support regarding actions.
- Refer clients to appropriate community resources.
- Use a combination of strategies to achieve outcomes.
- Monitor progress through follow-up contact.

Adapted from: U.S. Preventive Services Task Force: Guide to Clinical Preventive Services, 2nd ed. Baltimore: 1996, Williams and Wilkins, p. lxxvii-lxxx.

Clients requiring the same education program may demonstrate a wide range of learning, cognitive, experiential, and communication diversity, which may require adaption to maximize learning. Clients also will differ in their intellectual curiosity, learning preferences, motivation for learning, learning styles, and rate of learning.

Teaching and counseling initiatives related to health promotion need to be safe, timely, effective, client centered, equitable, and efficient. Health promotion programs should be designed to empower clients through an emphasis on the active role of the client as a stakeholder and inclusion in all aspects of the health promotion process.

Education and counseling for health promotion can include information on risk factors or behaviors impacting on health and ways to address negative social, economic, and environmental determinants of health. A health promotion format considers a person's personal values and beliefs about his or her ability to achieve health behavior changes (self-efficacy) as part of client assessment.

Evaluation of health promotion activities is essential. In addition to evaluating immediate program effects, longitudinal evaluation of the impact of health promotion activities on morbidity, mortality, and quality of life is desirable. Keep in mind that what constitutes quality of life is a subjective reality for each client and may differ from person to person (Fagerlind et al., 2010).

EMPOWERMENT STRATEGIES

There seems to be little question of a "direct relationship between an individual's level of health and the amount of perceived control the individual has in life situations" (Sheinfeld-Gorin & Arnold, 2006, p. 135). Empowering people to take the initiative with their own health and well-being is the cornerstone of health promotion and disease prevention strategies.

Information to empower clients in learning about healthy lifestyles, treatment, and potential side effects is readily available through the Internet (Coward, 2006). For many illnesses and health problems, clients and families can find specific information, regardless of the stage of their illness. Online support groups, chat rooms, and sharing of patient and family stories provide additional social support and practical learning tips for people who live in areas that are not geographically convenient to person-to-person contact. In the community, support groups are available for a wide variety of diagnoses. If the client or family does not use the Internet, flyers, fact sheets, and direct dialogue with opportunity for questions and follow-up can be helpful.

Active involvement of the learner enhances learning. Most people learn best when they engage more than one sense in the learning process and have an opportunity to practice essential skills. A highly participatory learning format, one that encourages different ways of thinking and opportunities to try out new behaviors, is far more effective than giving simple instructions to a client or family, or demonstration without teach back feedback (Willison, Mitmaker, & Andrews, 2005).

Case Example

Soon Mrs. Hixon began learning how to dress herself. At first she took an hour to complete this task. But with guidance and practice, she eventually dressed herself in 25 minutes. Even so, I practically had to sit on my hands as I watched her struggle. I could have done it so much faster for her, but she had to learn, and I had to let her (Collier, 1992, p. 63).

Strategies should demonstrate a sensitive appraisal and choice of targeted strategies, matched to the relevant needs of the individual, family, or group. When time is short, you will need to focus on the health teaching that addresses the most pressing of health needs. Many of the teaching learning strategies presented in Chapter 16 can be used or modified for health promotion health teaching. Exercise 15-5 provides an opportunity to use Maslow's theory in structuring health promotion activities.

Community Empowerment

Social and political action to enhance health services can augment educational efforts using a PRECEDE-PROCEED framework at the community level. Community empowerment strategies are used to help identify and address environmental and social issues needed to improve the overall health of the community.

Empowerment at the community level is sometimes referred to as "capacity building." Community-focused empowerment strategies build on the personal strengths, community resources, and problem-solving capabilities already existing in individuals and communities that can be used to address potential and actual health problems (Leddy, 2005). Capacity building

| EXERCISE 15-5 | Applying Maslow's Theory to Learning Readiness |

Purpose: To develop skill in facilitating learning readiness.

Procedure:
Students will break into four groups and receive a case scenario that depicts a client learning need. Using Maslow's hierarchy of needs, prioritize the client's needs and plan your teaching approach based on the client's current level. Include in your plan the supportive measures that would be necessary to foster readiness to learn.

Discussion:
Each group will present their case and plan. Discuss how the use of Maslow's hierarchy can be effective in addressing learning needs and determining nursing approach. Discuss factors that contribute to resistance to learning and noncompliance. Discuss the supportive measures that nurses must include as part of the learning process with clients.

requires the inclusion of informal and formal community leaders as valued stakeholders. Networking, partnering, and creating joint ventures with indigenous and local religious infrastructures is a powerful consensus building strategy needed for effective health promotional education planning and implementation. Box 15-3 outlines a process for engaging the community in health promotion activities.

Health Literacy

Parker, Ratzan, and Lurie (2003) define **health literacy** as "the degree to which people have the capacity to obtain, process, and understand basic health information and services needed to make appropriate health decisions" (p. 194). Approximately 21% of U.S. adults would be classified as functionally illiterate, which means they read at or below a ninth grade level and would have trouble comprehending written instructions on medication bottles, negotiating the health care system, and fully understanding consent forms (Davis et al., 1998). Health literacy can be further compromised with visual or auditory impairment, or diminished mental alertness, acute illness, limited education, and cultural differences. Health literacy is

| BOX 15-3 | Guiding Principles for Community Engagement |

Before starting a community engagement effort:
- Be clear about the purposes or goals of the engagement effort and the populations and/or communities you want to engage.
- Become knowledgeable about the community in terms of its economic conditions, political structures, norms and values, demographic trends, history, and experience with engagement efforts. Learn about the community's perceptions of those initiating the engagement activities.

For engagement to occur, it is necessary to:
- Go into the community, establish relationships, build trust, work with the formal and informal leadership, and seek commitment from community organizations and leaders to create processes for mobilizing the community.
- Remember and accept that community self-determination is the responsibility and right of all people who make up a community. No external entity should assume it can bestow to a community the power to act in its own self-interest.

For engagement to succeed:
- Partnering with the community is necessary to create change and improve health.
- All aspects of community engagement must recognize and respect community diversity. Awareness of the various cultures of a community and other factors of diversity must be paramount in designing and implementing community engagement approaches.
- Community engagement can be sustained only by identifying and mobilizing community assets, and by developing capacities and resources for community health decisions and action.
- An engaging organization or individual change agent must be prepared to release control of actions or interventions to the community, and be flexible enough to meet the changing needs of the community.
- Community collaboration requires long-term commitment by the engaging organization and its partners.

From CDC/ATSDR Committee on Community Engagement: *Principles of community engagement,* Atlanta, 1997, Centers for Disease Control and Prevention Program Office; available online: http://www.cdc.gov/phppo/pce/part3.htm. Accessed, July 28, 2010.

more than the capacity to read. It also includes medical knowledge, system navigational skills and initiative (Dewalt & Pignone, 2005).

Low health literacy is associated with medication nonadherence, increased incidence of side effects, and inadequate understanding of the impact of a medication on health outcomes (Ownby, 2006). People with inadequate health literacy tend to have worse health status, and functional physical and mental health. They also are less likely to seek preventive health care (Baker et al., 2002; Cutilli, 2007).

Low health literacy is not the same as having below average intelligence. People with inadequate health literacy may be highly intelligent, but functionally unable to fully grasp medical terminology. People with English as a second language can exhibit a much lower level of functional health literacy that is directly attributable to language limitations. Others demonstrate a lower level of functional literacy related to limited education or learning disabilities.

A persistent stigma about low literacy and learning disabilities exists even though it is unfounded. For this reason, many people try to hide the fact that they cannot read or do not know the meaning of complex words. They feel ashamed, so they fake their inability to understand by appearing to agree with the nurse educator, by saying they will read the instructions later, or by not asking questions. Functional illiteracy influences the type of questions a client might ask of a health professional and the adequacy of their descriptions about their illness or disability. Some of the problems clients with low literacy skills have in accessing health information include the following:

- Taking instructions literally
- Having a limited ability to generalize information to new situations
- Decoding one word at a time rather than reading a passage as a whole
- Skipping over uncommon or hard words
- Thinking in individual rather than categorical terms (Doak, Doak, & Root, 1996)

Educationally disadvantaged or functionally illiterate people are interested in learning, but nurses should adapt teaching situations to accommodate literacy learning differences. Marks (2009) suggests having written materials modified to six- to eighth-grade reading levels, and providing lists of key instructions for use after visits.

Using symbols and images with which the client is familiar helps overcome the barriers of low literacy. Taking the time to understand the client's use of words and phrases provides the nurse with concrete words and ideas that can be used as building blocks in helping the client understand difficult health-related concepts. Otherwise, the client may misunderstand what the nurse is saying.

Case Example

The discharge nurse said to a new mother, "Now you know to watch the baby's stools to be sure they're normal. You do know what normal stools look like, don't you?" The mother replied, "Oh, yeah, sure...I've got four of them in my kitchen" (Doak, Doak, & Root, 1985).

Safeer and Keenan (2005) suggest that clients can understand medical information better when a small amount of information is presented slowly, in easily understood everyday words. . Box 15-4 identifies guidelines for teaching low-literacy clients. Nurses should keep instructions as simple as possible, presenting ideas in an uncomplicated, step-by-step format. Advance organizers help low-literacy clients remember important concepts (see Chapter 16). Familiar words supplemented by common related pictures provide an extrasensory input for the client and improve retention. Drawings, diagrams, and photographs provide additional cues, allowing the client to understand meanings he or she would be unable to grasp through words alone.

BOX 15-4	Guidelines for Teaching Low-Literacy Clients

- Teach the smallest amount necessary to do the job for each session.
- Sequence key behavior information first.
- Use common concrete words and short sentences
- Make your point as vividly as you can (e.g., use visual aids and examples for emphasis).
- Incorporate as many senses as possible in the learning process.
- Break complex tasks into smaller sub-tasks that the client will find easy to achieve.
- Include interaction; have the client restate and demonstrate the information.
- Review repeatedly.

Adapted from Doak CC, Doak LG, Root JH, editors: *Teaching patients with low literacy skills*, ed 2, Philadelphia, 1996, JB Lippincott.

Use common concrete words rather than abstract or medical terminology and examples, for example, "Call the doctor on Monday if you still have pain or swelling in your knee." In addition to using simple words and literal interpretations, the nurse should use the same words to describe the same thing. For example, if you use "insulin" in one instance and "medicine" or "drug" later to describe the same medication, the client may become confused. The same instructions, written exactly as they were spoken, act as a reminder once the person leaves the actual teaching situation.

Sequence the content logically beginning with a core concept. Remember that the client with low health literacy may not be able to read or interpret the label instructions on the bottle. You can use the following question sequence to teach a client about taking a new medication.

- What do I take?
- How much do I take?
- When do I take it?
- What will it do for me?
- What do I do if I get a side effect?

Apply simple concrete common words such as "You should take your medicine with your meals," or "Call your doctor if you have stomach pain." Teach a little at a time. Select small, related pieces of data and structure them into informational chunks so that the client can remember the information through association, even if one fact is forgotten.

Whenever possible, link new information and tasks with what the client already knows. This strategy builds on previous knowledge and reinforces self-efficacy in mastering new concepts. Keeping sentences short and precise, and using active verbs helps clients understand what is being taught. When technical words are necessary for clients to communicate about their condition with other health professionals, clients may need direct instruction or coaching about appropriate words to use. Table 15-5 presents core constructs of health literacy.

Developmental Level

Developmental level affects both teaching strategies and subject content. You will find that clients are at all levels of the learning spectrum with regard to their social, emotional, and cognitive development. Developmental learning capacity is not always age related. It is easily influenced by culture and stress. Social and emotional development does not always parallel cognitive maturity. Mirroring the client's communication style and framing messages that reflect developmental characteristics helps improve comprehension and understanding. Parents can provide useful information about their child's immediate life experiences and commonly used words to incorporate in health teaching.

Culture

Culture adds to the complexity of health promotion strategies in health care. Values, norms, and beliefs are an integral part of a person and heavily influence collective community lifestyles (See Chapter 11). Culture helps explain assumptions about health and illness, the causes of and treatments for different types of illnesses, and traditionally accepted health actions or practices to prevent or treat illness. Incorporating health-related cultural beliefs in health teaching promotes better acceptance.

TABLE 15-5	Core Constructs of Health Literacy
I. Basic Literacy or Comprehension	Reading information, appointment cards
	Interpreting medical tests, dosages, and instructions, side effects, contraindications
	Understanding brochures, medication labels, informed consent, insurance documents
II. Interactive and Participatory Literacy (able to engage in two way Interactions)	Provision of appropriate and usable information Comprehension and ability to carry out information Mutual decision making Remembering and carrying out information
III. Critical literacy	Ability to weigh critical scientific facts Capacity to assess competing treatment options

Adapted from Marks R: Ethics and patient education: Health literacy and cultural dilemmas, *Health Promot Pract* 10(3):328–332, 2009.

In many cultures, the family assumes a primary role in the care of the client even when the client is physically and emotionally capable of self-care. All parties needing information, especially those expected to support the learning process of the client, should be included from the outset in all aspects of health teaching for health promotion. "Empowering ethnocultural communities through informal care may be the most culturally appropriate approach for improving the health status of ethnocultural populations" (Chiu, Balneaves, & Barroetavena 2006, p. 3)

Client motivation and participation increase with the use of indigenous teachers and cultural recognition of learning needs. If health literacy is related to language, qualified interpreters should be used for translation and preparation of written materials.

The culturally sensitive nurse develops knowledge of the preferred communication style of different cultural groups and uses this knowledge in choosing teaching strategies. For example, Native Americans like stories. Their tradition of telling stories orally is a primary means of teaching that the nurse can use as a teaching methodology for health promotion purposes.

Self-Awareness

Nurses have an ethical and legal responsibility in health teaching to maintain the appropriate expertise and interpersonal sensitivity to client needs required for effective learning. It is easy enough to remain engaged and to provide interesting teaching formats for the self-directed, highly motivated learner. It takes much more energy and imagination to impart hope to clients and to stimulate their emotions and interest when they see little reason to participate in learning about lifestyle changes and self-care management. Although the nurse is responsible for the quality of health teaching, only the client can assure the outcome. At all times, the nurse respects the client's autonomy. Some clients want symptom relief, whereas others want more in-depth teaching. Nurses have an ethical responsibility to provide appropriate health teaching and the right to hope that if the information is not used now, perhaps later it will be.

SUMMARY

This chapter focuses on health promotion as the basis for health education that can be applied at all practice levels. The WHO describes health promotion as a process of enabling people to increase control over and improve their health. Optimal health and well-being are considered the desired outcomes of health promotion activities. A health promotion/disease prevention focus views the client as an informed consumer and a valued partner in health care. Theory models relevant to health promotion include Pender's health promotion model, Prochaska's transtheoretical model, Miller's MI, and Bandura's social learning theory.

Learner variables important to the success of health promotion activities can be categorized as readiness to learn and ability to learn. Physical factors, level of anxiety, level of social support, active involvement of the learner, and inclusion of family members are identified as elements of readiness to learn. Lack of appropriate supports, physical barriers, health literacy, culture, and developmental status are factors that may influence the client's ability to learn.

Nurses participate routinely in community health promotion and disease prevention activities. They have an ethical and legal responsibility in health teaching to maintain the appropriate expertise and interpersonal sensitivity to client needs required for effective learning.

ETHICAL DILEMMA What Would You Do?

Jack Marks is a 16-year-old boy who comes to the clinic complaining of symptoms of a sexually transmitted disease (STD). He receives antibiotics, and you give him information about safe sex and preventing STDs. Two months later, he returns to the clinic with similar symptoms. It is clear that he has not followed instructions and has no intention of doing so. He tells you he's a regular jock and just can't get used to the idea of condoms. He really can't tell you the names of his partners—there are just too many of them. What are your ethical responsibilities as his nurse in caring for Jack?

REFERENCES

American Association of Colleges of Nursing: *The essentials of baccalaureate education for professional nursing practice*, 2008, Washington DC, Author.

Bandura A: *Self-efficacy: the exercise of control*, New York, 1997, WH Freeman.

Baker DW, Gazmararian JA, Williams MV, et al: Functional health literacy and the risk of hospital admission among medicare managed care enrollees, *Am J Public Health* 92(8):1278–1283, 2002.

Beckford-Ball J: The essence of care benchmark for patient health promotion, *Nurs Times* 102(14):23–24, 2006.

Bernard M: Health promotion/disease prevention: tempering the giant geriatric tsunami, *Geriatrics* 61(2):5–7, 2006.

Blumenthal DS: Clinical community health: revisiting "the community as patient, *Educ Health* 22(2):1–8, 2009. available online http://www.educationforhealth.net.

Brainy Quotes: Frederick Douglas, : available online http://www.brainyquote.com/quotes/quotes/f/frederickd201574.html Accessed, August 2, 2010.

Carels R, Darby L, Cacciapaglia H, et al: Using motivational interviewing as a supplement to obesity treatment: a stepped-care approach, *Health Psychol* 26(3):369–374, 2007.

Centers for Disease Control: CDC: our story, (2006): available online http://www.cdc.gov/about/ourstory.htm.

Chapman L, Lesch N, Aitken S: *WELCOA Special report: Resilience*, Omaha NE, 2005, Wellness Councils of America www.welcoa.org/freeresources/pdf/resilience_case_study.pdf Accessed August 2, 2010.

Chiu L, Balneaves L, Barroetavena M, et al: Use of complementary and alternative medicine by Chinese individuals living with cancer in British Columbia, *J Compl Integr Med* 3(1):1–21, 2006.

Cody W: *Philosophical and theoretical perspectives for advanced practice nursing*, ed 4, Sudbury MA, 2006, Jones and Bartlett Publishers, pp 183–190.

Collier S: Mrs. Hixon was more than "the C.V.A. in 251, *Nursing* 22(5):62–64, 1992.

Committee on Assuring the Health of the Public in the 21st Century (Institute of Medicine): *The future of the public's health in the 21st century*, Washington, DC, 2003, National Academies Press.

Coward D: Supporting health promotion in adults with cancer, *Fam Community Health* 29(Suppl 1):S52–S60, 2006.

Cutilli C: Health literacy in geriatric patients: an integrative review of the literature, *Orthop Nurs* 26(1):43–48, 2007.

Daley L, Fish A, Frid D, Mitchell L: Stage specific education/counseling intervention in women with elevated blood pressure, *Prog Cardiovasc Nurs* 24(2):45–52, 2009.

Davis T, Michielutte R, Askov E, et al: Practical assessment of adult literacy in health care, *Health Educ Behav* 22(5):613–624, 1998.

Dewalt DK, Pignone M: The role of literacy in health and health care, *Am Fam Physician* 72(3):387–388, 2005.

DiClemente C, Schlundt B, Gemmell B: Readiness and stages of change in addiction treatment, *Am J Addict* 13(2):103–119, 2004.

Doak CC, Doak LG, Root JH: *Teaching patients with low literacy skills*, Philadelphia, 1985, JB Lippincott.

Doak CC, Doak LG, Root JH: *Teaching patients with low literacy skills*, ed 2, Philadelphia, 1996, JB Lippincott.

Edelman C, Mandel C: *Health promotion throughout the lifespan*, ed 4, St Louis, 1998, Mosby Year Book.

Edlin G, Golanty E: *Health and wellness*, ed 10, Sudbury, MA, 2009, Jones & Bartlett Publishers.

Fagerlind H, Ring L, Brulde B, Feltelius N, Lindblad A: Patients' understanding of the concepts of health and quality of life, *Patient Educ Couns* 78:104–110, 2010.

Frankish CJ, Moulton G, Rootman I, et al: Setting a foundation: underlying values and structures of health promotion in primary health care settings, *Prim Health Care Res Dev* 7:172–182, 2006.

Freedman R: Coping, resilience, and outcome, *Am J Psychiatry* 165(12):1505–1506, 2008.

Gance-Cleveland B: Motivational interviewing: improving patient education, *J Pediatr Health Care* 21:81–88, 2007.

Goodwin A, Bar B, Reid G, Ashford S: Knowledge of motivational interviewing, *J Holist Nurs* 27(3):203–209, 2009.

Green J: Health education—the case for rehabilitation, *Crit Public Health* 18(4):447–456, 2008.

Green L, Kreuter M: *Health program planning: an educational and ecological approach*, ed 4, New York, 2005, McGraw Hill.

Hoving C, Visser A, Mullen PD, van den Borne B: A history of patient education by health professionals in Europe and North America, *Patient Educ Couns* 78(3):275–281, 2010.

Institute of Medicine (IOM): *Crossing the quality chasm: A new health system for the 21st century*, Washington DC, 2001, National Academy Press.

Institute of Medicine (IOM): *Improving the quality of health care for mental and substance-use conditions: The quality chasm series*, Washington DC, 2006, National Academy Press.

Kirk A, Mutrie N, Macintyre P, Fisher M: Promoting and maintaining physical activity in people with type 2 diabetes, *Am J Prevent Med* 27:289–296, 2004.

Kline M, Huff R: *Health promotion in multicultural populations: a handbook for practitioners and students*, ed 2, Thousand Oaks, CA, 2008, Sage Publications.

Leddy S: *Integrative health promotion: conceptual bases for nursing practice*, Sudbury, MA, 2005, Jones and Bartlett Publishers.

Levensky E, Forcehimes A, O'Donohue W, Beitz K: Motivational interviewing: an evidence-based approach to counseling helps patients follow treatment recommendations, *Am J Nurs* 107(10):50–58, 2007.

Maltby H, Robinson S: The role of baccalaureate nursing students in the matrix of health promotion, *J Community Health Nurs* 15(3):135–142, 1998.

Markle-Reid M, Weir R, Browne G, et al: Health promotion for frail older home care clients, *J Adv Nurs* 54(3):381–395, 2006.

Marks R: Ethics and patient education: health literacy and cultural dilemmas, *Health Promot Pract* 10(3):328–332, 2009.

Messias D, De Jong M, McLoughlin K: Being involved and making a difference: empowerment and well-being among women living in poverty, *J Holist Nurs* 23(1):70–88, 2005.

Miller W: Values and motivational interviewing: a symposium, *Minuet* 11(3):19–20, 2004.

Miller W, Rollnick S: *Motivational interviewing: preparing people for change*, ed 2, New York, 2002, Guilford Press.

Milio N: A framework for prevention: changing health-damaging to health-generating life patterns, *Am J Public Health* 66:435–439, 1976.

Ochieng B: Factors affecting choice of a healthy lifestyle: implications for nurses, *Br J Community Nurs* 11(2):78–81, 2006.

Ownby L: Medication adherence and cognition: medical, personal and economic factors influence level of adherence in older adults, *Geriatrics* 61(2):30–35, 2006.

Parker R, Ratzan S, Lurie N: Health illiteracy: a policy challenge for advancing high-quality health care, *Health Aff* 22(4):147–153, 2003.

Pender N, Murdaugh C, Parsons M: *Health promotion in nursing practice*, ed 4, Upper Saddle River, NJ, 2006, Prentice Hall.

Prochaska J, DiClemente C, Norcross J: In search of how people change: applications to addictive behaviors, *Am Psychol* 47(9):1102–1114, 1992.

Redman B: *Patient self management of chronic disease: the health care provider's challenge*, Sudbury, MA, 2004, Jones and Bartlett Publishers.

Rollnick S, Miller W, Butler C: *Motivational interviewing in health care: helping patients change behavior*, New York, 2008, Guilford Press.

Safeer RS, Keenan J: Health literacy: the gap between physicians and patients, *Am Fam Physician* 72:463–468, 2005.

Sandelowski M, DeVellis B, Campbell M: Variations in meanings of the personal core value "health"*Patient Educ Couns* 73(2):347–353, 2008.

Saylor C: The circle of health: a health definition model, *J Holist Nurs* 22(2):98–115, 2004.

Schieveld J: On grief and despair versus resilience and personal growth in critical illness, *Intens Care Med* 35:779–780, 2009.

Sheinfeld-Gorin S, Arnold J: *Health promotion in practice*, San Francisco, CA, 2006, Josey Bass.

Srof B, Velsor-Friedrich B: Health promotion in adolescents: a review of Pender's health promotion model, *Nurs Sci Q* 19(4):366–373, 2006.

U.S. Department of Health and Human Services (HHS): *Healthy people 2010*, Washington, DC, 2000, U.S. Government Printing Office.

U.S. Department of Health and Human Services (HHS): Healthy people 2020, available at: www.healthypeople.gov/HP2020. Accessed April 18, 2010.

U.S. Preventive Services Task Force: *Guide to Clinical Preventive Services*, 2nd ed. Baltimore, 1996, Williams and Wilkins.

Willison K, Mitmaker L, Andrews G: Integrating complementary and alternative medicine with primary health care through public health

to improve chronic disease management, *J Complement Integr Med* 2(1):1–24, 2005.

World Health Organization: *Health promotion glossary, Geneva, Switzerland*, 1998, Author.

World Health Organization: *Jakarta declaration on leading health promotion into the 21st century*, 1997, available online <www.who.int/hpr/NPH/docs/jakarta_declaration_en.pdf> Accessed, October 3, 2009.

World Health Organization (WHO): *Ottawa Charter for Health Promotion: First International Conference on Health Promotion, Ottawa, Ontario, Canada, November 21, 1986, available online http://www.who.int/healthpromotion/conferences/previous/ottawa/en/ Accessed September 21, 2009.*

World Health Organization (WHO) and World Organization of Family Doctors (WONCA) (2008): *Integrating mental health into primary care: a global perspective*, Geneva, Switzerland, 2008, WHO Press.

Yoo S, Weed N, Lempa M, et al: Collaborative community empowerment: an illustration of a six-step process, *Health Promotion Pract* 5(3):256–265, 2004.

Zubialde J, Mold J, Eubank D: Outcomes that matter in chronic illness: a taxonomy informed by self-determination and adult-learning theory, *Fam Syst Health* 27(30):193–200, 2009.

CHAPTER 16

Health Teaching in the Nurse-Client Relationship

Elizabeth C. Arnold

OBJECTIVES

At the end of the chapter, the reader will be able to:

1. Define health teaching and client education.
2. Identify the domains of learning.
3. Discuss theoretical frameworks used in client-centered health teaching.
4. Apply the nursing process in health teaching.
5. Discuss health teaching applications in different settings.
6. Describe applications in different care settings.

This chapter focuses on specialized communication strategies for health teaching and client education. The chapter explores theories of teaching and learning as the basis for effective health teaching and client education. It describes instructional principles and strategies that nurses can use with clients and families to help them make sound judgments about their health, learn technical skills needed to self-manage chronic illness, and work effectively with community resources to maximize health and well-being.

BASIC CONCEPTS

DEFINITIONS

Taylor, Lillis, and Lemone (2005) define teaching as "a planned method or series of methods used to help someone learn" (p. 477). **Health teaching** is a specialized form of teaching, defined as a focused, creative, interpersonal nursing intervention in which the nurse provides information, emotional support, and health-related skills training. Although health teaching has many definitions,

most do not address the complexity of the teaching process in health care (Wellard, Turner, & Bethune, 1998). For example, the "learner" in a health care setting can be a client, the client's family, a caregiver, or a community. Whereas other teaching situations instruct learners having a similar level of education and knowledge, health-teaching formats must be designed to meet the diverse learning needs of individuals from different socioeconomic, educational, and experiential backgrounds. A highly educated client, a noncompliant client, and a low-literacy client with the same medical condition have similar content requirements for health teaching but may demonstrate very different learning needs.

Masters (2008) describes **client (patient) education** as a set of planned educational activities, resulting in changes in health-related behaviors and attitudes, as well as knowledge. Health teaching is a highly participatory process involving multilevel interventions, linked by a common goal of maximizing client health and well-being. Specific teaching strategies, the type of involvement of others, and the level of content will necessarily reflect each client's unique learning needs.

CONTEMPORARY CONTEXTS OF HEALTH TEACHING

The context of health teaching shapes how knowledge is constructed and delivered. Although health teaching has always been an integral part of the nurse-client relationship, it is even more prominent in a managed-care health care delivery system with mandated limitations on time and resources (Greiner & Valiga, 1998). Nurses carry larger caseloads and generally have less time to spend with their clients. They must help clients achieve favorable health outcomes with fewer visits. This requires a stronger emphasis on helping clients to develop critical thinking skills, and encouragement of greater client responsibility for the self-care management of complex health problems. The realities of a managed health care environment requires a practical approach to health teaching with additional opportunities for critical questions specifically related to the situation.

An evolving paradigm shift in health care delivery from a medical hospital-based model of health care to a community-based, public health emphasis creates new learning conditions and challenges. Today's health care requirements mandate a broader content base for health teaching that includes primary prevention and quality-of-life issues (Ragland, 1997). Structured learning situations have yielded to a dynamic context-based format for health teaching, with a greater emphasis on the coaching components of health care teaching. Short, clear instructions, coupled with reflective prompts to elicit client feedback, create critical thinking opportunities.

Opportunities for health teaching occur can anywhere, for example, in the community, schools, parish nursing, the home, the hospital, and in clinics. Health teaching can be formal or informal. Ideally, it is a continuous process beginning in the community and extending across health care settings and systems. Even emergency departments provide opportunities for "teachable moments" for clients (Szpiro, Harrison, Van Den Kerkhof, & Lougheed, 2008).

Health teaching can take place under less-than-ideal circumstances. For many clients, the hospital or medical office is an anxiety-producing environment in which only part of what is said gets heard. Time constraints can limit the amount of material that can be covered in an individual session. Follow-up instructions or contacts, and written backup materials are useful adjuncts to onsite teaching. Physical and/or mental

symptoms, difficulty with concentration or memory, and hearing and vision loss can further compromise the ability of a client to receive or process information. Health teaching can occur during home visits as the nurse observes clients having specific difficulties with aspects of health care. Referred to as guided care, this type of on the spot health teaching is targeted to specific health issues as they appear (Doherty, 2009).

Health teaching formats range from informal one-to-one relationships, formal structured group sessions, and family conferences. The media provides health teaching guidelines related to primary prevention (e.g., safe sex and drug abuse prevention commercials) to targeted community groups.

Technology is rewriting virtually every form of education. Advances have expanded the depth and breadth of health information available to the health consumer and are an important resource for nurses. Telehealth formats work by telecasting health information through video or interactive computers. This type of health teaching is becoming increasingly important in rural areas, where distance precludes onsite nursing health teaching and support.

The Internet provides instant health information, with a wide range of learning resources to accommodate different levels of knowledge and learning styles. People can also learn from the experience of others with similar health conditions through chat rooms and blogs.

Information on the Internet is searchable, up to date, inexpensive to obtain, and accessible at any time of day. For example, the American Diabetes Association and the American Cancer Society have online tools to help clients understand their disease and related treatment options. Although the Internet is a powerful learning tool, it has limitations as an accurate information resource. Not all information is relevant or credible. Helping clients to interpret content as it applies to their health situation and to differentiate appropriate information from misinformation is a vital component of health teaching using this instructional modality.

PROFESSIONAL, LEGAL, AND ETHICAL MANDATES

Health teaching is not an option. It is a legal and ethical responsibility. The Joint Commission has established educational standards *requiring* health care agencies to provide systematic health education and training for clients that is:

- Specific to the client's needs
- Sufficient for clients to make informed decisions and to take responsibility for self-management activities related to their needs
- Provided to clients in an understandable manner, and designed to accommodate various learning styles
- Reflected in documented evidence of the client's understanding and response to the medical information

Professional nursing standards, developed by the American Nurses Association (ANA), reinforce the importance of health teaching as an essential nursing intervention (ANA, 2004). State Nurse Practice Acts mandate health teaching as an independent professional nursing function. Medicare requirements portray health teaching as a skilled nursing intervention for reimbursement purposes. The ANA Credentialing Center's Magnet Recognition Program (2005) devotes an entire section to the role of the nurse related to client education. Educating clients about their health conditions and treatment options is a legal and ethical responsibility of the nurse related to informed consent.

DOMAINS OF LEARNING

Health teaching is a dynamic process that involves making relevant connections to meaning within three domains initially described by Benjamin Bloom as *cognitive* (understanding content), *affective* (changing attitudes and promoting acceptance), and *psychomotor* (hands-on skill development). The domains are interrelated. When people learn about and practice a skill, they also develop "cognitive knowledge" about the factors that contribute to its success. As they become more proficient in performing a skill, people accept and value the skill and knowledge. Bloom's taxonomy describes a hierarchy of learning objectives ranging from the least to the most complex that are applicable to learning in each domain.

The **cognitive domain** is the focus when the client has a knowledge deficit. For example, objectives in the cognitive domain for a client with a recent diagnosis of diabetes would include understanding the disease; the role of diet, exercise, and insulin in diabetic control; and trouble signs that would require immediate attention. Learning outcomes would consist of having a basic understanding of the disease process and

treatment protocols, and being able to apply new information to meet personal health needs. A certain level of cognitive knowledge is an essential prerequisite for learning in the affective and psychomotor domains.

The information clients and families need related to informed consent falls into the cognitive domain. **Cognitive learning** formats allow for clarification of information and correction of misinformation that may have been received from other providers, family, friends, or the Internet.

Appealing to the cognitive domain, the nurse would provide concrete explicit information verbally, in writing, and/or with related pictures to explain the desired outcome and steps needed to achieve it. . Avoid the use of general abstract terms. "You must lose 7 pounds" is better that "you must lose weight" (Redman, 2007, p. 14).

Bloom's levels of knowledge acquisition (in ascending order) were revised in the 21st century to represent verbs rather than nouns. The hierarchy of synthesis and evaluation was reversed. The revised Bloom's taxonomy for the cognitive domain now consists of:

- Knowledge ➡ Remembering: recognizing, recalling information and facts
- Comprehension ➡ Understanding: interpreting, explaining, or constructing meaning
- Application ➡ Applying: carrying out or executing a procedure; using information in a new way
- Analysis ➡ Analyzing: considering constituent parts and how they relate to each other, and the whole
- Evaluation ➡ Evaluating: making judgments, critiquing, prioritizing, selecting, verifying
- Synthesis ➡ Creating: putting material together in a coherent whole, reorganizing material into a new pattern, creating something new (Anderson & Krathwohl, 2001)

The **affective domain** is concerned with emotional attitudes related to acceptance, compliance, valuing, and taking personal responsibility. Affective learning is essential when the client has issues that interfere with compliance or has reservations about treatment or self-efficacy. Health teaching targeted at the affective domain is more complex because of its association with values and beliefs. It usually takes longer than learning in the cognitive domain (Leahy & Kizilay, 1998).

Case Example

Jack cognitively understands that adhering to his diabetic diet is essential to control of his diabetes. He can tell you everything there is to know about the relationship of diet to diabetic control. Although he follows his diet at home, he eats snack foods at work and insists on extra helpings at dinner. His problem with compliance lies in the affective domain, because he resents having a lifelong condition that limits his food selections. Desired outcomes for Jack's learning in the affective domain include his accepting responsibility for treatment compliance despite his reservations. The nurse will need to allow him time to vent his frustration and help him figure out ways to cope with a chronic illness in less self-destructive ways. If you were Jack's nurse, what health teaching strategies could you use to help him become more comfortable with the changes he needs to make to promote his health and well-being?

BOX 16-1	Characteristics of Different Learning Styles

Visual
- Learns best by seeing
- Likes to watch demonstrations
- Organizes thoughts by writing them down
- Needs detail
- Looks around; examines situation

Auditory
- Learns best with verbal instructions
- Likes to talk things through
- Detail is not as important
- Talks about situation and pros and cons

Kinetic
- Learns best by doing
- Hands-on involvement
- Needs action and likes to touch, feel
- Loses interest with detailed instructions
- Tries things out

The **psychomotor domain** refers to learning a skill through *hands-on practice*. Performance learning promotes greater understanding than reading or hearing about a skill and is more likely to be remembered. Many skills required for effective self-care management require hands-on training, and supervised practice of a skill is one of the best ways for the nurse to evaluate the client's mastery of essential skills required for self-care management. Usually psychomotor learning involves demonstration of the skill by the nurse, followed by the client's return demonstration. Desired outcomes relate to proficiency in performing the motor skill, developing personal confidence, and the ability to adjust the performance of the skill when challenged with new situations.

Another factor to consider is how people learn best. Box 16-1 presents characteristics of different learning styles.

THEORETICAL FRAMEWORKS

CLIENT-CENTERED HEALTH TEACHING

Carl Rogers' (1983) ideas provide a theoretical foundation for the use of teaching methodologies in client-centered health teaching. Rogers emphasizes the primacy of the teacher-learner relationship as the means through which learning occurs. He describes learner-centered teaching as an interactive process. Applied to health care, a learner-centered approach involves engaging clients as active partners in the learning process and helping them take responsibility for their own learning, to whatever extent is possible. Rogers insists that the teacher must start where the learner is, structuring the learning process to support the learner's natural desire to learn, and being mindful of learner characteristics that enable or impede the process.

The same conditions of unconditional positive regard related to empathy, authenticity, and respect that are required for a successful therapeutic relationship apply to health teaching. Through a teaching relationship, clients begin to challenge old, unworkable ideas and habits; transform unproductive understandings and actions; and act on new perspectives (Hansen & Fisher, 1998).

Client-centered strategies place the learner in charge of his or her learning and build on personal strengths to achieve learning objectives. A highly participative learning environment, in which the nurse provides the teaching while the learner assumes primary responsibility for the learning process, encourages empowerment (Post-White, 1998). Empowerment strategies include providing sufficient information, specific instructions, and emotional support—but no more than is required—to allow each client to take charge of his or her health care to whatever extent is possible. The following case example illustrates the impact of a client-centered teaching encounter on a client.

Case Example

There was Nadine, who was an excellent preoperative teacher. She was the first person who clearly explained what a bladder augmentation entailed. She described different tubes I'd have and the purpose of each. When I returned from surgery, she helped me cope with my body image by teaching me how to use my bladder and by being a compassionate listener (Manning, 1992, p. 47).

Providing health information in unambiguous, concrete, objective terms using the client's terminology allows the client to integrate the health teaching in his or her unique way.

ANDRAGOGY AND PEDAGOGY

Andragogy refers to the "art and science of helping adults learn" (Knowles, Holton & Swanson, 1998). According to Knowles, who applied the term andragogy to adult learning, adult learners are self-directed and goal oriented. The adult's orientation to learning is practical and action oriented. Adult learners want to see the practicality of what they are learning. They favor a problem-focused approach to learning, and learn best when directly engaged in learning the skills and knowledge to help them master immediate life problems. The adult client learner expects the nurse to inquire about previous life experience and to incorporate this knowledge into the teaching plan. Figure 16-1 identifies Knowles' model of adult learning.

Pedagogy refers to the processes used to help children learn. A key difference between pedagogy and andragogy is the need to provide the child learner with additional direct guidance and structure in learning content. Children come to the learning experience with far less life experience that can be tapped as resources for learning. Recommended teaching strategies for learners at different developmental levels are presented in Table 16-1.

BEHAVIORAL MODELS

Behavioral approaches are based on the theoretical framework of B. F. Skinner (1971). He believed that behavior is learned, and that it is possible to change behavior by altering the predictable consequence or response to the behavior. Behavioral approaches use a structured learning format in which learning occurs by linking a desired behavior with reinforcement for performing the behavior. Behavior modification is used to teach people skills, to get children to assume a responsibility, and to curb or break an undesired behavior or habit.

Reinforcement, which refers to the consequences of performing targeted behaviors, is a central concept. Behaviorists believe that reinforcement strengthens learner responses. Behaviors that are rewarded (positive reinforcement) tend to be repeated. Ignored behaviors tend to diminish or disappear (extinction). When undesired behaviors are penalized, by having a reward removed or by a negative consequence, they tend to decrease. Different types of reinforcement with examples are found in Table 16-2. Research demonstrates that positive reinforcement produces the best results. As a person begins to routinely do desired behaviors, material or tangible rewards are gradually replaced with social reinforcement such as praise.

Reinforcement schedules refer to the timing of rewards. Schedules are identified as being continuous with rewards given for each success or interval schedules in which the reward is not given for each performance; instead, the reinforcement is given after a certain number of successful attempts (fixed interval) or after a random number of responses (variable ratio).

Selecting rewards (reinforcers) that have meaning to the learner is critical because what is reinforcing to one person may not be so for another. Referred to as the **Premack principle**, the choice of reinforcer should always be something of value to the individual learner. Initially, reinforcement is given immediately after each successful performance. Once a behavioral outcome is achieved, new content is introduced and rewards are distributed less frequently. Variable ratio reinforcement schedules are the most effective for maintaining behaviors.

Behavioral Strategies

Modeling is a behavioral strategy that describes learning by observing another person performing a behavior. Nurses model behaviors both unconsciously and consciously in their normal conduct of nursing activities and teaching situations. Bathing an infant, feeding an older person, and talking to a scared child in front of significant caregivers provide opportunities for informal teaching through modeling behaviors.

Shaping refers to the reinforcement of successive approximations of the target behavior. The long-term goal is broken down into smaller steps. The person is

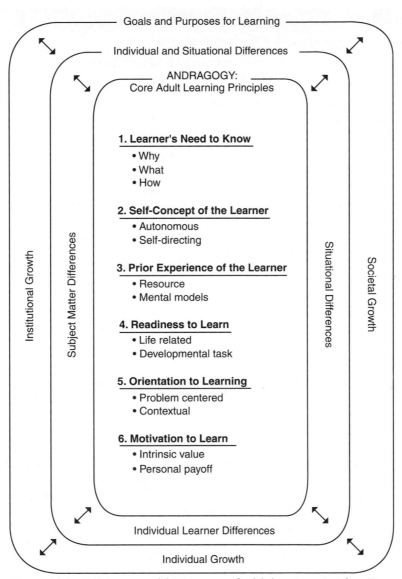

Figure 16-1 **Andragogy model: a core set of adult learning principles.** *(From Knowles M, Holton E, Swanson R: The adult learner: the definitive classic on adult education and training (p. 182), Terre Haute, IL, 1998, Butterworth-Heinemann.)*

reinforced for any behavior that gets him or her closer to accomplishing the desired behavior. Rewarding specific behaviors that move the person in the direction of the desired behavior (successive approximations) motivates the person to engage in the desired behavior. Steps build one upon the other, moving learners from the familiar to the unfamiliar as they progress toward meeting treatment goals.

Chaining refers to linking single behaviors together in a series of steps leading to the targeted desired behavior, for example, having a client with diabetes draw up insulin in the syringe. Once this task is mastered, the client can be instructed to inject an orange, followed by learning body sites for injection, and finally to inject the medication into identified sites. Prompts are faded as the single action tasks are mastered.

TABLE 16-1	Recommended Teaching Strategies at Different Development Levels

Developmental Level	Recommended Teaching Strategies
Preschool	Allow child to touch and play with safe equipment. Relate teaching to child's immediate experience. Use child's vocabulary whenever possible. Involve parents in teaching.
School-age	Give factual information in simple, concrete terms. Focus teaching on developing competency. Use simple drawings and models to emphasize points. Answer questions honestly and factually.
Adolescent	Use metaphors and analogies in teaching. Give choices and multiple perspectives. Incorporate the client's norm group values and personal identity issues in teaching strategies.
Adult	Involve client as an active partner in learning process. Encourage self-directed learning. Keep content and strategies relevant and practical. Incorporate previous life experience into teaching.
Elderly	Explain why the information should be important to the client. Incorporate previous life experience into teaching. Accommodate for sensory and dexterity deficits. Use short, frequent learning sessions (<1 hour).

TABLE 16-2	Types of Reinforcement

Concept	Purpose	Example
Positive reinforcer	Increases probability of behavior through reward	Stars on a board, smiling, verbal praise, candy, tokens to "purchase" items
Negative reinforcer	Increases probability of behavior by removing aversive consequence	Restoring privileges when client performs desired behavior
Punishment	Decreases behavior by presenting a negative consequence or removing a positive one	Time-outs, denial of privileges
Ignoring	Decreases behavior by not reinforcing it	Not paying attention to whining, tantrums, or provocative behaviors

Implementing a Behavioral Approach

A behavioral approach starts with a careful description and quantification of a concrete behavior requiring change. Describe each action as a single behavioral unit (e.g., failing to take a medication, cheating on a diet, or not participating in unit activities). It is important to start small so the client will experience success. Counting the number of times the client engages in a behavior as a baseline before implementing the behavioral approach allows the nurse and the client to monitor progress.

The next step in the process is to define the problem in behavioral terms and to validate the problem statement with the client (e.g., "The client does not take his medication as prescribed," or "The client does not attend any unit activities."). A behavioral approach requires the cooperation of the client and a mutual understanding of the problem on the part of the nurse and the client. Active listening skills can alert the nurse to any concerns or barriers to implementation.

Next, the nurse and client reframe the problem as a solution statement (e.g., "The client will attend all scheduled unit activities."). If the problem and solution are complex, you can break them down into simpler definitions, beginning with the simplest and most likely behavior to stimulate client interest. Identify the tasks in sequential order; define specific consequences, positive and negative, for behavioral responses; and solicit the client's cooperation.

Once these data are complete, the next step is to establish a learning contract with the client that serves as a formal commitment to the learning process. Contracts spell out the responsibilities of each party and the consequences if positive behaviors are completed or, in the case of undesired behaviors, negative consequences if behaviors persist. The contract should include:

- Behavioral changes that are to occur
- Conditions under which they are to occur
- Reinforcement schedule
- Time frame

Initially, each instance of expected behavior should be rewarded. If the client is noncompliant or needs to pay more attention to a particular aspect of behavior, the nurse can say, "This *(name the behavior or skill)* needs a little more work." One advantage of a behavioral approach is that it never considers the client as bad or unworthy.

Case Example

Peggy Braddock, a student nurse, was working with a seriously mentally ill client with diabetes. All types of strategies were used to help the client take responsibility for collecting and testing her urine. Regardless of whether she was punished or pushed into performing these activities, the client remained resistant. To avoid taking insulin injections, this client would take urine from the toilets or would simply refuse to produce a urine sample. Peggy decided to use a behavioral approach with her. She observed that the client liked sweets. Consequently, the reward she chose was artificially sweetened Jell-O cubes. To earn a Jell-O cube, the client had to bring her urine to Peggy. After some initial testing of Peggy's resolve to give the cubes only for appropriate behavior, the client began bringing her urine on a regular basis. Once this behavior was firmly established, Peggy began to teach the client how to give her own insulin. The reward remained the same, except that now the client received praise for what she had accomplished to date, and she had to achieve more complex tasks to receive the reward. Peggy used the time she spent with the client to build trust and acceptance. She became the client's coach and supporter. She wrote her plan in the Kardex, so other nurses could use the same approach with the client. Over time, this client took full responsibility for testing her urine and administering her own insulin. The intervention also increased the client's sense of independence and self-esteem.

Exercise 16-1 provides practice with a behavioral learning approach.

Developing an Evidence-Based Practice

Ruffolo M, Kuhn M, Evans M: Support, empowerment and education: a study of multiple family group psychoeducation, *J Emot Behav Disord* 13(4):200–212, 2005.

This quasi-experimental study was designed to evaluate a multiple family group psychoeducation intervention (MFGPI) for parents and primary caregivers of children with serious emotional disturbance who were enrolled in a community-based case management program. Parents and primary caregivers (N = 94) were randomly assigned to one of two treatment conditions (intensive case management plus adjunctive MFGPI or the usual treatment of intensive case management). Parent problem-solving skills, parental coping skills, perceived social support resources, and child behavior were measured initially, at 9 months, and at 18 months.

Results: At the 9-month measurement point, parents and primary caregivers in the treatment group reported significantly more people in their lives to turn to for help and significantly more coping resources. There were no significant differences between the two groups at the 18-month marker. The children in both groups demonstrated behavioral improvements, leading the authors to draw the conclusion that the parental involvement in both the case management and teaching sessions and the social support received was the most important element in behavioral change.

Application to Your Clinical Practice: As a profession, nurses need to develop effective strategies for involving parents and caregivers in the care of their children. How could you incorporate support and education as a way of empowering the clients that you see in your clinical practice?

APPLICATIONS

APPLYING THE NURSING PROCESS IN HEALTH TEACHING

Patient education consists of clinical teaching, which is provided in all clinical settings and health education, which focuses on wellness, health promotion and disease prevention (Dreeben, 2010). As people assume greater responsibility for managing their own health, client and health education become increasingly important as a vital nursing function, Nurses assume different roles in health teaching. Depending on the situation

| EXERCISE 16-1 | Using a Behavioral Approach |

Purpose: To help students gain an appreciation of the behavioral approach in the learning process.

Procedure:
Think about a relationship you have with one or more people that you would like to improve. The person you choose may be a friend, teacher, supervisor, peer worker, parent, or sibling.
1. Set a goal for improving that relationship.
2. Develop a problem statement as the basis for establishing your goal.
3. Identify the behaviors that will indicate you have achieved your goal.
4. Identify the specific behaviors you will have to perform to accomplish your goal.
5. Identify the personal strengths you will use to accomplish your goal.
6. Identify potential barriers to achieving your goal.
7. In groups of four or five students, present your goal-setting agenda and solicit feedback.

Discussion:
1. Do any of your peers have ideas or information that might help you reach your goals?
2. Are there any common themes, strengths, or behaviors related to goal setting that are found across student groups?
3. What did you learn about yourself that might be useful in helping clients develop goals using a behavioral approach?

and specific client needs, the nurse can act as a guide, an information provider, or as a resource and emotional support. As a *guide,* you can coach clients on actions they can take to improve their health and offer suggestions on the modifications needed as their condition changes. As *information provider,* you can help clients become more aware of why, what, and how they can learn to take better care of themselves. As *resource support,* you can help the client connect with appropriate community and health supports. By providing emotional support and appropriate descriptive, evaluative feedback, you can encourage positive learning efforts and help clients minimize the impact of negative events or temporary setbacks. Helping clients to anticipate actual and potential effects of a medication or treatment reduces anxiety and the incidence of errors. Health teaching responsibilities can be categorized into three broad categories: information gathering, information giving, and relationship building, as presented in Figure 16-2. Before beginning the education process, you should learn about all aspects of care for the client's condition (Bonaldi-Moore, 2009).

ASSESSMENT

Health teaching formats follow the nursing process, beginning with an assessment of client learning needs, strengths, and limitations. Bastable (2008) notes, "Learners are usually the most important source of needs assessment data about themselves" (p. 98).

Clients enter a learning situation with a story model of their illness or disability that helps them make sense of what is happening to them. Understanding the story forms the basis for intervention. Physical symptoms have an emotional, relational, and social context that

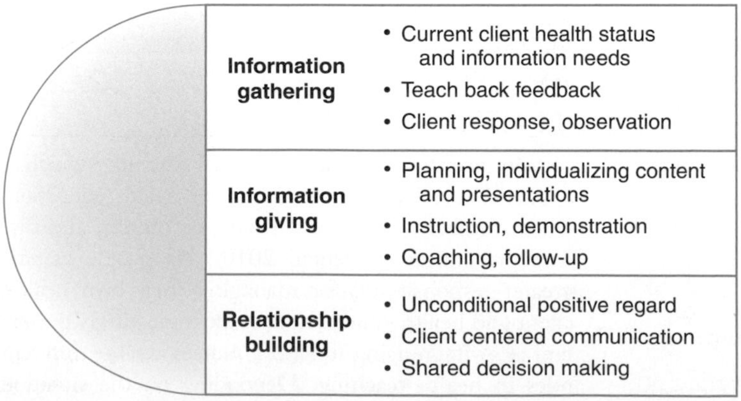

Information gathering	• Current client health status and information needs
	• Teach back feedback
	• Client response, observation
Information giving	• Planning, individualizing content and presentations
	• Instruction, demonstration
	• Coaching, follow-up
Relationship building	• Unconditional positive regard
	• Client centered communication
	• Shared decision making

Figure 16-2   Health teaching categories.

have important diagnostic value for health teaching focus. They can have an effect on relationships, work, and engagement in activities, which can be of considerable concern to the client and/or others involved with the client.

Broad, open-ended questions help nurses understand the learning needs of individual clients and families in a practical way, for example, "Tell me what this illness has been like for you so far," or "Tell me what your doctor has told you about your treatment." Asking questions demonstrates a genuine interest in what is important to clients and families, and helps tailor teaching responses to each client's unique needs. Box 16-2 provides other questions nurses can use to assess client learning needs.

Probing the learner's beliefs about his or her illness and proposed treatment is important because beliefs and values influence learning. For example, the client who believes that *any* drugs taken into the body are harmful will have a hard time learning about the insulin injection he needs to take every day. The same would be true of a client with depression, who views taking antidepressant medication as a "crutch," and not as a necessary treatment of a mental disorder. Finding out what the client feels is his or her primary health concern is important. This may differ from the reason that the client is seeking treatment.

Assessment of client learning needs should include the client's knowledge level, motivation, and ability to learn (see Chapter 15). A sometimes overlooked component in a learning assessment involves potential

---

BOX 16-2	Questions to Assess Learning Needs

- What does the client already know about his or her condition and treatment?
- In what ways is the client affected by it?
- In what ways are those persons intimately involved with the client affected by the client's condition or treatment?
- What does the client idtentify as his or her most important learning need?
- To what extent is the client willing to take personal responsibility for seeking solutions?
- What goals would the client like to achieve?
- What will the client need to do to achieve those goals?
- What resources are available to the client and family that might affect the learning process?
- What barriers to learning exist?

---

environmental barriers, such as limited health insurance, transportation difficulties, lack of follow-up facilities, and cultural dietary considerations and poverty. People may not have the money for medication, or a visit to the pediatrician for an ear infection may have a co-pay that the mother cannot afford. Health illiteracy can be a product of poverty, as well as culture (Lowenstein, Foord-May, & Romano, 2009). Failure to consider these factors can impact the effectiveness of health teaching and produce dangerous outcomes.

Case Example

"Everything was happening so fast and everybody was so busy," and that is why Mitch Winston, 66 years old and suffering from atrial fibrillation, did not ask his doctor to clarify the complex and potentially dangerous medication regimen that had been prescribed for him on leaving the hospital emergency department.

When he returned to the emergency department via ambulance, bleeding internally from an overdose of Coumadin, his doctor was surprised to learn that Mitch had not understood the verbal instructions he had received, and that he had ignored the written instructions and orders for follow-up visits that the doctor had provided. In fact, these had never been retrieved from Mitch's wallet. Despite their importance, they were useless pieces of paper. Mitch cannot read (Joint Commission, 2007, p. 5)

When processing assessment data as the basis for planning teaching interventions, it is appropriate to ask yourself the following questions:

- What specific *information* does the client need to enhance self-management and/or compliance with treatment?
- What *attitudes* does the client hold that potentially could enable or hinder the learning process?
- What specific *skills* does this client need for self-management?

Learner variables important in the teaching/learning process generally fall into two categories: readiness to learn and ability to learn. Incorporation of cultural values and the nurse's self-awareness of bias are other important features of effective client education at individual, family, community, and society levels.

LEARNING READINESS

Teaching cannot begin until the client is ready. The teachable moment takes place when the learner feels that there is a need to know the information and has the capacity to learn it. Two of the most important variables affecting learning new behaviors involve readiness and ability to learn. **Learning readiness** refers to a person's mind-set and openness to engaging in a learning or counseling process for the purpose of adopting new behaviors.

FACTORS THAT AFFECT READINESS TO LEARN

Readiness to learn is not the same as the cognitive ability to learn. Nurses need to remember that learning is never smooth or linear in its development. Rather than challenge the client's learning pattern, the nurse needs to understand it and incorporate it into new opportunities for learning (Blackie, Gregg, & Freeth, 1998). This is the art of health teaching. For example, a statement "I notice that we don't seem to be making much headway with the dietary changes required by your high cholesterol. I wonder if there are some issues that we have not addressed that may be getting in the way" is empathetic, and directly focused on what needs to happen next.." Psychosocial and physical factors that can affect the learner's ability to learn include previous knowledge and experience about the illness, as well as its personal and cultural meaning.

Level of Anxiety

High anxiety can compromise the teaching/learning process by interfering with the client's ability to focus attention and comprehend the material. Accurately assessing and managing a client's level of anxiety before health teaching is essential, as is choosing a time when the client is most likely to be receptive (Stephenson, 2006). Developing a relationship with the client helps establish credibility and trust, and decreases anxiety. Active listening and eliciting the expectations of clients help the nurse get a more complete picture of a situation and can illuminate less obvious apprehension.

FACTORS THAT AFFECT ABILITY TO LEARN

Many factors affect a client's capacity to learn new information and ways of behaving. Some clients are ready to learn but are unable to do so with traditional learning formats (Hemmings, 1998). Assessing the client's ability to learn and adapting the learning format to the learner's unique characteristics makes a difference. If the client cannot understand what is being taught, learning does not take place.

Physical Barriers

A client's physical condition or emotional state can temporarily preclude teaching. A client in pain can focus on little else. A client emerging from the shock of a difficult diagnosis may require teaching in small segments or postponement of serious teaching sessions until time to absorb the diagnosis has elapsed. Certain physical and mental conditions limit attention or compromise cognitive processing abilities. The client with significant thought disorders may need very concrete instructions and frequent prompts to perform adequately. Nausea, weakness, or speech or motor impairments may make it difficult for the client to maintain motivation. Medications or the period of disorientation after a diagnostic test or surgical procedure can influence the level of the client's ability to participate in learning. Careful assessment will usually reveal when the client's physical or emotional condition is a barrier to learning.

Comorbid health problems that could interfere with the goals or process of teaching are important pieces of data that influence what can and should be taught. For example, an exercise program might be useful for an overweight person, but if the client also has a cardiac condition or other problem that would limit activity, this information has a direct impact on the goals and strategies of the intervention.

Other physical or emotional issues favor learning. Mezirow (1990) notes that crisis and life transitions provide a format for the most significant adult learning because the anxiety associated with the crisis situation (if it is not extreme) can create the need to learn, and attention is likely to be more intense. Crisis learning is particularly effective with homeless and immigrant clients, who may not voluntarily seek health care or want to engage in health teaching at any other time. Health teaching for these clients should be immediate, practical, designed to resolve the crisis situation, and carefully organized to maximize client attention.

Assessment is an interactive process in which clients should be encouraged to ask questions. By introducing the idea that most people have questions, clients feel freer to question data or to ask for more explanation. At the end of an assessment interview, you can summarize important points and ask for validation. This helps to ensure a common understanding of the issues and identify any misinformation. It also reinforces the idea of a reciprocal relationship as the basis for health teaching.

Family Support and Teaching Needs

Health teaching can involve family members in either a supportive role or as a primary recipient. Comprehensive health teaching is required for those actively involved as a primary caregiver, for example, with children, or clients with significant mobility, sensory deficits, or cognitive deficits. Content presentations to these family members would be the same as those given to the client.

When family members take supportive roles, for example, with teenagers, clients in crisis, and frail elder or critically ill clients with intact cognitive abilities, health teaching should focus on what they need to know to support the client. Family caregivers need to be in a position to support the client's efforts to implement new behaviors. Information and anticipatory guidance about what to expect when the client goes home and early warning signs of complications or potential problems should be given to family support members, as well as to clients. Knowing when to seek professional assistance and resource support is critical information.

Family support is an important dimension of health maintenance for frail elders, and individuals who depend on others for direction and oversight of treatment for a chronic condition. Any change in the level of support from primary caregivers can affect a client's willingness or ability to learn. When these supports are no longer available through death or incapacity, the client may lack not only motivation but the skills to cope with complex health problems.

Case Example

Edward Flanigan, an 82-year-old man who was recently widowed, has moderately severe diabetes. There is no evidence of memory problems, but there are some significant emotional components to his current health care needs. All his life, his wife pampered him and did everything for him, from meal preparation to monitoring his diabetes. Now that his wife is dead, Edward takes no interest in controlling his diabetes. The home care nurse who visits him on a regular basis is discouraged because, despite careful instruction and seeming comprehension, Edward appears unwilling to follow the prescribed diabetic diet and is not consistent in taking his medication. Predictably, he goes into diabetic crisis. His family worries about him, but he is unwilling to consider leaving his home of 42 years.

Emotional issues of loss and change complicate the learning needs of this client. Edward could function and maintain his health when he could rely on his wife for support. To enhance Edward's learning readiness, the nurse might initially have to assess for depression and then help him find alternative ways to meet his dependency needs, for example, by expanding his social support system.

PLANNING

Health teaching is not a static process or one-time event. Stephenson (2006) notes that nurses need to consider the following questions:

What does the client understand so far?

What is the most important to learn about now?

What is the amount of information desired, prioritization preferred, and method of learning? (p. 243)

Planning requires more than knowledge of current client status. Each learning situation has a past and a present reality. Past experience and beliefs about illness, medications, certain treatments, cultural values, and the reactions of others produce assumptions that influence motivation and the acceptance of health teaching. Sample nursing diagnoses amenable to health teaching are presented in Box 16-3.

Nurses need to know what previous information the client has received and to whom the client looks for health information. Focusing on accurate information without destroying the credibility of well-meaning and influential informal health informants in the client's life is part of the art of health teaching. Nothing is gained by injuring the reputation of the person who gave the client the information. Instead, you could say, "There have been some new findings that I think you might be interested in. Current thinking suggests that *(give example)* works well in situations like this." With this statement, the nurse can introduce a different way of thinking without challenging the person identified in the client's mind as expert.

BOX 16-3	Sample Nursing Diagnoses Amenable to Health Teaching

- Risk for injury or violence
- Ineffective coping
- Alternations in parenting or family process
- Self-care deficits
- Anxiety
- Noncompliance
- Impaired home maintenance
- Deficient knowledge

Although too much information puts the learner into informational overload so that critical content is not learned, not enough direction can also prove harmful.

Case Example

A nurse on the evening shift instructed an 85-year-old man to keep his arm in an upright position after a treatment procedure. The nurse neglected to tell him that he could release his arm once the needle was securely in place. The man called his wife at 5 a.m. the next day to tell her he did not think he could hold his arm in that position any longer. The man had been awake all night, his arm felt numb, and he was at his wits' end because of incomplete health teaching. Had the nurse told him to keep his arm elevated for a specific period of time (e.g., 30 minutes), the outcome and level of client satisfaction could have been different.

Organized planning is pivotal to the purpose and methodology of health teaching. Timely comprehensive health information presented in an orderly fashion is a critical component of successful coping and treatment compliance. For example, a person with a recent myocardial infarction will need to learn about:

- The disease process
- The medications, diet, and exercise regimens needed to improve cardiac function
- Lifestyle changes to reduce stress and improve cardiac function
- Warning signs and symptoms requiring medical follow-up

In addition to giving complete information, the nurse can ask, "Do you have any questions for me?" and suggest that if things come up that the client has questions about later, the client should ask for further clarification.

Often hours or days after the teaching takes place clients will have questions or concerns about the information they received. Planning should include additional opportunities for discussion after the client has had time to absorb the initial information. You can encourage the client to jot down questions that may develop as they occur.

Developing Learning Goals

Setting mutual goals with clients with periodic reviews helps to motivate clients and serves as a benchmark for evaluating change. It is important to establish goals *with* your client rather than *for* your client. Clear

learning goals that the client is interested in meeting, and has the necessary ability and resources to achieve increase the chances that the information will be understood and applied (London, 2001). Prioritizing goals and objectives that are important to client health and well-being helps nurses and clients focus on the most relevant specifics.

Identify outcome goals with a general statement about what the client needs to achieve as a result of the teaching. (e.g., "After health teaching, the client will maintain dietary control of her diabetes."). An interim goal might be, "After health teaching, the client will develop an appropriate diet plan for 1 week."). Setting realistic goals prevents disappointment. Box 16-4 summarizes guidelines to use in the development of effective health teaching goals and objectives. Exercise 16-2 provides experience with developing relevant behavioral outcome goals.

Developing Measurable Objectives

Objectives are powerful guides to organizing content and suggesting appropriate planning activities. Each objective should describe an immediate action step that the client should take to accomplish relevant treatment outcomes. Teaching objectives should be modest and achievable in the time frame allotted. They should be logically organized and build on one another for maximum effectiveness. To determine whether an objective is achievable, consider the client's level of experience, educational level, resources, and motivation. Then define each learning objective needed to achieve the health goal in specific measurable behavioral terms.

Objectives should support the overall health outcome and directly relate to the nursing diagnosis. For example, the nursing diagnosis for a client with newly diagnosed diabetes might read, "knowledge deficit

BOX 16-4	Guidelines for Developing Effective Goals and Objectives

- Link goals to the nursing diagnosis.
- Make goals action-oriented.
- Make goals specific and measurable.
- Define objectives as behavioral outcomes.
- Design objectives with a specific time frame for achievement.
- Show a logical progression with established priorities.
- Review periodically and modify goals as needed.

EXERCISE 16-2	Developing Behavioral Goals

Purpose: To provide practical experience with developing teaching goals.

Procedure:
Establish a nursing diagnosis related to health teaching and a teaching goal that supports the diagnosis in each of the following situations:
1. Jimmy is a 15-year-old adolescent who has been admitted to a mental health unit with disorders associated with impulse control and conduct. He wants to lie on his bed and read Stephen King novels. He refuses to attend unit therapy activities.
2. Maria, a 19-year-old single woman, is in the clinic for the first time because of cramping. She is seven months pregnant and has had no prenatal care.
3. Jennifer is overweight and desperately wants to lose weight. However, she cannot walk past the refrigerator without stopping, and she finds it difficult to resist the snack machines at work. She wants a plan to help her lose weight and resist her impulses to eat.

Discussion:
1. What factors did you have to consider in developing the most appropriate diagnosis and teaching goals for each client?
2. In considering the diagnosis and teaching goals for each situation, what common themes did you find?
3. What differences in each situation contributed to variations in diagnosis and teaching goals? What contributed to these differences?
4. In what ways can you use the information in this exercise in your future nursing practice?

related to diabetic diet." Examples of appropriate progressive learning objectives required for mastering diabetic control might occur as follows:

- First teaching session: The client will identify the purpose of a diabetic diet and appropriate foods.
- Second teaching session: The client will identify appropriate foods and serving sizes allowed on a diabetic diet.
- Third teaching session: The client will demonstrate actions for urine/blood testing for glucose at home.
- Fourth teaching session: The client will identify foods to avoid on the diabetic diet and the rationale for compliance.
- Fifth teaching session: The client will describe symptoms and actions to take for hyperglycemia and hypoglycemia.

Timing

Health teaching is not an add-on; it is an essential nursing intervention. Factors involved in timing are presented in Box 16-5. Teaching interventions should

BOX 16-5	Factors Involved in Timing

- Client readiness
- Time needed to learn skill or body of knowledge
- Possible need for attitude change by client
- Time constraints of nurse
- Client priorities about information or skill
- Client's energy level
- Atmosphere of trust

never be eliminated because the nurse lacks time, but they can be streamlined. Even in the most limited situation, schedule a block of time for health teaching. You will need to consider how much time is required to learn a particular skill or body of knowledge, and build this into the learning situation. Complicated and/or essential skill development needs blocks of time and repeated practice with feedback.

Pick times for teaching when energy levels are high, the client is not distracted by other things, it is not visiting time, and the client is not in pain. Careful observation of the client will help determine the most appropriate times for learning.

People have saturation points as to how much they can learn in one time period. Because even under the best of circumstances, people can absorb only so many details and fine points, limit information to two or three points at a time. Keep the teaching session short, interesting, and to the point. Ideally, teaching sessions should last no longer than about 20 minutes, including time for questions. Otherwise, the client may tire or lose interest. Scheduling shorter sessions with time in between to process information helps prevent sensory overload and reinforces teaching points.

In addition to scheduled teaching sessions, nurses have many opportunities for informal teaching that occur during the course of providing care. Simple, spontaneous health teaching takes minutes, yet it can be highly effective. The following case example, taken from *Heartsounds* (Lear, 1980), illustrates this point.

Case Example

A nurse came in while he was eating dinner. "Dr. Lear," she said, "after angiography the patients always seem to have the same complaints, and I thought you might want to know about them. It might help." (This was a good nurse. I didn't know it then, because I didn't know how scared he was. But later I understood that this was a darned good nurse.)

"Thanks, it would help," he said.

"It's mostly two things. The first is, they say that during the test, they feel a tremendous flush. It's very sudden and it can be scary."

He responds to the nurse, "Okay, the flush. And what's the other thing?"

"It's…well, they say that at a certain point, they feel as though they are about to die. But that feeling passes quickly." He thanked her again. He was very grateful.

(Later, during the actual procedure, Dr. Lear remembered the nurse's words and found comfort.) "Easy. Easy. You're supposed to feel this way. This is precisely what the nurse described. The moment you feel you are dying." (Lear, 1980, pp. 120–121)

This teaching intervention probably took less than 5 minutes, yet its effect was long-lasting and healing. There are countless opportunities for informal health teaching in clinical practice if the nurse consciously looks for them.

IMPLEMENTATION

Each teaching session should demonstrate a thorough knowledge of the topic, a keen understanding of the client's learning needs, and a genuine interest in the client. The client must be actively involved in the

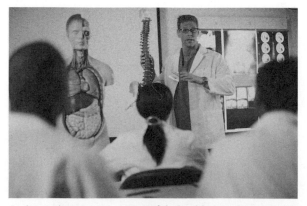

A key element in successful health teaching is an enthusiastic presentation.

process. Effective teaching involves not only a healthy exchange of information, but plenty of opportunities to ask questions and to receive feedback.

Health Teaching Format

No one teaching strategy can meet the needs of all clients (Rycroft-Malone et al., 2000), but people learn best when there is a logical flow and building of information from simple to complex. Begin by presenting a simple overview of what will be taught and why the information is important to learn. Include only essential information in your overview; for example, give a brief explanation of the health care problem, risk factors, treatment, and self-care skills the client will need to manage at home (Lee et al., 1998). Incorporate or ask about previous related experience. Introductory content that builds on the person's experiences, abilities, interests, motivation, and skills is more likely to engage the learner's attention.

Deliver key points and allow regular opportunities for client feedback and questions. If the material is complex, it can be broken down into smaller learning segments. For example, diabetic teaching could include the following segments:

- Introduction, including what the client does know
- Basic pathophysiology of diabetes (keep description simple and short)
- Diet and exercise
- Demonstration of insulin injection with return demonstration
- Recognizing signs and symptoms of hyperglycemia and hypoglycemia
- Care of skin and feet
- How to talk to the doctor

A strong closing statement summarizing major points reinforces the learning process. Exercise 16-3 provides practice with developing a mini teaching plan.

Using Clear Language

Use clear precise language. Choice of words should be familiar to the client. Whenever possible, avoid the use of nonessential adjectives. Place words with more than one meaning in context as many words have more than one connotation. Consider the word *cold*. It can refer to temperature, an illness, an emotional tone, or a missed opportunity. Using too general or vague language leaves the learner wondering what the nurse actually meant. For example, "Call the doctor if you

EXERCISE 16-3	Developing Teaching Plans

Purpose: To provide practice with developing teaching plans.

Procedure:
1. Develop a mini teaching plan for one of the following client situations:
   a. Jim Dolan feels stressed and is requesting health teaching on stress management and relaxation techniques.
   b. Adrienne Parker is a newly diagnosed diabetic. Her grandfather had diabetes.
   c. Vera Carter is scheduled to have an appendectomy in the morning.
   d. Marion Hill just gave birth to her first child. She wants to breast-feed her infant, but she does not think she has enough milk.
   e. Barbara Scott weighs 210 pounds and wants to lose weight.
2. Use guidelines presented in Chapter 15 and this chapter in the development of your teaching plan. Include the following data: a brief statement of client learning needs and a list of related nursing diagnoses in order of priority.
3. For one nursing diagnosis, develop an educative/supportive teaching plan outline that includes specific client-focused objectives, topical content outline, planned teaching strategies, time frame for planned activities, and evaluation criteria.

have any problems" has more than one meaning. "Problems" can refer to side effects of the medication, a return of symptoms, problems with family acceptance, changed relationships, and even alterations in self-concept. In this case, clear descriptors should cover the following:

- Identification of specific behaviors warranting attention
- What needs to happen if problems arise and under what specific circumstances
- Who needs to be contacted (with contact information) if something goes wrong

A clear statement that the nurse might use is, "If you should develop a headache or feel dizzy in the next 24 hours, call the emergency room doctor right away."

Note that comprehension involves more than simply hearing or decoding written words. It includes understanding language nuances and being able to put underlying themes together in ways that make sense of the message as a unified whole. Verbally checking in with clients to confirm a common understanding of words and concepts is critical to knowledge transfer in health teaching. Doak, Doak, Gordon, and Lorig (2001) suggest asking the client, "What does this material tell you about_____ [subject]? What does it tell you to do?" (p. 188).

Visual Aids

Visual aids can be used to reinforce a message by providing concrete images. Simple images and few words work better than complex visual aids (Huntsman & Binger, 1981). For example, the nurse might show a new mother pictures of common infant rashes. A chart or model showing the heart might help another client understand the anatomy and physiology of a heart disorder. Perdue, Degazon, and Lunny (1999) suggest that DVD tapes are useful in teaching clients with limited reading skills. They have the advantage of allowing clients to watch them again at their convenience. Related discussions help to correct misinterpretations and emphasize pertinent points.

Preparing Written Handouts

Written backup materials to which clients can refer when needed reinforce learning. Attention to the client's reading level and health care literacy helps ensure that the pamphlets can be read. Most reading materials should be geared to a sixth-grade reading level. Even people with adequate health literacy comprehend information better when the language is simple and clear. Incorporating relevant line drawings or pictures can be useful with clients who have language issues. Large-print pamphlets and audiotapes are helpful learning aids for those with sight problems.

Guidelines for preparing effective written materials include the following:
- Present the most important information first.
- Illustrations and diagrams should be designed to enhance clarity and appeal.
- Make sure that the content is current, accurate, objective, and consistent with information provided by other health providers.

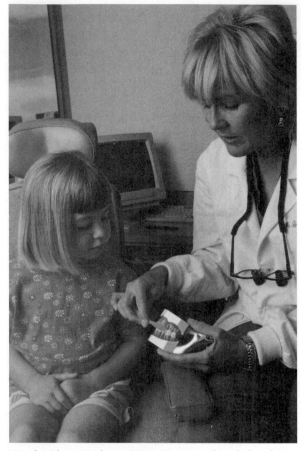

Visual aids provide concrete images that help clients remember essential information.

- Use appropriate language at a literacy level that the reader can understand.
- Use a 12-point font and avoid using all capital letters for reading ease.
- Define technical terms in lay language and avoid medical jargon.
- Check for spelling errors and stay away from complicated sentences.
- Include resources with contact information that the client can refer to for further information or for help with problems.

Using Advance Organizers

Advance organizers, sometimes called a mnemonic, consist of cue words, phrases, or letters related to more complex data. They are designed to help people remember and recall difficult concepts. For example,

the letters in the word *diabetes* can help a client remember key concepts about diabetes:

D = diet
I = infections
A = administering medications
B = basic pathophysiology
E = eating schedules
T = treatment for hyperglycemia or hypoglycemia
E = exercise
S = symptom recognition

Each letter stands for a concept or action needed to control diabetes. Taken together, the client has a useful tool for remembering *all* related concepts.

Nursing students can use mnemonics to help them remember key points. Word associations promote remembering in much the same way that linking new information to previously learned information does. For example, the four F's (fat, forty, female, family history) can help students remember risk factors for gallbladder disorder. Developing mnemonics can be fun and creative.

Accommodating Special Learning Needs

The level of information and amount of time for health teaching should reflect differences and changes in client circumstances. Clients experiencing a recent diagnosis will need more detailed basic information than clients having an unanswered question or requiring follow-up information. If a client's condition worsens, becomes stable, or improves, you will need to modify teaching goals, content, and strategies to reflect relevant changes.

Accommodating for Cultural Diversity. Clients with English as a second language or a strong ethnic background usually require learning accommodations. Health teaching and educational programs that take into consideration the cultural health practices of individuals and families are likely to be more successful. Whenever possible, include cultural values or beliefs about health in teaching content and delivery. Use culturally relevant terminology.

Use fewer, rather than more words to explain a concept and allow extra time to practice psychomotor skills with feedback. When teaching a client with English as a second language, keep in mind that words from one language do not necessarily translate with the same meaning into another. Words for certain concepts either do not exist or the phrases used for expressing and describing them can differ.

Sometimes there is a tendency for people to speak louder when instructing someone from a different culture. This is not necessary. People with health literacy issues because of language are neither deaf nor unable to grasp information, if their special needs are taken into account. Speak slowly in a normal conversational tone. Lorig (2001) suggests that in preparing teaching materials for translation, the following are important:

- Use nouns rather than pronouns, and simple unambiguous language
- Use short simple sentences of less than 16 words each
- Avoid the use of metaphors and informal slang
- Avoid verb forms that have more than one meaning, or include would or could (p. 181).

If the client still is unable to understand important concepts with accommodations, enlisting the services of a trained medical interpreter becomes an essential intervention.

Learners handicapped by memory deficits, lack of insight, poor judgment, and limited problem-solving abilities also require special accommodations. Special needs learners respond best when the content is presented in a consistent, concrete, and patient manner, with clear and frequent cues to action. Clients with limited literacy skills may benefit from using audiotapes in addition to or instead of written materials.

Giving Feedback

Feedback is an essential component of successful health teaching programs. To appreciate its significance, consider the effect on your performance if you never received feedback from your instructor. Feedback about how the client is accomplishing teaching goals should be descriptive, and include areas of accomplishment and need for growth. Effective feedback is honest and based on concrete data. When providing feedback, keep it simple and focus only on behaviors that can be changed. Behavioral statements on a continuum (e.g., "You seem skilled with drawing up the medication, but you may need a little more practice with selecting sites.") are more effective than absolute statements (e.g., "You still are not doing this correctly.").

Feedback given as soon as possible after an observation is more likely to be accepted by the client. Indirect feedback—provided through nodding, smiling,

and sharing information about the process and experiences of others—reinforces learning. Exercise 16-4 provides practice with giving feedback in health teaching.

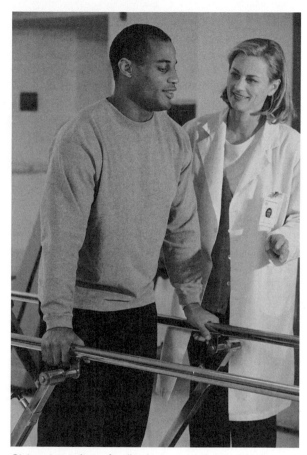

Giving immediate feedback is important with learning psychomotor tasks.

TEACHING SELF-MANAGEMENT AND CAREGIVING SKILLS

The subject of health teaching would be incomplete without a discussion of strategies focused on the development of self-management and caregiving skills needed by an increasing number of people coping with chronic illness and disability in the community. Although a lot of self-management strategies are disease or disability specific, common to most chronic conditions are issues of fatigue, pain, sleep management, lifestyle adjustments, limitations in social/role activities, self-efficacy, and identity issues.

EXERCISE 16-4	Giving Teaching Feedback

Purpose: To give students perspective and experience in giving usable feedback.

Procedure:
1. Divide the class into working groups of three or four students.
2. Present a 3-minute sketch of some aspect of your current learning situation that you find difficult (e.g., writing a paper, speaking in class, coordinating study schedules, or studying certain material).
3. Each person, in turn, offers one piece of usable informative feedback to the presenter. In making suggestions, use the guidelines on feedback given in this chapter.
4. Place feedback suggestions on a flip chart or chalkboard.

Discussion:
1. What were your thoughts and feelings about the feedback you heard in relation to resolving the problem you presented to the group?
2. What were your thoughts and feelings in giving feedback to each presenter?
3. Was it harder to give feedback in some cases than in others? In what ways?
4. What common themes emerged in your group?
5. In what ways can you use the self-exploration about feedback in this exercise in teaching conversations with clients?

Using a Problem-Solving Teaching Approach

Teaching about medications is a critical example of self-management education related to client safety where you can use a problem-solving approach. Begin by providing the client with both generic and commercial names of medications. Many medications look alike, so correctly labeling them and having clients/family caregivers visually identify the medication is helpful. Medication reconciliation is extremely important for elderly clients who usually are taking multiple medications, with the potential for getting them mixed up. Make sure that the client has the finances to obtain medication on a regular basis. If equipment is used, for example, syringes for insulin, make sure the client can read the calibrations and is injecting in appropriate areas.

You will need to clearly identify the purpose of the medication, expected therapeutic response, and side effects of the medications the client is receiving. Discuss what happens if the client misses a dose or decides to stop the medication. For example, doubling up on the next dose or stopping a medication abruptly may create significant issues for clients. Missing birth control pills even for a short period may result in an unwanted pregnancy. If blood tests are required to determine the efficacy or toxicity of the prescribed drug, the rationale and timing should be explained. Talk about symptoms that could require immediate medical attention and what to do in case of emergency. As with other forms of health teaching, summarize key points at the

conclusion of the teaching session. Family members need to be given enough information to support client adherence to the treatment protocol. Box 16-6 provides medication teaching tips developed by the Institute for Safe Medication Practices.

The Center for the Advancement of Health (2002) has identified problem solving, decision making, utilization of resources, development of client/provider partnerships, and taking action as essential self-management skills. Key caregiving skills identified in the literature are those involving "monitoring,

BOX 16-6	Medication Teaching Tips

- Provide clients with written drug information, particularly for metered-dose inhalants and high-alert medications such as insulin.
- Include family or caregivers in the teaching sessions for clients who need extra support or reminders.
- Do not wait until discharge to begin education about complex drug regimens.
- Clearly explain directions for using each medication.
- Always require repeat demonstrations or explanations about medications to be taken at home, particularly for those requiring special drug administration techniques.
- Use the time you already spend with clients during assessments and daily care to evaluate their level of understanding about their medications.
- Keep medication administration schedule as simple and easy to follow as possible.

Adapted from Institute for Safe Medication Practices: Patient medication teaching tips, Huntingdon Valley, PA, 2006, Author.

interpreting, making decisions, taking actions, making adjustments, accessing resources, providing hands-on care, working together with the ill person, and navigating the health care system" (Schumacher & Marren, 2004, p. 460).

Not all of these skills can be taught simultaneously. Development of self-management and caregiving skills requires a contextual, problem-based teaching approach. In addition to medical management of chronic conditions, people need coaching and support to integrate health-related changes into life roles, and management of the emotions created by having a chronic condition (Lorig & Holman, 2003). *Repetition is important*, as is careful inquiry with open-ended questions about any issues that might compromise compliance.

Clients and families should be advised of what to expect from treatment and medications, as well as risks, benefits, prognosis, and options for treatment. This information allows them to make better health care decisions. They should understand why an action is important, what they can expect from following a treatment protocol, and how aspects of treatment can help them.

Clients and families need to know the danger signals to watch for that would require a prompt call for assistance. They should be coached on the types of circumstances requiring a call to their health care provider.

Teach-Back Method

Allowing extra time for the client to talk about and do return demonstrations of tasks reinforces learning (Bohny, 1997). Teach back or show back is a teaching strategy used to evaluate and verify a client's understanding of health teaching and/or ability to execute

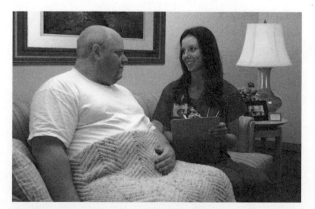

Health teaching can take place in the home, as well as in the hospital.

self-management skills. It involves asking the learner to repeat back relevant information and treatment instructions in his or her own words (Lorenzen, Melby, & Earles, 2008). Asking the learner to describe actions that would need to be taken if a protocol or procedure cannot be followed exactly or if the actions a client takes fails to produce the desired effect can be included. The method provides the nurse with valuable data about areas of skill learning that may need additional attention. Using it as you go along reinforces each piece of information and eliminates the problem of delivering a comprehensive teaching plan only to discover that the client lost your train of thought after the first few sentences.

Coaching Clients

Coaching is an effective teaching strategy used to teach self-management and problem-solving skills to clients and families experiencing unfamiliar tasks and procedures (Lewis & Zahlis, 1997). For example, coaching can help clients distinguish between which symptoms require immediate medical attention and which ones can be handled with self-management strategies.

Coaching clients as they negotiate a complex health care system can prove invaluable. For example, the nurse might assist the client or family in opening a communication with a health agency and choosing the appropriate questions to ask. Or, it may be as simple as coaching people to seek information from several sources rather than calling only one and waiting for a response (Lorig & Holman, 2003).

Coaching emphasizes the client's autonomy in developing appropriate solutions, as the client is always in charge of the pace and direction of the learning. Through a coaching dialogue, you can encourage a client to critically think about the elements of a situation, consider multiple options, and evaluate the appropriateness of choosing one option over another. Assessment for coaching purposes starts with an exploration of how the client is experiencing the fundamental patterns of a situation. This assessment assists clients to challenge obstructive perceptions, connect past experience with current knowledge about the context of a situation, look for cues in a situation, and consider the consequences of taking different actions.

In the coaching role, nurses can present different perspectives that the client may not have considered. Coaching can include role-playing and value clarification. The process can inform the client about timing of actions, potential outcomes, areas that need special attention, and contextual issues that might not otherwise emerge in a teaching situation. In addition to giving appropriate information, coaching involves taking the client step by step through a procedure or activities in which the client takes the lead in choice of actions. The secret of successful coaching is to provide enough information to help the client take the next step without taking over. Coaching involves a number of skills presented Figure 16-3. Exercise 16-5 provides practice with coaching as a teaching strategy.

Providing Transitional Cues

Directions for self-management of illness or disability may seem simple and obvious to you, but clients or families may have difficulty with material simply because they do not know how the information fits together in their particular circumstances. Instead of using generic explanations of skills and medication management, use language and concepts specific to the client's situation. For example, connecting the

purpose of taking a medication with the actual actions you want the client to take helps fix the process in a person's mind and makes it easier to remember related instructions. Ask clients how they will implement an essential medical management strategy such as using an inhaler or adhering to a therapeutic diet. This discussion requires clients to seriously consider how an application directly affects them and any changes in lifestyle behaviors needed to accommodate for it.

HEALTH TEACHING APPLICATIONS IN DIFFERENT SETTINGS

GROUP PRESENTATIONS

Group presentations offer the advantage of being able to teach a number of people at one time. The format allows people to learn from each other, as well as from the teacher. Health teaching topics that lend themselves to a group format include care of the newborn,

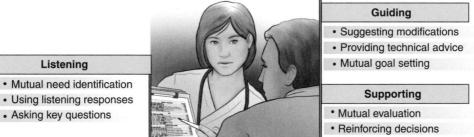

Figure 16-3   The nurse's role in coaching clients.

EXERCISE 16-5 | Coaching

Purpose: To help students understand the process of coaching.

Procedure:
Identify the steps you would use to coach clients in each of the following situations. Use Figure 16-1 as a guide to develop your plan.
1. A client returning from surgery, with pain medication ordered "as needed"
2. A client newly admitted to a cardiac care unit
3. A client with a newly inserted intravenous catheter for antibiotic medications

4. A child and his parents coming for a preoperative visit to the hospital before surgery
   Share your suggestions with your classmates.

Discussion:
1. What were some of the different coaching strategies you used with each of these clients?
2. In what ways were your coaching strategies similar to or unlike those of your classmates?
3. How could you use the information you gained from this exercise to improve the quality of your helping?

diabetes, oncology, and prenatal and postnatal care (Redman, 2007).

Formal group teaching should be structured in a space large enough to accommodate all participants. The learner should be able to hear and see the instructor and visual aids without strain. Technical equipment should be available and in working order. Should the equipment not work, it is better to eliminate the planned teaching aid completely than to spend a portion of the teaching session trying to fix it.

Preparation and practice can ensure that your presentation is clear, concise, and well spoken. In a group presentation, you will need to establish rapport with your audience. Make eye contact immediately and continue to do so throughout the presentation. Extension of eye contact to all participants communicates acceptance and inclusion. A quote at the beginning capturing the meaning of the presentation or a humorous opening grabs the audience's attention. Strengthen content statements with careful use of specific examples. Citing a specific problem and the ways another person dealt with it gives general statements credibility. Repeating key points and summarizing them again at the conclusion of the session helps reinforce learning.

If you plan to use PowerPoint, use a font that is large enough to see from a distance (32 point is recommended) and include no more than four or five items per slide. Use the slides wisely to identify key points, not as the primary content for the presentation. Face the audience, not the slides. Practice your presentation to ensure that you keep within the time frame and allot time for short discussion points. The key points can help you stay on track and move through the agenda. It is up to you as the presenter to set the pace. No matter how interesting the presentation and dialogue that it stimulates, running out of time can be frustrating for the audience and presenter.

Anticipate questions and be on the alert for blank looks. No matter how good a teacher you are, you will from time to time experience the blank look. When this occurs, it is appropriate to ask, "Does anyone have any questions about what I just said?" Give reinforcement for participation verbally, "I'm so glad you brought that up," or "That's a really interesting question (or comment)." Smiling and nodding your head are nonverbal reinforcers. If a participant has a question that you cannot answer, do not bluff it. Instead, say, "That is a good question. I don't have an answer at this moment, but I will get back to you with it." Sometimes another person will have the required information and will share it.

Handouts and other materials provide additional reinforcement. Make sure that the information is accurate, complete, easy to understand, logical, and very important, that you have enough for all participants. Exercise 16-6 provides an opportunity to practice health teaching in a group setting.

Health Teaching in the Home

Preparing for discharge has specialized teaching/learning needs that nurses need to consider in caring for clients and families (see also Chapter 24). Relevant areas of learning needs to assess are identified in Box 16-7.

In home care, the nurse is a guest in the client's home. Part of the teaching assessment includes appraisal of the home environment, family supports, and resources, as well as client needs. Although teaching aids and structured teaching strategies available in the hospital setting may not be available, in many ways the home offers a teaching laboratory unparalleled in the hospital. The nurse can actually "see" improvisations in equipment and technique that are possible in the home environment. Family members may have ideas that the nurse would not have

---

EXERCISE 16-6   Group Health Teaching

Purpose: To provide practice with presenting a health topic in a group setting.

Procedure:
1. Plan a 15- to 20-minute health presentation on a health topic of interest to you, including teaching aids and methods for evaluation.
   Suggested topics:

Nutrition	Weight control
Drinking and driving	Mammograms
High blood pressure	Safe sex
Dental care	

2. Present your topic to your class group.

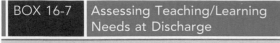

BOX 16-7	Assessing Teaching/Learning Needs at Discharge

- What potential problems are likely to prevent a safe discharge?
- What potential problems are likely to cause complications or readmission?
- What prior knowledge or experience does the patient and family have with this problem?
- What skills and equipment are needed to manage the problem at home?
- Who (what agency) will assume responsibility for continuing care?

thought of, and the nurse can see the obstacles the family face.

Always call before going to the client's home. This is common courtesy; it also protects the nurse's time if the client is going to be out. Teaching in home care settings is rewarding. Often, the nurse is the client's only visitor. Family members often display a curiosity and willingness to be a part of the learning group, particularly if the nurse actively uses knowledge of the home environment to make suggestions about needed modifications.

When in the home, it is important to model appropriate behaviors (e.g., washing hands in the bathroom sink before touching the client). Simple strategies, like not washing one's hands in the kitchen sink where food is prepared, encourage the client to do likewise.

Teaching in home care settings has to be short-term and comprehensive, because most insurance companies will provide third-party reimbursement only for intermittent, episodic care. Nurses need to plan teaching sessions realistically so that they can be delivered in the shortest time possible. Content must reflect specific information the client and family need to provide immediate effective care for the client, *nothing more and nothing less*. Sometimes it is tempting to include more than what is essential to know. Because there are so many regulations regarding the length and scope of skilled nursing interventions imposed by third-party reimbursement guidelines, the nurse needs to pay careful attention to health teaching content and formats. At the same time, reviewing medications with clients and families at every visit is useful.

Helping clients access supportive services can be extremely helpful to families who would not otherwise do so even with the appropriate written information. Having knowledge of community resources is essential. This knowledge allows you to help clients and families select from a number of existing resources and create new ones through novel uses of family and community support systems. Expert nurses know that clients often can be a source of information about resources they may not know about. An understanding of Medicare, Medicaid, and other insurance matters (e.g., regulations, required documentation, and reimbursement schedules) is factored into the management of health care teaching in home health care.

EVALUATION

Regardless of the setting in which health teaching takes place, the Joint Commission on Accreditation of Healthcare Organizations (JCAHO) *requires* written documentation of client health teaching. Notes about the initial assessment should be detailed, comprehensive, and objective. Teaching content and delivery should be related to assessment data, including client preferences, previous knowledge, and values. Included in the documentation are the teaching actions, the client response, and any clinical issues or barriers to compliance. If family members are involved, this information should be acknowledged. Accurate documentation serves a critical purpose in health teaching, helps ensure continuity, and prevents duplication of teaching efforts. The client's record informs other health care providers of what has been taught and what areas need to be addressed in future teaching sessions. See the following example for documentation of home health teaching:

4/8/Blood glucose check normal. Vital signs stable. Client on insulin for 10 years; has difficulty prefilling syringes. Lives with son who works. Nursing diagnosis: knowledge deficit related to prefilling syringes and ineffective coping in self-medication related to poor eyesight. Nurse prefilled syringes, wrote out med schedule, and discussed in detail with client. Client receptive to medication instruction, but may have difficulty with insulin prefill secondary to poor vision. Instructed client on medications, signs and symptoms to report to MD, diet and safety measures. Client able to repeat instructions. Spoke with son regarding medication supervision.

M. Haggerty, RN

SUMMARY

This chapter describes the nurse's role in health teaching. Theoretical frameworks, client-centered teaching, critical thinking, and behavioral approaches guide the nurse in implementing health teaching. Teaching is designed to access one or more of the three domains of learning: cognitive, affective, and psychomotor. Assessment for purposes of constructing a teaching plan centers on three areas: What does the client already know? What is important for the client to know? What is the client ready to know?

Essential content in all teaching plans includes information about the health care problem, risk factors, and self-care skills needed to manage at home. No one teaching strategy can meet the needs of all individual clients. The learning needs of the client will help define relevant teaching strategies. Several teaching strategies, such as coaching, use of mnemonics, and visual aids, are described. Repetition of key concepts and frequent feedback make the difference between simple instruction and teaching that informs. Documentation of the learning process is essential. The client's record becomes a vehicle of communication, informing other health care workers what has been taught and what areas need to be addressed in future teaching sessions.

REFERENCES

American Nurses Association: *Scope and standards of practice*, Washington, DC, 2004, Author.

American Nurses Credentialing Center: *The magnet recognition program. Recognizing excellence in nursing service. Application manual*, Silver Spring, MD, 2005, Author.

Anderson LW, Krathwohl DR, Bloom B, editors: *A taxonomy for learning, teaching and assessing: a revision of Bloom's Taxonomy of educational objectives: Complete edition*, New York, 2001, Longman.

Bastable SB: *Nurse as educator: principles of teaching and learning for nursing practice*, ed 3, Sudbury, MA, 2008, Jones and Bartlett Publishers.

Blackie C, Gregg R, Freeth D: Promoting health in young people, *Nurs Stand* 12(36):39–46, 1998.

Bohny B: A time for self-care: role of the home healthcare nurse, *Home Healthc Nurse* 15(4):281–286, 1997.

Bonaldi-Moore L: The nurse's role in educating postmastectomy breast cancer patients, *Plastic Surgical Nursing* 29(4):212–219, 2009.

Center for the Advancement of Health: *Essential elements of self-management interventions*, Washington, DC, 2002, Author.

Doherty D: Guided care nurses help chronically ill patients, *Patient Educ Manag* 16(12):139–141, 2009.

Doak C, Doak L, Gordon L, Lorig K: Selecting, preparing and using materials. In Lorig K, editor: *Patient education: a practical approach*, ed 3, Thousand Oaks, CA, 2001, Sage Publications.

Dreeben O: *Patient Education in Rehabilitation*, Sudbury MA, 2010, Jones and Bartlett Publishers.

Greiner P, Valiga T: Creative educational strategies for health promotion, *Holist Nurs Pract* 12(2):73–83, 1998.

Hansen M, Fisher JC: Patient teaching: patient-centered teaching from theory to practice, *Am J Nurs* 98(1):56–60, 1998.

Hemmings D: Health promotion for people with learning disabilities in the community, *Nurs Times* 94(24):58–59, 1998.

Huntsman A, Binger J: *Communicating effectively*, Wakefield, MA, 1981, Nursing Resources.

Joint Commission: What did the doctor say? Improving health literacy to promote patient safety. In *Health Care at the Crossroads Reports*, Oakbrook Terrace, IL, 2007, Joint Commission Resources, Inc.

Knowles M, Holton E, Swanson R: *The adult learner: the definitive classic on adult education and training*, Terre Haute, IL, 1998.

Leahy J, Kizilay P: *Fundamentals of nursing practice: a nursing process approach*, Philadelphia, 1998, WB Saunders.

Lear MW: *Heartsounds*, New York, 1980, Pocket Books, Simon & Schuster.

Lee N, Wasson D, Anderson M, et al: A survey of patient education post discharge, *J Nurs Care Qual* 13(1):63–70, 1998.

Lewis F, Zahlis E: The nurse as coach: a conceptual framework for clinical practice, *Oncol Nurs Forum* 24(10):1695–1702, 1997.

London F: Take the frustration out of patient education, *Home Healthc Nurse* 19(3):158–160, 2001.

Lorenzen B, Melby C, Earles B: Using principles of health literacy to enhance the informed consent process, *AORN J* 88(1):23–29, 2008.

Lorig K: *Patient education: a practical approach*, ed 3, Thousand Oaks, CA, 2001, Sage Publications.

Lorig K, Holman H: Self-management education: history, definition, outcomes and mechanisms, *Ann Behav Med* 26(1):1–7, 2003.

Lowenstein A, Foord-May L, Romano J: *Teaching strategies for health education and health promotion*, Sudbury, MA, 2009, Jones and Bartlett.

Manning S: The nurses I'll never forget, *Nursing* 22(8):47, 1992.

Masters K: *Role development in professional nursing*, Sudbury MA, 2008, Jones and Bartlett Publishers, Inc.

Mezirow J: *Fostering critical reflection in adulthood: a guide to transformative and emancipatory learning*, San Francisco, CA, 1990, Jossey-Bass.

Perdue B, Degazon C, Lunny M: Diagnoses and interventions with low literacy, *Nurs Diagn* 10(1):36–39, 1999.

Post-White J: Wind behind the sails: empowering our patients and ourselves, *Oncol Nurs Forum* 25(6):1011–1017, 1998.

Ragland G: *Instant teaching treasures for patient education*, St Louis, 1997, Mosby.

Redman BK: *The practice of patient education: a case study approach*, ed 10, St. Louis, 2007, Mosby.

Rogers C: *Freedom to learn for the '80s*, Columbus, OH, 1983, Merrill.

Rycroft-Malone J, Latter S, Yerrell P, et al: Nursing and medication education, *Nurs Stand* 14(50):35–39, 2000.

Skinner BF: *Beyond freedom and dignity*, New York, 1971, Knopf.

Schumacher K, Marren J: Home care nursing for older adults: state of the science, *Nurs Clin North Am* 39:443–471, 2004.

Stephenson P: Before the teaching begins: managing patient anxiety prior to providing education, *Clin J Oncol Nurs* 10(2):241–245, 2006.

Szpiro K, Harrison M, Van Den Kerkhof, Loutheed MD: Patient education in the emergency department, *Adv Emerg Nurs J* 30(1): 34–49, 2008.

Taylor C, Lillis C, Lemone P: *Fundamentals of nursing: the art and science of nursing care*, ed 5, Philadelphia, 2005, Lippincott Williams & Wilkins.

Wellard S, Turner D, Bethune E: Nurses as patient-teachers: exploring current expressions of the role, *Contemp Nurse* 7(1):12–14, 1998.

CHAPTER 17

Communicating with Clients with Communication Disabilities

Kathleen Underman Boggs

OBJECTIVES

At the end of the chapter, the reader will be able to:
1. Identify common communication deficits.
2. Describe nursing strategies for communicating with clients experiencing communication deficits secondary to visual, auditory, cognitive, or stimuli-related disabilities.
3. Discuss application of research findings to your clinical practice.

This chapter presents an overview of communication difficulties commonly encountered when caring for clients with sensory or cognitive deficits. Strategies for enhancing communication are described. The World Health Organization's (WHO's; 2001) International Classification of Functioning, Disability and Health shifted away from a medical diagnosis model to a functional model (i.e., how the person with a sensory impairment functions in his or her everyday life). Under this model, a communication disability definition includes any client who has any impairment in body structure or function that interferes with communication. Specifically, the client has a communication difficulty because of impaired functioning of one or more of his five senses, or he has impaired cognitive functioning. Examples include hearing loss, blindness, aphasia, or mental disorders. Communication deficits can also arise from the kind of sensory deprivation that occurs in some intensive care hospital units. The degree of difficulty in communicating is an interaction between the client's type of functional impairment, his personal adaptability, and the healthcare environment (i.e., body factors, personal factors, and environmental factors as stated in WHO's model).

Any impairment of a client's ability to send and/or receive information from health care providers may compromise his or her health, health care, and rights to make decisions. When working with these clients, you may need to modify communication strategies presented earlier in this textbook. Assess your client's communication. Two individuals can have the same sensory impairment but not be equally communication disabled. Each person compensates for their impairment in different ways. Our primary nursing goal is to maximize our client's ability to successfully interact with the health care system. This chapter focuses on suggested strategies for communication.

BASIC CONCEPTS

Clients with communication deficits are known to encounter barriers in obtaining adequate health care (Levy-Storms, 2008; O'Halloran, 2008). Studies show that when their nurses are unable to understand them, clients with communication disabilities become frustrated, angry, depressed, or uncertain. Some clients become so frustrated that they omit needed care. Even when care is accessed, communication deficits interfere with the therapeutic relationship and delivery of optimum care (McDonald, 2008). The client's deficit is one barrier. But other barriers may be staff's negative attitude or failure to adapt communication.

LEGAL MANDATES

In the legal system, the standard of "effective communication" is based on several statutes. The Americans with Disabilities Act (ADA) prohibits discrimination on the basis of a disability. Thus, physician offices are required to provide reasonable accommodations to ensure effective communication. The Rehabilitation Act bars discrimination by those providers receiving federal monies, including Medicare. Title VI of the 1964 Civil Rights Act prohibits discrimination on the basis of national origin. Health care agencies are required to develop a plan for accommodating non–English-speaking clients.

TYPES OF DEFICITS

HEARING LOSS

Nearly 28 million Americans have some problem hearing. Loss can be conductive, sensorineural, or functional. Nurses have both a legal and ethical obligation to provide appropriate care. Yet, deaf people are less likely to seek health-related information from care providers. Title III of the ADA delineates rights of the deaf and applies to communication between deaf clients and medical services (Lieu, Sadler, & Stohlmann, 2007).

People's sense of hearing alerts them to changes in the environment so they can respond effectively. The listener hears sounds and words, and also a speaker's vocal pitch, loudness, and intricate inflections accompanying the verbalization. Subtle variations can completely change the sense of the communication. Combined with the sound and intensity, the organization of the verbal symbols allows the client to perceive and interpret the meaning of the sender's message. The extent of your client's loss is not always appreciated because they often look and act in a normal fashion. Deprived of a primary means of receiving signals from the environment, clients with hearing loss may try to hide deficits, may withdraw from relationships, become depressed, or be less likely to seek information from health care providers.

Children

Nearly 3 of every 1,000 newborns are deaf or have hearing loss. Fortunately, many of these deficits are diagnosed at birth. Newborn hearing is tested in the nursery via auditory brainstem response tests (National Institute on Deafness and Other Communication Disorders, www.nidc.nih.gov/. **Hearing screening** is recommended for all newborn children by U.S. Preventive Services Task Force (USPSTF, online) and American Academy of Pediatrics.

Older Adults

As we age, we have an increased likelihood for experiencing sensory deficits related to the aging process. *Presbycusis,* or degeneration of ear structures, is a sensorineural dysfunction that normally occurs as we age. British studies found that older adults, as a group, have significant decreases in hearing, poorer consonant discrimination, and changes in their conversational styles, especially in those older than 75 years.

VISION LOSS

Humans rely more heavily on vision than do most species. More than 21 million adult Americans are blind or have low vision (Pleis & Lethbridge-Cejku, 2007). Clients who lack vision loose a primary method to decode the meaning of messages. All of the nonverbal cues that accompany speech communication (e.g., facial expression, nodding, and leaning toward the client) are lost to blind clients.

Children

Children with visual impairments lack access to visual cues, such as the facial expressions that encourage them to develop communication skills (Parker, Grimmett, & Summers, 2008). The USPSTF (2008) recommends testing children younger than 5 years for amblyopia, strabismus, and acuity. But traditional vision screening requires a verbal child and cannot be done reliably until age 3 (Rosenberg & Sperazza, 2008).

Older Adults

As your clients age, they are more likely to have vision problems that may interfere with the communication process. As we age, the lens of the eye becomes less flexible, making it difficult to accommodate shifts from far to near vision; this is a condition known as *presbyopia.* A British study found substantial decreases in visual acuity in older adults. These decreases ranged from 3% at age 65 to more than 35% in those older than 85 (van der Pols et al., 2000). Macular degeneration has become a major cause of vision loss in older adults.

IMPAIRED VERBAL COMMUNICATION SECONDARY TO SPEECH AND LANGUAGE DEFICITS

Clients who have speech and language deficits resulting from neurologic trauma present a different type of communication problem. Normal communication allows people to perceive and interact with the world in an organized and systematic manner. People use language to express self-needs and to control environmental events. Language is the system people rely on to represent what they know about the world. Early identification of children with at-risk prelinguistic skills may allow intervention to improve communication competencies (Crais, Watson, & Baranek, 2009). Clients unable to speak, even temporarily because of intubation or ventilator dependency, incur feelings of frustration, anxiety, fear, or even panic (Braun-Janzen, Sarchuk, & Murray, 2009).

When the ability to process and express language is disrupted, many areas of functioning are assaulted simultaneously. *Aphasia* is a neurologic linguistic deficit, such as occurs after a stroke. Aphasia can present as primarily an expressive or receptive disorder. The client with *expressive aphasia* can understand what is being said but cannot express thoughts or feelings in words. *Receptive aphasia* creates difficulties in receiving and processing written and oral messages. With *global aphasia,* the client has difficulty with both expressive

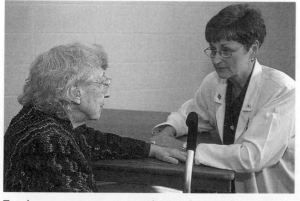

Touch, eye movements, and sounds can be used to communicate with clients experiencing aphasia.

language and reception of messages. Your client may have feelings of loss and social isolation imposed by the communication impairment. Although there may be no cognitive impairment, the client may need more "think time" for cognitive processing during a conversation.

IMPAIRED COGNITION

Impaired cognition can interfere with the communication process. The responsibility for assessing ability to understand, to give consent, and to overcome communication difficulties rests with both social services and health care workers. At times staff fail to determine the extent to which the client can understand or fail to effectively use alternative communication aids (O'Halloran et al., 2008).

Children

Atypical communication is often the first behavioral clue to cognitive impairment in young children, associated with conditions such as mental retardation, autism, and affective disorders. As these children grow, subtle distortions in communication may exist. For example, children with Down syndrome, have been shown to judge nonverbal facial expressions more positively than other children, which could lead to a misinterpretation of the nurses' messages.

Older Adults

Older cognitively impaired clients also have altered communication pathways (Magee & Bowen, 2008). While older adults retain their mental acuity, a study by Naylor and colleagues (2005) found cognitive deficits in 35% of 145 adults older than 70 years who were hospitalized for routine medical or surgical events. Memory loss, for example, interfered with client ability to correctly take prescribed medications.

COMMUNICATION DEFICITS ASSOCIATED WITH SOME MENTAL DISORDERS

Clients with serious mental disorders have a different type of communication deficit resulting from a malfunctioning of the neurotransmitters that normally transmit and make sense out of messages in the brain. Social isolation and impaired coping may accompany the client's inability to receive or express language signals.

Other communication problems occur with different mental disorders. As an example, some clients with mental disorders can have intact sensory channels, but they cannot process and respond appropriately to what they hear, see, smell, or touch. In some forms of *schizophrenia* there are alterations in the biochemical neurotransmitters in the brain, which normally conduct messages between nerve cells and help orchestrate the person's response to the external environment. Messages have distorted meanings. It is beyond the scope of this text to discuss the psychotic client's management. Basic communications strategies are described.

Some clients with mental disorders present with a poverty of speech and limited content. Speech appears blocked, reflecting disturbed patterns of perception, thought, emotions, and motivation. You may notice a lack of vocal inflection and an unchanging facial expression. A "flat affect" makes it difficult to truly understand your client. Illogical thinking processes may manifest in the form of illusions, hallucinations, and delusions. Common words assume new meanings known only to the person experiencing them.

ENVIRONMENTAL DEPRIVATION AS RELATED TO ILLNESS

Communication is particularly important in nursing situations characterized by sensory deprivation, physical immobility, limited environmental stimuli, or excessive, constant stimuli (Figure 17-1). Nurses need to show concern for the client in bewildering situations, such as emergency departments or intensive care units (ICUs). Clients may be frightened, in pain, and may by unable to communicate easily with others, because of intubation or other complications. Research indicates that the absence of interpersonal stimulation and the subsequent gradual decline of cognitive abilities are related. Clients with normal intellectual capacity can appear dull, uninterested, and lacking in problem-solving abilities if they do not have frequent interpersonal stimulation.

Developing an Evidence-Based Practice

Lindenmayer JP, Liu-Seifert H, Kulkarni PM et al.: Medication nonadherence and treatment outcome in patients with schizophrenia of schizoaffective disorder with suboptimal prior response, *J Clin Psychiatry* 70(7):990–997, 2009.

In an extensive review of research dealing with health care issues and clients with communication disabilities, O'Halloran et al. (2008) reported an astonishing lack of available studies. Schizophrenic clients with better symptom control are better able to communicate.

This large, randomized, 8-week study of antipsychotic medication compliance in 599 schizophrenic clients was conducted in 55 centers. In the post hoc analysis, (partial) nonadherence was determined by daily pill count and, in some, by plasma levels of medication. Baseline behaviors and treatment outcomes were assessed using multiple measurement tools.

Results: Thirty-four percent of subjects were nonadherent at least once during the study. Nonadherence was significantly related to reduced likelihood of treatment response (control of schizophrenic symptoms). No baseline characteristics were predictive of nonadherence to medication treatment except depression level. Higher depressive symptom scores (more sadness, concentration difficulties, and pessimistic thoughts as measured on the Montgomery–Asberg Depression Rating Scale MADRS]) were significantly related to greater nonadherence. A lower response rate was notable by Week 2.

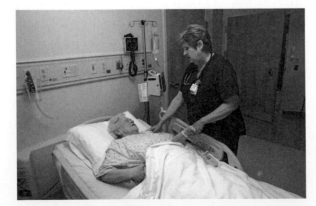

Figure 17-1 Situational Factors that Affect Client Responses to Critical Care Hospital Situations.
- Anxiety/fear
- Pain
- Altered stimuli - too much/too little [includes unusual noises, isolation]
- Sleep deprivation
- Unmet physiological needs such as thirst
- Losing track of time
- Multiple life changes
- Multiple care providers
- Immobility
- Frequent diagnostic procedures
- Lack of easily understood information

Application to Your Clinical Practice: Clients who receive antipsychotic prescriptions should be assessed for (and treated for) depression. Clients who show poor control of their schizophrenic symptoms by the second week of treatment should be specifically, carefully assessed for medication full compliance. Targeting clients at greater risk for nonadherence and devising appropriate early interventions may improve medication adherence, and thus improve symptom control/treatment outcome.

APPLICATIONS

Communication deficits may be developmental or acquired. Some nurse authors are redefining our nursing role from caregiver to care partner. This embodies the idea that clients living with communication disabilities need to be active participants in their care (Boyles, Bailey, & Mossey, 2008). All staff needs to be aware of the client's communication disability, using a sign or symbol on the door, and so on. In a number of studies, nurses lacked abilities to communicate effectively with these clients (Braun-Janzen et al., 2009; Gordon, Ellis-Hill, & Ashburn, 2009).

Nursing *goals* are to enable our clients to communicate effectively with a variety of health professionals. The following section should give you some basic strategies for fostering communication with these clients. Aspects of your nurse role include assessment, development of strategies to facilitate communication, education, provision of psychological support, and advocacy.

EARLY RECOGNITION OF COMMUNICATION DEFICITS

Identification of communication deficit is one aspect of your role. For example, if your 4-year-old client fails to speak at all or uses a noticeably limited vocabulary for his or her age, cannot name objects or follow your directions, would you recognize the need for further assessment? Given this history, you could make a referral for speech and language evaluation.

ASSESSMENT OF CURRENT COMMUNICATION ABILITIES

You need to assess each client's communication problems. Your plan of care can then be tailored to help meet identified communication needs. Provision of alternative communication methods is required by law.

COMMUNICATION STRATEGIES

Evidence-based practice suggests you create a quiet environment, allocate more of your time to facilitate communication, take time to listen, ask yes/no questions, observe nonverbal cues, repeat back comments, effectively use communication equipment, assign same staff for care continuity, and encourage family members to be present to assist in communications (Finke, Light, & Kitko, 2008; O'Halloran et al., 2008).

CLIENTS WITH HEARING LOSS

Assessment of functional hearing ability is recommended for all your clients. Assessment of auditory sensory losses can provide an opportunity for referral. Your assessment should include the age of onset and the severity of the deficit. Hearing loss that occurs after the development of speech means that the client has access to word symbols and language skills. Deafness in children can cause developmental delays, which may need to be taken into account in planning the most appropriate communication strategies. Clues to hearing loss occur when clients appear unresponsive to sound or respond only when the speaker is directly facing them. Ask clients whether they use a hearing aid and whether it is working properly.

Strategies for communicating with clients who have a hearing loss depend on the severity of the deafness. Covering your face with a mask or speaking with an accent may make it impossible for a lip reader to understand you. Communication-assisting equipment should be available. We need to know how to operate auditory amplifiers such as assisted listening devices, hearing aids, and telephone attachments. Often, clients have hearing aids but fail to use them because they do not fit well or are hard to insert. Some complain that the hearing aid amplifies all sounds indiscriminately, not just the voices of people in conversation. O'Halloran et al. (2008) cautions about the attitude displayed by providers. The client may have had a prior experience in which the provider viewed his deafness as sign of lack of intelligence or treated him with a lack of respect. Exercises 17-1 and 17-2 will help you understand what it is like to have a sensory deficit.

Refer to Box 17-1 to adapt your communication techniques. American Sign Language has been a standard communication tool for many years; however, few care providers were able to use it. Basic strategies include use of paper and pencil, use of hand signals or

EXERCISE 17-1	Loss of Sensory Function in Geriatric Clients

Purpose: To assist students in getting in touch with the feelings often experienced by older adults as they lose sensory function. If the younger individual is able to "walk in the older person's shoes," he or she will be more sensitive to the losses and needs created by those losses in the older person.

Procedure:
1. Students separate into three groups.
2. Group A: Place cotton balls in your ears. Group B: Cover your eyes with a plastic bag. Group C: Place cotton balls in your ears and cover your eyes with a plastic bag.
3. A student from Group B should be approached by a student from Group A. The student from Group B is to talk to the student from Group A using a whispered voice. The Group A student is to verify the message heard with the student who spoke. The student from Group B is then to identify the student from Group A.
4. The students in Group C are expected to identify at least one person in the group and describe to that

person what he or she is wearing. Each student who does not do the description is to make a statement to the other person and have that individual reveal what he or she was told.
5. Having identified and conversed with each other, hold hands or remain next to each other and remove the plastic bags and cotton balls (to facilitate verification of what was heard and described).

Discussion:
1. How did the loss you experienced make you feel?
2. Were you comfortable performing the function expected of you with your limitation?
3. What do you think could have been done to make you feel less handicapped?
4. How did you feel when your "normal" level of functioning was restored?
5. How would you feel if you knew the loss you just simulated was to be permanent?
6. What impact do you think this experience might have on your future interactions with older individuals with such sensory losses?

Courtesy B. J. Glenn, former member of the North Carolina State Health Coordinating Council Acute Care Committee, 1998.

EXERCISE 17-2	Sensory Loss: Hearing or Vision

Purpose: To help raise consciousness regarding loss of a sensory function.

Procedure:
- Pair up with another student. One student should be blindfolded. The other student should guide the "blind" student on a walk around the campus.
- During a 5- to 10-minute walk, the student guide should converse with the "blind" student about the route they are taking.
  or
- Watch the first 2 minutes of a television show with the sound turned off. All students should watch the

same show (e.g., the news report or a rerun of a situation comedy).
- In class, students share observations and answer the following questions.

Discussion:
1. Were perceptual differences noted? What implications do you think these differences have in working with blind or deaf clients?
2. How frustrating was it for you to be sensory deprived? How did it make you feel?
3. What did you learn about yourself from this exercise that you can apply to your nursing clinical practice?

gestures, and use of technologic communication assistance devices such as:
- *Speech amplifiers* such as the pocket talker
- Spelling boards or communication boards
- **Wireless text communication** (text messaging) on cell phones: deaf clients use handheld electronics to exchange e-mail and receive instant alphanumeric messaging, paging, and so on.
- The **Optacon**: a reading device that converts printed letters into a vibration that can be felt by the client who is both deaf and blind

- Pictographs: laminated **cards** that show drawings of common foods and activities; products such as the "AT&T Picture Guide" are commercially available and help you get your point across; these may be useful also with clients whose language you do not speak, as well as those clients with aphasia or altered hearing
- **Pagers**: vibrate to alert the deaf person to an incoming message, convert voice mail into e-mail that can be read

| BOX 17-1 | Suggestions for Helping the Client with Sensory Loss |

- Always maximize use of sensory aids, such as hearing aid, pictures, sign language, regular or laser cane (which vibrates a warning if an obstacle is within 5 feet).
- Pick the means of available communication best suited to your client.
- Help elderly clients adjust hearing aids. Lacking fine motor dexterity, the elderly client may not be able to insert aids to amplify hearing.

For Hearing-Impaired Clients
- Stand or sit so that you face the client and the client can see your facial expression and mouthing of words. Communicate in a well-lighted room.
- Use facial expressions and gestures that reinforce verbal content.
- Speak distinctly without exaggerating words. Partially deaf clients respond best to well-articulated words spoken in a moderate, even tone.
- Write important ideas and allow the client the same option to increase the chances of communication. Always have a writing pad available.
- Always face the client when communicating so the client can see your lips move.
- Tap on the floor or table to get client's attention via the vibration.

- Arrange for TTY (amplified telephone handset) for client with partial hearing loss.
- If unable to hear, rely primarily on visual materials.
- Arrange for closed-captioned television.
- Use text messaging on client's cell phone or e-mail at his or her computer.
- Encourage the client with hearing loss to verbalize speech, even if the person uses only a few words or the words are difficult to understand at first.
- Use an intermediary, such as a family member who knows sign language, to facilitate communication with deaf clients who sign.

For Vision-Impaired Clients
- Let the person know when you approach by a simple touch, and always indicate when you are leaving.
- Adapt teaching for low vision by using large print, audiotaped information, or Braille.
- Do not lead or hold the client's arm when walking; instead, allow the person to take your arm.
- Use touch and close physical proximity while you are with the client; give the person something substantial to touch in your absence.
- Develop and use signals to indicate changes in pace or direction while walking.

- **Real-time captioning devices**: allow spoken words to be typed simultaneously onto a screen
- **Interactive videodiscs**: have signing avatars, which are on-screen figures that sign words pre-programmed into bar codes that you select or that you speak into a microphone
- **Speech-generating devices** are also available, including laptop computers, fax machines, and PDAs (electronic personal digital assistant computers small enough to be held in one hand)
- Devices such as hearing-amplified stethoscopes also allow hearing-impaired nurses to care for clients

Case Example

Two student nurses were assigned to care for 9-year-old Timmy, who is deaf and mute. When they went into his room for assessment, he was alone and appeared anxious. No information was available as to his ability to read lips, the nurses were not sure what reading skills he had, and they did not know sign language. So, instead of using a pad and paper for communication, they decided to role-play taking vital signs by using some funny facial expressions and demonstrating on a doll.

CLIENTS WITH VISION LOSS

Vision assessment for impairment is recommended for all clients routinely. Nurses caring for any client with vision limitations should perform some evaluation and ensure that glasses and other equipment are available to hospitalized clients. Use of prompting and reinforcement are recommended (Parker et al., 2008).

Case Example

You can use words to supply additional information to counterbalance the missing visual cues. Ms. Sue Shu is a blind, elderly client who commented to Ruth, her student nurse, that she felt Ruth was uncomfortable talking with her and perhaps did not like her. Not being able to see Ruth, Ms. Shu interpreted the hesitant uneasiness in Ruth's voice as evidence that Ruth did not wish to be with her. Ruth agreed with Ms. Shu that she was quite uncomfortable but did not explain further. Had Ms. Shu been able to see Ruth's apprehensive body posture, she would have realized that Ruth was quite shy and ill at ease with *any* interpersonal relationship. To avoid this serious error in communication, Ruth might have clarified the reasons for her discomfort, and the relationship could have moved forward.

Refer to Box 17-1 for strategies of use in caring for vision-impaired clients. Use of vocal cues (e.g., speaking as you approach) helps prevent startling the blind client. Because clients cannot see our faces or observe our non-verbal signals, we need to use words to express what the client cannot see in the message. It also is helpful to mention your name as you enter the client's presence. Even people who are partially blind appreciate hearing the name of the person to whom they are speaking. Vision enhancing equipment includes:

- Electronic magnifier machines
- Auditory teaching materials, such as on an audio-cassette
- Computer screen readers with voice synthesizers
- Braille keypads
- The Braille Alphabet Card (letters in both print and Braille, so both nurse and client can understand)
- The **Tellatouch**, a portable machine into which the nurse types a message that emerges in Braille on a punched-out paper in Braille format
- Large print materials
- **Voice synthesizers** (available in a wide variety of household appliances such as talking scales)
- **Telemicroscopes**: handheld telescopes
- **Video magnifying machines**
- Enhanced lighting, light filters that reduce glare and enhance contrast

When caring for clients with macular degeneration, remember to stand to their side, an exception to the "face them directly" rule applied with clients with hearing loss. Macular degeneration clients often still have some peripheral vision.

Use of Touch

The social isolation experienced by blind clients can be profound, and the need for human contact is important. Touching the client lightly as you speak alerts the client to your presence. Voice tones and pauses that reinforce the verbal content are helpful. The client needs to be informed when the nurse is leaving the room. Compensatory interventions for the blind include a plentiful assortment of auditory stimuli, such as books on tape and music, as well as tactile stimuli.

ORIENTATION TO ENVIRONMENTAL HAZARDS

When a blind client is being introduced to a new environmental setting, you should orient the client by describing the size of the room and the position of the furniture and equipment. When placing their food tray, describe the position of items, perhaps using a clock face analogy (i.e., "Carrots are at 2 o'clock, potatoes at 11 o'clock, etc.). If other people are present, you could name each person. A good communication strategy is to ask the other people in the room to introduce themselves to the client. In this way, the client gains an appreciation for their voice configurations. You should avoid any tendency to speak with a blind client in a louder voice than usual or to enunciate words in an exaggerated manner. This may be perceived by some clients as condescending or insensitive to the nature of the handicap. Voice tones should be kept natural.

The blind client needs guidance in moving around in unfamiliar surroundings. For example, surveyed blind clients said they needed assistance getting to and from their bathroom. One way of preserving the client's autonomy is to offer your arm to the client instead of taking the client's arm. Mention steps and changes in movement as they are about to occur to help the client navigate new places and differences in terrain.

IMPAIRED VERBAL COMMUNICATION SECONDARY TO SPEECH AND LANGUAGE DEFICITS

Assessment of speech and language is part of the initial evaluation. For adults with aphasia, an assessment of the type your client is experiencing will aid in selecting the most appropriate intervention. Expressive language problems are evidenced in an inability to find words or to associate ideas with accurate word symbols. Some clients with expressive aphasia can find the correct word if given enough time and support. Other clients have difficulty organizing their words into meaningful sentences or describing a sequence of events. Clients with receptive communication deficits have trouble following directions, reading information, writing, or relating data to previous knowledge. Even when your client appears not to understand, you should explain in very simple terms what is happening. Using touch, gestures, eye movements, and squeezing of the hand should be attempted. Clients appreciate nurses who take the time to respond to communication attempts.

Refer to Box 17-2 for strategies to use with clients having speech deficits. Clients who lose both expressive and receptive communication abilities have *global*

BOX 17-2	Strategies to Assist the Client with Speech and Language Difficulties

- Avoid prolonged, continuous conversations; instead, use frequent, short talks. Present small amounts of information at a time.
- When clients falter in written or oral expression, supply needed compensatory support.
- Praise efforts to communicate.
- Provide regular mental stimulation in a nontaxing way.
- Help clients focus on the faculties still available to them for communication.
- Allow extra time for delays in cognitive processing of information.
- For print materials, use short, bulleted lists.

aphasia. These clients can become frustrated when they are not understood. Struggling to speak causes fatigue. Short, positive sessions are used to communicate. Otherwise, the client may become nonverbal as a way of regaining energy and composure. Changes in self-image occasioned by physical changes, the uncertain recovery course and outcome of strokes, shifts in family roles, and the disruption of free-flowing verbal interaction among family members all make the loss of functional communication particularly agonizing for clients. Any language skills that are preserved should be exploited. Other means of communication (e.g., pointing, gesturing, using pictures, and repeating phrases) can be used.

Case Example

Your client Mr. Lopez is totally paralyzed immediately after a rupture of a blood vessel in his brain, except he can still blink his eyes. You tell him, "Blink once for yes and twice for no." You point out familiar objects in his immediate environment.

CLIENTS WITH IMPAIRED COGNITION OR LEARNING DELAY

As a nurse providing care to learning delay (LD) clients, you need to adapt your messages to an understandable level. This is crucial when you are seeking to gain informed consent for treatment. The rules outlining who can give informed consent were discussed in Chapter 2. To what extent should you involve your cognitively impaired client? Sowney and Barr (2007) note that emergency department nurses tend to overlook involving LD patients when explaining treatments

and making care decisions, not just when obtaining informed consent. They recommend that nurses make the effort to involve cognitively impaired clients.

A good strategy is to enhance social interaction by emphasizing any activity that can be shared between nurse and client and between caregiver and client. Communication adaptations include simple explanations, touch, and use of familiar objects. Alternative methods of communication include music, *communication boards*, picture *card*, and use of *picture pain rating scales*.

COMMUNICATION DEFICITS ASSOCIATED WITH SOME MENTAL DISORDERS

When working with some clients with mental disorders, you will face a formidable challenge in trying to establish a relationship. Clients with altered reality discrimination have both verbal and nonverbal communication deficits. Rarely will this client approach you directly. The client generally responds to questions, but the answers are likely to be brief, and the client does not elaborate without further probes. Although the client appears to rebuff any social interaction, it is important to keep trying to connect. People with mental disorders such as schizophrenia are easily overwhelmed by the external environment. Tremeau and colleagues (2005) demonstrate that schizophrenic clients have the same expressive deficits as do depressed clients. Keeping in mind that the client's unresponsiveness to words, failure to make eye contact, unchanging facial expression, and monotonic voice are parts of the disorder and not a commentary on your communication skills helps you to continue to engage with the client.

If your client is hallucinating or using delusions as a primary form of communication, you should neither challenge their validity directly nor enter into a prolonged discussion of illogical thinking. Often you can identify the underlying theme the client is trying to convey with the delusional statement. For example, when your client says, "Voices are telling me to do...," you might reply, "It sounds as though you feel powerless and afraid at this moment." Listening to your client carefully, using alert posture, nodding to demonstrate active listening, and trying to make sense out of his underlying feelings models effective communication and helps you decode nonsensical

EXERCISE 17-3	Schizophrenia Communication Simulation

Purpose: To gain insight into communication deficits encountered by clients with schizophrenia.

Procedure:
1. Break class into groups of three (triads) by counting off 1, 2, 3.
2. Person 1 (the nurse) reads a paragraph of rules to the client and then quizzes him or her afterward about the content.
3. Person 2 (the client with schizophrenia) listens to everything and tries to answer the nurse's questions correctly to get 100% on the test.

4. Person 3 (representing the mental illness) speaks loudly and continuously in the client's ear while the nurse is communicating, saying things like "You are so stupid," "You have done bad things," and "It is coming to get you" over and over.

Discussion:
Did any client have 100% recall? Ask the client to share how difficult is it to communicate to the nurse when you are "hearing voices."

Courtesy Ann Newman, PhD, University of North Carolina, Charlotte.

messages. Exercise 17-3 may help you gain some understanding of communication problems experienced by the client with schizophrenia.

CLIENTS EXPERIENCING TREATMENT-RELATED COMMUNICATION DISABILITIES

Communication disabilities can stem from sedative medications, mechanical ventilation, isolation in an ICU, or isolation such as occurs when older adults are in long-term care facilities. A number of recent studies of client communication in intensive care show that they are very dependent on their nurse to institute communication. Specific recommended skills include asking many questions, asking questions your client can answer with yes or no, reading lips, using a communication board, offering pen and paper, and assessing whether your communication was successful. When a client is not fully alert, it is not uncommon for nurses to speak in his presence in ways they would not if they thought the client could fully understand what is being said, forgetting that hearing can remain acute. Good practice suggests you never say anything you would not want the client to hear.

In addition to conveying a caring, compassionate attitude, you may use several of the strategies for communicating listed in Box 17-3. Giving orienting cues is recommended, such as labeling of meals as breakfast, lunch, or dinner, and linking events to routines (e.g., saying, "The x-ray technician will take your chest x-ray right after lunch") helps secure the client in time and space. When clients are unable or unwilling to engage in a dialogue, you should continue to initiate communication in a one-way mode.

BOX 17-3	Strategies for Communicating with Clients in the Intensive Care Unit

- Encourage the client to display pictures or a simple object from home.
- Orient the client to the environment.
- Frequently provide information about the client's condition and progress.
- Reassure the client that cognitive and psychological disturbances are common.
- Give explanations before procedures by providing information about the sounds, sights, and feelings the client is experiencing.
- Provide the client with frequent orienting cues to time and place.

Case Example

Nurse: I am going to give you your bath now. The water will feel a little warm to you. After your bath, your wife will be in to see you. She stayed in the waiting room last night because she wanted to be with you. (No answer is necessary if the client is unable to talk, but the sound of a human voice and attention to the client's unspoken concerns can be very healing.)

Your client should be called by name. We need to identify our name and explain procedures in simple language even if our client does not appear particularly alert. Clients who are awake or even semi-alert should not be allowed to stare at a blank ceiling for extended periods. Changing the client's position frequently benefits the person physiologically and offers us something to talk about. Our efforts to create a more stimulating environment, to offer reassurance and support have later been reported to have been meaningful to the client. If clients in ICUs become temporarily delusional or experiences hallucinations, you can use strategies similar to those used with the psychotic client. The client is reassured if you are able to confirm to him that experiencing strange sensations, thoughts, and feelings is a common occurrence in the ICU.

CLIENT ADVOCACY

Our nurse role also includes acting as an advocate for our clients who have communication disabilities. Too often these clients are discounted. Medical treatment decisions may be made without seeking input from them. Appropriate communication aids may be withheld while the client is hospitalized. In the larger community, we need to advocate for community services designed to foster communication, including referrals to speech and language therapists.

SUMMARY

This chapter discusses the specialized communication needs of clients with communication deficits. Adapting our communication skills and projecting a caring, positive attitude are important in overcoming barriers. Basic issues and applications for communicating with clients experiencing sensory loss of hearing and sight are outlined. Sensory stimulation and compensatory channels of communication are needed for clients with sensory deprivation. All workers who come in contact with the client need to be aware of their communication impairments. We need to learn how to operate and fit equipment such as hearing aids, because hospitalized clients often need help with devices. The mentally ill client has intact senses, but information processing and language are affected by the disorder. It is important for you to develop a proactive communication approach with clients who are learning impaired or who suffer from mental disorders. For clients such as those with aphasia, you can develop alternative methods of communicating. Other clients can experience communication isolation and temporary distortion of reality. Such clients need frequent cues that orient them to time and place, as well as providing sensory stimulation. Evidence shows that we need to be careful not to associate communication disability with intellectual dysfunction. Our skill in adapting communication is important to the client.

ETHICAL DILEMMA What Would You Do?

Working in a health department clinic, the nurse—through a Spanish-speaking translator—interviews a 46-year-old married woman about the missing results of her recent breast biopsy for suspected cancer. Because the translator is of the same culture as the client and holds the same cultural belief that suicide is shameful, he chooses to withhold from the nurse information he obtained about a recent suicide attempt. If this information remains hidden from the nurse and doctor, could this adversely affect the client? What ethical principle is being violated?

REFERENCES

Boyles CM, Bailey PH, Mossey S: Representations of disability in nursing and healthcare literature: an integrative review, *J Adv Nurs* 62(4):428–437, 2008.

Braun-Janzen, Sarchuk L, Murray RP: Roles of speech-language pathologists and nurses in providing communication intervention for nonspeaking adults in acute care: a regional pilot study, *Can J Speech Lang Pathol Audiol* 33(1):5–23, 2009.

Crais ER, Watson LR, Baranek GT: Use of gesture development in profiling children's prelinguistic communication skills, *Am J Speech Lang Pathol* 18:95–108, 2009.

Finke EH, Light J, Kitko L: A systematic review of the effectiveness of nurse communication with patients with complex communication needs with a focus on the use of augmentative and alternative communication, *J Clin Nurs* 17:2102–2115, 2008.

Gordon C, Ellis-Hill C, Ashburn A: The use if conversational analysis: nurse-patient interaction in communication disability after stroke, *J Adv Nurs* 65(3):544–553, 2009.

Levy-Storms L: Therapeutic communication training in long-term care institutions: recommendations for future research, *Patient Educ Couns* 73(1):8–21, 2008.

Lieu CC, Sadler GR, Stohlmann PD: Communication strategies for nurses interacting with patients who are deaf, *Dermatol Nurs* 19(6): 541–544, 549–551, 2007.

Magee WL, Bowen C: Using music in leisure to enhance social relationships with patients with complex disabilities, *NeuroRehabilitation* 23(4):305–311, 2008.

McDonald HL: Inpatients with cerebral palsy and complex communication needs identified barriers to communicating, *Evid Based Nurs* 11(1):30, 2008.

Naylor MD, Stephens C, Bowles KH, et al: Cognitively impaired older adults: from hospital to home, *Am J Nurs* 105(2):52–61, 2005.

O'Halloran R, Hickson L, Worrall L: Environmental factors that influence communication between people with communication disability and their healthcare providers in hospital: a review of the literature within the International Classification of Functioning, Disability, and Health (ICF) framework, *Int J Lang Commun Disord* 43(6):601–632, 2008.

Parker AT, Grimmett ES, Summers S: Evidence-based communication practices for children with visual impairments and additional disabilities: an examination of single-subject design studies, *J Vis Impair Blind* 102(9):540–552, 2008.

Pleis JR, Lethbridge-Cejku M: Summary health statistics for US adults: National Health Interview Survey, 2006. National Center for Health Statistics, *Vital Health Stat* 10:235, 2007.

Rosenberg EA, Sperazza LC: The visually impaired patient, *Am Fam Physician* 77(100):1431–1436, 2008.

Sowney M, Barr O: The challenges for nurses communicating with cognitively impaired, *J Clin Nurs* 16(9):1678–1686, 2007.

Tremeau F, Malaspina D, Duval F, et al: Facial expressiveness in patients with schizophrenia compared to depressed patients and nonpatient comparison subjects, *Am J Psychiatry* 162(1):92–101, 2005.

van der Pols JC, Bates CJ, McGraw PV, et al: Visual acuity measurements in a national sample of British elderly people, *Br J Ophthalmol* 84(2):165–170, 2000.

World Health Organization: *International classification of functioning, disability, and health*, Geneva, Switzerland, 2001, Author.

USPSTF [United States Preventive Health Services Task Force]: Agency for Healthcare Research and Quality. *The Guide to Clinical Preventive Services: Recommendations of the US Preventive Services Task Force*, author, 2008. http://epss.ahrq.gov/ePSS/ accessed 5/20/09.

CHAPTER 18

Communicating with Children

Kathleen Underman Boggs

OBJECTIVES

At the end of the chapter, the reader will be able to:

1. Identify how developmental levels impact the child's ability to participate in interpersonal relationships with caregivers.
2. Briefly discuss one research-based application in communicating with a child.
3. Describe modifications in communication strategies to meet the specialized needs of children.
4. Describe interpersonal techniques needed to interact with concerned parents of ill children.
5. Discuss application on one research study results to clinical practice.

This chapter is designed to help you recognize and apply communication concepts related to the nurse-client relationship in pediatric clinical situations. Each nursing situation represents a unique application of communication strategies. Tools needed by caregivers to provide effective and ethical care are attitudinal, cognitive, developmentally appropriate, and interpersonal. For each of these domains, the child's and family's socioeconomic status and cultural background must be considered.

Communicating with children at different age levels requires modifications of the skills learned in previous chapters. By understanding the child's cognitive and functional level, you are able to select the most appropriate communication strategies. Children undergo significant age-related changes in the ability to process cognitive information and in the capacity to interact effectively with the environment. To have an effective therapeutic relationship with a child, you need to understand the feelings and thought processes from the child's perspective and convey honesty, respect, and acceptance of feelings.

Communicating with parents of seriously ill children requires a deliberate effort. Hong, Murphy, and Connolly's (2008) study found that less than half of parents surveyed rated communication with nurses as excellent. Parents need explanations they can understand, need to have established trust with the nurse, and need to feel they have some control over what is happening to their child. This chapter identifies strategies to enhance communication with parents.

BASIC CONCEPTS

LOCATION

More than 70% of pediatric care occurs in ambulatory settings. Quality of care studies indicate that in all settings children receive only half to two thirds of "best evidence" interventions (Mangione-Smith et al., 2007). These deficits may compromise child safety.

ATTITUDE

Major changes in society are mirrored in changing health care for children. Involving children in their own health care decision making is seen as desirable. Yet few care providers give real choices (Coad & Shaw, 2008). Serious consideration needs to be given to educating care providers about the need to involve children in their care, to devolve adult control and give the child some choices. Making the child a (limited) partner might lead to better health outcomes than the current attitude of treating him as a target for our delivery of care.

COGNITION

Childhood is very different from adulthood. A child has fewer life experiences from which to draw and is still in the process of developing skills needed for reasoning and communicating. Every child's concept of health and illness must be considered within a developmental framework. Erikson's (1963) concepts of ego development and Piaget's (1972) description of the progressive development of the child's cognitive thought processes together form the theoretical basis for the child-centered nursing interventions described in this chapter. Both theorists say that the child's thought processes, ways of perceiving the world, judgments, and emotional responses to life situations are different from those of the adult. Cognitive and psychosocial development unfold according to an ordered hierarchical scheme, increasing in depth and complexity as the child matures.

DEVELOPMENTALLY APPROPRIATE

Piaget's descriptions of stages of cognitive development provide a valuable contribution toward understanding the dimensions of a child's perceptions. Cognitive development and early language development are integrally related. Although current developmental theorists expand on Piaget's theoretical model by recognizing the effects of the parent-child relationship and a stimulating environment on developing communication abilities, his work forms the foundation for the understanding of childhood cognitive development. Piaget observed cognitive development occurring in sequential stages (Table 18-1). The ages are only approximated, because Piaget himself was not specific.

Wide individual differences exist in the intellectual functioning of same-age children. Variations also occur across situations, so that the child under stress or in a different environment may process information at a lower level than he would under normal conditions. Because two children of the same chronologic age may have quite different skills as information processors, we need to assess level of functioning. Language alternatives familiar to one child because of

TABLE 18-1		Stages of Cognitive Development	
Age	**Piaget's Stage**	**Characteristics**	**Language Development**
Birth to 2 years	**Sensorimotor**	Infant learns by manipulating objects At birth, reflexive communication, then moves through six stages to reach actual thinking	**Presymbolic** Communication largely nonverbal Vocabulary of more than 4 words by 12 months, increases to >200 words and use of short sentences before age 2 years
2–6 years	**Preoperational**	Beginning use of symbolic thinking Imaginative play Masters reversibility	**Symbolic** Actual use of structured grammar and language to communicate Uses pronouns Average vocabulary >10,000 words by age 6 years
7–11 years	**Concrete operations**	Logical thinking Masters use of numbers and other concrete ideas such as classification and conservation	Mastery of passive tense by age 7 years and complex grammatical skills by age 10 years
12+ years	**Formal operations**	Abstract thinking. Futuristic; takes a broader, more theoretical perspective	Near adult-like skills

Adapted from Piaget J: *The child's conception of the world,* Savage, MD, 1972, Littlefield, Adams.

certain life experiences may not be useful in providing health care and teaching with another. Integrating cognitive and psychosocial developmental approaches into communication with children at different ages enhances effectiveness.

INTERPERSONAL

GENDER DIFFERENCES IN COMMUNICATION

Some studies show school-age children are more satisfied if their health care provider is the same sex. Woman providers tend to engage in more social conversation, spend more time giving encouragement and reassurance, and more often speak directly to children when gathering information. Use of good age-appropriate communication strategies probably outweighs gender as a factor in successful communication with a child, but gender cannot be excluded as a factor affecting this communication.

UNDERSTANDING THE ILL CHILD'S NEEDS

Difficulties arise in adult-child communication, in part, because of the child's limited experience in interpreting subtle nuances of facial expression, inflection, and word meanings. When illness and physical or developmental disabilities occur during formative years, situational stressors are added that affect the way children perceive themselves and the environment. Illness may lead to significant alterations in role relationships with family and peers. You need to assess not only the physical care needs of the child but the impact of the illness on the child's self-esteem and on his or her relationships with family and friends. Responses to hospitalization vary with the individual according to his or her age. Negative responses may include separation anxiety, night terrors, feeding disturbances, or regression to earlier developmental stage behavior. Things that affect a child's response may include the chronicity of illness, its impact on lifestyle, the child's cognitive understanding of the disease process, and the family's ability to cope with care demands.

Children with Special Health Care Needs

Some children have chronic physical, developmental, behavioral, or emotional conditions that require health services. In the United States, 1 in every 5 households has a child with a chronic condition, totaling more than 10 million children (Looman, O'Connor-Von, & Lindeke, 2008). Many of these children previously would have died but were saved by current technology. Some are left with chronic problems (see discussion in Chapter 17).

FAMILY-CENTERED CARE

The trend toward family-centered health care of children will continue with attention to family diversity and family processes in "successful" families. A growing body of research is documenting relationships between such processes and child health outcomes. If the child needs to be hospitalized, this is a *situational crisis* for the child and the entire family. Hospitalization is always stressful. Hospitalized children have to contend not only with physical changes but with possible separation from family and friends, as well as living in a strange, frightening, and probably hurtful environment. Nurses need to assist parents to meet their hospitalized child's needs. The family needs to learn new interactional patterns and coping strategies that take into consideration the meaning of an illness and disability in family life. *Prehospitalization preparation* needs to be done to decrease the child's anxiety. Before elective procedures, many hospitals now offer orientation education tours to youngsters. There are many good books designed to prepare children for their hospitalization available in most public libraries. In the case of hospitalization for critical illness, good communication between staff and family is viewed as most important. A key component of this communication is sharing decision making with the child.

Developing an Evidence-Based Practice

Hong SS, Murphy SO, Connolly PM: Parental satisfaction with nurses' communication and pain management in a pediatric unit, Pediatr Nurs 34(4):289–293, 2008.

To test the hypothesis that parental satisfaction with communication with nurses caring for their child would increase after an intervention, 50 parents randomly selected from a total of 400 whose child was treated on one pediatric unit were surveyed in a pretest and post-test study. The intervention consisted of a 30-minute educational inservice for 20 nurses and distribution of a written brochure to parents explaining pain management.

Results: Mean satisfaction scores for nurses' communication increased from 81.6 to 85.3; satisfaction with explanations of treatment increased from 78 to 82, and satisfaction with pain management increased from 80.8 to 82.4. These increases show a positive trend, but none was statistically significant.

Application to Your Clinical Practice: Lack of significant findings limits application. Both presurvey and postsurvey scores show that there are still parents with needs for improved communication. Specifically, they need better explanations about treatments, tests, and pain management. All parents need clear communication from nursing staff. Written materials can successfully be used to reinforce this communication.

APPLICATIONS

Although children historically have not been the subjects of study, research has contributed to our knowledge of child learning and development. Children are more vulnerable, and thus are entitled to extra protection as research subjects, though Pieper (2008) argues that some would want to participate and are entitled to. Findings are limited because of over-reliance on what parents have told us. Agencies see children as similar, without consideration of differences because of age, gender, race, or culture. To give one example, many of the medicines we use to treat children have been tested only on adults by pharmaceutical companies.

Major sources of stress for parents of critically ill children include uncertainty about current condition or prognosis, lack of control, and lack of knowledge about how to best help their hospitalized child or how to deal with their child's response. Although more nursing research is being conducted on effective communication with both parents and their ill children, many of the applications we discuss are based more on experience than on research.

ASSESSMENT

Assessing a child's reaction to illness requires knowing the child's normal patterns of communication. Interactions are observed between parent and child. The child's behavioral responses to the entire interpersonal environment (including nurse and peers) are assessed. Are the child's interactions age-appropriate? Are behaviors organized, or is the child unable to complete activities? Does the child act out an entire play sequence, or is such play fragmented and disorganized? Do the child's interactions with others suggest imagination and a broad repertoire of relating behaviors, or is communication devoid of possibilities? Because children cannot communicate fully with us,

we have a special responsibility to assess for problems. For example, nearly a million American children are victims of neglect, physical abuse, psychological abuse, or even sexual abuse (Taylor, Guteman, Lee, & Rathouz, 2009). Once baseline data have been collected, you can plan specific communication strategies to meet the specialized needs of the child client (Figure 18-1). An overview of nursing adaptations needed to communicate effectively with children is summarized in Box 18-1.

REGRESSION AS A FORM OF CHILDHOOD COMMUNICATION

A severe illness can cause a child to show behaviors that are reminiscent of an earlier stage of development. A certain amount of regression is normal. Common behaviors include whining, demanding undue attention, withdrawal, or having toileting "accidents." These behaviors might stem from the powerlessness the child feels in attempting to cope with an overwhelming, frightening environment. Reassuring the parent that this is a common response to the stress of illness can be helpful.

Because children have limited life experience to draw from, they exhibit a narrower range of behaviors in coping with threat. The quiet, overly compliant child who does not complain may be more frightened than the child who screams or cries. This should alert you to the child's emotional distress. You need to obtain detailed information regarding the usual behavioral responses of the family and child. Some behaviors that look regressive may be a typical behavioral response for the child (e.g., the 2-year-old who wants a bedtime bottle). A complete baseline history offers a good counterpoint for assessing the meaning of current behaviors.

AGE-APPROPRIATE COMMUNICATION

An assessment of vocabulary and understanding is essential in fostering communications. Whenever possible, you should communicate using words familiar to the child. Parents are valuable resources in helping interpret behavioral data. You might assist a child who is having difficulty finding the right words by reframing what he said and repeating it in a slightly different way.

The ill child's peers often have difficulty accepting individual differences created by health deviations. They lack the knowledge and sensitivity to deal with physical changes that they do not understand, as evidenced by "bald" jokes about the child receiving

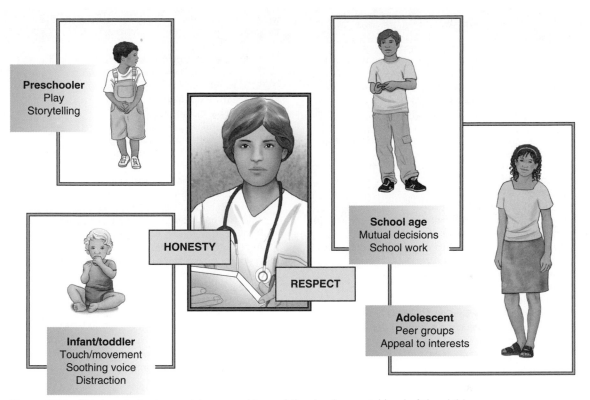

Figure 18-1 Nursing strategies must be geared toward the developmental level of the child.

chemotherapy. Children with hidden disorders such as diabetes, some forms of epilepsy, or minimal brain dysfunction are particularly susceptible to interpersonal distress. For example, it may be difficult for diabetics to regulate their intake of fast foods when all of their friends are able to eat what they want. When peer pressure is at its peak in adolescence, a teenager with a newly diagnosed convulsive seizure disorder may find it difficult to tell peers he no longer can ride his bicycle or drive a car. Unless the family and nurse provide appropriate interpersonal support, such children have to cope with an indistinct assault to their self-concept alone. A summary of age-appropriate strategies is provided in Box 18-2.

COMMUNICATING WITH CHILDREN WITH PSYCHOLOGICAL BEHAVIORAL PROBLEMS

One out of 10 adolescents and children in our society suffer from a mental illness These illnesses lead to some level of interactional problems, which may be encountered by nurses in schools, hospitals, or clinics treating common physical illnesses. Discussion of mental illness and appropriate interventions is beyond the scope of this textbook. Please refer to a multitude of hot links available through U.S. Health and Human Services Web site in the Maternal Child Health Library (Online Resources: MCH, www.hhs. gov/mch).

COMMUNICATING WITH PHYSICALLY ILL CHILDREN IN THE HOSPITAL AND AMBULATORY CLINIC

Overestimating a child's understanding of information about illness results in confusion, increased anxiety, anger, or sadness. Beyond physiologic care, ill children of all ages need support from every member of the health team—support that they normally would receive from parents. The nurse must provide stimulation to talk, listen, and play. Play is their language, especially because children have major difficulties verbalizing their true

BOX 18-1	Nurse-Child Communication Strategies: Adapting Communication to Meet the Needs of the Ill Child

- Develop an understanding of age-related norms of development
- Let the child know you are interested in him or her; convey respect and authenticity.
- Let the child know how to summon you (call bell, etc.).
- Develop trust through honesty and consistency in meeting the child's needs.
- Use "transitional objects" such as familiar pictures or toys from home.
- Assess:
  - Level of understandings
  - The child's needs in relation to the immediate situation
  - The child's capacity to cope successfully with change
- Observe for nonverbal cues.
- Use *nonverbal* communication:
  - Tactile (soothing strokes)
  - Kinesthetic (rocking)
  - get down to the child's height; don't tower over him or her
  - Make eye contact and use reassuring facial expressions
  - Interpret the child's nonverbal cues verbally back to him

- Instead of conversation, use some indirect age-appropriate communication techniques (e.g., storytelling, picture drawing, music, creative writing)
- Use *verbal* communication:
  - Use familiar vocabulary
  - Listen without interrupting
  - Humor and active listening to foster the relationship
  - Use open-ended questions
  - Use "I" statements
  - Help child to clarify his ideas and feelings ("Tell me more...," "You got scared when...")
- Respect the child's privacy.
- Accept child's emotions.
- Help child with the difference between thoughts and actions.
- Increase coping skills by providing play opportunities; use creative, unstructured play, medical role-play, and pantomime.
- Use alternative, supplementary communication devices for children with specialized needs (e.g., sign language and computer-enhanced communication programs).

Revisions include limited material from University of California Library Systems: "Communicating with Your Child," 2007; see online references, www.mdconsult.com/das/patient/body/115729442-4/788918080/10068/18752.html.

BOX 18-2	Key Points in Communicating with Children According to Age Group

INFANTS
- Nonverbal communication is a primary mode.
- Infants are biologically "wired" to pay close attention to words. In first year, infants are able to distinguish all conversational sounds.
- Infants are bonded to primary caregivers only. Those older than 8 months may display separation anxiety when separated from parent or when approached by strangers.

Use Kinesthetic Communication
- Use stroking, soft touching, and holding.
- Use motion (e.g., rocking) to reassure. Allow freedom of movement, and avoid restraining when possible.
- Learn specifically how the primary caregiver provides care in terms of sleeping, bathing, and feeding, and attempt to mimic these approaches.

Hold Close to Adapt to Limited Vision (20/200–20/ 300 at Birth)
- Encourage the infant's caregivers (parents) to use a lot of intimate space interaction (e.g., 8–18 inches). Mimic the same when trust is established.

Talk with Infants
- Talk with infants in normal conversational tones; soothe them with crooning voice tone.

Establish Trust
- Use parents to give care. Arrange for one or both parents to remain within the child's sight.

Shorten Your Stature
- Sit down on chair, stool, or carpet to decrease posture superiority, so as to look less imposing.

Continued

| BOX 18-2 | Key Points in Communicating with Children According to Age Group—cont'd |

Handle Separation Anxiety When Primary Caregiver Is Absent

- Establish rapport with the caregiver (parent) and encourage them to be with child and reassure child that staff will be there if they are away. At first keep at least 2 feet between nurse and infant. Talk to and touch the infant and initially smile often. Provide for kinesthetic approaches; offer self while infant is protesting (e.g., stay with the child; pick the child up and rock or walk; talk to the child about Mommy and Daddy and how much the child cares for them).

1- TO 3-YEAR-OLDS

- Child begins to talk around 1 year of age; learns nine new words a day after 18 months.
- By age 2, child begins to use phrases; should be able to respond to "what" and "where" type questions.
- By age 3, child uses and understands sentences.

Adapt to Limited Vocabulary and Verbal Skills

- Make explanations brief and clear. Use the child's own vocabulary words for basic care activities (e.g., use the child's words for defecate [poop, goodies] and urinate [pee-pee, tinkle]). Learn and use self-name of the child.
- Rephrase the child's message in a simple, complete sentence; avoid baby talk. Child should be able to follow two simple directions.

Continue to Use Kinesthetic Communication

- Allow ambulating where possible (e.g., using toddler chairs or walkers). Pull the child in a wagon often if child cannot achieve mobility.

Facilitate Child's Struggle with Issues of Autonomy and Control

- Allow the child some control (e.g., "Do you want a half a glass or a whole glass of milk?").
- Reassure the child if he or she displays some regressive behavior (e.g., if child wets pants, say, "We will get a dry pair of pants and let you find something fun to do.").
- Allow the child to express anger and to protest about his or her care (e.g., "It's okay to cry when you are angry or hurt.").
- Allow the child to sit up or walk as often as possible and as soon as possible after intrusive or hurtful procedures (e.g., "It's all over and we can do something more fun.").
- Use nondirective modes, such as reflecting an aspect of appearance or temperament (e.g., "You smile so often."), or playing with a toy and slowly coming closer to and including the child in play.

Recognize Fear of Bodily Injury

- Show hands (free of hurtful items) and say, "There is nothing to hurt you. I came to play/talk."

Accept Egocentrism and Possible Regression

- Allow child to be self-oriented. Use distraction if another child wants the same item or toy rather than expect the child to share. Some children cope with stress of hospitalization by regressing to an earlier mode of behavior, such as wanting to suck on a bottle, and so forth.

Redirect Behavior to a Verbal Level

- Use a nondirective approach. Sit down and join the parallel play of the child. Reflect messages sent by toddler (nonverbally) in a verbal and nonverbal manner (e.g., "Yes, that toy does lots of interesting and fun things.").

Deal with Separation Anxiety

- Accept protesting when parent(s) leave. Hug, rock the child, and say, "You miss Mommy and Daddy! They miss you too." Play peek-a-boo games with the child. Make a big deal about saying, "Now I am here."
- Show an interest in one of the child's favorite toys. Say, "I wonder what it does" or the like. If the child responds with actions, reflect them back.

3- TO 5-YEAR-OLDS

- Most children this age can make themselves understood to strangers.
- They speak in sentences but are unable to comprehend abstract ideas.
- Unable to recognize their own anxiety, at this age some will somaticize (i.e., complain only of stomachache, etc.).
- They begin to understand cause-and-effect relationships; should be able to understand "If you do. . ., then we can. . ."
- Can follow a series of up to four directions, unless anxious about being hurt, and so on.

Use Age-Appropriate, Simple Vocabulary

- Use simple vocabulary; avoid lengthy explanations. Focus on the present, not the distant future; use concrete, meaningful references. For example, say, "Mommy will be back after you eat your lunch" (instead of "at 1 o'clock").

Behave in a Culturally Sensitive Manner

- In some cultures, child is unable to tolerate direct eye-to-eye contact, so use some eye contact and

Continued

| BOX 18-2 | Key Points in Communicating with Children According to Age Group—cont'd |

attending posture. Sit or stoop, and use a slow, soft tone of voice.

Attempt to Decrease Anxiety about Being Hurt

- Use brief, concrete, simple explanations. Delays and long explanations before a painful procedure increase anxiety.
- Be quick to complete the procedure; give explanations about its purpose afterward. For example, say, "Jimmy, I'm going to give you a shot," then quickly administer the injection. Then say, "There. All done. It's okay to cry when you hurt. I'd complain too. This medicine will make your tummy feel better." Some experts suggest you create a "safe zone" in the child's bed by doing all painful procedures elsewhere, perhaps in a treatment room.

Use Play Therapy

- Explanations and education can be done using imagination (puppetry, drama with dress-ups), music, or drawings.
- Allow the child to play with safe equipment used in treatment. Talk about the needed procedure happening to a doll or teddy bear, and state simply how it will occur and be experienced. Use sensory data (e.g., "The teddy bear will hear a buzzing sound.").

Use Distraction and a Sense of Humor

- Tell corny jokes and laugh with the child.

Allow for Child's Continuing Need to Have Control

- Provide for many choices (e.g., "Do you want to get dressed now or after breakfast?").

5- TO 10-YEAR-OLDS

- They are developing their ability to comprehend. Can understand sequencing of events if clearly explained: "First this happens..., then..."
- They can use written materials to learn.

Facilitate Child to Assume Increased Responsibility for Own Health Care Practices

- Include the child in concrete explanations about condition, treatment, and protocols.
- Use draw-a-person to identify basic knowledge the child has and build on it.
- Use some of the same words the child uses in giving explanations.

- Use sensory information in giving explanations (e.g., "You will smell alcohol in the cast room.").
- Reinforce basic health self-care activities in teaching.

Respect Increased Need for Privacy

- Knock on the door before entering; tell the client when and for what reasons you will need to return to his or her room.

11-YEAR-OLDS AND OLDER

- Have an increased comprehension about possible negative threats to life or body integrity, yet some difficulty in adhering to long-term goals.
- Continue to use mainly concrete rather than abstract thinking.
- They are struggling to establish identity and be independent.

Verbalize Issues in Age-Appropriate Ways

- Talk about treatment protocols that require giving up immediate gratifications for long-term gain. Explore alternative options (e.g., tell a diabetic adolescent who must give up after-school fries with friends that he or she could save two breads and four fats exchanges to have a milkshake). If you use abstract thinking, look for nonverbal cues (e.g., puzzled face) that may indicate lack of understanding; then clarify in more concrete terms. Use humor or street slang, if appropriate.

Remember That Confidentiality May Be an Issue

- Reassure the adolescent about the confidentiality of your discussion, but clearly state the limits of this confidentiality. If, for example, the child should talk of killing himself, this information needs to be shared with parents and staff.

Allow Sense of Independence

- Allow participation in decision making, wearing own clothes. Avoid an authoritarian approach when possible. Avoid a judgmental approach. Use a clarifying and qualifying approach. Actively listen. Accept regression.

Assess Sexual Awareness and Maturation

- Offer self and a willingness to listen. Provide value-free, accurate information.

Updated 2010, from material originally supplied by Joyce Ruth, MSN, University of North Carolina Charlotte, College of Health Sciences.

feelings about the treatment experience. As nurses, we adapt our communication to meet the ill child's needs. Many agencies also have play therapists who serve as excellent resources for staff.

INFANTS

Cues to assessment of the preverbal infant include tone of the cry, facial appearance, and body movements. Because the infant uses the senses to receive information, nonverbal communication (e.g., touch) is an important tool for the pediatric nurse. Tone of voice, rocking motion, use of distraction, and a soothing touch can be used in addition to or in conjunction with verbal explanations. Face-to-face position, bending or moving to the child's eye level, maintaining eye contact, and making a reassuring facial expression further help in interactions with infants.

Anticipate developmental behaviors such as "stranger anxiety" in infants between 9 and 18 months of age. Rather than reaching to pick a child up immediately, the nurse might smile and extend a hand toward the child or stroke the child's arm before attempting to hold the child. In this way, the nurse acknowledges the infant's inability to generalize to unfamiliar caregivers. If the child is able to talk, asking the child his or her name and pointing out a notable pleasant physical characteristic conveys the impression that you see the child client as a unique person. To a tiny child, this treatment can be synonymous with caring.

TODDLERS

Almost all small children receiving invasive treatment feel some threat to their safety and security, one of Maslow's hierarchies of human needs. This need is exaggerated in toddlers and young children, who cannot articulate their needs or understand why they are ill. To help the child's comprehension, use phrases rather than long sentences and repeat words for emphasis. Because the toddler has a limited vocabulary, you may need to put into words the feelings that the ill child is conveying nonverbally.

Evaluate the Agency Environment

Is it safe? Does it allow for some independence and autonomy? Care in the ambulatory setting is facilitated if a parent or caregiver is present. Agency policies should promote parent-child contact (e.g., unlimited visiting hours, rooming in, or use of audiocassettes of a parent's voice). Familiar objects make the environment feel safer. Use transitional objects such as a teddy bear, blanket, or favorite toy to remind the alone or frightened child that the security of the parent is still available even when he is not physically present. Some hospitals offer a prehospitalization orientation.

Distraction is a successful strategy with toddlers in ambulatory settings. Use of stuffed animals, wind-up toys, or "magic" exam lights that blow out "like a birthday candle" can turn fright into delight. The author wears a small toy bear on her stethoscope and asks the child to help listen for a heart sound from the bear, so the child focuses on the toy, making it easier to listen to the child's heart.

PRESCHOOLERS

Throughout the preoperational period, young children tend to interpret language in a literal way. For example, the child who is told that he will be "put to sleep" during the operation tomorrow may think it means the same as the action recently taken for a pet dog who was too ill to live. Children do not ask for clarification, so messages can be misunderstood quite easily.

Preschool children have limited auditory recall and are unable to process auditory information quickly. They have a short attention span. Verbal communication with the preschool child should be clear, succinct, and easy to understand.

Before the age of 7 years, most children cannot make a clear distinction between fantasy and reality. Everything is "real," and anything strange is perceived as potentially harmful. In the hospital, preschool children need frequent concrete reminders to reinforce reality. Assigning the same caregiver reduces insecurity. Visiting the preschooler at the same time each day and posting family pictures are simple strategies to reduce the child's fears of abandonment. You can link information to activities of daily living. For example, saying, "Your mother will come after you take your nap," rather than "at 2 o'clock" is much more understandable to the preschool client.

Children need to be assessed for misconceptions and troubling problems, preferably using free play and fantasy storytelling exercises. Egocentrism can be a normal developmental process that may prevent children from understanding why they cannot have a drink when they are fasting before a scheduled test. Explanations given a long time beforehand may not be remembered. If something is going to hurt, you should be forthright about it, while at the same time reassuring the child that he will have the appropriate support. Simple explanations reduce the child's anxiety. No child should ever be left to figure out what is happening without some type of simple explanation. Reinforce the child's communication by praising the willingness to tell you how he feels. Avoid judging or censuring the child who yells such things as "I hate you," or "You are mean for hurting me." Not being able to recognize or communicate anxiety, the child may just complain of a physical symptom, like a headache or stomachache (Emslie, 2008). Box 18-2 can help you focus on specific communication strategies with the hospitalized preschooler.

Play as a Communication Strategy

The preschooler lacks a suitable vocabulary to express complex thoughts and feelings. Small children cannot picture what they have never experienced. Play is an effective means by which a puzzling and sometimes painful real world can be approached. Play allows the child to create a concrete experience of something unknown and potentially frightening. By constructing a situation in play, the child is able to put together the components of the situation in ways that promote recognition and make it a concrete reality. When the child can deal with things that are small or inanimate, the child masters situations that might otherwise be overwhelming. Cartoons, pictures, or puppets can be used to demonstrate actions and terminology. Dolls with removable cloth organs help children understand scheduled operations.

Preschoolers tend to think of their illness, their separation from parents, and any painful treatments as punishment. Play can be used to help children express their feelings about an illness and to role-play coping strategies. Allowing the young child to manipulate syringes and give "shots" to a doll, or put a bandage or restraint on a teddy bear's arm allows the child to act out his feelings. The child becomes "the aggressor." Play can be a major channel for communication in the nurse-client relationship involving a young child. Preschool children develop communication themes through their play and work through conflict situations in their own good time; the process cannot be rushed.

Play materials vary with the age and developmental status of the child. Simple, large toys are used with young children; more intricate playthings are used with older preschoolers. Clay, crayons, and paper become modes of expression for important feelings and thoughts about problems.

Play can be your primary tool for assessing preschool children's perceptions about their hospital experience, their anxieties, and their fears. Play can increase their coping ability. Preschoolers love jokes, puns, and riddles; the cornier, the better. Using jokes during the physical assessment, such as "Let me hear your lunch," or, "Golly, could that be a potato in your ear?" helps form the bonds needed for a successful relationship with the preschool client.

Storytelling as a Communication Strategy

A communication strategy often used with young children is the use of story plots. As early as 1986, Gardner described a mutual storytelling technique. You ask the child whether he would like to help make up a story. If the child is a little reluctant, you may begin, as described in Exercise 18-1. At the end of the story, the child is asked to indicate what lesson might be learned from the story. If the child seems a little reluctant to give a moral to the story, you might suggest that all stories have something that can be learned from them. Analyze the themes presented by the child, which usually reveal important feelings. Is the story fearful? Are the characters scary or pleasing? The child should be praised for telling the story. The next step in the process is to ask yourself what would be a healthier resolution than the one used by the child. Then suggest an alternative ending. In your version of the story, the characters and other details remain the same initially, but the story contains a more positive solution or suggests alternative answers to problems. The object of mutual storytelling is to offer the child an opportunity to explore different alternatives in a neutral communication process with a helping person. Exercise 18-1 provides an opportunity to experiment with a mutual storytelling strategy.

SCHOOL-AGE CHILDREN

As children move into concrete operational thinking, they begin to internalize the reasons for illness: illness is caused by germs, or you have cavities because you ate too much candy or did not brush your teeth. In later childhood, most children become better able to work with you verbally. It still is important to prepare responses carefully and to anticipate problems, but the child is capable of expressing feelings and venting frustration more directly through words. Use Exercise 18-2 to reformulate medical technology into age-appropriate expressions.

| EXERCISE 18-1 | Using a Mutual Storytelling Technique |

Purpose: To give practical experience with the mutual storytelling technique.

Procedure:
1. Use the mutual storytelling process described in the text with a 5- to 8-year-old child in your neighborhood.
2. Write down the story the child told and suggest alternate endings.
3. Share your stories in turn during the next class period.

Discussion:
1. How difficult was it for you to engage the child? If you had trouble, what alternate actions would you incorporate in using the technique again?
2. Were you surprised at the story the child produced? If so, in what ways?
3. What did you learn about the child when using this technique?
4. What conclusions might you draw from hearing the other students relate their experiences about the use of this technique? In what situations was it most effective? Least effective?

5. What did you learn about yourself as a helping person in using this technique?

Sample Answer:

Nurse: Once upon a time in a land far away, there lived a...
Child: Dragon.
Nurse: A dragon who ate...
Child: Carrots.
Nurse: The dragon ate carrots and slept...
Child: In a cave.
Nurse: One day he left the cave to go out and find many sweet carrots to eat, but as he walked along he ran into a...
Child: Bike.
Nurse: He was afraid of the bike and so he...
Child: Kicked it and ran away.
Nurse: After he ran away, is there any more to the story?
Child (upset): He got hit with a stick.
Nurse: What is the message to this story? What does it tell us?
Child: About running away not to be punished.

| EXERCISE 18-2 | Age-Appropriate Medical Terminology |

Purpose: To help students think of terminology appropriate to use with young clients.

Procedure:
This can be fun if the instructor quickly asks students, going around the room.
   Reformulate the following expressions using words a child can understand:

Anesthesia

Cardiac catheterization

Inflammation

Injection

NPO

Operating room

Disease

Dressings

Enema

Infection

Intake and output

Isolation

IV needle

Nausea

Sedation

Urine specimen

Vital signs

Discussion:
Think of any experiences you might have had as a child client or may have observed. What were some of the troublesome words you remember from these experiences?

Assessment of the child's cognitive level of understanding continues to be essential. Search for concrete examples to which the child can relate rather than giving abstract examples. If children are to learn from a model, they must see the model performing the skill to be learned. School-age children thrive on explanations of how their bodies work and enjoy understanding the scientific rationales for their treatment. Ask questions directly to the child, consulting the parent for validation.

Using Audiovisual Aids as a Communication Strategy

Audiovisual aids and reading material geared to the child's level of understanding may supplement verbal explanations and diagrams. Details about what the child will hear, see, smell, and feel are important. For the younger school-age child, expressive art can be a useful method to convey feelings and to open up communication. The older school-age child or adolescent might best convey feelings by writing a poem, a short story, or a letter. This written material can assist you in understanding hidden thoughts or emotions.

Mutuality in Decision Making

Children of this age need to be involved in discussions of their illness and in planning for their care. Explanations giving the rationale for care are useful. Involving the child in decision making may decrease fears about the illness, the treatment, or the effect on family life. Videos and written materials may be useful in involving the child in the management phase of care.

ADOLESCENTS

An understanding of adolescent developmental principles is essential in working with teens. Adolescence is the time when we clinicians encourage a shift in responsibility for health-related decisions from parent to the teen. Even teens enjoying good health are forced to deal with new health issues such as acne, menstrual problems, or sexual activity. The adolescent vacillates between childhood and adulthood, and is emotionally vulnerable. The ambivalence of the adolescent period may be normally expressed through withdrawal, rebellion, lost motivation, and rapid mood changes. A teen may look adult-like, but in illness especially may be unable to communicate easily with care providers. Identity issues become more difficult to resolve when the normal opportunities for physical independence, privacy, and social contacts are compromised by illness or handicap. All adolescents have questions about their developing body and sexuality. Ill teens have the same longings, but problems may be greater because the natural outlets for their expression with peers are curtailed by the disorder or by hospitalization. Use of peer groups, adolescent lounges (separate from the small children's playroom), and telephones, as well as provisions for wearing one's own clothes, fixing one's hair, or attending hospital school, may help teenagers adjust to hospitalization. When the developmental identity crisis becomes too uncomfortable, adolescents may project their fury and frustration onto family or staff. Identifying rage as a normal response to a difficult situation can be reassuring.

Assessment of the adolescent should occur in a private setting. Attention to his comfort and space will have a tremendous impact on the quality of the interaction. To the teenager, the nurse represents an authority figure. The need for compassion, concern, and respect is perhaps greater during adolescence than at any other time in the life span. Often lacking the verbal skills of adults, yet wishing to appear in control, adolescents do well with direct questions. Innocuous questions are used first to allow the teenager enough space to check the validity of his reactions to the nurse. In caring for a teen in an ambulatory office or clinic, conduct part of the history interview without the parent present. If the parent will not leave the exam room, this can be done while walking the teen down to the laboratory. Questions about substance use, sexual activity, and so on demand confidentiality.

To assess a teen's cognitive level, find out about his ability to make long-term plans. An easy way to do this is the "three wishes question." Ask the teen to name three things he would expect to have in 5 years. Answers can be analyzed for factors such as concreteness, realism, and goal-directness.

Some teens lack sufficient experience to recognize that life has ups and downs, and that things will eventually be better. Suicide is the second leading cause of death in teenagers, and many experts think that the actual rate is greater because many deaths from the number one cause, motor vehicle accidents, may actually be attributed to this cause. Be aware of danger signs such as apathy, persistent depression, or self-destructive behavior. When faced with a tragedy, teens tend to mourn in doses, with wide mood swings. Grieving teens may need periods of privacy, but also need the opportunity for relief through distracting activities, music, and games. In communicating with an ill adolescent, remember to listen. When a teen asks a direct question, he or she is ready to hear the answer. Answer directly and honestly. In an analysis of pediatric nursing interventions, one category identified as a recurrent activity was helping the child find meaning, a form of spiritual nurturance (Zengerle-Levy, 2006).

Using Hobbies as a Communication Strategy

Adolescents still rely primarily on feedback from adults and from friends to judge their own competency. A teen may not yet have developed proficiency and comfort in carrying on verbal conversations with adults. The teen may respond best if the nurse uses several modalities to communicate. Using empathy, conveying acceptance, and using open-ended questions are three useful strategies. Sometimes more innovative communication strategies are needed. In the following case example, the teen has a difficult time talking, so the use of another modality is appropriate.

Case Example

Ashley, a first-year student nurse, becomes frustrated during the course of her conversation with her assigned client, 17-year-old Cary, admitted 5 days ago to the psychiatric unit. Despite a genuine desire to engage him in a therapeutic alliance, the client would not talk. Attempts to get to know him on a verbal level seemed to increase rather than decrease his anxiety. The nurse correctly inferred that, despite his age, this adolescent needed a more tangible approach. Knowing that the client likes cars, Ashley brought in an automotive magazine. Together, they looked at the magazine; the publication soon became their special vehicle for communication, bridging the gap between the client's inner reality and his ability to express himself verbally in a meaningful way. Feelings about cars gradually generalized to verbal expressions about other situations, and Cary quickly began describing his life dreams, disappointments, and attitudes about himself. When Ashley left the unit, he asked to keep the magazine and frequently spoke of her with fondness. This simple recognition of his awkwardness in verbal communication and use of another tool to facilitate the relationship had a positive effect.

DEALING WITH CARE PROBLEMS
Pain

The literature has identified a lack of understanding about pain in children, as well as nurses' personal beliefs that children over-report their pain, as a barrier to giving optimal nursing care (Van Hulle Vincent, 2005). For years, children's ability to feel pain has been underrated by adult caregivers. For example, male newborns were routinely circumcised in the last century without pain relief. Since 1999, the American Academy of Pediatrics no longer recommends circumcision, but it takes years for evidenced-based information to become accepted common practice. When circumcision is performed now, pain interventions are recommended. Lack of adequate pain relief may, in part, be due to fears of oversedating a child, but more likely are due to the child's limited capacity to communicate the nature of his or her discomfort. Infants indicate pain with physiologic changes (e.g., diaphoresis, pallor, increased heart rate, increased respirations, and decreased oxygen saturation). Migdal and associates (2005) found lidocaine, a local anesthetic, effective in reducing the pain associated with venipuncture. Effective nonpharmacologic interventions for pain include pacifiers, rocking, physical contact, and sometimes even swaddling. We now use age-specific pain assessment instruments, such as smiley faces or poker chips with toddlers and preschoolers, to evaluate levels of pain with our pediatric clients. Exercise 18-3 will stimulate discussion about care for children in pain.

Anxiety

Illness is often an unanticipated event. Uncertainty and even anxiety should be expected when both treatment and outcome are unknown. Young children react to unexpected stimuli, to painful procedures, and even to the presence of strangers with fear. Older children fear separation from parents, but also may fear injury, loss of body function, or even just being perceived by friends as different because of their illness. Exercise 18-4 helps develop age-appropriate explanations that may reduce anxiety.

Acting-Out Behaviors

Behavior problems present a special challenge to the nurse. Clear communication of expectations, treatment protocols, and hospital rules is of value. As much as possible, adolescents should be allowed to act on their own behalf in making choices and judgments about their functioning. At the same time, limits need to be set on acting-out behavior. Limits define the boundaries of acceptable behaviors in a relationship. Initially determined by the parents or the nurse, limits can be

---

EXERCISE 18-3	Pediatric Nursing Procedures

Purpose: To give practice in preparing young clients for painful procedures.

Procedure:
Timmy, age 4, is going to have a bone marrow aspiration. (The insertion of a large needle into the hip is a painful procedure.) Answer the following questions:

1. What essential information does Timmy need?
2. If this is a frequently repeated procedure, how can you make him feel safe before and after the procedure?
3. How soon in advance should you prepare him?

| EXERCISE 18-4 | Preparing Children for Treatment Procedures |

Purpose: To help students apply developmental concepts to age-appropriate nursing interventions.

Procedure:
Students divide into four small groups and design an age-appropriate intervention for the following situation. As a large group, each small-group spokesperson writes the intervention on the board under the label for the age group.

Situation:
Jamie is scheduled to go to the surgical suite later today to have a central infusion catheter inserted for hyperalimentation. This is Jamie's first procedure on the first day of this first hospitalization experience.

Discussion:
Group focuses on comparing interventions across the age spans.
1. How does each intervention differ according to the age of the child? (Describe age-appropriate interventions for preschooler, school-age child, and adolescent.)
2. What concept themes are common across the age spans? (education components; assessing initial level of knowledge; assessing ability to comprehend information, readiness to receive information; adapting information to cognitive level of child)
3. What formats might be best used for each age group? (Role-play with tools such as dolls, pictures, comic books, educational pamphlets, and peer group sessions.)

developed mutually as an important part of the relationship as the child matures. Determining consequences has a positive value in that it provides the child with a model for handling frustrating situations in a more adult manner.

Once the conflict is resolved and the child has accepted the consequences of his behavior, the child should be given an opportunity to discuss attitudes and feelings that led up to the need for limits, as well as his reaction to the limits set. Serious symptoms such as substance abuse require specialist interventions. Estimates are that 75% of abusers have serious mental adjustment problems, especially depression (Griswold, Aronoff, Kernan, & Kahn, 2008).

Although communication about limits is necessary for the survival of the relationship, it needs to be balanced with time for interaction that is pleasant and positive. Sometimes with children who need limits set on a regular basis, discussion of the restrictions is the only conversation that takes place between nurse and client. When this is noted, nurses might ask themselves what feelings the child might be expressing through his or her actions. Putting into words the feelings that are being acted out helps children trust the nurse's competence and concern. Usually it is necessary for the entire staff to share this responsibility. Box 18-3 presents ideas for setting limits within the context of the nurse-client relationship.

| BOX 18-3 | Guidelines for Developing Workable Limit-Setting Plan |

1. Have the child describe his or her behavior.
   Key: Evaluate realistically.
2. Encourage the child to assess behavior. Is it helpful for others and himself or herself?
   Key: Evaluate realistically.
3. Encourage the child to develop an alternative plan for governing behavior.
   Key: Set reasonable goals.
4. Have the child sign a statement about his or her plan.
   Key: Commit to goals.
5. Consequences for unacceptable behavior are logical and fit the situation.
   Key: Consequences are known.
6. At the end of the appropriate time period, have the child assess his or her performance.
   Key: Evaluate realistically.
7. Consequences are applied in a matter-of-fact manner, without lengthy discussion.
   Key: Consequences immediately follow the transgression.
8. Provide positive reinforcement for those aspects of performance that were successful.*
   Key: Evaluate realistically.
9. Encourage the child to make a positive statement about his or her performance.
   Key: Teach self-praise.

*If the child's performance does not meet the criteria set in the plan, return to Step 3 and assist the child in modifying the plan so that success is more possible. If, on the other hand, the child's performance is successful, help him or her to develop a more ambitious plan (e.g., for a longer period or for a larger set of behaviors).

MORE HELPFUL STRATEGIES FOR COMMUNICATING WITH CHILDREN

Adapting the general communications strategies studied earlier in this book to interactions with children requires some imagination and creativity.

Active Listening

Knowing what a child truly needs and values is the heart of successful interpersonal relationships in health care settings. The process of active listening takes form initially from watching the behaviors of children as they play and interact with their environments. As a child's vocabulary increases and the capacity to engage with others develops, listening begins to approximate the communication process that occurs between adults, with one important difference: Because the perceptual world of the child is concrete, the nurse's feedback and informational messages should coincide with the child's developmental level.

Working with children is rewarding, hard work that sometimes must be evaluated indirectly. For instance, George was the primary care nurse who had worked very hard with a 13-year-old girl over a 6-month period while the girl was on a bone marrow transplant unit. He felt bad when, at discharge, the girl stated, "I never want to see any of you people again." However, just before leaving, the nurse found her sobbing on her bed. No words were spoken, but the child threw her arms around George and clung to him for comfort. For this nurse, the child's expression of grief was an acknowledgment of the meaning of the relationship. Children, even those who can use words, often communicate through behavior rather than verbally when under stress.

Authenticity and Veracity

Crises are an inevitable part of life. Many parents and health professionals ignore children's feelings or else deceive them about procedures, illness, or hospitalization in the mistaken belief that they will be overwhelmed by the truth. Just the opposite is true. Children, like adults, can cope with most stressors as long as they are presented in a manner they can understand and given enough time and support from the environment to cope. In fact, very ill children often are a source of inspiration to the adults working with them because of their courage in facing the truth about themselves and dealing with it constructively. Teens rate honesty, attention to pain, and respect as the three most important factors in their quality of care. Completing Exercise 18-5 may stimulate some discussion.

EXERCISE 18-5 | **Working with the Newly Diagnosed HIV-Positive Teenager**

Purpose: To stimulate class discussion about how to deal with the adolescent with whom it is difficult to communicate.

Procedure:
Read the case situation and answer the questions that follow. Questions can be done out of class, with class time used only for discussion.

Situation:
Bill, age 17, seeks treatment for gonorrhea. He is hospitalized for further testing after his initial workup reveals he is seropositive for human immunodeficiency virus (HIV) type 1. For 2 days on the unit he has cried, cursed, and been uncooperative. Staff tends to avoid him when possible. A team of residents begins a bone marrow aspiration procedure in the treatment room after obtaining his absent mother's permission. (She has expressed condemnation and has not yet been to visit.) A technician walks in and out of the room to obtain supplies while the doctors concentrate on completing the procedure. A student nurse is asked to come in to help restrain Bill, who is alternately screaming, crying, and being very quiet.

1. What communication strategies could this student use while squeezing into this small room? (Clue: Verbal and nonverbal directed to the client and to the doctors)
2. What assessment might the nurse want to make? (Clue: What are Bill's feelings about his diagnosis?)
3. What can be inferred about Bill's current behavior?
4. What interventions would you suggest for initiating interaction with his single mom?
5. What additional data are needed before attempting any teaching about acquired immunodeficiency syndrome (AIDS)?

Discussion:
May be discussed in small groups.

You should never allow any individual, even a parent, to threaten a child. For example, a few parents have been heard to say, "You be good or I'll have the nurse give you a shot." It is appropriate to interrupt this parent. Children respect honest expression of emotions in adults. Being truthful and trustworthy with children is a crucial factor in the development of a therapeutic relationship.

Case Example

In a community setting, an older student nurse, with a family of her own, was monitoring a family in which the mother had terminal cancer. There were three children in the family, and the identified client of the student was a 13-year-old boy. He was abnormally quiet, and it was difficult to draw him out. Halfway through the semester, the boy's father died unexpectedly of a heart attack. When the boy and student nurse next met, the nurse asked the boy whether there was anything special that had happened between father and son that the boy would remember about his father. The boy replied that the day before his father's death he had received a letter of acceptance to the same school his father had attended, and he had shared this with his father. He said his father was very proud that he had been accepted. The student nurse could feel her eyes fill as the boy revealed himself to her in this special way. Her sharing of honest emotion was a significant turning point in what became a very important relationship for both participants. It was a moment of shared meaning for both of them and, from that time on, the needed common ground for communication existed.

Being authentic does not mean being overly familiar. Trying to interact with older children and adolescents as though the nurse is a buddy is confusing to the client. What the child wants is an emotionally available, calm, caring, competent resource who can protect, care about, and above all, listen to him or her.

Conveying Respect

It is easy for adults to impose their own wishes on a child. Respecting a child's right to feel and to express his or her feelings appropriately is important. Providing truthful answers is a hallmark of respect. When interacting with the older child, using the concept of mutuality will promote respect and should foster more positive and lasting health care outcomes. Confidentiality needs to be maintained unless the nurse judges that revealing information is necessary to prevent harm to the child or adolescent. In such cases, the child needs to be advised of the disclosure.

Providing Anticipatory Guidance to the Child

The nursing profession advocates client education. A physician would call similar preventive education anticipatory guidance. As more clinics become located within schools, more emphasis is being placed on anticipatory guidance. The American Academy of Pediatrics has published guidelines for health care providers working with well children in the community. These suggestions focus on health promotion information to be given to caretakers at appropriate ages. Managed care has brought an increased focus on the role a child can assume in being responsible for his or her own health care. It is never too early to begin. For example, McCarthy and Hobbie (1997) provide very clear written handouts for incorporating violence prevention into well-child visits made to nurse practitioners. This shift in placing responsibility for good health practices onto the individual is in line with recommendations in *Healthy People 2010* (Online Resources, http://hp2010. nhlbihin.net/).

INTERACTING WITH PARENTS OF ILL CHILDREN

Having an ill child is stressful for parents. Many research studies have shown that loss of the ability to act as the child's parent, to alleviate the child's pain, and to comfort the child is more stressful than factors connected with the illness, including coping with uncertainty over the outcome. Other stressors include financial and marital strains. Studies pointed to a lack of needed information and support from professionals as being a top stressor, exacerbating already existing family problems and resulting in feelings of fear and helplessness. Parents want to participate in their child's care during acute hospitalizations but need information, advice, and clarification as to their role—that is, what is okay to do. They need to feel valued but not pressured into doing tasks they are uncomfortable with or do not want to do.

Parents often have questions about discussing their child's illness or disability with others. Telling siblings and friends the truth is important. For one thing, it provides a role model for the siblings to follow in answering the curious questions of their friends. Issues such as overprotectiveness, discipline, time out for parents to replenish commitment and energy, and the quality and quantity of interactions with the hospitalized child have a powerful impact on the child's growth and development. However, older children have a need for confidentiality and respond better if the nurse interviews and treats them away from parents' presence. Consider the ethical dilemma provided.

More frustrating to nurses are parents who are critical of the nurse's interventions, displacing the anger they feel about their own powerlessness onto the nurse (Box 18-4). The nurse may be tempted to become defensive or sarcastic, or simply to dismiss the comments of the parent as irrational. However, a more helpful response would be to place oneself in the parents' shoes and to consider the possible issues. Asking the parents what information they have or might need, simply listening in a nondefensive way, and allowing the parents to vent some of their frustrations facilitate the possibility of dialogue about the underlying feelings. The listening strategies given in Chapter 10 are helpful. Sometimes a listening response that acknowledges the legitimacy of the parent's feeling is helpful: "I'm sorry that you feel so bad," or "It must be difficult for you to see your child in such pain." These simple comments acknowledge the very real anguish parents experience in health care situations having few palatable options. If possible, parental venting of feeling should occur in a private

---

BOX 18-4 Representative Nursing Problem: Dealing with a Frightened Parent

During report, the night nurse relates an incident that occurred between Mrs. Smith, the mother of an 8-year-old admitted for possible acute lymphocytic leukemia, and the night supervisor. Mrs. Smith told the supervisor that her son was receiving poor care from the nurses, and that they frequently ignored her and refused to answer her questions. While you are making rounds after the report, Mrs. Smith corners you outside her son's room and begins to tell you about all the things that went wrong during the night. She goes on to say, "If you people think I'm going to stand around and allow my son to be treated this way, you are sadly mistaken."

Problem
Frustration and anger caused by a sense of powerlessness and fear related to the son's possible diagnosis

Nursing Diagnosis
Ineffective coping related to hospitalization of son and possible diagnosis of leukemia

Nursing Goals
Increase the mother's sense of control and problem-solving capabilities; help the mother develop adaptive coping behaviors.

Method of Assistance
Guiding; supporting; providing developmental environment

Interventions
1. Actively listen to the client's concerns with as much objectivity as possible; maintain eye contact with the client; use minimal verbal activity, allowing the client the opportunity to express her concerns and fears freely.
2. Use reflective questioning to determine the client's level of understanding and the extent of information obtained from health team members.
3. Listen for repetitive words or phrases that may serve to identify problem areas or provide insight into fears and concerns.
4. Reassure the mother when appropriate that her child's hospitalization is indeed frightening and it is all right to be scared; remember to demonstrate interest in the client as a person; use listening responses (e.g., "It must be hard not knowing the results of all these tests.") to create an atmosphere of concern.
5. Avoid communication blocks, such as giving false reassurance, telling the client what to do, or ignoring the concerns; such behavior effectively cuts off therapeutic communication.
6. Keep the client continually informed regarding her child's progress.
7. Involve the client in her son's care; do not overwhelm her or make her feel she has to do this; watch for cues that tell you she is ready "to do more."
8. Acknowledge the impact this illness may have on the family; involve the health team in identifying ways to reduce the client's fears and provide for continuity in the type of information presented to her and to other family members.
9. Assign a primary nurse to care for the client's son and serve as a resource to the client. Identify support systems in the community that might provide help and support to the client.

From M. Michaels, University of Maryland School of Nursing, Baltimore.

setting out of hearing range from the child. It is very upsetting to children to experience splitting in the parent-nurse relationship.

You can reduce parents' stress by educating them about their child's condition. When the child has a chronic illness, the family is called on to continually adjust the family system to adapt to changing demands in the child's health. Because nursing care is largely moving to care in the home, nurses will have an increasing need to help families cope with seriously chronically ill children. At times, the nurse will be called on to act as the child's advocate in giving parents helpful information, anticipatory guidance, and complex technical assistance in caring for the health and developmental needs of their child. Guidelines for communicating with parents are presented in Box 18-5.

COMMUNICATING WITH PARENTS OF SPECIAL HEALTH CARE NEEDS CHILDREN

Approximately 29% of American children have a chronic health condition requiring additional services. Caring for these children requires parental time and alters family communication patterns. Studies show these families have less time for communication (Bransletter et al., 2008). Nurses need to provide care and information about the child's condition, time for discussions about balancing family needs with care

| BOX 18-5 | Guidelines for Communicating with Parents |

- Present complex information in informational chunks.
- Repeat information and allow plenty of time for questions.
- Keep parents continually informed of progress and changes in condition.
- Involve parents in determining goals; anticipate possible reactions and difficulties.
- Discuss problems with parents directly and honestly.
- Explore all alternative options with parents.
- Share knowledge of community supports; help parents role-play responses to others.
- Acknowledge the impact of the illness on finances; on emotions; and especially on the family, including siblings.
- Use other staff for support in personally coping with the emotional drain created by working with very ill children and their parents.

for this child, suggest strategies for moving the child toward future independence, and refer parents to community resources. We need to recognize that as the child reaches developmental milestones, this can be a time of increased family stress, requiring additional support from us.

ANTICIPATORY GUIDANCE IN THE COMMUNITY

Every parent is entitled to a full explanation of his child's condition and treatment. Because the parents usually assume responsibility for the child's care after they leave the hospital, it is essential to encourage active involvement from the very beginning of treatment. Many parents look to the nurse for guidance and support in this process. All parents need facts about normal development and milestones to expect, as well as information about prevention of illness.

COMMUNITY, FAMILY, AND NURSE PARTNERSHIPS

FORMING A NURSE-PARENT PARTNERSHIP

Partnering with the family can be the best method you have to address the complex health care needs of children. Parents' participation in the care of their child, and active involvement in decision making regarding the youngster's treatment, ensure a more stable environment for the child. Providing family support is important for those caring for chronically ill children.

The focus of care is shifting to parents, who are the central figures in care planning. They need information about which community agencies, networks, and professionals will be mobilized to provide care to their child. Successful collaboration requires active commitment to meet client needs by all parties involved. School nurses are often crucial to the ability of the child with a chronic illness to maintain school attendance. In addition, school nurses often act as case managers by communicating about the child's needs among parent, care providers, teachers, and other resource personnel. By law in the United States, children with special needs in the educational system are required to have an Individualized Education Plan. A part of this may be the health plan for children who need medical intervention/treatment during school.

SUPPORT GROUPS

Community groups have organized to assist families. Often information about the group's meeting times can be obtained from health care providers, from the national or local organization, or even from the phone book. For parents who cannot travel to meetings, a new form of support may be available via the Internet, as described in Chapter 26.

NURSE AS ADVOCATE FOR CHILDREN IN THE COMMUNITY

Because children cannot communicate their needs, we need to broaden our advocacy to fight for better child health at local and national levels. For example, *Healthy People 2010* (online, http://hp2010.nhlbihin.net/) has designated obesity and physical activity as 2 of 10 priorities for action. Nurse researchers such as Kubic (2008) have signaled concern about an epidemic of childhood obesity and have piloted school intervention programs. Child obesity is causing a huge increase in related health problems such as diabetes (Lawlor & Chaturvedi, 2006; "Hospitalizations for Obese Kids Double," 2009). Poor and low-income children more often lack parks, safe neighborhoods for exercising, and tend to have an abundance of fast-food restaurants selling high-calorie foods (Blacksher, 2008). Examples of nursing advocacy interventions include organizing campaigns to eliminate sale of junk food in schools, reinstituting recess and physical education opportunities, joining community activist groups advocating restructuring of community neighborhoods to allow for increased exercise with sidewalks to school and safe bike paths.

SUMMARY

Working with children requires patience, imagination, and creative applications of therapeutic communication strategies. Children's ability to understand and communicate with nurses is largely influenced by their cognitive developmental level and their limited life experiences. Nurses need to develop an understanding of feelings and thought processes from the child's perspective, and communication strategies with children should reflect these understandings. Various strategies for communicating with children of different ages are suggested, as are strategies for communicating with their parents. A marvelous characteristic of children is how well they respond to caregivers who make an effort to understand their needs and take the time to relate to them.

ETHICAL DILEMMA   What Would You Do?
You are caring for Mika Soon, a 15-year-old adolescent. She has confided to you that she is being treated for chlamydia. Her mother approaches you privately and demands to know if Mika has told you if she is sexually active with her boyfriend. Since Mika is a minor and Mrs. Soon is paying for this clinic visit, are you obligated to tell her the truth?

REFERENCES

Blacksher E: Children's health inequalities: ethical and political challenges to seeking social justice, The Hastings Center available online: http://www.the hastingscenter.org/Publications/HCR/Detail.aspx?id=1750. Accessed November 18, 2008.

Bransletter JE, Domain EW, Williams PD, et al: Communication themes in families of children with chronic conditions, *Issues Compr Pediatr Nurs* 31(4):171–184, 2008.

Coad JE, Shaw KL: Is children's choice in health care rhetoric of reality: a scoping review, *J Adv Nurs* 64(4):318–327, 2008.

Emslie GJ: Pediatric anxiety-under recognized and under treated, *N Engl J Med* 359(26):2835–2836, 2008.

Erickson EH: *Childhood and society*, New York, 1963, Norton.

Gardner R: *Therapeutic communication with children*, ed 2, New York, 1986, Science Books.

Griswold KS, Aronoff H, Kernan JB, Kahn LS: Adolescent substance use and abuse: recognition and management, *Am Fam Physician* 77(3):331–336, 2008.

Hong SS, Murphy SO, Connolly PM: Parental satisfaction with nurses' communication and pain management in a pediatric unit, *Pediatr Nurs* 34(4):289–293, 2008.

Hospitalizations for obese kids double, *USA Today* 6D, July 9, 2009.

Kubic M: *Personal interview*, 2008, University of Minnesota May 23.

Lawlor DA, Chaturvedi N: Treatment and prevention of obesity-are there critical periods for intervention? *Int J Epidemiol* 35:3–9, 2006.

Looman WS, O'Connor-Von S, Lindeke LL: Caring for children with special healthcare needs and their families: what advanced practice nurses need to know, *J Nurse Pract* 4:512–517, 2008.

Mangione-Smith R, DeCristofaro AH, Setodji CM, et al: The quality of ambulatory care delivered to children in the United States, *N Engl J Med* 35715:1515–1523, 2007.

McCarthy V, Hobbie C: Incorporating violence prevention into anticipatory guidance for well child visits, *J Pediatric Health Care* 11(5):222–226, 1997.

Migdal M, Chudzynska-Pomianowska E, Vause E, et al: Rapid, needle-free delivery of lidocaine for reducing the pain of venipuncture among pediatric subjects, *Pediatrics* 115(4):e393–e398, 2005; available online: http://pediatrics.aappublications.org/cgi/content/full/115/4/e393.

Piaget J: *The child's conception of the world*, Savage, MD, 1972, Littlefield, Adams.

Pieper P: Ethical perspectives of children's assent for research participation: deontology and utilitarianism, *Pediatr Nurs* 34(4):319–323, 2008.

Taylor CA, Guteman NB, Lee SJ, Rathouz PJ: Intimate partner violence, maternal stress, nativity, and risk for maternal maltreatment of young children, *Am J Public Health* 1–25, 2009; available online www.medscape.com/viewarticle/702408_print. Accessed May 20, 2009.

Van Hulle Vincent C: Nurses' knowledge, attitudes and practices regarding children's pain, *MCN Am J Matern Child Nurs* 30(3): 177–183, 2005.

Zengerle-Levy K: Nursing the child who is alone in the hospital, *Pediatr Nurs* 32(3):226–231, 2006.

Communicating with Older Adults

Elizabeth C. Arnold

OBJECTIVES

At the end of the chapter, the reader will be able to:

1. Discuss concepts of normal aging.
2. Identify the use of theoretical frameworks used in the care of older adult clients.
3. Describe assessment strategies with older adults.
4. Describe supportive nursing care strategies with older adults.
5. Discuss assessment and support interventions for cognitively impaired older adults.

This chapter focuses on assessment and communication strategies related to client-centered relationships with older adults. The chapter presents basic concepts about aging as part of the life process and explores age-related changes that can affect communication. Developmental frameworks and the nursing process form a structural foundation for providing care to older adults. Communication strategies to support successful aging and to use with clients demonstrating cognitive impairment are included. Effective communication is critical to the health and well-being of older adults.

BASIC CONCEPTS

CONCEPTS OF NORMAL AGING

Effective communication with older adult adults requires a thorough understanding of the normal health-related changes associated with aging. **Aging** is a term used to describe "advancing through the life cycle, beginning at birth and ending at death" (Pankow & Solotoroff, 2007, p. 19). Although aging is a lifelong process, the most common interpretation refers to physiologic decline, and associated mental and social changes occurring in late adulthood.

Aging is a normal physiologic process, accompanied to a greater or lesser degree by changes in appearance and energy levels, degenerative changes in organs and tissues, a weaker immune system, sensory losses, and decreased functional capacity related to mobility. Aging affects physical strength, stamina, and flexibility, and ultimately, an individual's ability to negotiate the physical environment. Cotter and Gonzalez (2009) define "*successful aging* as the ability to adapt flexibly to age-related changes without relinquishing the central components of self-definition" (p. 335).

Older adults are often treated as if they represent a single cohort, when, in fact, there are huge differences in their life experiences, opportunities, capabilities, interests, and relationships. As people live longer, the term *older adult* or *senior* is broken down into three age cohorts: young old (65–74 years), old-old (75–84 years), and oldest-old (85 years and older) (Moody, 2010). A lot of older adults are frail and can have reduced function because of age-related disease, but many will retain a high level of physical and intellectual function until close to their death.

Each person's experience of the aging process is unique, reflecting his or her genetic makeup, personality, life experiences, as well as environmental and cultural factors. Aging is a life process influenced by many factors, some of which are preventable or reversible. Although genetic and physiologic factors are not totally within an older person's control, learning adaptive self-management strategies can make a major difference in an older adult's overall health and quality of life.

Aging need not be a negative experience. Healthy older adults generally have more time and less responsibilities. There is time to travel, engage in activities one didn't have time for previously, develop new interests, take a course, take an active role in community activities, share their talents with others, and enjoy family and grandchildren. Our attitude toward aging can become a self-fulfilling prophecy. Bortz (1990) states:

> If we dread growing old, thinking of it as a time of forgetfulness and physical deterioration, then it is likely to be just that. On the other hand, if we expect it to be full of energy and anticipate that our lives will be rich with new adventures and insight; then that is the likely reality. We prescribe who we are. We prescribe what we are to become. (p. 55)

Biggs (2001) notes that positive stories of aging need to be told and incorporated into contemporary social policy. Older adults often lack the developmental supports provided earlier in life. People take pride in teaching and supporting children and young adults to achieve the life building skills they need as their developmental needs change. Articles detail the signs and symptoms of degenerative changes, with less attention paid to what older adults need to enhance quality of health and well-being.

Aging has direct and indirect effects on communication and interpersonal relationships. Nurses working with older clients need to have a thorough understanding of the aging process and positive respect for their struggles. Exercise 19-1 provides you with an opportunity to explore your personal ideas about aging.

AGING AND HEALTH

Sowers and Rowe (2007) note, "By 2050, the number of persons aged 60 and over is projected to increase from 600 million to almost 2 billion (p. 11). Four- and five-generation families are becoming common as life span increases. Family-based assistance as the primary source of long-term care for the frail elderly will continue to increase (Gavan, 2003).

Older adults are not a homogenous population with similar health needs. Individual differences in the aging process allow many to experience relatively few health problems even into their eighties. But it is true that after the age of 60, people are more vulnerable to a variety of age-related diseases, such as cancer, cardiac and circulatory problems, stroke, and degenerative bone loss. Older people may gradually lose control over some of their bodily functions and movements, which interferes with their sense of dignity and self-image (Franklin, Ternestedt, & Nordenfelt, 2006). Older adults disproportionately experience a

EXERCISE 19-1	What Is It Like to Be Old?

Purpose: To stimulate personal awareness and feelings about the aging process.

Procedure:
Think about and write down the answers to the following questions about your own aging process:
1. What do you think will be important to you when you are 65?
2. Prepare a list of the traits, qualities, and attributes you hope you will have when you are this age.
3. What do you think will be different for you in terms of physical, emotional, spiritual, and social perceptions and activities?
4. How would you like people to treat you when you are an older adult?

Discussion:
In groups of three to four students, share your thoughts. Have one person act as a scribe and write down common themes. Students should ask questions about anything they don't understand.
1. In what ways did doing this exercise give you some insight into what the issues of aging might be for your age group?
2. In what ways might the issues be different for people in your age group and for people currently classified as older adults?
3. How could you use this exercise to better understand the needs of older adults in the hospital, long-term setting, or home?

larger number of chronic conditions and diseases. As a cohort, they are the largest users of health services (Scholder, Kagan, & Schumann, 2004).

Older adults can experience subtle discrimination in accessing health care, level of screening and choice of treatment options. Physicians are less likely to use extensive diagnostic testing or aggressive treatment with older adults and they are underrepresented in clinical trials in part because of co-existing medical conditions. Medicare does not pay for experimental drugs. Other obstacles include navigating the complexity of the medical system, and limitations and gaps in services for chronic health care conditions. The decreasing number of physicians and other health care providers accepting elderly clients and/or suboptimal Medicare reimbursement for chronic care conditions is another factor.

CONTEMPORARY OLDER ADULTS

Our view of the elderly is changing as people live longer and experience less disability for shorter periods before death. Our perception of quality of life for older adults is changing and is likely to continue to evolve.

Contemporary "older adults" are not the same as they were even a few decades ago. They have been exposed to different opportunities than their parents had, related to economics, health, information technology, gender roles, and so on (Curtis & Dixon, 2005). As baby boomers "come of age," they represent a highly educated cohort who is more health conscious and better informed about health matters than in previous generations. By 2030, the baby boomers will have all reached the age of 65, double the number of older adults at the beginning of the 21st century (Mellor & Rehr, 2005). To date, this cohort represents the future

for health care needs of older adults. Very shortly, it will become the present. Exercise 19-2 offers an opportunity to think about the implications of planning health care for contemporary older adults (baby boomers).

Older adults are generally healthier in terms of less severe functional problems and chronic disability. They are living longer with a more robust quality of life (Maples & Abney, 2006). With current recessionary trends and Social Security changes, people are retiring later, and many remain actively engaged in the community. With many more people living into their 90's, living adult children in their fifties and sixties are likely to become primary caregivers for very old relatives. Health care reform, long-term care, the future of Medicare, and new images of health and well-being in older adults are important issues that health care professionals will need to consider.

The literature, anchored by Rowe and Kahn (1998), identifies three fundamental characteristics associated with successful aging:

- Low risk for disease and disease-related disability
- High mental and physical function
- Active engagement with life (p. 38)

THEORETICAL FRAMEWORKS USED IN THE CARE OF OLDER ADULT CLIENTS

ERIK ERIKSON'S EGO DEVELOPMENT MODEL

Erikson's (1982) model of psychosocial development is one of the only developmental models that specifically addresses later adulthood (>60 years) as a stage of

---

EXERCISE 19-2 | **Quality Health Care for Baby Boomers**

Purpose: To provide an understanding of changes needed to provide quality health care for baby boomers.

Procedure:
Break into groups of four to six students. Allow yourself to go beyond the facts and think about your personal response.
   Answer the following questions:
1. How do you think the influx of baby boomers will affect health care?

2. What should be the focus of health care for the baby boomer generation?
3. What types of challenges do you see the health care system facing with the anticipated dramatic increase in numbers of older adults?
4. What are your ideas as a health professional to resolve the health care issues of the future related to care of older adults.

ego development. Erikson portrays the maturational crisis of old age as that of ego integrity versus ego despair. Awareness of one's personal mortality leads to the psychosocial crisis identified with this last stage of ego development.

Ego integrity relates to the capacity of older adults to look back on their lives with satisfaction and few regrets, coupled with a willingness to let the next generation carry on their legacy. Integrity involves acceptance of "one's one and only life cycle as something that had to be and that by necessity permitted of no substitution" (Erikson, 1950, p. 268). Acceptance develops through self-reflection and dialogue with others about the meaning of one's life. Nursing strategies encourage life review, and reminiscence groups facilitate the process. **Ego despair** describes the failure of a person to accept one's life as appropriate and meaningful. Left unresolved, despair leads to feelings of emotional desolation and bitterness.

Wisdom, the virtue associated with Erikson's eighth and final stage of ego development, represents an integrated system of "knowing" about the meaning and conduct of life. It involves a general knowledge about human nature and specific knowledge about its variations. (Kunzmann & Baltes, 2003). Sharing one's wisdom with others enhances the experience of ego integrity. Wisdom includes deep understanding of self and others, good judgment, and the insights that people have about living a life filled with courage, purpose, and meaning.

Le (2008) discusses two forms of wisdom: practical wisdom and transcendent wisdom. Practical wisdom emphasizes good judgment and the capacity to resolve complex human problems in the real world. Transcendent wisdom focuses on existential concerns and development of the self-knowledge that allows a person to transcend subjectivity, bias, and self-centeredness. Wisdom encourages older adults to share their understanding of life with those who will follow. Erikson (Erikson, Erikson, & Kivnick, 1986) believed that wisdom develops from confronting and successfully resolving life's psychosocial crises. Sharing wisdom in the form of personal stories creates a strong legacy for those in the next generation. Exercise 19-3 explores the relationship of life experiences with wisdom.

ABRAHAM MASLOW'S BASIC NEEDS MODEL

Maslow's (1954) hierarchy of needs (see Chapter 1) helps nurses prioritize nursing actions, beginning with basic survival needs. Physiologic integrity, followed by safety and security, emerge as the most basic critical issues for aging adults and need to be addressed first. Love and belonging needs are challenged by increased losses associated with death of important people. Esteem needs, especially those associated with meaningful purpose, and independence remain important issues in later life. Abraham Maslow believed that self-actualization occurs more often in middle-aged and older adults (Moody, 2010).

EXERCISE 19-3	The Wisdom of Aging

Purpose: To promote an understanding of the sources of wisdom in the older adult.

Procedure:
1. Interview an older adult (75 years or older) who, in your opinion, has had a fulfilling life. Ask the person to describe his or her most satisfying life events, and what he or she did to accomplish them. Ask the person to identify his or her most meaningful life experience or accomplishment. Immediately after the interview, write down your impressions, with direct quotes if possible to support your impressions.
2. Reflect on the person's comments and your ideas of what strengths this person had that allowed him

or her to achieve a sense of well-being, and to value his or her accomplishments.

Discussion:
1. Were you surprised at any of older adults' responses to the question about most satisfying experiences? Most meaningful experiences?
2. On a blackboard or flip chart, identify the accomplishments that people have identified. Classify them as work-related or people-related.
3. What common themes emerged in the overall class responses that speak to the strengths in the life experience of older adults?
4. How can you apply what you learned from doing this exercise in your future nursing practice?

Developing an Evidence-Based Practice

Weman K, Fagerberg I: Registered nurses working together with family members of older people, *J Clin Nurs* 15(3):281–289, 2006.

Murray LM, Boyd S: Protecting personhood and achieving quality of life for older adults with dementia in the U.S. health care system, *J Aging Health* 21:350–373, 2009.

This aim of this study was to explore the perceptions of nurses working in elder care about the difficulties and problems encountered in working with families of elder clients. Positive and negative aspects of working with family members to ensure quality care of their elderly family member were examined using a latent content analysis methodology of responses to open-ended questions related to the topic.

Results: Findings stressed the need for family members and nurses to work together cooperatively as a team in their care of the elderly.

Application to Your Clinical Practice: Family members are and can be an important resource for older adults. Keeping family members informed and having a good relationship with them is essential in building the type of cooperative working relationship needed for quality care, especially when time and/or resources are needed. As a professional nurse, what factors do you see as being most important in building an effective working relationship with family members of older adults? How would you involve the client's family in clinical decision making?

APPLICATIONS

ASSESSMENT STRATEGIES WITH OLDER ADULT CLIENTS

New situations can cause transitory confusion for older adults, apart from cognitive impairment. Many clients are aware of the stereotypes associated with aging and are reluctant to expose themselves as inadequate in any way. Knowing what to expect helps decrease anxiety and build trust. Continuity of care with one primary caregiver, when possible, helps foster the development of a comfortable nurse-client relationship.

Older adults are likely to be more responsive when time is taken to establish a supportive environment before conducting a formal assessment. Otherwise, it can be difficult for clients to discuss emotional issues associated with the aging process or their physical ailments. Sensitive issues such as loneliness, abuse and neglect, caregiver burden, fears about death or frailty, memory loss, incontinence, alcohol abuse, and sexual

---

BOX 19-1 | Communication Guidelines for Assessment Interviews

- Establish rapport.
- Use open-ended questions first, followed by focused questions.
- Ask one question at a time.
- Elicit client perspectives first.
- Elicit family perspectives, if indicated.
- Invite ideas and feelings about diagnosis and treatment.
- Acknowledge feelings and emotions.
- Communicate a willingness to help.
- Provide information in small segments.
- Summarize the problem or condition discussed in the interview.
- Validate with the client and/or family for accuracy.
- Provide contact information for further questions or concerns.

---

dysfunction will only be discussed within a trustworthy relationship (Adelman, Greene, & Ory, 2000).

Older adults appreciate having the nurse provide structure to the history-taking interview by explaining the reasons for it and what it will involve (Cochran, 2005). Asking clients to share something about themselves and their life history, apart from the reasons for the health visit or admission, helps to establish rapport and increases the client's comfort level.

By relating their life stories and exploring options relevant to their current health situation, older adults are able to step back and look at their situation in the present from a broader perspective. Nurses get to know the client as a person, rather than categorically as an "older adult." Box 19-1 identifies communication guidelines for assessment interviews.

Moody (2010) maintains that old age "is shaped by a life time of experience" (p. 2). Assessment of older adult clients begins with their story. As they relate their story, look for value-laden psychosocial issues (e.g., independence, fears about being a burden, role changes, and vulnerability) and client preferences. These are significant issues for older adults clients that may not be directly expressed.

Case Example

Nurse: You seem concerned that your stroke will have a major impact on your life.

Client: Yes, I am. I'm an old woman now, and I don't want to be a burden to my family.

Nurse: In what ways do you think you might be a burden?

> *Client:* Well, I obviously can't move around as I did. I can't go back to doing what I used to do, but that doesn't mean I'm ready for a nursing home.
>
> *Nurse:* What were some of the things you used to do?
>
> *Client:* Well, I raised three children, and they're all married now with good jobs. That's hard to do in this day and age. I did a lot for the church. I held a job as a secretary for 32 years, and I got several awards for my work.
>
> *Nurse:* It sounds as though you were very productive and were able to cope with a lot of things. Those coping skills are still a part of you, and can be used in a different way now."

Helping clients identify sources of social support, personal resources, and coping strategies helps soften the impact of physical and emotional stressors associated with age-related transitions (Gilmer & Aldwin, 2003). Exercise 19-4 provides a glimpse into the life stories of older adults.

ASSESSING AGE-RELATED SENSORY CHANGES

Sensory changes occur with normal aging. In particular, hearing and vision changes can have a direct and significant impact on communication and cognitive processing (Gonsalves & Pichora-Fuller, 2008). Vision and hearing enhancements are essential to ensuring client safety and staying connected with people in their environment. Anderson (2005) notes that addressing common causes of sensory impairment and providing sensory cues can help reduce confusion.

Hearing

According to the National Institute on Deafness and Other Communication Disorders (NIDCD, 2010), one in three people older than 60 and half of those older than 85 will experience hearing loss. Hearing loss associated with normal aging begins after age 50 years and is due to loss of hair cells (which are not replaced) in the organ of Corti in the inner ear. This change leads initially to a loss in the ability to hear high-frequency sounds (e.g., f, s, th, sh, ch) and is called presbycusis (Gallo, 2000). Lower frequency sounds of vowels are preserved longer. Older adults have special difficulty in distinguishing sounds against background noises and in understanding fast-paced speech. Hearing problems can diminish an older person's ability to interact with others, attend concerts and other social functions, and understand medical directions.

Adaptive Strategies for Hearing Loss. With a little planning in modifying communication with the hearing-impaired older adult, the relationship should not be any different from one with a client who does not have this disability. Ideally, you should position yourself at the same level as the client. It is important to speak with a normal or slightly louder than normal voice tone. You do not need to shout. Other strategies include the following:

- Address the person by name before beginning to speak. It focuses attention.
- If the person has a "better" ear, sit or stand on the side with the more functional ear.
- Speak slowly and distinctly.
- If your voice is high-pitched, lower it.
- If older adults doesn't understand certain words, rephrase rather than repeat the words.
- Face older adults so they can see your facial expression and/or read your lips to enhance comprehension. Keep the client's view of your mouth unobstructed.

| EXERCISE 19-4 | The Story of Aging |

Purpose: To promote an understanding of older adults.

Procedure:
1. Interview an older adult in your family (minimum age, 65 years). If there are no older adults in your family, interview a family friend whose lifestyle is similar to your family's.
2. Ask this person to describe what growing up was like, what is different today from the way it was when he or she was your age, what are the important values held, and if there have been any changes in them over the years. Ask this person what advice

he or she would give you about how to achieve satisfaction in life. If this person could change one thing about our society today, what would it be?

Discussion:
1. Were you surprised at any of the answers older adults gave you?
2. What are some common themes you and your classmates found that related to values and the type of advice older adults gave each of you?
3. What implications do the findings from this exercise have for your future nursing practice?

- Help older adults adjust hearing aids. Lacking fine-motor dexterity, older adults may not be able to insert aids correctly to amplify hearing. Make sure hearing aids are turned on. If difficulties persist, check the batteries.
- Keep background noise to a minimum (e.g., radio or television).
- Solicit feedback to monitor how much and what the person has heard.

Vision

Vision normally declines as a person ages (Whiteside, Wallhagen, & Pettengill, 2006). Colors become dimmer, and images are less distinct. Even with corrective lenses, blurring occurs, and words are harder to read in soft lighting. Brighter lighting and larger print help immensely. More serious age-related vision problems such as cataracts, glaucoma, and age-related macular degeneration can cause blindness.

Vision has implications for effective communication and functional ability. Older adults with progressive vision loss may not see you shaking your head or nodding. They may see changes in emotional facial expressions. Loss of vision can affect a person's ability to perform everyday activities (e.g., dressing, preparing meals, taking medication, driving, handling the checkbook, and seeing phone numbers). Vision affects functional ability to engage in hobbies or leisure activities (e.g., reading, doing handwork, and watching television). Poor vision is a major safety issue related to falls.

Adaptive Strategies for Vision Loss. Nurses can play a vital role in supporting the independence of the visually impaired client with a few simple strategies.

- If eyeglasses are worn, make sure they are clean, and in place.
- Stand in front of the client.
- Verbally explain all written information, allowing time for the client to ask questions.
- Provide bright lighting with no glare.
- When using written materials, consider font and letter size for readability. Use upper and lower-case letters rather than all capitals. Use solid paper, with sharp contrasting writing, and a lot of white space.

ASSESSMENT OF COGNITIVE CHANGES

Age-related changes in cognition for healthy adults are minimal and should not require major modifications in communication, although mental processing and reaction times may be slower (Moody, 2010). Without the ravages of disease, older adults show little loss of intelligence but may require more time in completing verbal tasks or in retrieving information from long-term memory (Wilson, Bennet, & Swartzendruber, 1997). Older adults are less likely to make guesses when they are presented with ambiguous testing items in mental status examinations. They may hesitate or not respond as well if they are under time pressure to perform. Otherwise, there should be no difference in functioning.

Approximately 6% to 8% of the population older than 65 years and more than 30% of those who reach the age of 85 will experience profound progressive cognitive changes associated with dementia (Yuhas et al., 2006). Dementia is characterized by memory loss, personality changes, and a deterioration in intellectual functioning that affects every aspect of the person's life. A small percentage of abnormal cognitive changes are caused by other organic problems (e.g., drug toxicity, metabolic disorders, and depression) and may be reversed with treatment.

Appraisal of serious cognitive changes is critical to assessment of older adults, because it has the most impact on a person's ability to perform activities of daily living (Moody, 2010). When the nurse has concern about a client's cognitive capability, it is prudent to perform a mental status assessment early in the interview to avoid obtaining questionable data. The Mini-Mental State Examination (Folstein, Folstein, & McHugh, 1975) measures several dimensions of cognition (e.g., orientation, memory, abstraction, and language). Guidelines for mental status testing with older adults are presented in Box 19-2.

Another useful assessment tool is the clock drawing test (CDT). The client is asked to draw a clock with numbers and a selected time; for example, 20 minutes after 8. A normal score is given if the numbers are presented in the correct sequence and position, and the clock displays the requested time. An abnormal score suggests dementia, and further evaluation is recommended.

ASSESSMENT OF FUNCTIONAL STATUS

More than any other factor, impaired functional status is associated with an older adult's inability to live independently. **Functional status** refers to a broad

| BOX 19-2 | Guide for Mental Status Testing with Older adults |

1. Select a standardized test such as the Mini-Mental State Examination (MMSE), which can be completed in 5 minutes.
2. Administer the test in a quiet, nondistracting environment at a time when the client is not anxious, agitated, or tired.
3. Make sure the client has eyeglasses or hearing aids, if needed, before testing.
4. Ask easier questions first and provide frequent reassurance that the client is doing well with the testing.

5. Determine the client's level of formal education. If the client never learned to spell, it will be impossible to spell "world" backward. Saying the days of the week backward is a good alternative.
6. Document your findings clearly in the client's record, including the client's response to the testing process, so that future comparisons can be made.

range of purposeful abilities related to physical health maintenance, role performance, cognitive or intellectual abilities, social activities, and level of emotional functioning. Stress, acute and chronic illness, and age-related physiologic changes influence a person's ability to function (Zisberg, Zysberg, Young, & Schepp, 2009).

Functional status rather than chronologic age should be the stronger indicator of disability-related needs in older adults. Chronologic age is somewhat of a misnomer, in that functional impairment is not associated solely with age. Burke and Laramie (2004) note that a chronically ill 50-year-old with no support system may have more disabling symptoms of aging than a healthy, active 75-year-old with a strong social support system in place.

Although age typically robs some of life's vigor from older adults, most healthy cognitively intact older adults are able to perform activities of daily living (ADLs) independently, or with a little assistance. Instrumental activities of daily living (IADLs) are more complex than basic ADLs. IADLs refer to tasks older adults have to cope with on a daily basis, include cooking, cleaning, shopping, managing medications, getting to places beyond walking, using a telephone, and paying bills (Kleinpell, 2007).

From a basic health perspective, function relates to a person's ability to perform essential ADLs. Essential ADLs refer to six areas of essential function: "toileting, feeding, dressing, grooming, bathing, and ambulation" (Miller, 2009, p. 96).

Evaluation of functional abilities helps determine the type and level of care an older adult requires. Functional abilities in older adults can range from vigorous, active, and independent, to frail and highly dependent, with serious physical, cognitive, psychological, and sensory deficits (Bonder & Bello-Haas, 2009).

ASSESSMENT OF PAIN

Persistent pain is a common concern of older adults, related to chronic conditions such as osteoarthritis, diabetic peripheral neuropathy, constipation, among others (Jansen, 2008). Both client and health care professionals can assume that moderate or episodic pain associated with chronic disorders of aging is a natural part of growing old. Pain limits an older adult's functional ability and compromises well-being; it should not be considered a normal consequence of aging. There is no more reason for an older adult client to suffer with chronic pain than there is for the younger client.

Chronic coexisting disorders such as depression or dementia can limit an older adult's ability to report or to correctly interpret underlying causes of pain. For example, undiagnosed depression may present as neck or shoulder pain, severe enough to interfere with sleep or activity. Liberal dispensing of analgesics to older adults for pain relief without full assessment of the nature of the pain and considering compliance issues can lead to undesired outcomes. Rowan and Faul (2007) label prescription drug abuse as one of the fastest growing public health problems among older adults in the United States.

Older adults, even those who are cognitively intact, can have trouble interpreting the level of their pain with the commonly used Faces Pain Scale. Although they can report whether their pain interferes with daily functioning, identifying pain levels on a linear scale is more of a challenge (Gloth, 2004).

A comprehensive pain assessment for older adults should ask the client to

- Describe the quality and nature of the pain, for example, aching, burning, pressure, acute, or stabbing. (Some older adults will use the word *discomfort* instead of *pain.*)
- Identify when the pain occurs and under what circumstances.
- Identify specific pain patterns and/or changes in pain intensity.
- Describe how the pain affects the client's physical, psychological, and social functioning (Feldt, 2008).
- Define the area of the body where the pain occurs, whether it is deep or superficial, localized or radiating.

Assessment of pain in cognitively impaired clients and in those who cannot communicate verbally, for example, a stroke victim with receptive aphasia, is accomplished through behavioral observation. Behaviors suggestive of pain include grimacing, tightened muscles, groaning, crying, agitation, lethargy, and unwillingness to move.

PSYCHOSOCIAL ASSESSMENT

Windsor and Anstey (2008) cite several studies indicating that older adults experience higher psychosocial well-being compared with younger counterparts. Older adults are more likely to seek emotionally meaningful activities in the moment and are less concerned with future achievements.

Loss is a reoccurring issue for older adults. Most will suffer more meaningful losses of people, activities, and functions that were important to them than earlier in life.

Although most people weather the necessary losses of life, late-life depression is an often untreated problem in older adults. Unlike symptoms of depression in younger people, somatization with vague physical complaints may be its first presenting sign (Arnold, 2005). Whenever the nurse senses a loss of emotional energy in life and feelings of desolation about their situation, it is important to seek additional data from the client. Statements warranting further exploration include:

"I am just useless."

"Life doesn't hold much for me anymore."

"I'd never do anything to myself, but sometimes I wish I wasn't here."

Age is a strong risk factor for suicide, among older white men (Groh & Whall, 2001). Statements reflecting helplessness and hopelessness should never be taken lightly.

SUPPORTIVE PLANNING AND INTERVENTION STRATEGIES IN NURSE-CLIENT RELATIONSHIPS

Personal strengths form the basis for planning and interventions. Although older adults face many negative situational stressors, they also possess a lifetime of strengths that can be temporarily forgotten. Many older adults can live independently with social, spiritual, and environmental supports, with a good quality of life.

General nursing care for cognitively intact older adult clients, with the exception of acute care, centers around providing supports related to self-management of chronic illness and promoting healthy lifestyles. The level of support people need depends on personal, financial, and social resources that the older adult has at his or her disposal, and is willing and able to use. Asking questions such as "Can you tell me who visits you, or whom you have visited in the last month?" "If you needed immediate help, whom are you able to call?" and "Do you have enough sources of income to meet your basic needs?" gives nurses important data needed for planning and intervention.

PSYCHOSOCIAL COMMUNICATION SUPPORTS

Older adults who are institutionalized in nursing homes appreciate short, frequent conversations. Like everyone else, the need to be acknowledged is paramount to older adults' sense of self-esteem. Heliker (2009) describes a story sharing intervention identified as "a reciprocal give-and-take process of respectful telling and listening that focuses on what matters to the individual and minimizes the power of one over another" (p. 44). Conducted in long-term care facilities, this strategy emphasizes simple one-on-one human conversations with older adults about topics of interest to them.

Everyone has a story to tell. The use of short stories to frame conversation as a shared experience reminds clients that they have a valued social identity that goes beyond descriptions of their health. Each time an older adult tells their story, they remember when they saw themselves as a valued, productive member of society and that someone cares to listen. Nurses can teach and model this communication strategy with nursing assistants.

The conversational world for older adults can narrow for many reasons, for example, mobility, death of friends, and transportation. Spontaneous current events to draw from as a means of starting a conversation are not as available. A limited conversation repertoire happens with cognitively intact older adults, and they may repeat stories.

Repetitive stories can be frustrating for nurses. Rather than thinking, "Oh my, here he goes again with that old 'Model T' car story," it is better to respond to the story and enter the conversation as fully as possible. Each conversation is an opportunity to gain insight into the person who he or she was, what aspirations and dreams were fulfilled or unfulfilled, what contributions are valued, and what goals are yet to be attained.

Life Review

Life review is a useful intervention with older adult clients. Gentle prompts and relevant questions for clarification are required. Sharing recollections from youth or early adulthood days with a compassionate listener helps older adults review their life, establish its meaning, and confront their conflicts, as well as pleasures. Sometimes it provides opportunities for older adults to reconcile long-standing conflicts (Bohlmeijer et al., 2009).

Reminiscence Groups

The interpersonal contact in groups can be therapeutic for lonely, isolated older adults (Henderson &

Gladding, 2004). Guidelines for group communication with older adult clients in long-term care settings are presented in Box 19-3.

A specialized therapeutic form of group for older adults in long-term settings is the reminiscence group. Minardi and Hayes (2003) differentiate between life review, which explores life events in depth, and reminiscence groups, which focus on sharing life experiences from a socializing and a therapeutic perspective. They are powerful sources of self-esteem for older adult clients.

Reminiscence groups follow a structured format, with themes decided beforehand. Examples include special times in childhood or adolescence, child-rearing or work experience, and handling of a crisis. The leader guides the group in telling their stories, asking questions, and points out common themes to stimulate further reflections. Members create for themselves a shared reality by revealing to one another what life has meant and can be for them. In the process of remembering critical incidents, people can reconnect with sometimes forgotten parts of their life that held meaning for them. Jonsdottir, Jonsdottir, Steingrimsdottir and Tryggvadottir, 2001) note, "Recalling the past helps people to adjust to life's changes and thus provides a sense of continuity, integrity and purpose within the person's current life context" (p. 80).

SOCIAL AND SPIRITUAL SUPPORTS

Social isolation compromises the health and well-being of older adults (Strine, Chapman, Balluz, & Mokdad, 2008). Staying engaged with life to whatever extent is possible and stimulating the mind are two critical strategies healthy older adults can use on a daily basis to promote health and well-being as they grow older.

BOX 19-3	**Working with Older Adult Groups**

- Affirm the dignity, intelligence, and pride of elderly group members.
- Ask group members to introduce themselves and ask how they would like to be called.
- Make use of humor, but never at the expense of an individual group member.
- Keep the communication simple, but at an adult level.
- Ask relevant questions at important points in a client's story.

- Call attention to the range of life experiences and personal strengths when they occur.
- Allow group members to voice their complaints, even when nothing can be done about them, and then refocus on the group task.
- Avoid probing for the release of strong emotions that neither you nor they can handle effectively in the group sessions.
- Thank each person for contributing to the group and summarize the group activity for that session.

Adapted from Corey M, Corey G: *Groups for the elderly* (p. 406), ed 7, Belmont, CA, 2006, Thompson/Brooks Cole.

Quality friendship is an incomparable resource for older adults. Social support for older adults may need to be more proactive and wide-ranging than for younger people, because the older adults' physical or intellectual vulnerability. They may require instrumental support with self-management of IADLs from family and friends. Helping family members and friends balance necessary assistance with the client's need for autonomy is a delicate art.

Bishop (2008) notes, "Social and spiritual ties share an interdependent link to positive psychological well-being in late adulthood (p. 2). For people who have lost a "people" support system, connection with a personal God or faith can be a very important source of support. Older adults express their spirituality through prayer, reading their bible, and engaging in religious or spiritual practices.

Awareness of a shortened life span promotes thinking about existential issues, death, and for some, the need to work through unresolved life issues. Spiritual interventions relevant to the care of older adults include instilling hope, prayer, and talking about the client's spiritual concerns. Helping clients cope with unfinished business and find forgiveness for self and others is identified as an important nursing intervention (Delgado, 2007). Clients with advanced dementia will often respond positively to spiritual hymns remembered from the past and to Bible readings.

Case Example

Lois visited an elderly patient with dementia in a nursing home on a weekly basis. The woman was mostly mute except for occasional words. One day Lois read her the 23rd Psalm. The woman spontaneously repeated the psalm from a different version, following Lois's reading in its entirety. She could not respond in the present; she could in the past when something was meaningful to her.

ENVIRONMENTAL SUPPORTS

Maintaining independence for as long as possible with a good quality of life should be a goal for older adults. Independence is something most people take for granted as a younger adult, but it becomes a significant issue for older adults and their caregivers. Corey and Corey (2006) note, "As we age, we have to adjust to an increasingly external locus of control when confronted with losses over which we have little control" (p. 403).

The nurse plays a critical role in helping older adults maintain their autonomy. For older clients,

being independent means that they are still in charge of their lives. As nurses assist clients to clarify values, make choices, and take action, a stronger understanding of their unique needs and strengths emerges. Older adults need to take as much responsibility for their choices and goal setting in health care as is possible.

Case Example

Nurse: Mr. Matturo, it sounds as if being in charge of your life is very important to you.

Client: Yes, it is. I grew up on a farm and was always taught that I should pull my own weight. You have to on a farm. I've lived my entire life that way. I've never asked anyone for anything.

Nurse: I can hear how important that is to you. What else has been important?

Client: Well, I was a Marine sergeant in World War II, and I led many a platoon into battle. My men depended on me, and I never let them down. My wife says I've been a good provider, and I've always taught my children to value honor and the simple way of life.

Nurse: It sounds as though you have led a very interesting and productive life. Tell me more about what you mean by honor and the simple way of life.

Dialogues linking successful past coping experiences with present situations make it easier for the client to imagine possible individualized coping skills in the present. At the end of the dialogue, the nurse might summarize what the client has expressed and follow up with, "I enjoyed talking with you. You've had a fascinating life. What do you think is next for you?"

Nurses need to be sensitive to the unexpressed fears of older adults around surrendering their independence. Formal support services in the community, home health aides, and informal family supports can be critical factors in enabling frail older adults to remain independent.

You may need to directly observe environmental supports, bearing in mind a potential association in the older adults' mind between accepting help and relinquishing independent living. For example, an older adult in cardiac rehabilitation told his nurse that he had a bedside commode and no stairs in his home. When the nurse visited the home, there was no commode, and the client's home had a significant number of stairs. He told the nurse that he was afraid she would take steps to make him move if these facts were known.

SAFETY SUPPORTS

Although there will always be a delicate balance between the client's needs and restrictions or supports needed for safety, usually at least some areas can be negotiated. Simple interventions to promote independence include the following:

- Allowing elders personal choices about their bedtime, within reason
- Respecting choices in food selection
- Providing chair risers that help elders raise themselves from sitting to standing position
- Safety modifications in the home (e.g., bathtub rails, scatter rug removal, night lights)
- Including elder clients in decision making about health care and giving them the information they need to make responsible choices

Modern technology presents new possibilities to support the independence of older adults. Telehealth assistive services encompass virtual health visits, reminder systems, home security, social and health alarm monitors, and compensatory supports for failing functional abilities (Magnusson, Hanson, & Borg, 2004). Although telehealth is currently unavailable in many areas, innovative technology is likely to become an increasingly important component of support care for independent older adults.

Medication Supports

Polypharmacy is a fact of life for older adults. As people age, many need multiple medications to maintain a healthy lifestyle. Polypharmacy places older adults at risk for side effects and drug interactions because of age-related changes in metabolism (Cochran, 2005).

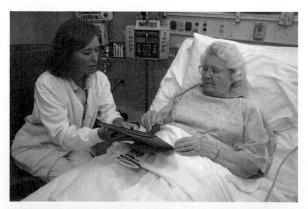

Health teaching for older adults is critical if they are to achieve and maintain their health.

Medications in general have a stronger effect on the older population and take longer to eliminate from the body.

Keeping track of medications can be challenging for older adults. Usually there is more than one provider. Prescriptions from different providers can create adverse reactions. When a provider lacks access to the complete client profile of medications, or does not have knowledge that the client is taking over-the-counter medications, the client suffers. Encouraging clients or a family to keep a written list of all medications to be shared with each provider helps prevent adverse drug interactions.

Healthy People 2010 objectives (Department of Health and Human Services [USDHHS], 2000) identify polypharmacy among older adults with chronic illness as a key safety issue. Medication mismanagement is associated not only with adverse drug reactions, but with hospital and nursing home admission. It is a major contributor to falls and hip fractures. Factors associated with poor self-management of medications include complexity of taking multiple medications, using incorrect techniques, improper medication storage, level of health literacy, cost of medications factors, and poor eyesight. Nurses should use every opportunity, informal as well as formal, to help clients establish and maintain appropriate self-management of medications (Curry, Walker, Hogstel, & Burns, 2005). The adage "start low, and go slow" (Miller, 2009, p. 129), which is a basic principle of geriatric drug prescription and regular communication with prescribers, is essential. Simplifying the older adult's medication regimen and regular checking of expiration dates enhance medication management and lessen the possibility of adverse reactions.

During an assessment interview, and on each subsequent home or primary care visit, you should ask specifically about medication and treatment implementation. Ownby (2006) recommends using an open-ended question, such as "Tell me how you take your medications," rather than asking, "Are you taking your medication as prescribed?" (p. 33). Box 19-4 covers key areas for medication assessment. Visually checking medications with the client and talking about how the medication is working with the client and/or primary caretaker is useful in home care.

Careful instruction as to the purpose, dosage, anticipated outcomes, and side effects can increase medication compliance. Establish a system with the client or family for medication administration, for

BOX 19-4 | Teaching Medication Self-Management

Areas of Assessment:
- List of current and previously taken medications, herbal and over-the-counter medications
- Medications taken episodically for insomnia, pain, intestinal upsets, colds, and coughs
- Allergies (include exact symptoms)
- Does the client know what each medication is for, storage, what to do for missed doses, drug interactions, side effects
- Ability to read medication labels or printed instructions
- Motor difficulties with appropriate medication administration
- Expiration dates, brown bag syndrome (having older adult bring all medications in a brown bag for clinic visit observation)
- Determination of family responsibility, and availability if medication administration support is needed

example, prefilled medication dispensers or a medication calendar. Use a teach-back strategy to ensure that instructions are understood, and the client or family feels comfortable with their knowledge and capacity to implement administration.

Elder Abuse

Elder abuse represents a major threat to the safety and well-being of older adults. The term refers to the mistreatment of vulnerable older adults, usually at the hands of caregivers, including professional personnel. The most common form of elder abuse is neglect, both passive and active. Active neglect is deliberate. Passive neglect occurs when clients, most notably those with dementia, do not receive properly supervised care.

Elder abuse is a difficult problem to identify and treat. Diminished mental capacity compromises an older adult's ability to even understand what is happening, let alone take constructive actions to stop the abuse, or to use any community services available to them (Nerenberg, 2008). Alternative options for older adults are not readily available, and older adults are reluctant to consider a nursing home as an option. Pride, embarrassment, and a desire to protect family members prevent vulnerable older adults from wanting to prosecute a family member for abuse or neglect. If the nurse identifies abuse or neglect, it must be reported to appropriate social and legal protective services.

ADVOCACY SUPPORT

Fundamental rights of older adults in health care settings are identified in Box 19-5. Nurses play an important service in explaining treatment to clients and families, and helping them frame questions for physicians and hospitalists. Nurses assume advocate roles with older adults around the following issues:
- Referrals and home care
- Right to refuse medication or treatment
- Informed consent
- End-of-life decisions about care and life support issues
- Liaison between an older adult client and other health professionals
- Mediator with family and client concern around treatment, level of care, and placement issues
- Third-party reimbursement
- Suspected cases of elder abuse
- Balancing an older adult's need for freedom with necessary protections

Role modeling is an indirect form of advocacy, affecting the interpersonal relationships older adults

BOX 19-5 | Fundamental Older Adult Rights

Older adults need to be able to:
- Live in safe and appropriate living environments.
- Establish and maintain meaningful relationships and social networks.
- Have equal access to health care, legal, and social services consistent with their needs.
- Have the right to make decisions about their care and quality of life.
- Have their rights, autonomy, and assets protected.
- Have appropriate information to make reasoned decisions.

- Have their personal, cultural, and spiritual values, beliefs, and preferences respected.
- Participate in all aspects of their care plan, including care decisions to the fullest extent possible.
- Expect confidentiality of all communication and clinical records related to their care.
- Be involved in advocacy and the formulation of policies that directly impact their health and well-being.

have with their caregivers. Nursing assistants or professional caregivers provide the majority of care for older adult clients. Role-modeling excellent care and respect for the dignity of the older client, regardless of medical condition, is important. It is noted by family and nonprofessional staff, and has a ripple effect on the care that they provide.

Nurses can refer client family members to local Alzheimer's disease and related dementia support groups. Support groups provide a place to talk about the challenges of caring for their family member. The *36-Hour Day* (Mace & Rabins, 2006), developed from the insights of family members coping with dementia in a loved one, is an excellent resource.

Advocating for Legal Protections

Frail older adults and particularly clients with dementia usually need legal protection to safeguard their personal and financial affairs, and to allow others by proxy to make health care decisions when they are unable to do so. Nurses can be invaluable resources and advocates for clients and families in discussing health-related personal legal matters. Advance directives and a durable power of attorney for health care (proxy) provide direction for the client's health care wishes should the person become incapacitated. For financial and property manners, the client needs to have a durable power of attorney, a living trust, and/or a will. Power of attorney documents are subject to state laws and are only in effect when people are unable to manage their own affairs. Under broad federal guidelines, state laws determine qualifications for Medicaid and property distribution if a person dies with no will or trust. Guidelines vary from state to state. Medicaid qualifications may be important for families requiring long-term care for a family member.

The time to execute legal documents to client rights is *before* clients become unable to cognitively assign decision-making authority to someone they trust. Clients in the early stages of dementia usually have sufficient mental competence to participate in legal decisions regarding their health care and finances. Later, they may not be able to execute the documents. Consultation with a lawyer regarding wills, durable and health powers of attorney, and living wills should be initiated at this time (Arnold, 2005).

Once cognitive capacity is lost, a court procedure is necessary to establish a conservatorship or guardianship. This action is more costly and emotionally painful for most families, as it requires legally certifying the person as incompetent. Mental incompetence is a medicolegal determination that identifies a person's inability to manage his or her personal affairs because of injury, disease, or disability.

Clinical incompetence refers to a person's inability to make appropriate health care decisions or to carry them out, as determined by a physician or qualified health care practitioner. Nurses can help clients make their wishes known and feel more comfortable about allowing trusted people in their lives to act on their behalf.

HEALTH PROMOTION FOR OLDER ADULTS

The CDC maintains that health-damaging behaviors such as poor nutrition, inactivity, and alcohol and tobacco abuse contribute heavily to the onset of disability in the elderly. They recommend an integrated health promotion approach to address common risk factors and comorbidities in older adults (Lang et al., 2005).

Older adults are much more health conscious today. They benefit from health promotion activities tailored to their stage of life. It is never too late to practice good nutrition; engage in healthful exercise such as strength training, walking, and yoga; connect with social relationships on a regular basis; and improve safety factors.

At the same time, healthy older adults are not young people. Their nutrition, exercise, and other health needs are different. Health promotion strategies need to be modified to meet the unique requirements of this population (Nakasato & Carnes, 2006). Box 19-6 identifies areas of relevant health promotion activities for older adults.

BOX 19-6	Areas of Relevant Health Promotion Activities

- Health protection: public health approaches promoting flu vaccines
- Health prevention: environmental or home assessments to prevent falls
- Health education: information about healthy eating and exercise
- Health preservation: promoting optimal levels of functioning by increasing the control older adults have over their lives and health

Adapted from Sanders K: Developing practice for healthy aging, *Nurs Older People* 18(3):18–21, 2006; Bernard M: *Promoting health in old age,* Buckingham, England, 2000, Open University Press.

Through regularly scheduled health promotion activities, nurses can assist clients in learning about a healthier lifestyle. Nurses can engage older adults in health promotion activities by appealing to their interests and by incorporating cultural values in the presentation. Examples of relevant activities can include:

- Preparing examples of healthy ethnic food (e.g., "soul cooking the healthy way")
- Assigning blocks of time for preventive screening, specifically for older adults
- Combining multiple prevention services into one clinical visit
- Providing free flu and pneumonia immunizations at convenient times in traditional and nontraditional settings (Lang et al., 2005; Penprase, 2006)

Health Teaching

Moody (2010) notes that health teaching for the elderly is critical if they are to master the tasks of old age and maintain their health. Healthy older adult clients are similar to other adult learners, except that they may need more time to think about how they want to handle a situation. The sensitive nurse observes the client before implementing teaching and gears teaching strategies to meet the individual learning needs of each client.

Assuming that older adult clients lack the capacity to understand instructions is a common error. Health care providers often direct instruction to the older adult client's younger companion, even when the client has no cognitive impairment. This action invalidates the client and diminishes self-worth. Mauk (2006) identifies simple modifications to reduce age-related barriers to learning when teaching older adults. Suggestions include:

- Explain why the information is important to the client.
- Use familiar words and examples in providing information.
- Draw on the client's experiences and interests in planning your teaching.
- Make teaching sessions short enough to avoid tiring the client and frequent enough for continuous learning support.

- Speak slowly, naturally, and clearly.

ASSESSMENT AND SUPPORT INTERVENTIONS FOR COGNITIVELY IMPAIRED OLDER ADULTS

Assessment of cognitive function should occur early in the client relationship. Dementia is a neurologic syndrome characterized by a progressive decline in intellectual and behavioral functioning that ends in death. Alzheimer's disease is the most common form, followed by vascular dementia and rare forms of dementia.

Symptoms of cognitive impairment and communication difficulties in older adults can be similar in clients suffering from depression, delirium, and dementia. Diagnosis has important implications for treatment. Communicating with a client suffering from dementia requires a different set of strategies than for the client with depression. Clients with depression can still communicate normally. Table 19-1 identifies important differences between these three common disorders in late adulthood. Secondary clinical depression and/or delirium can be superimposed on dementia, making a difficult situation even more challenging. Exercise 19-5 provides an opportunity to distinguish between dementia, delirium, and depression, using a case study.

SUPPORTING ADAPTATION TO DAILY LIFE

Box 19-7 outlines early cognitive changes seen with dementia. Memory loss is a consistent finding. Structure and consistency in the environment are important themes to consider. In the early stages, nurses can help clients develop reminder strategies such as making notes to themselves and using colored labels, alarms, or calendars. Focusing on what the client can do, rather than on deficits, does not change the course of the dementia. This strategy taps into the functions still available to the client and decreases feelings of hopelessness (Cotter, 2009).

Apraxia, defined as the loss of the ability to take purposeful action even when the muscles, senses, and

TABLE 19-1	Sorting Out the Three D's: Delirium, Dementia, Depression		
Disorder	**Delirium**	**Dementia**	**Depression**
Onset	Acute, over hours, days	Insidious, over months, years	Relatively rapid, over weeks to months
Acuity	Acute symptoms, medical emergency	Chronic symptoms, progresses slowly	Episodic symptoms, coincides with losses
Course	Short term; resolves with identification of cause, treatment	Gradual, progressive deterioration, memory loss	Self-limiting; recurrent symptoms; resolves with treatment
Duration	Lasts hours to weeks, resolves with treatment	Progressive and irreversible, ends in death	At least 2 weeks, may last months to years, responds to treatment
Alertness or consciousness	Fluctuates, intervals of lucidity and confusion, worse at night	Clear, stable during day, sundown syndrome	Clear, thinking may appear slowed; decreased alertness because of lack of motivation
Attention	Trouble focusing, short attention span, fluctuates	Usually unaffected	Minimal deficit, difficulty concentrating
Orientation	Disoriented to time and place, but not to person	Impaired as disease progresses; inability to recognize familiar people or objects, including self	Selective disorientation
Memory	Recent and immediate impaired	Impaired memory for immediate/recent events; unconcerned about memory deficits	Selective impairment, concerned about memory deficits
Thinking	Incoherent, global disorganization	Impoverished, inability to learn, trouble word finding	Intact, negative themes
Perception	Gross distortions; illusions, visual, tactile hallucinations	Prone to hallucinations as disease progresses	Intact, but colored by negative themes
Speech	Incoherent, disorganized, loud, belligerent	Impoverished, tangential, repetitive, superficial, confabulations	Quiet, decreased, can be irritable, language skills intact
Sleep/Wake cycle	Disturbed; changes hourly	Disturbed; day/night reversal	Disturbed; early-morning wakening, hypersomnia during day
Contributing factors	Underlying medical cause; toxicity, fever, tumor, infection, drugs	Degenerative disorder associated with age, cardiovascular deficits, substance dependence	Significant or cumulative loss; drug toxicity, diabetes, myocardial infarction

Adapted from Arnold E: Sorting out the three D's: delirium, depression, dementia, *Holist Nurs Pract* 19(3):99–104, 2005.

vocabulary seem intact is a common feature of dementia. The person appears to register on a command but acts in ways that suggest he or she has little understanding of what transpired verbally. In the following case example, the caregiver observes the client's difficulty. Notice how her response supports his ability to function. The client in the example had been the president of his company before being diagnosed with dementia.

EXERCISE 19-5	Distinguishing Between Dementia, Delirium, and Depression in the Older Adult

Purpose: To differentiate between the 3 D's.

Mrs. S. is a recently widowed 78-year-old woman living alone in a senior apartment complex in a suburban community. Her son and his wife live nearby and visit weekly. Over the last month, the family has noticed that Mrs. S. "has not been herself." Once a meticulous dresser, she shows no current interest in dressing and grooming. She has had difficulty keeping doctor appointments and getting medications refilled. When approached by the family regarding her change in behavior, Mrs. S. says that she "doesn't know—if I could just get a good night's sleep, I would feel better."

Discussion:

What distinguishing alterations in cognition does Mrs. S exhibit to suggest a depression or a dementia?

What additional questions would you like to ask to support your observations?

What screening tools are appropriate?

What approaches would you suggest for communicating with Mrs. S?

Identify ways to improve ability to function safely and independently for Mrs. S.

What sources of support can you identify to help Mrs. S and her family cope?

Developed by A. M. Spellbring, PhD, RN, FAAN, February 9, 2010.

BOX 19-7	Signs of Early Cognitive Changes with Dementia

- Difficulty remembering appointments
- Difficulty recalling the names of friends, neighbors, and family members
- Using the wrong word when talking
- Jumbling words: mixing up or missing letters in words when talking
- Not following the conversation of friends or coworkers
- Not understanding an explanation or story
- Difficulty recalling whether a task was just completed the day or week before
- Difficulty keeping up with all the steps to a task
- Difficulty planning and doing an activity such as a board meeting or family reunion
- New difficulty filling out complicated forms such as income tax forms
- Different behavior: restless, quick to get angry, constant hunger (especially for sweets), quiet or withdrawn, etc.
- Buying items and forgetting there is plenty at home
- Struggling with work or home tasks that used to be routine and easy
- Loss of interest in meeting with friends or doing activities

Case Example

The care staff member noticed IA's restlessness as he struggled to figure out which shoes to put on. IA began looking around with darting eyes, quickly shifting his gaze from here to there. The care staff member said, "I am sorry. I have put two pairs of shoes here and it is confusing. Please put these on." IA looked relieved, put on the shoes, and moved to a table where the care staff member placed a box that had many small articles brought from IA's company. The care staff member said, "Would you help us, president?" IA smiled and said, "Okay...I can see you need help here," as he began to organize the articles into piles. He did not wander on that day (Ito, Takahashi, & Liehr, 2007, p. 14).

SUPPORTING COMMUNICATION

Difficulty with communication is a hallmark of dementia. The dementia client's loss of communication is a gradual process initially and most clients can maintain superficial conversation, with empathetic support. Miller (2008) notes that dementia affects basic receptive (decoding and understanding) and expressive (conveying information) forms of communication. These deficits impact the person's capacity to think abstractly and solve problems. Clients may have more difficulty with communication when stressed or tired. Identify yourself and address the client by name before beginning each conversation. Clients benefit from frequent orientations, word sharing, and redundancy. Box 19-8 summarizes communication guidelines.

The use of cues in communication is helpful to the older adult with short-term memory impairment. Word retrieval to express ideas diminishes *(aphasia)* over time. The dementia client, unable to continue, stops in mid-sentence or continues with phrases that have little to do

| **BOX 19-8** | Communication Do's and Don'ts with Dementia Clients |

Communication Do's

1. Simplify environmental stimuli before beginning to converse.
2. Look directly at the client when talking.
3. Refer to the client by surname (Mrs. Jones rather than Mary).
4. Try to identify the emotions behind the client's words or behavior.
5. Identify and minimize anything in the environment that creates anxiety for the client
6. Watch your body language; convey interest and acceptance.
7. Repeat simple messages slowly, calmly, and patiently.
8. Give clear, simple directions one at a time in a step-by-step manner.
9. Direct conversation toward concrete, familiar objects.
10. Communicate with touch, smiles, calmness, and gentle redirection.
11. Structure the environment and routines, to allow freedom within limits
12. Use soft music or hymns when the client seems agitated.

Communication Don'ts

1. Don't argue or reason with the client; instead, use distraction.
2. Avoid confrontation.
3. Don't use slang, jargon, or abstract terms.
4. If attention lapses, don't persist. Let the client rest a few minutes before trying to regain his or her attention.
5. Don't focus on difficult behavior; look for the underlying anxiety and redirect.
6. Avoid hand restraints if at all possible.
7. Avoid small objects that could be a choking hazard.

with the intended meaning (Mace & Rabins, 2006). Allow extra time for clients to decode the material.

Anything to help reduce the client's anxiety about groping for thoughts that do not come easily is useful. Helping clients put words or thoughts together allow the conversation to continue. Nurses can support clients by filling in missing words, or supplying a logical meaning, and then asking the client if this is what he or she meant. Another strategy is to almost finish a sentence and have the client supply the last word. If there are terms the client typically substitutes for common words or phrases, for example, the word "clock" for asking about time, use the client's term. You also can ask the client to point to an object or describe something similar if you don't understand what the client is referencing (Miller, 2008). As dementia progresses, clients become increasingly unable to understand and express complete thoughts. Eventually the client with dementia cannot carry on even simple conversations. Use questions that can be answered with a yes or no for clients with less verbal skill. Note whether the client's behavior is consistent with the yes or no answer, and follow up if the behavior is incongruent with the words.

Restate ideas using the same words and sequence, and validate the meaning of a client's response. Instead of using abstract prompts (like a specific time), use words directly applicable to the client's daily routine, such as "before lunch" to anchor the client's

recognition of time frames. If a client rambles, you can refocus attention by selecting a single relevant thought from the stream of loosely connected ideas.

Cognitively impaired clients often are unable to follow instructions that consist of multiple steps. Breaking instructions down into single smaller steps helps mildly impaired clients master tasks that otherwise are beyond their comprehension.

Case Example

A young woman in a dementia support group for family members spoke of a meaningful experience with her grandmother. As she went to make a tuna fish sandwich for her grandmother, she decided to involve her in the process. She gave her grandmother step-by-step verbal instructions (e.g., "Get the tuna fish out of the cabinet," "Get the knife from the drawer," etc.), all of which her grandmother was able to do with her verbal guidance. As the granddaughter was spreading the mayonnaise, her grandmother said, "Now don't forget the onions." It was a priceless moment of connection for the granddaughter.

Asking mild to early moderate cognitively impaired older adults about their past life experiences serves as a way to connect verbally with those who might have difficulty telling you what they had for breakfast 2 hours ago. Nurses should appreciate that when cognitively impaired adults share memories they are giving a gift to the nurse by sharing part of themselves when they may have very little else to give.

Remote memory (recall of past events) is retained longer than memory for recent events. Family members can be encouraged to reminisce with dementia clients. This can be a meaningful experience for the family member even when the client cannot actively engage in the discussion, as it is a means of connecting. It is not uncommon for a dementia client to show through facial expression or garbled words that he or she too experiences the connection, even if only for a fleeting moment. Or it may come later.

Case Example

Mary was visiting her sister with dementia in the nursing home. She had traveled from Ohio to to Maryland to visit her. Her sister was unresponsive to her and Mary was upset that she didn't seem to realize that she was her sister. A few days after Mary returned home, her sister told the nurse, "You know, my sister Mary was here last week." Things register with dementia clients that are not always visible.

Touch

Touch is something clients with dementia can no longer ask for, create for themselves, or tell another of its meaning. Touch is a form of communication, used to reinforce simple verbal instructions with cognitively impaired adults, and as a primary form of communication. It is experienced "not only physically as sensation, but also affectively as emotion and behavior" (Kim & Buschmann, 2004, p. 35). As dementia progresses, gentle touch can anchor an anxious or disoriented person in present time, space, and humanity. When used to gain a client's attention, or to guide a person toward an activity, touch can acknowledge a client's stress, calm an agitated client, or provide a sense of security. In general, clients with dementia appreciate the use of touch. But to some, it can be frightening if the client perceives the caregiver as threatening. You can usually tell when a client thinks you are entering his or her personal space by looking at facial expression. Before using touch, make sure that the client is open to it.

Putting lotion on dry skin, giving back rubs, and warming cold hands or feet can be meaningful to the dementia client, as is something as simple as holding the client's hand. When a person is no longer able to recognize familiar caregivers by name, nurturing touch provides a touchstone with the physical reality of someone who cares about the client. It may be his or her only remaining opportunity for human interaction.

REALITY ORIENTATION GROUPS

Reality orientation groups are used with older adults experiencing moderate-to-severe cognitive impairment. Focusing on their personal environment, these groups keep people in touch with time, place, and person. Topics can include landmarks in the dining room, routes to the dining room or bathroom, the date, time and weather, what people would like to wear, and so on. Reality orientation groups may be conducted daily or weekly with three to four clients (Minardi & Hayes, 2003).

VALIDATION THERAPY

Validation describes a therapeutic communication process used in later stages of dementia. Developed by Naomi Feil, validation recognizes that a client is responding to a different reality related to time, place, or person (Minardi & Hayes, 2003). Rather than confronting dementia clients with "facts"—that people they knew or places they have lived are no longer available to them—the nurse focuses on the personal meaning events and people hold for the client. For example, you might say, "Tell me about Mary," or "What was it like living on M street?"

DEFUSING CATASTROPHIC REACTIONS

Older adults with memory loss lack the cognitive ability to develop alternatives. They emotionally overreact to situations, and can have what look like temper tantrums in response to real or perceived frustration. Older adult tantrums are called **catastrophic reactions**, and they represent a completely disorganized set of responses. Usually there is something in the immediate environment that precipitates the reaction. Fatigue, multiple demands, overstimulation, misinterpretations, or an inability to meet expectations are contributing factors (Mace & Rabins, 2006).

The emotion may be appropriate, even if its behavioral manifestation is not. Warning signs of an impending catastrophic reaction include restlessness, body stiffening, verbal or nonverbal refusals, and general uncooperativeness.

Instead of focusing on the behavior, try to identify and eliminate the cause(s) (Hilgers, 2003). Use distraction to move older adults away from the offending stimuli in the environment; use postponement. For example, you could say, "We will do that later; right now, let's go out on the porch," while gently leading the person away. Direct confrontation and an appeal for more civilized behavior usually serve to escalate rather than diminish the episode.

Sundowning is the term used to describe episodic agitated behavior occurring in the late afternoon or early evening with clients in the middle stages of dementia. Common childlike behaviors of whining, agitation, and temper tantrums characterize the syndrome. Small doses of medication are used to alleviate symptoms. Caution is needed to avoid over-sedating the client.

CARING FOR CLIENTS WITH ADVANCED DEMENTIA

As the dementia progresses, people lose control over most of their body functions and will experience one or more psychopsychiatric symptoms. They will require total care, which, in many cases, will include formal and informal caregiving strategies. Table 19-2 identifies common neuropsychiatric symptoms associated with advanced dementia, with suggested behavioral communication interventions.

TABLE 19-2	Neuropsychiatric Symptoms with Suggested Behavioral Communication Interventions
Neuropsychiatric Symptom Pattern	**Suggested Intervention**
Agitation	Identify and remove cause Assess for physical problems Reduce stimuli, suggest a walk Use simple repetitive activities: folding towels, rolling socks Use soothing music, Bible verses Look for patterns that trigger agitation
Aggression: grabbing, hitting	Recognize that the client is frightened Decrease stimuli, move client to a quiet place Don't take the client's behavior personally Respect and enlarge the client's personal space Identify and minimize cause Make eye contact; speak in a calm voice Acknowledge frustration; don't reprimand Check medications
Withdrawal: decreased socialization, apathy, social isolation	Use simple activities Find simple socialization opportunities, and support client involvement
Refusal/resistance to suggestions	Drop the topic/activity and reintroduce later
Disturbed motor activity: wandering, pacing, raiding waste cans, shadowing caregiver	Keep the environment safe Remove trash Use medical alert bracelets Label drawers, room (photos help) Use locks on doors at home
Sleep disturbances: Day/night sleep reversal, calling out/moaning in sleep	Keep active during the day Toilet client as needed during night without conversation Control wandering at night; lead back to bed; avoid use of restraints
Hallucinations, delusions, illusions	Respond to the emotion, not content Reduce stimuli Use good nonglare lighting Use distraction, e.g., walk, simple activity Use touch, reassurance, postponement
Disinhibition: inappropriate speech, touching, improper body exposure, entering other people's space	Don't reprimand Respond to the emotion Redirect client

TABLE 19-2	Neuropsychiatric Symptoms with Suggested Behavioral Communication Interventions—cont'd	
Neuropsychiatric Symptom Pattern	**Suggested Intervention**
Incontinence: urine, feces, eliminating in wrong places	Check for bladder infection, fecal impaction Note elimination pattern; establish corresponding toileting timetable Schedule toileting at frequent intervals Toilet before bedtime Take client to bathroom, verbally cue Use washable clothing, Velcro closings
Swallowing difficulty: choking, stuffing mouth, not swallowing	Cut food into small pieces, offer small quantities of liquid at one time Check medications for size, modify as needed Sit with client while eating Verbally cue to chew and swallow
Agnosia: difficulty recognizing faces, including one's own	Remove or cover mirrors if client is frightened by self-image Verbally identify familiar people and their relationship to the client

Treatment goals for clients with advanced dementia should emphasize dignity, quality of life, and supportive comfort strategies, rather than focusing on prolonging life (Rabins, Lyketsos, & Steele, 2006).

SUMMARY

This chapter discusses concepts of aging and presents supportive communication strategies nurses can use in client-centered relationships with older adults. Aging is associated with a decline in sensory and motor functions for most people, but contemporary older adults can expect to live longer and enjoy a better quality of life than in previous generations.

Erikson's theory of psychosocial development identifies wisdom as the virtue associated with his last stage of ego development, integrity versus despair. Supportive strategies to assist clients maximize their health and well-being during this important stage of life focus on communication, social and spiritual structure, the environment, safety, and medication management.

Assessment of depression, delirium, and dementia is important, as some symptoms are hard to differentiate. Guidelines for communicating with clients with dementia emphasize touch, as well as verbal supports. Strategies such as reminiscing, promoting client autonomy, using a proactive approach, acting as a client advocate, and treating older adults with dignity are proposed. Health promotion activities that take into account the unique needs and cultural values of older adults are more likely to be successful. As a primary provider in long-term care and in the community, the nurse is in a unique role to support and meet the communication needs of older adult clients.

ETHICAL DILEMMA   What Would You Do?

Mrs. Porter's mother, Eileen O'Connor, is a feisty, independent, 86-year-old. She lives alone and treasures her independence. Mrs. O'Connor is in your urgent care clinic for suturing of a lesion on her leg, which was injured in a fall. Mrs. Porter accompanies her mother and you listen to them argue; it is clear to you that Mrs. Porter wants to commit her mother to a long-term care facility. While you are alone with Mrs. O'Connor in the examination room, taking her history, she swears you to silence and confides in you that she is having increasingly frequent lapses in memory, sometimes forgetting to eat. You are aware of the need to maintain client confidentiality, but you also recognize that to ignore the ethical concept of beneficence and keep silent may well endanger Mrs. O'Connor's life. What would you do?

Courtesy Elaine Cloud, MD, 2002.

REFERENCES

Adelman RD, Greene M, Ory M, et al: Communication between older patients and their physicians, *Clin Geriatr Med* 16(1):1–24, 2000.

Anderson D: Preventing delirium in older people, *Br Med J* 73(74): 25–34, 2005.

Arnold E: Sorting out the 3 D's: delirium, dementia, depression, *Holist Nurs Pract* 19(3):99–104, 2005.

Biggs S: Toward critical narrativity: stories of aging in contemporary social policy, *J Aging Stud* 15(4):301–316, 2001.

Bishop A: Stress and depression among older residents in religious monasteries: do friends and God matter? *Int J Aging Hum Dev* 67(1):1–23, 2008.

Bohlmeijer E, Kramer J, Smit F, et al: The effects of integrative reminiscence on depressive symptomatology and mastery of older adults, *Community Ment Health J* 45:476–484, 2009.

Bonder BR, Bello-Haas V, editors: *Functional performance in older adults*, ed 3, Philadelphia, 2009, FA Davis.

Bortz W: Use it or lose it, *Runner's World* 25:55–58, 1990.

Burke M, Laramie J: *Primary care of the older adult: a multidisciplinary approach*, ed 2, St. Louis, 2004, Mosby.

Cochran P: Acute care for elders prevents functional decline, *Nursing* 35(10):70–71, 2005.

Corey M, Corey G: Groups for the elderly. In *Groups: process and practice*, ed 7, Belmont, CA, 2006, Thompson Brooks/Cole.

Cotter V: Hope in early-stage dementia: a concept analysis, *Holist Nurs Pract* 23(5):297–301, 2009.

Cotter V, Gonzalez E: Self-concept in older adults: an integrative review of empirical literature, *Holist Nurs Pract* 23(6):335–348, 2009.

Curry L, Walker C, Hogstel M, et al: Teaching older adults to self-manage medications: preventing adverse drug reactions, *J Gerontol Nurs* 31(4):32–42, 2005.

Curtis E, Dixon M: Family therapy and systemic practice with older people: where are we now? *J Fam Ther* 27(1):43–64, 2005.

Delgado C: Meeting clients' spiritual needs, *Nurs Clin North Am* 42(2):279–293, 2007.

Department of Health and Human Services (USDHHS): *Healthy people 2010*, Washington, DC, 2000, U.S. Government Printing Office.

Erikson EH: *Children and Society*, New York, 1950, Norton.

Erikson E: *The life cycle completed*, New York, 1982, Norton.

Erikson E, Erikson J, Kivnick H, et al: *Vital involvement in old age: the experience of old age in our time*, New York, 1986, WW Norton & Company.

Feldt K: Pain assessment in older adults. In Jansen M, editor: *Managing pain in older adults*, New York, 2008, Springer, pp 35–54.

Folstein MF, Folstein S, McHugh PR, et al: Mini-mental state: a practical method for grading cognition state of patients for the clinician, *J Psychiatr Res* 12:189–198, 1975.

Franklin L, Ternestedt B, Nordenfelt L, et al: Views on dignity of elderly nursing home residents, *Nurs Ethics* 13(2):130–146, 2006.

Gallo JJ: *Handbook of geriatric assessment*, ed 3, Gaithersburg, MD, 2000, Aspen.

Gavan CS: Successful aging families—a challenge for nurses, *Holistic Nurs Pract* 17(1):11–18, 2003.

Gilmer D, Aldwin C: *Health, illness, and optimal ageing: biological and psychosocial perspectives*, Thousand Oaks, CA, 2003, Sage Publications.

Gloth FM: *Handbook of pain relief in older adults*, Totowa, NJ, 2004, Humana Press.

Gonsalves G, Pichora-Fuller M: The effect of hearing loss and hearing aides on the use of information and communication technologies by community-living older adults, *Can J Aging* 27(2):145–157, 2008.

Groh CJ, Whall AL: Self-esteem disturbances. In Maas ML, Buckwalter KC, Hardy MD, et al, editors: *Nursing care of older adults: diagnoses, outcomes, & interventions*, St. Louis, 2001, Mosby.

Heliker D: Enhancing relationships in long-term care: through story sharing, *J Gerontol Nurs* 35(6):43–49, 2009.

Henderson DA, Gladding ST: Group counseling with older adults. In DeLucia-Waack JL, Gerrity DA, Kalodner CR, et al, editors: *Handbook of group counseling and psychotherapy*, Thousand Oaks, CA, 2004, Sage.

Hilgers J: Comforting a confused patient, *Nursing* 33(1):48–50, 2003.

Ito M, Takahashi R, Liehr P, et al: Heeding the behavioral message of elders with dementia in day care, *Holist Nurs Pract* 21(1):12–18, 2007.

Jansen M: Common pain syndromes in older adults. In Jansen M, editor: *Managing pain in older adults*, New York, 2008, Springer, pp 17–34.

Jonsdottir H, Jonsdottir G, Steingrimsdottir E, et al: Group reminiscence among people with end-stage chronic lung diseases, *J Adv Nurs* 35(1):79–87, 2001.

Kim E, Buschmann M: Touch—stress model and Alzheimer's disease, *J Gerontol Nurs* 30(12):33–39, 2004.

Kleinpell R: Supporting independence in hospitalized elders in acute care, *Crit Care Nurs Clin North AM* 19(3):247–252, 2007.

Kunzmann P, Baltes B: Wisdom-related knowledge: affective, motivational, and interpersonal correlates, *Pers Soc Psychol Bull* 29:1104–1119, 2003.

Lang J, Moore M, Harris A, et al: Healthy aging: priorities and programs of the Centers for Disease Control and Prevention, *Generations* 29(2):24–29, 2005.

Le T: Cultural values, life experiences, and wisdom, *Int J Aging Hum Dev* 66(4):259–281, 2008.

Mace NL, Rabins PV: *The 36-hour day: a family guide to caring for people with Alzheimer's disease, other dementias, and memory loss in later life*, ed 4, Baltimore, MD, 2006, The Johns Hopkins University.

Magnusson L, Hanson, Borg M, et al: A literature review study of information and communication technology as a support for frail older people living at home and their family carers, *Technol Disabil* 16:223–235, 2004.

Maples MF, Abney P: Baby boomers mature and gerontological counseling comes of age, *J Couns Dev* 84:3–9, 2006.

Maslow A: *Motivation and personality*, New York, 1954, Harper & Row.

Mauk KL: Healthier aging: reaching and teaching older adults, *Holist Nurs Pract* 20(3):158, 2006.

Mellor MJ, Rehr H: *Baby boomers: Can my eighties be like my fifties?*, New York, NY, 2005, Springer Publishing Co, Inc.

Miller C: Communication difficulties in hospitalized older adults with dementia, *Am J Nurs* 108(3):58–66, 2008.

Miller C: *Nursing for wellness in older adults*, ed 5, Philadelphia, 2009, Lippincott Williams & Wilkins.

Minardi H, Hayes N: Nursing older adults with mental health problems: therapeutic interventions—part 2, *Nurs Older People* 15(7):20–24, 2003.

Moody H: *Aging: concepts and controversies*, Thousand Oaks, CA, 2010, Pine Forge Press.

Nakasato Y, Carnes B: Health promotion in older adults: promoting successful aging in primary care settings, *Geriatrics* 61(4):27–31, 2006.

Nerenberg L: *Elder abuse prevention: emerging trends and promising strategies*, New York, 2008, Springer Publishing Co.

National Institute on Deafness and Other Communication Disorders (NIDCD): *Hearing loss and older adults.* Available at: www.nidcd.nih.gov/health/hearing/older.asp Accessed, August 16, 2010.

Ownby R: Medication adherence and cognition: medical, personal and economic factors influence level of adherence in older adults, *Geriatrics* 61(2):30–35, 2006.

Pankow L, Solotoroff J: Biological aspects and theories of aging. In *Handbook of gerontology: evidence-based approaches to theory, practice, and policy,* Hoboken NJ, 2007, John Wiley & Sons, Inc, pp 19–56.

Penprase B: Developing comprehensive health care for an underserved population, *Geriatr Nurs* 27(1):45–50, 2006.

Rabins PV, Lyketsos CG, Steele CD, et al: *Practical dementia care,* ed 2, New York, 2006, Oxford University Press.

Rowan N, Faul A: Substance abuse. In Blackburn J, Dulmus C, editors: *Handbook of gerontology: evidence-based approaches to theory, practice, and policy,* Hoboken, NJ, 2007, John Wiley & Sons, Inc, pp 309–332.

Rowe J, Kahn R: *Successful aging,* New York, 1998, Dell Publishing.

Scholder J, Kagan S, Schumann MJ, et al: Nursing competence in aging overview, *Nurs Clin North Am* 39:429–442, 2004.

Sowers K, Rowe W: Global aging. In Blackburn J, Dulmus C, editors: *Handbook of gerontology: evidence-based approaches to theory, practice, and policy,* Hoboken, NJ, 2007, John Wiley & Sons, Inc, pp 3–15.

Strine TW, Chapman DP, Balluz L, et al: Health-related quality of life and health behaviors by social and emotional support: their relevance to psychiatry and medicine, *Soc Psychiatry Psychiatr Epidemiol* 43:151–159, 2008.

Wilson RS, Bennet DA, Swartzendruber A, et al: Age-related change in cognitive function. In Nussbaum PD, editor: *Handbook of neuropsychology and aging,* New York, 1997, Plenum Press.

Whiteside M, Wallhagen M, Pettengill E, et al: Sensory impairment in older adults: part 2: vision loss, *Am J Nurs* 106(11):52–61, 2006.

Windsor T, Anstey K: Volunteering and psychological well-being among young-old adults: how much is too much, *Gerontologist* 48(1):59–70, 2008.

Yuhas N, McGowan B, Fontaine T, et al: Interventions for disruptive symptoms of dementia, *J Psychosoc Nurs* 44(11):34–42, 2006.

Zisberg A, Zysberg L, Young H, et al: Trait routinization, functional and cognitive status in older adults, *Int J Aging Hum Dev* 69(1):17–29, 2009.

CHAPTER 20

Communicating with Clients in Stressful Situations

Elizabeth C. Arnold

OBJECTIVES

At the end of the chapter, the reader will be able to:

1. Define stress and associate concepts.
2. Describe biological and psychosocial models of stress.
3. Identify concepts related to coping with stress.
4. Discuss stress assessment strategies.
5. Describe stress reduction strategies nurses can use in stressful situations.
6. Identify stress management therapies.
7. Address occupational stress in nurses.

This chapter provides a framework for understanding basic concepts of stress, and supporting client and family coping with stress through the nurse-client relationship. Included in the chapter are physiologic and psychological models of stress reactions, and descriptions of behaviors associated with stress reactions. The chapter addresses nursing interventions and communication strategies nurses can use to help people cope more effectively with stress.

BASIC CONCEPTS

DEFINITIONS

Stress represents a natural physiologic, psychological, and spiritual response to the presence of a stressor. Stress feelings set into motion an immediate emergency physiologic response to real or perceived threats. Normally, the stress response turns off when the immediate danger has passed.

A **stressor** is defined as a demand, situation, internal stimulus, or circumstance that threatens a person's personal security or self-integrity. Stressors can be catastrophic (war, hurricane, earthquake), related to a major life change (marriage, divorce, death, moving to a new area), or experienced as a minor hassle (traffic jam, child misbehavior, computer crashes).

Stressors can be potential, actual or imagined, and negative or positive. Illness, significant loss (e.g., job or relationship, home), a move to a different city, and loss of income can create negative stress. A job promotion, impending wedding and birth of a child are positive events that can be stressors. Box 20-1 lists personal sources of stress.

Stressors likely to stimulate an intense stress response are those in which a person has limited control over the situation, the situation is ambiguous, or the current situation resembles unresolved stressful events in the past. Concurrent and cumulative stressors increase the stress response level. The intensity and duration of stress varies according to the circumstances, level of social support, and the emotional state of the person. People have different tolerance levels for stress. Some people are highly sensitive to any stressor, others are more laid-back and have selective responses to stressful circumstances. Stress reduces the efficiency of cognitive functions and reduces access to previous knowledge. Caplan (1981) emphasizes the importance

BOX 20-1	Personal Sources of Stress

Physical Stressors
- Aging process
- Chronic illness
- Trauma or injury
- Pain
- Sleep deprivation
- Mental disorder

Psychological Stressors
- Loss of a job or job security
- Loss of a significant person or pet
- Significant change in residence, relationship, work
- Personal finances
- Work relationships
- High-stress work environment
- Caretaking (frail elderly, children)
- Loss of role

Spiritual Stressors
- Loss of purpose
- Loss of hope
- Questioning of values or meaning
- Disenchantment with religious affiliation

of community education, and socio-cultural support as a way to compensate for perceptual deficits and minimize the impact of negative stress.

CHARACTERISTICS OF STRESS

Hans Selye used the term **eustress** to describe a short-term, mild level of stress. It acts as a positive stress response with protective and adaptive functions, and is perceived as being within the person's ability to manage. **Distress** is defined as a negative stress that causes a higher level of anxiety, and is perceived as exceeding the person's coping abilities. It is experienced as being unpleasant and diminishes performance.

Current research suggests that men and women respond to stress differently. Men respond with patterns of "fight or flight," whereas women use a "tend and befriend" approach. Women use nurturing activities to reduce stress and promote safety for self and others. They seek social support from others, particularly from other women (Taylor, Klein, Lewis, Gruenewald et al. 2000). Children express stress through behavior, according to their stage of development, and family patterns. Acting out behaviors can mask a child's distress.

LEVELS OF STRESS

Mild stress can be beneficial. It helps people stay focused and alert. Mild stress serves as a motivator to develop skills to meet challenges and accomplish goals. Awareness of personal strengths and mastery of coping strategies learned in mastering a stressful situation helps people cope better in other life circumstances (Aldwin & Levenson, 2004).

Moderate stress occurs when people experience frustration or conflict over an inability to change a desired outcome through their own efforts. When people are stressed, they are more susceptible to illness (Dolbier, Smith & Steinhardt (2007). Chronic stress is implicated in the development and exacerbation of cardiac conditions, migraine, and digestive disorders. Stress create comorbidities between physical disease and mental disorder (Askew & Keyes, 2005).

High stress levels interfere with a person's ability to function because anxiety reduces a person's objectivity. People have trouble envisioning possibilities, weighing options, making choices, and taking action. They can exhibit anger, anxiety, and depressive symptoms. Severe or chronic stress weakens the immune system, thereby contributing to the development of stress-related illnesses (Martin, Lae, & Reece, 2007). Untreated, severe mental stress reactions associated with traumatic events can develop into post-traumatic syndrome, a clinical disorder. Stress and coping is said to account for up to 50% of the variation in psychological symptoms (Sinha & Watson, 2007).

BIOLOGICAL AND PSYCHOSOCIAL MODELS OF STRESS

PHYSIOLOGIC RESPONSE MODELS

Walter Cannon (1932) was the first to describe a scientific physiologic basis for an acute stress response. Cannon believed that when people feel physically well, emotionally centered, and personally secure, they are in a state of dynamic equilibrium or **homeostasis**. Stress disturbs homeostasis. Physiologically, the sympathetic-adrenal medulla system in the brain sets into motion an immediate hormonal cascade designed to mobilize the body's energy resources to cope with acute stress.

Cannon proposed that people attempt to adapt to stress with either a "fight or flight" response. The fight response refers to a person's inclination to take action against a threat if the threat appears to be resolvable, and the flight component, to flee, if it is unlikely that the threat can be overcome.

GENERAL ADAPTATION SYNDROME

Stress hormone levels generally revert to normal once the cause of the stress is resolved. Hans Selye (1950) expanded on Cannon's work in describing responses to longer term stress exposure. He described a three-stage progressive pattern of nonspecific physiologic responses, which he branded as alarm, resistance, and exhaustion. The alarm stage is similar to Cannon's acute stress response, characterized by increased activity in the hypothalamic-pituitary-adrenal (HPA) axis. Corticosteroids are released, which mobilizes the body's energy resources. If the stressor is not resolved in the initial alarm stage, a second adaptive phase referred to as "resistance" occurs as the body tries to accommodate for the stressor. In the resistance stage, the alarm symptoms subside as the immune system helps the body to adapt as best it can. Although the acute stress symptoms seem to disappear, the body functions less efficiently, and the resistance stage drains productive energy. If the body fails to adapt, or is still unable to resist the continued stress, it leads to "exhaustion." In the exhaustion stage, people are at high risk for stress-related illness or mental disorder.

The same physiologic response occurs regardless of whether a stressor is psychological or physical. Activation of the HPA axis occurs with the stress of critical illness, surgery, trauma, and emotional disorders (Johnson & Renn, 2006). The longer the physiologic responses remain elevated, the greater its negative effect on the organism.

ALLOSTASIS

A recent theory of stress response challenges the idea that physiologic systems respond to stressors as an attempt to achieve a fixed level of homeostasis (Sterling & Eyer, 1988). Allostasis describes how the organism achieves homeostasis through adaptation, referred to as "stability through change" (McEwen, 2000, p. 1219). The interaction between stressors and physical responses is ongoing such that individuals become more or less susceptible to the negative consequences of stress over time.

The brain serves as a "primary mediator" between the "current stressor exposure, internal regulation of bodily processes, and health outcomes" (Ganzel, Morris, &

Wethington, 2010, p. 134). The brain determines what experiences are threatening or nonthreatening, and the physiologic response requirements of each situation. It tries to find a new homeostasis that better fits the requirements of the environmental stressor, using a range of adaptive functioning (allostatic accommodation). The inclusion of genetic risk factors, early life events, and lifestyle behaviors in the model offers a way to understand the interaction between stressful events and physiologic adaptation processes (McEwen & Wingfield, 2003). Figure 20-1 identifies relationships in the allostasis model.

Stress hormones protect the body against short-term acute stress (allostasis). Stress mediators, such as social support, are capable of producing protective effects. When small or moderate levels of stressor exposure are encountered, and social support is available, the outcome is increased health and functioning. If a stressor continues, presents repeated challenges, or stress responses are ineffective, there is "wear and tear" on the body, which can have a damaging effect. McEwen (2007) terms this phenomena *allostatic load*. The allostatic load can be negligible or severe and protracted enough to result in significant illness or death.

STIMULUS STRESS MODEL

In 1967, Thomas Holmes and Richard Rahe developed a stress model that considered stressful life events such as marriage, divorce, death, losing a job, and so on as stimuli that threaten or disrupt homeostasis. The Holmes and Rahe scale gave each individual life event a weighted numerical score reflecting its stress impact on a person. Stressors requiring a significant change in the lifestyle of the individual have greater impact, as do cumulative stresses occurring within a short time. The quantity and severity of stressors influence a person's potential for developing later physical illness.

TRANSACTIONAL MODEL OF STRESS

Lazarus and Folkman's (1984) transactional model of stress is one of the most widely used to explain stress responses. It is based on the premise of a stressful experience is the result of a transaction between a situation or circumstance in the environment (stressor) and the individual experiencing the stressor. The transaction is the dynamic that accounts for a stressor's impact on a person. A person's perception of stressful events and interpretation of its meaning,

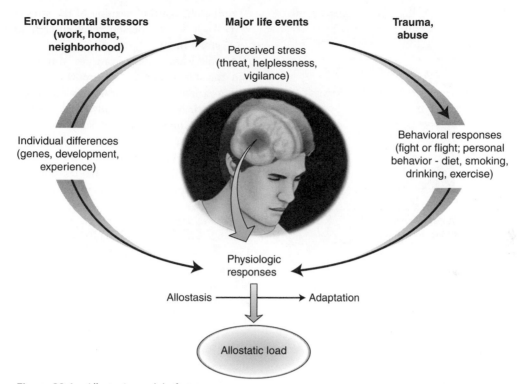

Figure 20-1   Allostasis model of stress.

and not the objective stress value of a stressor, determines the stress response.

Stress responses to cumulative daily stressors are a primary focus of the transactional model (Neale, Arentz, & Jones-Ellis, 2007). The model asserts that stress is as likely to occur with daily "hassles" as it is with major life events. The transactional model considers appraisal of stressors and coping strategies as a primary emphasis.

Primary and Secondary Appraisal

A person's interpretation of a stressful event is the result of two levels of cognitive appraisal. A primary appraisal initially evaluates the magnitude of the stressor, followed by a secondary appraisal evaluating an individual's perceived ability to cope with it (Figure 20-2). Both are required to determine whether a stressor will be appraised as harm, threat, or challenge (Folkman, 2008).

Primary appraisal focuses on the stressor or stressful event itself—its content and strength as a personal threat. A person determines whether an event is stressful and draws one of three conclusions: It is not stressful, it is a relatively benign stressor, or it poses a significant threat to self-integrity. Stressors perceived as a major threat to self elicit a stronger stress response, for example, losing an important relationship or being diagnosed with a serious illness. Primary stress appraisals can include threat of harm or losses that are anticipated but have not yet occurred.

When a primary cognitive appraisal determines a stressor to be a significant threat, the person automatically switches to a secondary appraisal related to coping skills. **Secondary appraisal** involves a person's perception of personal coping skills and the availability of resources in the environment to aid in reducing stressor impact.

COPING WITH STRESS

Knowledge of coping is essential to understanding how stress affects people (Skinner, Edge, Altman, & Sherwood, 2003). Coping strategies can reduce or increase the effects of stressors and the development of distress. In their classic work, Pearlin and Schooler (1978) define **coping** as "any response to external life strains that serves to prevent, avoid, or control emotional distress" (p. 2). They identify three purposes of coping strategies:

- To change the stressful situation

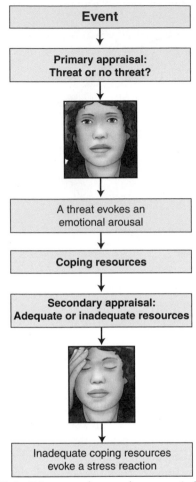

Figure 20-2 Primary and secondary appraisal in stress reactions.

- To change the meaning of the stressor
- To help the person relax enough to take the stress in stride

People learn coping strategies from parents, peers, and the circumstances life presents to them. Those with a variety of life opportunities and supportive people in their lives have an advantage over people who lack either opportunity or support system. People who have been overprotected or have been exposed to danger without support or mentoring generally lack experience with coping skills. Exercise 20-1 helps identify adaptive and maladaptive coping strategies in your life.

TYPES OF COPING STRATEGIES

Lazarus and Folkman (1984) identify two types of coping. **Problem-focused coping** strategies use approach behaviors, for example, confronting a problem directly, seeking social support, and constructive problem solving. Negotiation, directly confronting challenging issues, and taking action are deliberately used to change a stressful situation. Recognition of personal and outside resources can foster options, and people who have options generally are better able to cope with stress. Balancing coping resources include health, energy, problem-solving skills, the amount and availability of social supports and other material resources to cope effectively with the stressor. Individuals who are generally capable, have financial resources, and are by nature optimistic typically handle stress more easily.

Emotion-focused coping refers to avoidance behaviors that serve to distance the person from stress. They can be helpful alone or in combination with problem-solving strategies when people are faced with overwhelming irreversible situations.

EXERCISE 20-1	Identifying Adaptive and Maladaptive Coping Strategies

Purpose: To help students identify the wide range of adaptive and maladaptive coping strategies.

Procedure:
1. Identify all of the ways in which you handle stressful situations.
2. List three personal strategies that you have used successfully in coping with stress.
3. List one personal coping strategy that did not work, and identify your perceptions of the reasons it was inadequate or insufficient to reduce your stress level.

4. List on a chalkboard or flip chart the different coping strategies identified by students.

Discussion:
1. What common themes did you find in the ways people handle stress?
2. Were you surprised at the number and variety of ways in which people handle stress?
3. What new coping strategy might you use to reduce your stress level?
4. Are there any circumstances that increase or decrease your automatic reactions to stress?

Research suggests that constructive emotion-focused coping, featuring change in attitude, acceptance, and emotional respite from overthinking about a stressful situation, is associated with positive outcomes (Mohr, Goodkin, Gatto, & Van der Wende, 1997). Emotion-focused coping can be a positive realistic choice when a situation cannot be changed, and the person deliberately chooses to "let go" of negative feelings associated with it. Most people use both types of coping strategies, with the choice of strategy being somewhat dependent on the nature of the stressor.

Helping clients and families develop a different perspective can be just as important as the more traditional problem-solving strategies used to cope with stress (Michalenko, 1998).

Defensive Coping Strategies

People need time to absorb the meaning of a serious stressor. As a short-term coping strategy, defense mechanisms can be temporarily adaptive in minimizing the threat of a potentially overwhelming stressor (Richards & Steele, 2007). As a primary stress reducer, and over time, defense mechanisms are ineffective because they serve as a disincentive to action. **Ego defense mechanisms** represent a largely unconscious pattern of coping that people use to protect the self from full awareness of challenging conflict situations. They are designed to protect the ego from anxiety and loss of self-esteem by denying, avoiding, or attributing responsibility for a challenging conflict to an external source. Persistent use of ego defense mechanisms as a primary coping strategy generally is considered pathologic, although a few have positive value. Recent authors (Reich, Zautra and Hall, 2010; Vaillant and Mukamal, 2001) contend that healthy defense mechanisms; humor, anticipation, affiliation (asking for help) and sublimation can be adaptive and are associated with resilience. For example, sublimation is used to channel extreme anger impulses into acceptable behaviors, for example, by becoming a butcher or boxer. Table 20-1 provides definitions and examples of common defense mechanisms.

It is important to remember most ego defense mechanisms are unconscious. Because a defensive reframing of a conflict in a person's mind is usually not under the conscious control of the client, it is difficult to help them consider alternative coping strategies

TABLE 20-1	Ego Defense Mechanisms
Ego Defense Mechanism	**Clinical Example**
Regression: returning to an earlier, more primitive form of behavior in the face of a threat to self-esteem	Julie was completely toilet trained by 2 years. When her younger brother was born, she began wetting her pants and wanting a pacifier at night.
Repression: unconscious forgetting of parts or all of an experience	Elizabeth has just lost her job. Her friends would not know from her behavior that she has any anxiety about it. She continues to spend money as if she were still getting a paycheck.
Denial: unconscious refusal to allow painful facts, feelings, or perceptions into awareness	Bill Marshall has had a massive heart attack. His physician advises him to exercise with caution. Bill continues to jog 6 miles a day.
Rationalization: offering a plausible explanation for unacceptable behavior	Annmarie tells her friends she is not an alcoholic even though she has blackouts, because she drinks only on weekends and when she is not working.
Projection: attributing unacceptable feelings, facts, behaviors, or attitudes to others; usually expressed as blame	Ruby just received a critical performance evaluation from her supervisor. She tells her friends that her supervisor does not like her and feels competitive with her.
Displacement: redirecting feelings onto an object or person considered less of a threat than the original object or person	Mrs. Jones took Mary to the doctor for bronchitis. She is not satisfied with the doctor's explanation and feels he was condescending, but says nothing. When she gets to the nurse's desk to make the appointment, she yells at her for not having the prescription ready and taking too much time to set the next appointment.

Continued

TABLE 20-1	Ego Defense Mechanisms—cont'd
Ego Defense Mechanism	**Clinical Example**
Intellectualization: unconscious focusing on only the intellectual and not the emotional aspects of a situation or circumstance	Johnnie has been badly hurt in a car accident. There is reason to believe he will not survive surgery. His father, waiting for his son to return to the intensive care unit, asks the nurse many questions about the equipment, and philosophizes about the meaning of life and death.
Reaction formation: unconscious assuming of traits opposite of undesirable behaviors	John has a strong family history of alcoholism on both sides. He abstains from liquor and is known in the community as an advocate of prohibition.
Sublimation: redirecting socially unacceptable unconscious thoughts and feelings into socially approved outlets	Bob has a lot of aggressive tendencies. He decided to become a butcher and thoroughly enjoys his work.
Undoing: verbal expression or actions representing one feeling, followed by expression of the direct opposite	Barbara criticizes her subordinate, Carol, before a large group of people. Later, she sees Carol on the street and tells her how important she is to the organization.

without support. Challenging defense mechanisms directly usually is not successful. The Prochaska model and motivational interviewing (see Chapter 15) offer guidelines for gently casting doubt, providing new information and introducing problem-solving strategies to assist clients in positively reframing secondary appraisals.

Case Example

Lynn was diagnosed as having a high cholesterol count and was advised to go on a low-fat diet. Basically, she knows she needs to do this, but Lynn says she sees no purpose in going on a low-fat diet because "it's all in the genes." Both her parents had high cholesterol and died of heart problems. Lynn claims there is nothing she can do about it, even though the physician has advised her differently. Her defensive interpretation prevents her from taking action needed to reduce her risk for cardiovascular disease and can result in a heart attack or death. Here the nurse might inquire about the client's health goals and provide the client with information about the link among diet, exercise, and heart disease. Linking the information to Lynn's stated life goals provides her with a different frame of reference.

SOCIAL SUPPORT

Social support is a key factor in alleviating stress and promoting the self-efficacy people need for successful coping and mastery of stress (Caplan, 1981). **Social support** is defined as the emotional comfort, advice,

and instrumental assistance that a person receives from other people in their social network (Taylor, Welch, Kim, & Sherman, 2007). Social support has three distinct functions: validation, emotional support, and correction of distorted thinking. Social support can refer to both the "perceived availability of help, or support actually received (Schwarzer & Knoll, 2007, p. 244). A person's social networks are drawn from family, friends, church, work, social groups, or school. Being able to contact family and friends when you need an emergency babysitter or an extra hand in a stressful situation immediately lessens stress.

Social support allows for honest sharing of feelings and concerns in an emotionally supportive relationship. Not only does sharing with others reduce stress by "externalizing" negative emotions, but family and friends can provide a sounding board, practical assistance, and tangible encouragement. Seeking help can empower both seeker and provider of emotional support. Sharing a laugh, eating a meal with others, and being in good company helps people feel more relaxed, which, in turn, reduces stress levels.

Social support does not have the same meaning for all cultures in terms of self-disclosure. Taylor et al. (2007) report that Asian American clients may be more comfortable with an implicit form of social support that does not require extensive sharing of thoughts. Examples of implicit social support include showing kindness, caring, acceptance, and positive regard for a client.

Developing an Evidence-Based Practice

Drageset S, Lindstrom T, Christine MA: Coping with a possible breast cancer diagnosis: demographic factors and social support, *J Adv Nurs* 51(3):217–226, 2005.

The authors completed an exploratory study examining the relationships between demographic characteristics, social support, anxiety, coping, and defense among women with a possible breast cancer diagnosis. A survey design was used to elicit data from a non-probabilistic convenience sample of 117 women who had recently undergone breast biopsy. Study instruments included the Social Provisions Scale, State-Trait Anxiety Scale, Utecht coping list, and Defense Mechanisms Inventory. Demographic data were also collected. Data were analyzed using stepwise linear regression and statistical analysis methods.

Results: Study results indicated high internal reliability for the instruments used in the study. The social provisions scale was positively related to instrumental-oriented and emotion-focused coping, and unrelated to cognitive defense and defensive hostility. Social support was most strongly correlated to coping style. There were positive correlations between education, attachment, and instrumental coping, with education emerging as the most important determinant. Family was also found to be an important source of social support. A defensive hostile style of relating was negatively related to social support.

Application to Your Clinical Practice: This study demonstrates the need to educate clients experiencing the stress of a new diagnosis about the benefits of social support. Defensive hostility is a behavior that often masks anxiety. How could you use this information to help clients experiencing the stress of a new diagnosis cope more effectively?

BOX 20-2	Factors That Influence the Impact of Stress

- Magnitude and demands of the stressor on self and others
- Multiple stressors occurring at the same time
- Suddenness or unpredictability of a stressful situation
- Accumulation of stressors and duration of the stress demand
- Level of social support available to the client and family
- Previous trauma, which can activate unresolved fears
- Presence of a co-occurring mental disorder
- Developmental level of the client
- Attitude and outlook
- Knowledge, expectations, and realistic picture

APPLICATIONS

STRESS ASSESSMENT

Stress can worsen almost any illness. Factors that influence the impact of stress are identified in Box 20-2. Addressing relevant issues and teaching clients related coping strategies as early as possible enhances recovery potential. Clients and family members usually welcome an opportunity to tell their story and talk about concerns beyond the concrete needs of a stressful situation.

Understanding how a stressful event relates to other life issues, including stressors from the past, and current financial or family concerns puts the current stressor in context. Ask open-ended questions about changes in daily routines, new roles and responsibilities, and the client/family's understanding of diagnosis and treatment options.

Pay attention to cultural values. What is a small stressor in one culture can be huge in another, and normal coping strategies can be quite different. When clients present with stress-related symptoms, an initial assessment should include:

- Identification of stress factors the person is experiencing, including which one(s) is causing the most stress
- Perception of stressor as being harmful, threatening, or challenging
- Value or meaning attached to the stressor
- Identification of usual coping strategies and methods used to cope with current stressors
- Assessment of linked or underlying issues such as developmental stage, culture, family understandings, and level of support

IDENTIFYING SOURCES OF STRESS IN HEALTH CARE

Disruptions in health status create stress, anxiety, and vulnerability. Health-related stressors for clients and families include fear of death, uncertainty about clinical outcome, changes in roles, disruption of family life, and financial concerns created by the hospitalization (Leske, 1998).

Hospitalization intensifies stress. Hospital-related stress can negatively impact client outcomes, level of satisfaction with care, and compliance with treatment.

Examples include physical discomfort, strange noises and lights, unfamiliar people asking personal questions, and strange equipment. Clients and their families experience anxiety with transfer to the intensive care unit, and again when they are preparing to a step-down or regular unit, and still again when they are transitioning to home (Chaboyer, James, & Kendall, 2005). Providing immediate practical and emotional support during each of these transitions can reduce unnecessary stress. Box 20-3 provides an assessment/intervention tool that you can use to organize assessment data and plan interventions.

A client-centered approach involves differentiating the type of stress a client is experiencing. For example, stress perceived as a threat provokes anxiety, whereas stress associated with loss presents as depression and grief. The strategies that nurses would use to help clients reduce their stress would differ based on the source of the stress. When stress presents as anxiety, the nurse might suggest problem-solving techniques. However, if the stress is related to a significant loss, the nurse would want to focus on the loss and work with the client from a grief perspective.

Behavioral Observations

Distress often presents through behavior rather than being communicated with words. Emotional distress in collectivistic cultures, for example, Hispanic and Asian, are commonly expressed through somatic symptoms (Lehrer, Woolfolk, & Sime, 2007). Physical and mental symptoms of stress include:

- Significant changes in eating or sleeping habits
- Headaches, gastric problems, muscular tension, aches and pains, tightness in the throat
- Restlessness and irritability
- Inability to cope with normal everyday concerns and obligations
- Inability to concentrate

Anger, hostility, shame, embarrassment, dread, and social withdrawal are behaviors associated with anxiety. Stress anxiety can present as emotional numbness, feelings of going crazy, a déjà vu experience, or night terrors. Other symptoms can include inability to recall information, blocked speech, and fear of losing control (Arnold, 1997).

Putting your observations into words helps clients link emotional states to specific stress reactions using

---

| **BOX 20-3** | **Assessment/Intervention Tool** |

Assessment

A. Perception of stressors
   1. Major stress area or health concern
   2. Present circumstances related to usual pattern
   3. Experienced similar problem? How was it handled?
   4. Anticipation of future consequences
   5. Expectations of self
   6. Expectations of caregivers

B. Intrapersonal factors
   1. Physical (mobility, body function)
   2. Psychosociocultural (attitudes, values, coping patterns)
   3. Developmental (age, factors related to present situation)
   4. Spiritual belief system (hope and sustaining factors)

C. Interpersonal factors
   1. Resources and relationship of family or significant other(s) as they relate to or influence interpersonal factors

D. Environmental factors
   1. Resources and relationships of community as they relate to or influence interpersonal factors

Prevention as Intervention

A. Primary
   1. Classify stressor
   2. Provide information to maintain or strengthen strengths
   3. Support positive coping mechanisms
   4. Educate client and family

B. Secondary
   1. Mobilize resources
   2. Motivate, educate, involve client in health care goals
   3. Facilitate appropriate interventions; refer to external resources as needed
   4. Provide information on primary prevention or intervention as needed

C. Tertiary
   1. Attain/maintain wellness
   2. Educate or reeducate as needed
   3. Coordinate resources
   4. Provide information about primary and secondary interventions

Developed by J. Conrad, University of Maryland School of Nursing, Baltimore, MD, 1993.

words rather than behavior. For example, you might say, "This (name stressor) must be very upsetting," or "It seems like you are pretty anxious about..." If individual clients feel uncomfortable about talking about stress initially, let them know that you will be there when they do feel like talking. When people can put their needs and behaviors in words, they experience less anxiety. They need additional information and frequent support delivered in a calm, competent manner.

Anger and Hostility

Anger and hostility are the most common stress emotions associated with feeling helpless or psychologically threatened. Blame is a frequent form of hostility. Family members angrily blame each other for an injury, blame the physician for operating (or not operating) on a loved one, and criticize the nurse for not responding quickly enough.

Anger projected on the nurse can temporarily threaten a nurse's involvement. Recognizing hostility as a cry for help in coping with escalating stress makes it easier to respond empathetically. Most outbursts have little to do with you, personally, other than that you are available, you are the one most involved with the care of the loved one, and you are least likely to retaliate.

Reflecting on how hostility relates to underlying anxiety helps nurses remain empathetic. Often, people become hostile when they don't understand what is happening or have little control over a treatment outcome. What a hostile anxious client or family needs most at that moment, despite their behavior, is understanding, comfort, and human caring. Listen, ask, and respond empathetically to contributory themes and feelings.

Case Example

Client: I'm paying a lot of money here and no one is willing to help me. The nursing care is terrible, and I just have to lie here in pain with no one to help me.

Nurse: I'm sorry you are feeling so bad. Can you tell me a little more what's going on with you so we can try to do something a little differently to help you.

Allow verbal venting within reason. Set limits if necessary, but do so with a calm attitude and manner. Carefully listening to a client's concerns goes a long way toward neutralizing anger and hostility. The client feels heard, even if the issues cannot be fully resolved to the client's satisfaction. In the course of the conversation, both nurse and client can sort out how the client perceptually experiences a stressor as a basis for focusing on productive solutions. Exploring anger and anxiety as a normal response to stress allows a conversational space to contradict false information. If client and/or family expectations are unrealistic, or can't be met in the current situation, alternative explanations and suggestions can be introduced. Exercise 20-2 is designed to address the relationship between anger and anxiety.

ASSESSMENT OF COPING SKILLS

Assessment of a client's coping behaviors and social support network is critical to understanding stress from a holistic perspective. Ask about coping strategies a client has used in the past and what the person is currently using to resolve stress. Relevant issues include those about the cultural meanings of stressors and typical family coping strategies. Sample questions might include:

- What kinds of things increase your stress?
- What leisure activities do you engage in?
- What do you do to relieve your stress?
- What are your usual methods of coping when you do not feel stress?

Nurses should ask these questions using an informal conversational format. Clients will feel more comfortable if their nurse presents an open, nonthreatening stance and a calm attitude. Appearing patient, being willing to listen, and being attentive without being intrusive is reassuring to anxious clients. The client's reactions will serve as a guide as to how much and how quickly the information can be gathered.

ASSESSMENT OF IMMEDIATE SOCIAL SUPPORT

Asking questions about how the client and family is coping with the current situation provides useful contextual data. Stress-related family assessments can include the following questions:

- Does the family perceive the stressors in the same way as the client?
- Have important issues been discussed fully?
- To what extent are family values challenged by the current situation?
- How might the family and client work together to improve their stress management skills?

EXERCISE 20-2	Relationship Between Anger and Anxiety

Purpose: To help students appreciate the links between anger and anxiety, and understand how anger is triggered.

Procedure:
1. Think of a time when you were really angry. It need not be a significant event or one that would necessarily make anyone else angry.
2. Identify your thoughts, feelings, and behavior in separate columns of a table you construct. For example, what were the thoughts that went through your head when you were feeling this anger? What were your physical and emotional responses to this experience? Write down words or phrases to express what you were feeling at the time. How did you respond when you were angry?
3. Identify what was going on with you before experiencing the anger. Sometimes it is not the event itself, but your feelings before the incident that make the event the straw that breaks the camel's back.
4. Identify underlying threats to your self-concept in the situation (e.g., you were not treated with respect, your opinion was discounted, you lost status, you were rejected, you feared the unknown).

Discussion:
1. In what ways were your answers similar to and different from those of your classmates?
2. What role did anxiety and threat to the self-concept play in the development of the anger response? What percentage of your anger related to the actual event and to self-concept?
3. In what ways did you see anger as a multidetermined behavioral response to threats toself-concept?
4. Did this exercise change any of your ideas about how you might handle your feelings and behavior in a similar situation?
5. What are the common threads in the events that made people in group angry?
6. In what ways could experiential knowledge of the close association between anger and anxiety be helpful in your nursing practice?

- Are family members and the client communicating with each other?

Because family members can be a major support for clients experiencing stress, nurses can inquire about their willingness to be involved with a different set of questions.

- What are the family's and client's expectations of care?
- In what ways, if any, are the expectations different?
- What does the family or client need from you as the nurse? From each other?
- Is there a family spokesperson?
- What are the client's cultural, religious, and family values concerning the meaning of the stressor?

IDENTIFYING SOURCES OF STRENGTH AND HOPE

In times of stress, people, particularly women, will reach out to others for solace, support, and direction (Taylor et al., 2000; Taylor, 2006). Some people turn to their God or Higher Power, others to family and friends. People without a social network should be linked with community resources, the point being that interpersonal connection is an essential buffer against stress. Community resources include support groups, social services, and other public health agencies that provide practical support, as well as social contacts. The more knowledgeable the nurse is about community resources, the better the client and family are served. Exercise 20-3 is designed to help you become better acquainted with resources in your community.

Stress challenges and/or strengthens people's spirituality. Health disruptions bring mortality and morbidity into sharper relief as personal issues. This is because before having a significant illness or a life-changing health-related crisis, people don't think about their personal death or the fact that a life can be changed completely. They haven't seen firsthand the effects of death or potentially lethal complications of disorders.

Belief in a personal God provides interested clients with an incomparable personal resource that helps them cope with shattered dreams and incomprehensible life crises. Some people rely on faith to facilitate their acceptance of a reality that cannot be changed. Stress can challenge a person's spiritual connections and it is not uncommon for people to experience a spiritual void in stressful times. Assessing and providing spiritual comfort to clients is an important consideration in caring for clients experiencing stress.

Community Resources for Stress Management

Purpose: To help students become aware of the community resources available in the community for stress management.

Procedure:

1. Contact a community agency, social services group, or support group in your community that you believe can help clients cope with a particularly stressful situation. Look in the newspaper for ideas.
2. Find out how a person might access the resource, what kinds of cases are treated, what types of treatment are offered, the costs involved, and what

you as a nurse can do to help people take advantage of the resource.

Discussion:

1. How did you decide which community agency to choose?
2. How difficult or easy was it to access the information about the agency?
3. What information about the community resource did you find out that surprised or perplexed you?
4. In what ways could you use this exercise in planning care for your clients?

ASSESSING IMPACT ON FAMILY RELATIONSHIPS

Nurses play an important role in helping client families reduce their own stress levels in health care situations. They can help families process complex information and address specific concerns. Topics can include what will happen next, how to explain the illness, or what the client or family could have done differently to

change the situation. For example, the nurse might say to the wife of a recent paraplegic, "Seeing your husband like this must be a terrible shock. I suspect you might be wondering how you are going to cope with his care at home." This type of statement normalizes feelings and introduces subjects that are difficult but necessary to talk about. Table 20-2 identifies interventions to decrease family stress.

TABLE 20-2	Nursing Interventions to Decrease Family Anxiety
Recommendation	**Specific Actions**
Identify a family spokesperson and support persons involved in decision making	Choose a person the family/client trusts; Establish mechanisms for contact
Identify a primary nursing contact for the family	If possible, choose the nurse most in contact with the client, Meet with the family within 24 hrs of admission to explain roles of each healthcare team member, Provide contact number to family spokesperson.
Discuss family access to the client	Arrange for visitation based on unit protocols, client condition/ needs, family preferences, Educate the family about visiting hours, how to reach the hospitalist, when rounds occur, Involve family in client care whenever possible and desired.
Call the family about any changes in client condition or treatment	Inform family of changes as they occur, Provide frequent status reports, Allow time for questions.
Provide complete data in easily understandable terms	Ask questions about what the client/family understands about the client's condition, how they are coping, what they fear, Check for misunderstandings, incomplete information, Provide information based on family needs, Respect cultural and personal desire for level of information disclosure.
Actively involve the client/family in all clinical decisions;	Hold formal care conferences for important care decisions, Take into account and respect client preferences, spiritual and cultural attitudes, Allow time for questions, Strive for consensus in decisions

Continued

TABLE 20-2	Nursing Interventions to Decrease Family Anxiety—cont'd
Recommendation	**Specific Actions**
Connect family with support services	Provide information about support groups, hospital based social, spiritual, medicare, hospice, home care, and other care services as needed.
Ensure collaborative rapport and support among health care team members.	Maintain clear communication among health care team members. Avoid conflicting messages to the family. Provide opportunities for staff to decompress and discuss difficult situations and feelings.

Data from: Davidson J, Powers K, Hedayat K, Tieszen M, Kon A. et. Al. Clinical practice guidelines for support of the family in the patient-centered intensive care unit: American College of Critical Care Medicine Task Force 2005-2005. *Critical Care Medicine.* 35(2): 605-622, 2007; Leske J: Interventions to decrease family anxiety, *Crit Care Nurs* 22(6):61–65, 2002.

CONSIDERING STRESS ISSUES FOR CHILDREN

Health disruptions create special problems for children because they lack the words and life experience to sort out the meaning of illness, either their own or that of a significant family member (Compas et al., 2001). Children express their stress through behavior. Signs of distress such as academic decline, gastric distress, and headaches can alert the nurse to unvoiced stress. In the hospital, children withdraw, demonstrate clinging behaviors, or have frequent meltdowns. Uncertainty creates stress for both parents and children (Stewart & Mishel, 2000).

Parents may need help with communicating information about serious illness to children, with thinking through their children's reactions, and with advice on ways to break bad news or set realistic limits with an ill child. Nurses should base their responses on detailed knowledge of the child's cognitive and psychosocial development, as well as concrete data. Children need to have their questions answered simply and honestly. Hearing information from someone they trust is important in modifying the uncertainty of a serious illness. Small children can be encouraged to express their stress feelings through drawings and manipulating puppets.

CONSIDERING STRESS ISSUES FOR OLDER ADULTS

Stress issues for older adults occur during a phase of life when health and loss of important personal supports are no longer the assets they were during other phases of adulthood. Changes in lifestyle and financial status after retirement are sources of stress, particularly for people who have not thought about necessary changes in the life cycle associated with retirement or loss of a spouse. Worries about finances, fears of not being able

to live independently, or of being moved to an assisted living or nursing home are common. Older adults living alone can feel vulnerable about their safety or ability to reach help should they experience a sudden physical change. The loss of significant people, isolation and loneliness can complicate treatment issues.

In addition to the normal stress reducers and coping strategies discussed in this and other chapters, nurses can help older clients develop tangible ways to promote physical and emotional safety, and to maximize their health situation. Sometimes all it takes is simple suggestions and well-timed questions about recreational activities or hobbies that the older adult has not considered.

Stress management strategies for the older adult from a health promotion perspective include maintaining an active social life and a healthy lifestyle that keeps mind and body active. Sharing concerns and developing leisure or volunteer interests help older adults develop a harmonious lifestyle that acts to release and reduce stress. Most communities have low-impact exercise activities, continuing education, and social outlets for older adults. Elderly caregivers of clients with dementia can benefit from some of the suggestions in Chapter 19 to reduce stress and balance their health and well-being with that of a family member with dementia.

STRESS REDUCTION STRATEGIES

PROVIDING INFORMATION

Information is an essential need for both clients and families, and an important stress reducer. Each family member's health and well-being is affected by the communication and actions of the health care team during a hospitalization (Davidson, 2009). Relevant information can range from providing basic data about visiting hours, the timing of tests and procedures, plans for discharge, to complex facts about the client's condition or treatment. Information sharing should begin with orienting clients and families to the health care situation or unit, and providing enough information to familiarize but not overwhelm them as to what they might expect from health care. Take time to briefly explain the following:

- What will happen during tests or surgery
- Who is likely to interview the client, and why
- How the client can best cooperate or assist in his or her treatment process

In stressful situations, the perceptual field narrows so most people hear only a fraction of what has been said. Information and directions given in the first 48 hours of an admission should be repeated, usually more than once, because this is the time of highest stress. A calm approach and repetition of instructions can help clients in stressful situations relax enough to hear important instructions. Providing written instructions that can be discussed at the time and then left with the client or family enhances understanding. Allow time to answer questions and provide the client's family with the health provider's contact numbers to call if other issues arise.

PROCESSING STRONG FEELINGS

Clients experiencing stress should be given the opportunity to express their feelings, thoughts, and worries. Crying, anger, and magical thinking are normal reactions to situations that one cannot control. Although aggression toward self or others cannot be tolerated, the client should be allowed to express anger and should be given the lead in how he or she wants to address stressors, if there is no immediate jeopardy to treatment.

Listen carefully and ask gentle, probing questions. Helpful statements can include, "This must be very difficult for you to absorb. Can you tell me what you are experiencing right now?" This listening response allows the client to put concerns into words. If the client tells the nurse, "I think I'm losing my mind," the nurse might respond, "Many people feel that way. It feels that way, but what is happening is that you are feeling disoriented because this situation is sudden and overwhelming. It's a normal response. Can you identify what worries you the most?" Notice in both probes, the nurse normalizes the client's "strange" feelings. Acknowledging the legitimacy of feelings as a normal response to an abnormal situation reinforces

the client's self-integrity and helps the client put boundaries on his or her anxiety.

Allowing clients to be in charge of areas and issues that are not at odds with a treatment protocol, and helping clients discover the real causes of their frustration can reduce stress through direct action. Encourage clients to take one day at a time in their expectations and recovery activities. Concrete assistance with negotiating appropriate referral resources is helpful.

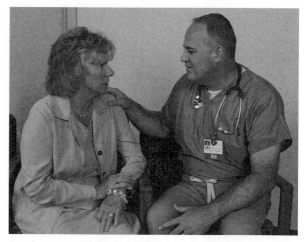

A calm approach and repetition of instructions can help clients in stressful situations relax enough to hear important instructions.

ANTICIPATORY GUIDANCE

Anticipatory guidance is a term used to describe the process of sharing information about a circumstance, concern, or situation before it occurs. Fear of the unknown intensifies the impact of a stressor. Knowing what lies ahead can often prevent the development of a crisis (Hoff & Hallisey, 2009). Your response to client/family anxiety should be tentative and reflect your level of knowledge about the unique concerns of the client, as well as the condition and situation. In framing a response, you might reflect on the following:

- What type of information would be most helpful to this particular client at this particular time, given what the client has told me?
- How would I feel if I was in this person's position, and what would I want to know that might bring me comfort in this situation?

It is difficult to directly answer stress-related questions about uncertainties, such as "If I take the chemotherapy, will I be cured, or am I going to die anyway?"

The reality is that there may be no single answer. It helps to ask the client what prompted the question, and to have a good idea of the client's level of knowledge before answering. Honest communication is essential, but sensitivity to the client's experience is critical.

Providing anticipatory guidance can put needless worry to rest. For example, you could use a simple statement such as "You've never had this procedure before. Let me explain how it works" (Keller & Baker, 2000).

When providing anticipatory guidance, do not offer more than what the situation dictates. Encourage the client to expand on suggestions rather than presenting a full plan. The growth in client ability to set priorities, to develop a plan that has meaning to them, and to establish milestones in the evaluation process stimulates self-confidence and decreases stress. Exercise 20-4 provides practice in helping clients handle stressful situations.

Anticipatory guidance can be helpful in preparing family members for their first visit with a client with a visible disfigurement, a marked physical or psychological deterioration, or the presence of life support machines. If you sense family awkwardness in how to approach a vulnerable or comatose client, you could say to a family member: "You might want to identify yourself and tell your father you are here with him."

Priority Setting

Clients need support and encouragement when coping with stress, but they don't always know where to start. Priority setting helps reduce hesitation and offers a stepwise framework for stress resolution. In addition to helping clients determine which task elements are critical and which can be addressed later, nurses can help clients break down tasks into smaller manageable segments. The most important tasks should be scheduled during times when the client or family has the most energy and freedom from interruption.

Nurses need to help clients identify the concrete tasks needed to achieve treatment goals, including the people involved, the necessary contacts, the amount of time each task will take, and specific hours or days for each task. Some tasks are more important than others in stressful situations, and not everything can be handled at once. A helpful suggestion might be, "Let's see what you need to do right now and what can wait until tomorrow." Tasks that someone else can do and those that are not essential to the achievement of goals should be delegated or ignored for the moment.

SUPPORTING CLIENT EFFORTS

Without command over the controllable parts of life, people feel helpless and stressed. Coping mechanisms such as negotiation, specific actions, seeking advice, and rearranging priorities can significantly diminish stress through direct action. Once stressors are named, nurses can use health teaching formats and coaching that help clients to:

- Develop a realistic plan to offset stress
- Deal directly with obstacles as they emerge

EXERCISE 20-4	Role-Play: Handling Stressful Situations

Purpose: To give students experience in responding to stressful situations.

Procedure:
Use the following case study as the basis for this exercise.

Dave is a 66-year-old man with colon cancer. In the past, he had a colostomy. Recently, he was readmitted to your unit and had an exploratory laparotomy for small-bowel obstruction. Very little can be done for him because the cancer has spread. He is in pain, and he has to have a feeding tube. His family has many questions for the nurse: "Why is he vomiting?" "How come the pain medication isn't working?" "Why isn't he feeling any better than he did before the surgery?" You have just entered the client's room; his family is sitting near him, and they want answers now.

1. Have different members of your group role-play the client, the nurse, the son, the daughter-in-law, and the wife. One person should act as observer.
2. Identify the factors that will need to be clarified in this situation to help the nurse provide the most appropriate intervention.
3. Using the strategies suggested in this chapter, intervene to help the client and the family reduce their anxiety.
4. Role-play the situation for 10 to 15 minutes.

Discussion:
1. Have each player identify the interventions that were most helpful.
2. From the nurse's perspective, which parts of the client and family stress were hardest to handle?
3. How could you use what you learned from doing this exercise in your clinical practice?

- Evaluate action steps
- Make needed modifications in the plan and often lifestyle

Case Example

Sam Hamilton received a diagnosis of prostate cancer on a routine physical examination. His way of coping included obtaining as much information on the disease as possible. He researched the most up-to-date material on treatment options and sought advice from physician friends as to which surgeons had the most experience with this type of surgery. As he shared his diagnosis with friends and colleagues, he found several men who had successfully survived without a cancer recurrence. Sam used the time between diagnosis and surgery to finish projects and delegate work responsibilities. He attended a support group with his wife and was able to obtain valuable advice on handling his emotional responses to what would happen. When the time came for his surgery, Sam was still apprehensive, but he felt as though he had done everything humanly possible to prepare for it. The actions he took before surgery reduced his stress.

PROMOTING A HEALTHY LIFESTYLE

Encouraging a healthy lifestyle is an essential but sometimes overlooked component of stress reduction strategies. Good health habits improve stress resistance. Eating a healthy diet, and avoiding emotional eating and the wrong foods give people a sense of control and well-being. Too much caffeine and alcohol can exacerbate stress. Laughter dissolves it.

Adequate quality sleep is restorative. Healthy nighttime habits, such as establishing a scheduled bedtime and having a small snack before bedtime, encourages sleep. Regular exercise helps the body release tension, as well as contributes to fitness. Exercise can be accomplished in a social setting, for example, hiking or biking. Certain exercise programs such as yoga or tai chi incorporate meditation, deep breathing, and muscle stretching, all of which are known to reduce stress.

Organizing time and doing activities that energize rather than stress, balancing work with leisure activities, restructuring priorities, and eliminating unnecessary obligations reduce stress.

HELPING FAMILIES HANDLE STRESS

Families can suffer potentially overwhelming stress when their family member is critically ill or injured. Contemporary health care environments with advanced technology, shorter stays, and multiple caregivers are complex and anxiety producing. Sources of stress for families can include "fear of death, uncertain outcome, emotional turmoil, financial concerns, role changes, disruption of routines, and unfamiliar hospital environments" (Leske, 2002, p. 61). Families look to nurses for support and direction. Consistent regular communication is key to family satisfaction and effective shared decisions. Direct family contact offers firsthand insight into client preferences, health care needs and resources especially when the client is unable to provide this information (Davidson, 2009).

It is helpful to put yourself in the family's position and to put into words how you might feel in a similar situation. Statements such as "Most people would feel anxious in this situation," or "It would be hard for anyone to have all the answers in a situation like this" help put stressors and stress responses into perspective.

Families have a strong need to remain physically close to the client in critical care situations and there is a strong correlation between proximity to the client and satisfaction with care (Davidson, 2009). When this need translates into constant attendance, family members can become physically and emotionally exhausted (Leske, 2000). A preventive strategy is to suggest that the family members take short breaks. Family members may need "permission" to go to a movie or eat in a restaurant outside the hospital. Usually, they will do so only with an assurance that they will be called should there be any change in the client's condition.

Being able to "do something" for the client helps family members defuse their anxiety. Family members want to provide support and comfort. Letting family members participate in the client's care to whatever extent is possible for the client and comfortable for the family can be a meaningful experience for both. On the other hand, it is important to ask family members about how they would like to participate, rather than making assumptions.

STRESS MANAGEMENT THERAPIES

MIND/BODY THERAPIES

Mind/body therapies are coping strategies designed to lessen the intensity of the stressor on a person once the stress response has occurred. Examples include meditation, relaxation techniques, yoga, and cognitive restructuring. Altering physiologic reactions such as blood pressure, heart rate, muscle tension, and respiratory rate helps people experience greater calm and peace of mind (Luskin et al., 1998). Regular practice of these techniques can improve physical and emotional well-being.

Meditation

Meditation is a stress-reduction strategy dating back to early Christian times. People use meditation to develop a sense of inner peace and tranquility, and to center themselves. Meditation allows people to decrease stress by focusing their attention on something other than the stress, and clears the mind of disturbing thoughts. This action helps to reduce the concentration of stress hormones attached to stressful thinking. A guide to meditation is provided in Box 20-4.

Mindfulness is a stress management tool that can be used at any point. It can be as simple as focusing on deep breathing. Focusing completely on your breathing, music, or what is happening in the current moment forces you to at least momentarily let go of stressful thoughts. It is an easy way of quieting the mind and decreasing the intensity of stressful feelings.

Biofeedback

Biofeedback plays an important role in management of clients with chronic stress responses affecting individual body systems (e.g., essential hypertension, migraine headaches, Raynaud's disease, and ulcerative colitis). People are trained to voluntarily take control over a variety of physiologic activities such as their brain activity, blood pressure, heart rate, pain, migraine or tension headaches, and other bodily functions as a means to improve their health. Biofeedback provides awareness of minute-by-minute changes in biologic activity. The goal is to lower physiologic arousal and promote relaxation (Grazzi & Andrasik, 2010). Equipment used with biofeedback includes the electroencephalogram, skin temperature devices; blood pressure measures; galvanic skin resistance measurements; and the electromyogram, which measures muscle tension.

Progressive Relaxation

Progressive relaxation is a technique that focuses the client's attention on conscious control of voluntary skeletal muscles. Originally developed by Edmund Jacobson (1938), a physiologist physician, the technique consists of alternately tensing and relaxing muscle groups. Each muscle group is worked with individually with the client sitting in a relaxed position in a chair with arm supports or lying down. Davis, Eshelman and McKay (2008) provide an excellent step-by-step description of the basic procedure for progressive relaxation.

A variant of progressive relaxation is deep breathing. This can be accomplished anywhere and at any time a person experiences stress.
- Deeply inhale to the count of 10, and hold your breath.
- Exhale slowly, again to the count of 10.
- Concentrate as you do this exercise only on your breathing.
- Feel the tension leave your body.

The person breathes 10 times in a row with each inhalation/exhalation counted as 1 breath. Focusing the mind on the continuous rhythm of inhaling and exhaling turns the mind away from thinking about specific stressors. To experience the progressive relaxation technique, see Exercise 20-5.

Yoga and Tai Chi

Yoga is a mind/body exercise practice rooted in ancient India. The practice of yoga emphasizes correct alignment, controlled postures or poses, and regulated breathing to help people relax and reduce stress. Controlling breathing helps to quiet the mind. Some forms of yoga place an emphasis on meditation and developing self-awareness.

BOX 20-4	Meditation Techniques

1. Choose a quiet, calm environment with as few distractions as possible.
2. Get in a comfortable position, preferably a sitting position.
3. To shift the mind from logical, externally oriented thought, use a constant stimulus: a sound, word, phrase, or object. The eyes are closed if a repetitive sound or word is used.
4. Pay attention to the rhythm of your breathing.
5. When distracting thoughts occur, they are discarded and attention is redirected to the repetition of the word or gazing at the object. Distracting thoughts will occur and do not mean you are performing the techniques incorrectly. Do not worry about how you are doing. Redirect your focus to the constant stimulus and assume a passive attitude.

Adapted from Benson H: *The relaxation response*, New York, 1975, Morrow.

EXERCISE 20-5	Progressive Relaxation

Purpose: To help students experience the beneficial effects of progressive relaxation in reducing tension.

Procedure:
This exercise consists of alternately tensing and relaxing skeletal muscles.
1. Sit in a comfortable chair with arm supports. Place the arms on the arm supports, and sit in a comfortable upright position with legs uncrossed and feet flat on the floor.
2. Close your eyes and take 10 deep breaths, concentrating on inhaling and exhaling.
3. Your instructor or a member of group should give the following instructions, and you should follow them exactly:
   • I want you to focus on your feet and to tense the muscles in your feet. Feel the tension in your feet. Hold it, and now let go. Feel the tension leaving your feet.
   • I would like you to tense the muscles in your calves. Feel the tension in your calves and hold it. Now let go and feel the tension leaving your calves. Experience how that feels.
   • Tense the muscles in your thighs. Most people do this by pressing their thighs against the chair. Feel the tension in your muscles and experience how that feels. Now release the tension and experience how that feels.
   • I would like you to feel the tension in your abdomen. Tense the muscles in your abdomen and hold it. Hold it for a few more seconds. Now release those muscles and experience how that feels.
   • Tense the muscles in your chest. The only way you can really do this is to take a very deep breath and hold it. (The guide counts to 10.) Concentrate on feeling how that feels. Now let it go and experience how that feels.

• I would like you to tense your muscles in your hands. Clench your fist and hold it as hard as you can. Harder, harder. Now release it and concentrate on how that feels.
• Tense the muscles in your arms. You can do this by pressing down as hard as you can on the arm supports. Feel the tension in your arms and continue pressing. Now let go and experience how that feels.
• I would like you to feel the tension in your shoulders. Tense your shoulders as hard as you can and hold it. Concentrate on how that feels. Now release your shoulder muscles and experience the feeling.
• Feel the tension in your jaw. Clench your jaw and teeth as hard as you can. Feel the tension in your jaw and hold it. Now let it go and feel the tension leave your jaw.
• Now that you are in this relaxed state, keep your eyes closed and think of a time when you were really happy. Let the images and sounds surround you. Imagine yourself back in that situation. What were you thinking? What are you feeling?
• Open your eyes. Students who feel comfortable may share the images that emerged in the relaxed state.

Discussion:
1. What are your impressions in doing this exercise?
2. Do you feel more relaxed after doing this exercise?
3. If applicable, after doing the exercise, in what ways do you feel differently?
4. Were you surprised at the images that emerged in your relaxed state?
5. In what ways do you think you could use this exercise in your nursing practice?

Tai chi is a system initially developed in China. It consists of posture or movements practiced in a slow, graceful manner. It involves stretching, rhythmic movements coordinated with controlled breathing. The concentration required for both yoga and tai chi require a person to forget distressing thoughts at least for the moment.

Guided Imagery

Guided imagery is a technique often used in combination with relaxation strategies for cancer pain and stress (Kwekkeboom, 2008). Imagery techniques use the client's imagination to stimulate healing mental images designed to promote stress relief. The process involves asking the client to imagine a scene, previously experienced as safe, peaceful, or beautiful. Supportive prompts to engage all of senses deepen the imagery experience. The healing scene can be used each time that the client begins to experience stress.

ADDRESSING OCCUPATIONAL STRESS IN NURSES
BURNOUT

Nurses face a greater risk for burnout than people in other lines of work. They work in high-stress service environments, helping people cope with serious life and death situations every day. Freudenberger (1980) defines **burnout** as "a state of fatigue or frustration brought about by devotion to a cause, way of life, or relationship that failed to produce an expected reward" (p. 13). It develops in individuals involved with "people work," and is characterized by emotional exhaustion, depersonalization, and a sense of diminished professional accomplishment (Maslach, 2001). Although burnout shares some characteristics with depression and anxiety, it is a different syndrome, clearly linked to a work environment, and personal expectations of self and others within that setting.

The development of burnout begins insidiously, particularly in nurses who strive for perfection. Unchecked, it is a progressive syndrome associated with emotional exhaustion and loss of meaning. Freudenberger (1980) refers to burnout as the "overachievement syndrome." People who are high achievers, committed, and passionate about their work are more at risk to develop burnout symptoms.

The need to be perfect does not allow for error, or the reserve needed to correct for unexpected events (Porter-O'Grady, 1998). A story about Babe Ruth offers an appropriate metaphor. Coaching a young, aspiring ball player, he asked the boy how he planned to pitch the ball. The boy answered, "I'm going to throw it with all my might and get it right where it needs to go. I'm going to give it 110 percent." Ruth had different advice: "Throw the ball with 80 percent of your might. You will need the reserve to correct for any mistakes." Nurses need the same reserve to correct for the inevitable curve balls inherent in clinical practice—and life in general. Contemporary thinking about burnout considers it as originating from combined factors in the work environment and within the person. Six areas of organizational contributors to burnout include workload, control, reward, community, fairness, and values (Freeney & Tiernan, 2009; Maslach & Leiter, 1997). Sources of work-related burnout for nurses include working too many hours or at an accelerated pace with no respite, feeling unappreciated, giving too much to needy clients, trying to meet multiple demands of administrators, lack of community with coworkers, and feeling resentment, in place of the meaning that work once held.

Symptoms of Burnout

A person experiencing burnout is always tired and preoccupied with work (Vernarec, 2001). People who are burned out feel disillusioned and lack zest for their work. Other signs include loss of motivation and ideals, boredom or dissatisfaction at work, irritability and cynicism, resentment of expectations, and avoidance of meaningful encounters with clients and families. Headaches, gastric disturbances, skipping meals or eating compulsively on the run, feeling irritated by the intrusion of others, and a lack of balance between a nurse's work and personal life can signal the onset of burnout. In a study of co-workers' perceptions of colleagues suffering from burnout, signs observed included a struggle to achieve unobtainable goals, wanting to manage alone, and becoming isolated from others (Ericson-Lidman & Strandberg, 2007). Figure 20-3 identifies common symptoms of burnout.

Burnout Prevention Strategies

The ABCs of burnout prevention (Arnold, 2008) are presented in Table 20-3. Reflecting on the sources of stress in your life puts boundaries on it. Think about your goals, and what is important to you. Rather than simply complaining, seek role models or trusted coworkers who can offer you the support and sensitivity you need to become aware of what is going on in your life. A useful exercise is to imagine yourself a year from now and ask yourself how important the issue would be a year from now.

Identifying realistic goals that are achievable and in line with your personal values is an excellent burnout prevention strategy. Goals should be aligned with purpose and values. Focusing on one thing at a time and finishing one project before starting another has several benefits. Achieving small related goals promotes self-efficacy and offers hope that more complex goals are achievable.

Maintaining a healthy balance among work, family, leisure, and lifelong learning activities enhances personal judgments, satisfaction, and productivity in all three spheres. Actively schedule a time for each of these activities and stick to it.

Remember that you always have choices. People experiencing burnout lose sight of this fact. Life is a series of choices and negotiations. The choices we make create the fabric of our lives. Refusing to delegate work because someone else cannot do it as well, or not going out to dinner with friends because you have too much work to do are choices—bad options that lead to burnout.

Detachment from ego and/or taking responsibility for outcomes is a critical component of burnout

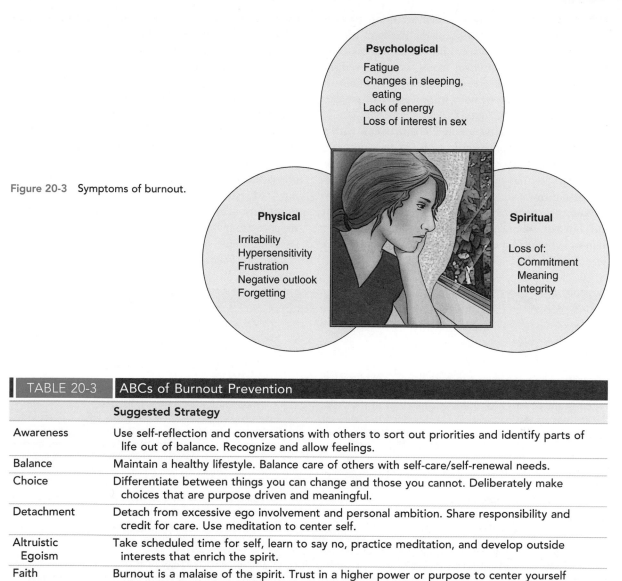

Figure 20-3   Symptoms of burnout.

TABLE 20-3	ABCs of Burnout Prevention
	Suggested Strategy
Awareness	Use self-reflection and conversations with others to sort out priorities and identify parts of life out of balance. Recognize and allow feelings.
Balance	Maintain a healthy lifestyle. Balance care of others with self-care/self-renewal needs.
Choice	Differentiate between things you can change and those you cannot. Deliberately make choices that are purpose driven and meaningful.
Detachment	Detach from excessive ego involvement and personal ambition. Share responsibility and credit for care. Use meditation to center self.
Altruistic Egoism	Take scheduled time for self, learn to say no, practice meditation, and develop outside interests that enrich the spirit.
Faith	Burnout is a malaise of the spirit. Trust in a higher power or purpose to center yourself when you do not know what will happen next.
Goals	Identify and develop realistic goals in line with personal strengths. Seek feedback and support.
Hope	Hope is nurtured through conversations with others that lighten the burden, and a belief in one's possibilities and personal worth in the greater scheme of things.
Integrity	Recognize that each of us is the only person who can determine the design and application of meaning in our lives.

Data from: Arnold E: Spirituality in educational and work environments (pp. 386–399). In Carson V, Harold Koenig, editors: *Spiritual dimensions of nursing practice*, revised edition, Conshohocken, PA, 2008, Templeton Foundation Press.

prevention. It means that you don't allow emotional involvement in a task or relationship to undermine your quality of life, values, or needs. Someone once asked Mother Teresa how she was able to remain so energetic and hopeful in the midst of suffering she encountered in Calcutta. She replied that it was because she did the best she could and didn't worry about the outcome because she couldn't control it.

It is important to pay as much attention to your own personal needs as you do to the needs of others. Although this seems obvious, nurses sometimes consider attention to their own needs as being selfish. However, one cannot give from an empty cupboard. Replenishing the self actually improves what one can give to others.

Faith is defined as an intangible connection with a larger purpose or higher power to guide and support a person during both good and bad times. Faith helps people develop an optimistic worldview and experience less distress.

Nurses experiencing burnout often feel helpless and hopeless about changing their situation, other than to leave it. Hope is a powerful antidote for burnout. Exercise 20-6 provides an opportunity to think about your personal burnout potential and ways to achieve better balance in your life.

Burnout challenges personal integrity in the sense that important values are ignored or devalued. When you begin to forget who you are and try to become what everyone else expects of you, you are in trouble. Reclaim yourself. Taking responsibility for yourself and doing what is important to you helps to reverse burnout. Take the risk to be all that you are, as well as all that you can be, without worrying about what others think. Seek professional supports such as training, staff retreats, staff support networks, and job rotation to stimulate new ideas and insights. Professional support groups are effective as a means of providing encouragement to nurses in acute settings (Parish, Bradley, & Franks, 1997).

EXERCISE 20-6   Burnout Assessment

Purpose: To help students understand the symptoms of burnout.

Procedure:

Consider your life over the past year. Complete the questionnaire by answering with a 5 if the situation is a constant occurrence, 4 if it occurs most of the time, 3 if it occurs occasionally, 2 if it has occurred once or twice during the last 6 months, and 1 if it is not a problem at all. Scores ranging from 60 to 75 indicate burnout. Scores ranging from 45 to 60 indicate you are stressed and in danger of developing burnout. Scores ranging from 20 to 44 indicate a normal stress level, and scores of less than 20 suggest you are not a candidate for burnout.

1. Do you find yourself taking on, or being overwhelmed by other people's problems?
2. Do you feel resentful about the amount or nature of claims on your time?
3. Do you find you have less time for social activities?
4. Have you lost your sense of humor?
5. Are you having trouble sleeping?
6. Do you find you are more impatient and less tolerant of others?
7. Is it difficult for you to say no?
8. Are the things that used to be important to you slipping away from you because you don't have time?
9. Do you feel a sense of urgency and not enough time to complete tasks?
10. Are you forgetting appointments, friends' birthdays?
11. Do you feel overwhelmed and unable to pace yourself?
12. Have you lost interest in intimacy?
13. Are you overeating, or have you begun to skip meals?
14. Is it difficult to feel enthusiastic about your work?
15. Do you feel it is difficult to connect on a meaningful level with others?

Tally up your scores and compare your scores with your classmates. Nursing school is a strong breeding ground for the development of burnout (demands exceed resources). To offset the possibility of developing burnout symptoms, do the following:

1. Think about the last time you took time for yourself. If you cannot think of a time, you really need to do this exercise.
2. Identify a leisure activity that you can do during the next week to break the cycle of burnout.
3. Describe the steps you will need to take to implement the activity.
4. Identify the time required for this activity and what other activities will need rearrangement to make it possible.
5. Describe any obstacles to implementing your activity and how you might resolve them.

Discussion:

1. Was it difficult for you to come up with an activity? If so, why?
2. Were you able to develop a logical way to implement your activity?
3. Were the activities chosen by others surprising or helpful to you in any way?
4. How might you be able to use this exercise in your future practice?

SUMMARY

This chapter focuses on the stress response in health care, and supporting client and family coping with stress through nurse-client relationships. Stress can negatively impact client outcomes, level of satisfaction with care, and compliance with treatment. A fundamental goal in the nurse-client relationship is to empower clients and families with the knowledge, support, and resources they need to cope effectively with stress.

Stress is a part of everyone's life. Mild stress can be beneficial, but greater stress levels can be unhealthy. Concurrent and cumulative stresses increase the response level. Theoretical models address stress as a physiologic response, as a stimulus, and as a transaction between person and environment. Factors that influence the development of a stress reaction include the nature of the stressor, personal interpretation of its meaning, number of previous and concurrent stressors, previous experiences with similar stressors, and availability of support systems and personal coping abilities.

People use problem- and emotion-focused coping strategies to minimize stress. Social support is key to effectively coping with stress. Assessment should focus on stress factors the person is experiencing, the context in which they occur, and identification of coping strategies. Supportive interventions include giving information, opportunities to express their feelings, thoughts, and worries, and anticipatory guidance.

Nurses are at the forefront of health care delivery to clients and families experiencing complex health and life issues. They too can experience stress and need support to do their job effectively. Burnout prevention requires recognition and resolution of organizational and personal factors contributing to job-related stress in professional nurses.

ETHICAL DILEMMA What Would You Do?

The mother of a client with AIDS does not know her son's diagnosis because her son does not want to worry her and fears her disapproval if she knows he is gay. The mother asks the nurse if the family should have an oncology consult because she does not understand why, if her son has leukemia, as he says he does, that an oncologist is not seeing him. What should the nurse do?

REFERENCES

Aldwin CM, Levenson MR: Posttraumatic growth: a developmental perspective, *Psychol Inq* 15(1):19–22, 2004.

Arnold E: Spirituality in educational and work environments. In Carson V, Koenig H, editors: *Spiritual dimensions of nursing practice*, revised edition, Conshohocken, PA, 2008, Templeton Foundation Press.

Arnold E: The stress connection: women and coronary heart disease, *Crit Care Nurs Clin North Am* 9(4):565–575, 1997.

Askew R, Keyes C: Stress and somatization: a sociocultural perspective. In Oxinton KV, editor: *Psychology of stress*, Hauppage, NY, 2005, Nova Biomedical Publishers, pp 129–144.

Benson H: *The relaxation response*, New York, 1975, Morrow.

Cannon WB: *The wisdom of the body*, New York, 1932, Norton Pub.

Caplan G: Mastery of stress: psychosocial aspects, *Am J Psychiatry* 13(8):41, 1981.

Chaboyer W, James H, Kendall M, et al: Transitional care after the intensive care unit, *Crit Care Nurse* 25(3):16–27, 2005.

Compas B, Connor-Smith JK, Saltzman H, et al: Coping with stress during childhood and adolescence: problems, progress, and potential in theory and research, *Psychol Bull* 127(1):87–127, 2001.

Davidson J: Family-centered care: meeting the needs of patients' families and helping families to critical illness, *Crit Care Nurse* 29(3):28–34, 2009.

Davidson J, Powers K, Hedayat K, Tieszen M, Kon A, et al: Clinical practice guidelines for support of the family in the patient-centered intensive care unit: American College of Critical Care Medicine Task Force 2005–2005, *Crit Care Med* 35(2):605–622, 2007.

Davis M, Eshelman E, McKay M, et al: *The relaxation and stress reduction workbook*, Oakland CA, 2008, New Harbinger Publications, Inc.

Dolbier C, Smith S, Steinhardt MA, et al: Relationships of protective factors to stress and symptoms of illness, *Am J Health Behav* 31(4): 423–433, 2007.

Erikson-Lidman E, Strandberg G: Burnout: co-workers' perceptions of signs preceding workmates' burnout, *J Adv Nurs* 60(2):199–208, 2007.

Folkman S: The case for positive emotions in the stress process, *Anxiety Stress Coping* 21(1):3–14, 2008.

Freeney Y, Tiernan J: Exploration of the facilitators of and barriers to work engagement in nursing, *Int J Nurs Stud* 46:1557–1565, 2009.

Freudenberger H: *Burn-out: the high cost of high achievement*, Garden City, NY, 1980, Doubleday.

Ganzel B, Morris P, Wethington E, et al: Allostasis and the human brain: integrating models of stress from the social and life sciences, *Psychol Rev* 117(1):134–174, 2010.

Grazzi L, Andrasik F: Non-pharmacological approaches in migraine prophylaxis: behavioral medicine, *Neurol Sci* 31(Suppl 1):S133–S135, 2010.

Hoff LA, Hallisey B, Hoff M, et al: *People in crisis: clinical diversity perspectives*, ed 6, New York, NY, 2009, Routledge.

Holmes T, Rahe R: The social readjustment rating scale, *J Psychosom Res* 11:213–218, 1967.

Jacobson E: *Progressive relaxation*, Chicago, 1938, University of Chicago Press.

Johnson K, Renn C: The hypothalamic-pituitary-adrenal axis in critical illness, *AACN Clin Issues* 17(1):30–40, 2006.

Keller V, Baker L: Communicate with care, *RN* 63(1):32–33, 2000.

Kwekkeboom K: Patients' perceptions of the effectiveness of guided imagery and progressive muscle relaxation, *Complement Ther Clin Pract* 14(3):185–194, 2008.

Lazarus R, Folkman S: *Stress, appraisal and coping*, New York, 1984, Springer.

Lehrer P, Woolfolk R, Sime W, et al: *Principles and practice of stress management*, New York, 2007, Guilford Press.

Leske J: Family stresses, strengths, and outcomes after critical injury, *Crit Care Nurs Clin North Am* 12(2):237–244, 2000.

Leske J: Interventions to decrease family anxiety, *Crit Care Nurs* 22(6): 61–65, 2002.

Leske J: Treatment for family members in crisis after critical injury, *AACN Clin Issues* 9(1):129–139, 1998.

Luskin F, Newell K, Griffith M, et al: A review of mind-body therapies in the treatment of cardiovascular disease, *Altern Ther Health Med* 4(3):46–61, 1998.

Martin P, Lae L, Reece J, et al: Stress as a trigger for headaches: relationship between exposure and sensitivity, *Anxiety Stress Coping* 20(4):393–407, 2007.

Maslach C: What have we learned about burnout and health? *Psychol Health* 16:607–611, 2001.

Maslach C, Leiter MP: *The truth about burnout: how organizations cause personal stress and what to do about it*, San Francisco, 1997, Jossey-Bass.

McEwen B: Allostasis, allostatic load, and the aging nervous system: role of excitatory amino acids and excitotoxity, *Neurochem Res* 9(10):1219–1231, 2000.

McEwen B: Physiology and neurobiology of stress and adaptation: central role of the brain, *Physiol Rev* 87(3):873–904, 2007.

McEwen BS, Wingfield JC: The concept of allostasis in biology and biomedicine, *Hormones Behav* 43:2–15, 2003.

Michalenko C: The odyssey of Marian the brave: a biopsychosocial fairy tale, *Clin Nurse Spec* 12(1):22–26, 1998.

Mohr DC, Goodkin DE, Gatto N, et al: Depression, coping and level of neurological impairment in multiple sclerosis, *Mult Scler* 3:254–258, 1997.

Neale DJ, Arentz A, Jones-Ellis J, et al: The negative event scale: measuring frequency and intensity of adult hassles, *Anxiety Stress Coping* 20(2):163–176, 2007.

Parish C, Bradley L, Franks V, et al: Managing the stress of caring in ITU: a reflective practice group, *Br J Nurs* 6(20):1192–1196, 1997.

Pearlin LI, Schooler C: The structure of coping, *J Health Soc Behav* 19:2–21, 1978.

Porter-O'Grady T: A glimpse over the horizon: choosing our future, *Orthop Nurse* 17(Supp 2):53–60, 1998.

Reich J, Zautra A, Hall J, et al: *Handbook of adult resilience*, New York, NY, 2010, The Guilford Press.

Richards M, Steele R: Children's self-reported coping strategies: the role of defensiveness and repressive adaptation, *Anxiety Stress Coping* 20(2):209–222, 2007.

Schwarzer R, Knoll N: Functional roles of social support within the stress and coping process: a theoretical and empirical overview, *Int J Psychol* 42(4):243–252, 2007.

Selye H: Stress and the general adaptation syndrome, *Br Med J* 4667: 1383–1392, 1950.

Sinha B, Watson D: Stress, coping and psychological illness: a cross-cultural study, *Int J Stress Manag* 14(4):386–397, 2007.

Skinner E, Edge K, Altman J, et al: Searching for the structure of coping: a review and critique of category systems for classifying ways of coping, *Psychol Bull* 129(2):216–269, 2003.

Sterling P, Eyer J: Allostasis: a new paradigm to explain arousal pathology. In Fisher S, Reason J, editors: *Handbook of life stress, cognition and health*, New York, 1988, Wiley, pp 629–649.

Stewart JL, Mishel MH: Uncertainty in childhood illness: a synthesis of the parent and child literature, *Sch Inq Nurs Pract* 14(4):299–319, 2000, discussion 321–326.

Taylor SE: Tend and befriend: biobehavioral bases of affiliation under stress, *Curr Dir Psychol Sci* 15:273–277, 2006.

Taylor SE, Welch WT, Kim HS, et al: Cultural differences in the impact of social support on psychological and biological stress responses, *Psychol Sci* 18:831–837, 2007.

Taylor S, Klein L, Lewis B, et al: Biobehavioral responses to stress in females: tend and befriend, not fight or flight, *Psychol Rev* 107 (3):411–429, 2000.

Valiant G, Mukamal K: Successful aging, *Am J Psychiatry* 158:839–847, 2001.

Vernarec E: How to cope with job stress, *RN* 64(3):44–46, 2001.

CHAPTER 21

Communicating with Clients in Crisis

Elizabeth C. Arnold

OBJECTIVES

At the end of the chapter, the reader will be able to:

1. Define crisis and related concepts.
2. Discuss theoretical frameworks related to crisis and crisis intervention.
3. Identify and apply structured crisis intervention strategies in the care of clients experiencing a crisis state.
4. Apply crisis intervention strategies to mental health emergencies.
5. Discuss crisis management strategies in disaster and mass trauma situations.

This chapter describes nurse-client relationships in crisis situations and discusses related communication strategies. The chapter focuses on the nature of crisis and presents crisis intervention guidelines nurses can use with clients and families in clinical and community settings. Included are theoretical frameworks that guide the process of crisis intervention. The application section provides practical guidelines nurses can use with clients in crisis, mental health emergencies, and disaster management.

BASIC CONCEPTS

DEFINITIONS

CRISIS

Flannery and Everly (2000) state, "A *crisis* occurs when a stressful life event overwhelms an individual's ability to cope effectively in the face of a perceived challenge or threat" (p. 119). People in crisis experience an actual or perceived overwhelming threat to self-concept, or a loss that conventional coping measures cannot handle.

Unabated, the resulting tension continues to increase, creating major personality disorganization and a crisis state.

The word *crisis* comes from the Greek root word *krisis,* meaning "turning point." The Chinese ideograph used to represent crisis consists of one character for danger and another for opportunity (Roberts, 2005). Personal responses to crisis can be adaptive or maladaptive. Successfully working through a crisis strengthens people's coping responses and sense of self-efficacy. People can learn new coping skills, expand their support system, and raise their level of functioning. Maladaptive responses can result in the development of acute or chronic psychiatric symptoms requiring professional treatment.

Crisis State

Everly (2000) defines a *crisis state* as an acute *normal* human response to severely abnormal circumstances; it is *not* a mental illness. Because a crisis state represents a personal response, two people experiencing the same crisis event will respond differently to it.

Understanding the *person* who is experiencing the crisis rather than an objective crisis stressor is critical to successful crisis intervention.

A crisis state creates a temporary disconnect from attachment to others, loss of meaning, and a disruption of previous mastery skills (Flannery & Everly, 2000). Individuals feel vulnerable. People in crisis are open to but also need a goal-directed approach to resolve a crisis state. Crisis intervention strategies are designed to help support people experiencing crisis achieve psychological homeostasis. A favorable outcome depends on the person's interpretation of the crisis, perception of coping ability, resources, and level of social support.

TYPES OF CRISIS
Developmental Crises

A crisis is commonly classified as developmental or situational. Erik Erikson's (1982) stage model of psychosocial development forms the basis for understanding developmental crisis. Each stage is associated with a psychosocial crisis to be resolved. Successful resolution of each maturational stage leaves a person better able to meet the interpersonal challenges and stressors of the next. Examples of critical incidents associated with developmental crises include marriage, pregnancy and birth of a child, midlife crisis, retirement, meaning in aging, and so on.

Erikson's (1982) descriptions of normative psychosocial crisis are used as benchmarks for assessing signs and symptoms of developmental crisis. When a situational crisis is superimposed on a normative developmental crisis, the crisis experience can be more intense. For example, a woman losing a spouse at the same time she is going through menopause experiences the double impact of a situational crisis and a normal maturational crisis associated with midlife.

Situational Crises

A situational crisis refers to an unusually stressful life event that exceeds a person's resources and coping skills. Examples include unexpected illness or injury, rape, car accident, loss of home, spouse, job, and so forth. In health care settings, most crises are situational.

A situational crisis is *not* defined by the life event itself (Hoff, 2009). Rather, it is the person's experience of the event—its origin and meaning to an individual, plus combined individual and social factors that influence a person's perception of the event as a

crisis. Common factors influencing how successfully a person responds to a crisis include:

- Previous experience with crises, coping, and problem solving
- Perception of the crisis event
- Level of help or obstruction from significant others
- Developmental level and ego maturity
- Concurrent stressors

Adventitious Crisis

An adventitious crisis is *not* a part of everyday experience. It is unplanned, unusual, horrific, and beyond anyone's control. Examples of adventitious crisis include:

- Natural disasters such as floods, earthquakes, fires, mudslides
- National disasters such as terrorism, riots, wars
- Crimes of violence such as rape, child abuse, assault, or murder (Boyd, 2008)

Disasters are catastrophic for large groups of people or whole communities simultaneously (Michalopoulos & Michalopoulos, 2009).

Other Classifications

Roberts and Yeager (2009) differentiate between a private and public crisis. A *private* crisis affects individuals and families, but not the community at large. Examples include suicide, terminal diagnosis, a car crash, rape, or the death of a family member. A *public* crisis event, more commonly referred to as a disaster, affects a whole community or large groups of people simultaneously. People are acutely aware of the precipitating events, for example, with Hurricane Katrina and terrorist attacks.

James (2008) describes two additional types of crisis. An *existential* crisis occurs when a person questions the meaning of his or her life, and whether it has any value. Midlife crisis falls into this category. *Environmental* crises are associated with major changes in the ecosystem, such as global warming, volcanic eruptions, disease epidemics, wars, and severe economic depression. Table 21-1 presents the Burgess and Roberts continuum of the different levels of crisis (Roberts & Yeager, 2009).

CRISIS INTERVENTION

Crisis intervention represents a systematic application of theory-based problem-solving strategies designed to help individuals and families resolve a crisis situation quickly and successfully, with an anticipated outcome of achieving precrisis level functional

TABLE 21-1	Burgess and Roberts' Stress-Crisis-Trauma Continuum	
Levels	**Type**	**Actions/Approach**
Levels 1 and 2	Somatic distress crisis and transitional stress crisis	Brief crisis intervention and primary outpatient mental health care/treatment
Level 3	Traumatic stress crisis	Traumatic and group crisis–oriented therapy
Level 4	Family crises	Individual, couple, or family therapy, case management, and crisis intervention focus with forensic intervention
Level 5	Mentally ill persons in crisis	Crisis intervention, psychopharmacology, case and medication monitoring, day treatment, and community support
Level 6	Psychiatric emergencies	Crisis stabilization, outpatient treatment, inpatient hospitalization, and/or legal intervention
Level 7	Catastrophic traumatic stress crises	Application of multiple levels of crisis/trauma intervention inclusive of all previously listed intervention strategies

From Roberts A, Yeager K: *Pocket guide to crisis intervention* (p. 15), New York, 2009, Oxford University Press.

capacity (Roberts & Yeager 2009). Each person's experience of a crisis is unique to that person and situation. Crisis intervention strategies should be adapted to fit each client's preferences, beliefs, values, and individual circumstances.

Crisis intervention is a *time-limited* treatment modality. Four to six weeks is considered the standard time frame for crisis resolution, although full recovery can take a much longer period of time, particularly from a disaster crisis (Callahan, 1998).

Strategies are focused on immediate problem solving and strengthening the personal resources of clients and their families. Nurses function as advocate, resource, partner, and guide in the crisis intervention process. There should be a strong focus on helping clients mobilize personal resources and use support resources effectively (Hoff, 2009). The goal of crisis intervention is to return the client to his or her previous level of functioning. Specific goals include:

- Stabilization of distress symptoms
- Reduction of distress symptoms
- Restoration of functional capabilities
- Referrals for follow-up support care, if indicated (Everly, 2000, pp. 1–2)

THEORETICAL FRAMEWORKS

Erich Lindemann (1944) and Gerald Caplan (1964, 1989) are considered primary contributors to the development of crisis theory. Lindemann's study of

bereavement in survivors coping with the crisis of death of a loved one or experiencing a disaster provided an initial frame of reference for understanding the stages involved in resolving emotional crisis and bereavement. His findings suggest, "Proper psychiatric management of grief reactions may prevent prolonged and serious alterations in the patient's social adjustment, as well as potential medical disease" (p. 147).

Caplan broadened Lindemann's model to include developmental crisis and personal crisis (Roberts, 2005). Although the direct focus of crisis intervention is on secondary prevention because the crisis state is already in motion, Caplan applied concepts of primary, secondary, and tertiary prevention to crisis intervention. His model of preventive psychiatry incorporates reducing the incidence of mental disorders in the community, limiting the duration of mental upset, and reducing impairment from clinical symptoms. Consistent with Caplan's ideas was the development of practical crisis intervention strategies related to crisis telephone lines, training for community workers, and crisis response strategies. Caplan viewed nurses as key service providers in crisis intervention.

Caplan (1964) described the initial response to a crisis situation as *shock*, with variations in emotions ranging from anger, laughing, hysterics, crying, and acute anxiety to social withdrawal. Then follows an extended period of adjustment, a period of *recoil*.

EXERCISE 21-1   Understanding the Nature of Crisis

Purpose: To help students understand crisis in preparation for assessing and planning communication strategies in crisis situations.

Procedure:

1. Describe a crisis you experienced in your life. There are no right or wrong definitions of a crisis, and it does not matter whether the crisis would be considered a crisis in someone else's life.
2. Identify how the crisis changed your roles, routines, relationships, and assumptions about yourself.

3. Apply a crisis model to the situation you are describing.
4. Identify the strategies you used to cope with the crisis.
5. Describe the ways in which your personal crisis strengthened or weakened your self-concept and increased your options and your understanding of life.

Discussion:

What did you learn from doing this exercise that you can use in your clinical practice?

This period can last from 2 to 3 weeks. Client behaviors can appear normal to outsiders, but the person often describes nightmares, phobic reactions, and flashbacks of the crisis event.

Caplan uses the term *restoration* or reconstruction to describe the final phase of crisis intervention. This phase involves taking constructive actions to face and resolve the reality issues present in a crisis situation. If successfully negotiated, the person achieves precrisis functioning or better. When people use self-destructive coping strategies such as drug or alcohol use, violence, or avoidance, restoration is delayed and/or the person is at risk for development of physical or mental symptoms.

Donna Aguilera (1998) developed a nursing model identifying how a crisis develops and corresponding factors needed for resolution. The model proposes that a crisis state occurs in response to a potentially life-changing event because of a distorted perception of a situation or because the client lacks the resources to cope successfully with it. Balancing factors include a realistic perception of the event, the client's internal resources (beliefs or attitudes), and the client's external (environmental) supports. These factors can reduce the impact of the stressor, leading to the resolution of the crisis, and can help minimize overreactions.

The absence of adequate situational support and coping skills and/or a distorted perception of the crisis event can result in a crisis state, leaving individuals and families feeling overwhelmed and unable to cope. Interventions are designed to increase the balancing factors needed to restore the person to precrisis functioning. Exercise 21-1 provides insight into the nature of crisis.

Developing an Evidence-Based Practice

Dirkzwager A, Kerssens J, Yzermans C: Health problems in children and adolescents before and after a man-made disaster, *J Am Acad Child Adolesc Psychiatry* 45(1):94–103, 2006.

The authors completed an exploratory study designed to examine the health problems of children ages 4 to 12 and adolescents ages 13 to 18 before and after exposure to a manmade fireworks disaster, and to compare these with a control group of children and adolescents who had not experienced this disaster. Longitudinal data were collected from electronic medical records of family practitioners related to health problems from 1 year before disaster until 2 years after disaster (N = 1,628 for victims; N = 2,856 for the control group). Prevalence rates of health problems were calculated for the two age groups related to psychological and social problems; medically unexplained physical symptoms; and gastrointestinal, musculoskeletal, respiratory, and skin problems.

Results: Study results indicated that postdisaster increases in health problems were significantly greater for the postdisaster group related to psychological and musculoskeletal problems and stress reactions. Children in the 4 to 12 age group experienced significantly greater rates of sleep problems than the control group, whereas adolescents 13 to 18 years old showed larger increases in anxiety problems than the control subjects. Significant predictors for postdisaster psychological problems included being relocated, low socioeconomic status, and having psychological problems before the disaster.

Application to Your Clinical Practice: This study strongly suggests that young victims of disaster experience significant and long-lasting sequelae following a disaster. Particularly at risk are those who must be relocated. What implications do you see in your nursing practice for promoting the health and well-being of children and adolescents exposed to a disaster?

APPLICATIONS

STRUCTURING CRISIS INTERVENTION STRATEGIES

Roberts (2005) provides a seven-stage sequential blue-print for clinical intervention, which can be used to structure the crisis intervention process in nurse-client relationships. This model is compatible with the nursing process sequencing of assessment, planning, implementation, and evaluation.

STEP 1 (ASSESSMENT): ASSESSING LETHALITY AND MENTAL STATUS

Safety should be the foremost assessment in any crisis situation. Assessment should focus on determining the severity of the crisis state, and the client's current danger potential—both to self and to others. If a person's crisis state is induced or complicated by physiologic factors, the person should be treated as a medical emergency first and then as a psychiatric emergency. Assessment for suicide and homicide should be part of every crisis care assessment.

Nurses need to evaluate the client's mental status if there is any reason to suspect unsafe or unusual thoughts and behaviors. Clients who are psychotic, under the influence of drugs, severely agitated, or temporarily out of control for medical reasons will require immediate triage to stabilize their physical condition. Close one-to-one observation is critical until the situation is brought under control. Table 21-2 provides guidelines for communicating with a client who is unable to cooperate with assessment or treatment. Family and significant others can provide additional assessment data related to the current crisis state (e.g., documenting changes in behavior, ingestion of drugs, or medical history) if the client is unable to do so.

STEP 2: ESTABLISHING RAPPORT AND ENGAGING THE CLIENT

- A simple introductory statement can quickly orient the client to the purpose of the crisis questions and how the information will be used. Health Insurance Portability and Accountability Act (HIPAA) of 1996 regulations require confidentiality. If clients expect family members to give or receive information to health providers when the client is not present, they will need to sign a consent form. Clients in crisis look to health professionals to structure interactions.
- Providing professional support to help the client and family feel more comfortable helps reduce anxiety in crisis situations. Clients and families experiencing a crisis state require a compassionate,

TABLE 21-2	Guidelines for Working with Uncooperative Clients in the Emergency Department	
Stage	**Client Behavior**	**Nurse Actions**
1. Environmental trigger	Stress response	Encourage venting: avoid challenge; speak calmly, clearly; offer alternative
2. Escalation period	Movement toward loss of control	Take control: maintain safe distance, acknowledge behavior, medicate if appropriate, remove to quiet area, "show force" if necessary
3. Crisis period	Emotional/physical discharge	Apply external control: implement emergency protocol, initiate confinement, give focused intensive care
4. Recovery	Cool down	Reassure: support; no retaliation; encourage to discuss behavior and alternative; release when in control; assess reaction to environment; conduct sessions for staff to process all areas of incident
5. Postcrisis and letdown	Reconciliatory	Demonstrate acceptance while continuing clarification of unit standards and expectations

From Steele RL: Staff attitudes toward seclusion and restraint: anything new? *Perspect Psychiatr Care* 29(3):28, 1993. Reprinted by permission of Nursecom, Inc.

flexible, but clearly directive calm approach from nurses. The client should be placed in a quiet, lighted room with no shadows, away from the mainstream of activity.

- Only a minimum number of people should be involved with the client, until he or she is stabilized. If the client is unable to cooperate, for safety reasons, more than one professional may be needed. Ideally, one nurse should be the primary contact for information. Depending on the nature of the crisis and client's personal responses, family members may be included or asked to return when the client is stabilized. The condition, as well as the preferences of the client, should be determining factors.

- In the early stages of crisis, people need to be listened to, rather than being given elaborate information (Artean & Williams, 1998). It is important to find out the client's perception of the crisis—how it developed, how it impacts on a person's life, is this a first encounter with a serious crisis, or one of many that the client has experienced? Questions to assess the client's perception of the client's emotional coping strength are important. James (2008) suggests asking question such as "How were you feeling about this before the crisis got so bad?"

"Where do you see yourself headed with this problem?" (p. 51).

Let clients tell you what they are experiencing. Listen for facts and associated feelings. Use a reflective listening response to identify applicable feelings (e.g., "It sounds as if you are feeling very sad [angry, lonely] right now."). You can help clients focus on relevant points by repeating a phrase found in the dialogue, asking for validation of its importance, or asking for clarification to focus further thought. Exercise 21-2 offers an opportunity to understand reflection as a listening response in crisis situations.

STEP 3 (ASSESSMENT): IDENTIFYING MAJOR PROBLEMS

The following are guidelines for identifying major problems:

- Ask for a general outline of how the client has experienced the crisis, and note the sequential order of the crisis.
- Keep the focus on the here and now. Questions should be short and relevant to the crisis.
- Request more specific details (e.g., ask who was involved, what happened, and when it happened) if this information is not easily forthcoming from the client.

| EXERCISE 21-2 | Interacting in Crisis Situations |

Purpose: To give students experience in using the three-stage model of crisis intervention.

Procedure:
1. Break up into groups of three. One student should take the role of the client and one the role of the nurse; the third functions as observer.
2. Using one of the following role-plays, or one from your current clinical setting, engage the client and use the crisis intervention strategies presented in this chapter to frame your interventions.
3. The observer should provide feedback.
   (This exercise can also be handled as discussion points rather than a role-play, with small-group or class feedback as to how students would have handled the situations.)

Role-Play:
Julie is a 23-year-old graduate student who has been dating Dan for the past 3 years. They plan to marry within the next 6 months. Last summer she had a brief affair with another graduate student while Dan was

away but never told him. She is seeing you in the clinic having just found out that she has herpes from that encounter.

Sally is a 59-year-old postmenopausal woman admitted for diagnostic testing and possible surgery. She has just found out that her tests reveal a malignancy in her colon with possible metastasis to her liver. You are the nurse responsible for caring for her.

Bill's mother was admitted last night to the ICU with sepsis. She is on life support and intravenous antibiotics. Bill had a close relationship with his mother earlier in his life, but he has not seen her in the past year. You are the nurse for the shift but do not yet know her well.

Discussion:
1. What would you want to do differently as a result of this exercise when communicating with the client in crisis?
2. What was the effect of using the three-stage model of crisis intervention as a way of organizing your approach to the crisis situation?

- Ask about the feelings associated with the immediate crisis.
- Responses to clients should be brief, empathetic, and clearly related to the client's story.
- Note changes in expression, body posture, and vocal inflections as clients tell their story and at what points they occur.
- Identify central emotional themes in the client's story (e.g., powerlessness, shame, hopelessness) to provide a focus for intervention.
- Periodically summarize content so that you and your client simultaneously arrive at the same place with a comprehensive understanding of major issues.

Dealing with Feelings

People do not necessarily link a crisis event to their feelings about it. Nurses can call the client's attention to the linkage by specifically connecting crisis data with observations about client response (e.g., "I wonder if because you think your son is using drugs *[precipitating event]*, you feel helpless and confused *[client emotional response]*, and it seems you don't know what to do next *[client behavioral reaction]*."). Checking in with clients helps ensure that your interpretations represent the client's truth.

Clients in crisis often feel that their emotional reactions to a situation are abnormal because they are intense or uncomfortable. It is helpful to point out that most people will experience a variety of powerful feelings in crisis situations.

Recognizing Personal Strengths

In a crisis, people have a tendency to focus on what is wrong, which stimulates negative thinking patterns. Empowering clients to identify existing personal strengths through compassionate witnessing is an important strategy. Compassionate witnessing is defined as "noticing and feeling empathy for others" (Powley, 2009, p. 1303). When combined with social supports and community resources, compassionate witnessing of personal strengths can significantly enhance coping skills. For example, having a job, financial resources, and knowledge about accessing health care services are critical assets people can use in crisis situations. In the heat of the moment, clients may not recognize their value. Reinforce strengths as you observe them or as the client identifies them. Exercise 21-3 provides an opportunity to experience the value of personal support systems in crisis situations.

Providing Truth in Information

Being truthful about what is known and unknown, and updating information as you learn about it is a critical strategy for building trust with clients in crisis. Explain what is going to happen, step by step. Letting clients know as much as possible about progress, treatment, and consequences of choosing different alternatives allows clients to make informed decisions and reduces the heightened anxiety associated with a crisis situation.

EXERCISE 21-3 | **Personal Support Systems**

Purpose: To help students appreciate the breadth and importance of personal support systems in stressful situations.

Procedure:
All of us have support systems we can use in times of stress (e.g., church, friends, family, coworkers, clubs, recreational groups).
1. Identify a support person or system you could or do use in times of stress.
2. What does this personal support system or person do for you (e.g., listen without judgment; provide honest, objective feedback; challenge you to think; broaden your perspective; give unconditional support; share your perceptions)? List everything you can think of.

3. What factors go into choosing your personal support system (e.g., availability, expertise, perception of support)? Which is the most important factor?
4. How did you develop your personal support system?

Discussion:
1. What types of support systems were most commonly used by class or group members?
2. What were the most common reasons for selecting a support person or system?
3. After doing this exercise, what strategies would you advise for enlarging a personal support system?
4. What applications do you see in this exercise for your nursing practice?

STEP 5 (PLANNING): EXPLORING ALTERNATIVE OPTIONS AND PARTIAL SOLUTIONS

People in crisis often develop tunnel vision (Dass-Brailsford, 2010) and feel they have no resolution of their problem. Finding viable solutions to seemingly impossible problems challenges this assumption, and helping clients to develop targeted alternative strategies increases self-efficacy. Problems not related to the crisis can be handled later.

Clients in crisis generally feel powerless. Nurses can introduce alternative methods that the client may not have considered. Helping a client examine the consequences of proposed solutions and breaking tasks down into small, achievable parts empowers clients. Proposed solutions should accommodate both the problem and client resources. Its helpful to assist clients in discussing the consequences, costs, and benefits of choosing of one action versus another (e.g., "What would happen if you choose this course of action as compared with. . .?" or "What is the worst that could happen if you decided to. . .?").

The locus of control for decision making should always remain with the client to whatever extent is possible. Making autonomous choices encourages clients to become invested in the solution-finding process and hopeful about finding a resolution to a crisis situation.

Involving Social Support Systems

Positive social supports and available community resources act as a buffer to the intensity of a crisis state. Evaluating the availability and ability of a client's support system to be involved is a critical assessment. Support networks provide practical advice and a sense of security. Equally important, they are a source of encouragement that can reaffirm a client's worth and help defuse anxiety associated with the uncertainty present in most crisis situations.

Not everyone in a client's support system holds equal or positive resource value for the client or family. It is important to ask not only about the number and variety of people in the client's support network, but "who does the client and/or family trust," and "who would they be most comfortable telling about their situation." In crisis situations, many clients and families temporarily withdraw from natural support systems and may need encouragement to reconnect.

STEP 6 (PLANNING): DEVELOPING A REALISTIC ACTION PLAN

Crisis intervention "is action-oriented and situation focused" (Dass-Brailsford, 2010, p. 56). Formulating a realistic action plan starts with prioritizing identified problems. An effective crisis plan should have a practical, here-and-now, therapeutic, short-term focus and should reflect the client's choices about best options. Keep in mind the overarching goal of crisis intervention: to restore the functional capabilities of the individuals to their precrisis state.

Introduce consideration of immediate small steps to encourage stabilization. Provide instructions as clearly and simply as possible, explain what is going to happen step by step, and have clients repeat instructions back to you to ensure mutual understanding.

Focusing on the Present

Help your clients to think in terms of short time intervals and immediate next steps (e.g., "What can you do with the rest of today just to get through it better"?) Examples include getting more information, gathering essential data, taking a walk, calling a family member, taking time for self. When people begin to take even the smallest step, they gain a sense of control, and this stimulates hope for future mastery of the crisis situation. Thinking about crisis resolution as a whole is counterproductive.

Incorporate Previously Successful Coping Strategies

People with a record of resiliency and creativity in other aspects of their lives are more likely to weather a crisis satisfactorily. Looking at past coping strategies can reveal skills that can be used in a current crisis situation and offer hope that the current crisis also is resolvable. Ask, "What do you usually do when you have a problem?" or "To whom do you turn when you are in trouble?"

Explore the nature of tension-reducing strategies the client has used in the past (e.g., aerobics, Bible study, calling a friend). If the client seems immobilized and unable to give an answer about usual coping strategies, the nurse can offer prompts such as "Some people talk to their friends, bang walls, pray, go to church. . ." Usually, with verbal encouragement, clients begin to identify successful coping mechanisms, which can be built on, for use in resolving the current crisis.

STEP 6 (IMPLEMENTATION): DEVELOPING AN ACTION PLAN
Developing Reasonable Goals

Developing realistic goals is a critical component of crisis intervention. This process includes becoming aware of choices, letting go of ideas that are toxic or self-defeating, and making the best choice among the viable options. Goal-directed activities should reflect the client's strengths, values, capabilities, beliefs, and preferences.

Achievable goals give clients and families hope that they can get to a different place with their emotional and physical pain. Goals that have meaning to the client are more likely to be accomplished. Crisis offers clients an opportunity to discover and develop new self-awareness about things that are important to them and skills.

Designing Achievable Tasks

Help clients choose tasks that are within their capabilities, circumstances, and energy level. Achievable tasks can be as simple as getting more information or making time for self. You can suggest, "What do you think needs to happen first?" or "Let's look at what you might be able to do quickly." Engaging clients in simple problem solving can help with crisis-related feelings of helplessness and hopelessness. Problem-solving tasks that strengthen the client's realistic perception of the crisis event, incorporate a client's beliefs and values, and integrate social and environmental supports offer the best chance for success. Greene, Lee, Trask and Rheinscheld (2005) suggest that helping clients tap into and use their personal resources to achieve goals facilitates crisis resolution and provides individuals with tools for further personal development.

Providing Structure and Encouragement

Clients need structure and encouragement as they perform the tasks that will move them forward. Making a commitment to achieve a small task related to crisis resolution helps clients see crisis resolution as a process they can master and stimulates hope. Setting time limits and monitoring task achievement is important.

Resolving a crisis state is not experienced as only steady movement forward. There will be setbacks. Clients need ongoing affirmation of their efforts. Supportive reinforcement includes validation of the struggles clients are coping with, anticipatory guidance

regarding what to expect, the normalcy of ambivalent feelings, uncertainty, and discussion of fears surrounding the process. Comparing current functioning with baseline admission presentations helps nurses and their clients mutually evaluate progress, foresee areas of necessary focus, and measure achievement of treatment goals.

Providing Support for Families

Part of crisis intervention strategies includes providing support for family members. Crisis for the family can be experienced collectively as a direct strike in a disaster, or as a secondary individual response to the illness or injury of a family member. Family members supporting individuals in crisis are coping not only with the acute emotional fallout brought about by the client's crisis, but with the management of an unstable home environment created by the client's absence or inability to function in previous roles. There may be legal or safety issues that family members have to address.

Bluhm (1987) suggests an image of a family in crisis as "a group of people standing together, with arms interlocked. What happens if one family member becomes seriously ill and can no longer stand? The other family members will attempt to carry their loved one, each person shifting his weight to accommodate the additional burden" (p. 44).

Individual family members will experience the crisis in diverse ways, so different levels of information and support will be required. Giving families an opportunity to talk about the meaning of the crisis for each family member, and offering practical guidance about resources they can use to support the client and take care of themselves are important strategies nurses can use with families. Communication strategies the nurse can use to help families in crisis are presented in Box 21-1.

STEP 7 (EVALUATION): DEVELOPING A TERMINATION AND FOLLOW-UP PROTOCOL

Kavan, Guck, and Barone (2006) note, "Follow up provides patients with a lifeline and improves the likelihood that they still follow through with the action plan (p. 1164). All clients should receive verbal instructions, and *written* discharge or follow-up directives, with phone numbers to call for added help or clarification. Although acute symptoms may subside

BOX 21-1   Interventions for Initial Family Responses to Crisis

Anxiety, Shock, Fear
- Give information that is brief, concise, explicit, and concrete.
- Repeat information and frequently reinforce; encourage families to record important facts in writing.
- Determine comprehension by asking family to repeat back to you what information they have been given.
- Provide for and encourage or allow expression of feelings, even if they are extreme.
- Maintain constant, nonanxious presence in the face of a highly anxious family.
- Inform family as to the potential range of behaviors and feelings that are within the "norm" for crisis.
- Maximize control within hospital environment, as possible.

Denial
- Identify what purpose denial is serving for family (e.g., Is it buying them "psychological time" for future coping and mobilization of resources?).
- Evaluate appropriateness of use of denial in terms of time; denial becomes inappropriate when it inhibits the family from taking necessary actions or when it is impinging on the course of treatment.
- Do not actively support denial, but don't dash hopes for the future (You might say, "It must be very difficult for you to believe your son is nonresponsive, and in a trauma unit.").
- If denial is prolonged and dysfunctional, more direct and specific factual representation may be essential.

Anger, Hostility, Distrust
- Allow for venting of angry feelings, clarifying what thoughts, fears, and beliefs are behind the anger; let the family know it is okay to be angry.
- Do not personalize family's expressions of these strong emotions.
- Institute family control within the hospital environment when possible (e.g., arrange for set times and set person to give them information in reference to the patient and answer their questions).
- Remain available to families during their venting of these emotions.

- Ask families how they can take the energy in their anger and put it to positive use for themselves, for the patient, and for the situation.

Remorse and Guilt
- Do not try to "rationalize away" guilt for families.
- Listen and support their expression of feeling and verbalizations (e.g., "I can understand how or why you might feel that way; however...").
- Follow the "however's" with careful, reality-oriented statements or questions (e.g., "None of us can truly control another's behavior"; "Kids make their own choices despite what parents think and want"; "How successful were you when you tried to control _____'s behavior with that before?"; "So many things happen for which there are no absolute answers").

Grief and Depression
- Acknowledge family's grief and depression.
- Encourage them to be precise about what it is they are grieving and depressed about; give grief and depression a context.
- Allow the family appropriate time for grief.
- Recognize that this is an essential step for future adaptation; do not try to rush the grief process.
- Remain sensitive to your own unfinished business, and hence comfort or discomfort with family's grieving and depression.

Hope
- Clarify with families their hopes, individually and with one another.
- Clarify with families their worst fears in reference to the situation. Are the hopes/fears congruent? Realistic? Unrealistic?
- Support realistic hope.
- Offer gentle factual information to reframe unrealistic hope (e.g., "With the information you have or the observations you have made, do you think that is still possible?").
- Assist families in reframing unrealistic hope in some other fashion (e.g., "What do you think others will have learned from _____ if he doesn't make it?" "How do you think _____ would like for you to remember him/her?").

Adapted from Kleeman K: Families in crisis due to multiple trauma, *Crit Care Nurs Clin North Am* 1(1):25, 1989.

with standard crisis intervention strategies, some clients will need follow-up for residual clinical issues. Many agencies include a follow-up call to the client or family to check on how things are going after crisis discharge.

Mobilizing resources in the community often is necessary in helping clients maintain continued mastery of health care situations. Community agency resources can provide clients with essential supports. An important piece of assessment data is whether

EXERCISE 21-4	Using Reflective Responses in a Crisis Situation

Purpose: To provide students with a means of appreciating the multipurpose uses of reflection as a listening response in crisis situations.

Procedure:

Have one student role-play a client in an emergency department situation involving a common crisis situation (e.g., fire, heart attack, auto accident). After this person talks about the crisis situation for 3 to 4 minutes, have each student write down a reflective listening response that they would use with the client in crisis. Have each student read their reflective response

to the class. (This can also be done in small groups of students if the class is large.)

Discussion:

1. Were you surprised at the variety of reflective themes found in the students' responses?
2. In what ways could differences in the wording or emphasis of a reflective response influence the flow of information?
3. In what ways do reflective responses validate the client's experience?
4. How could you use what you learned from doing this exercise in your clinical practice?

the client is willing to use outside resources, and if so, which ones. Some clients are reluctant to use social services, medications, or mental health services, even short term, because of the stigma they feel about their use. Nurses can help clients and families sort out their concerns, assess their practicality, and develop viable contacts.

If indicated, nurses can facilitate the referral process by sharing information with community agencies and by giving clients enough information to follow through on getting additional assistance. Having written referral information available regarding eligibility requirements, location, cost, and accessibility can make a difference in compliance. Exercise 21-4 provides an opportunity to practice crisis intervention skills.

MENTAL HEALTH EMERGENCIES

Mental health emergencies present significant challenges for nurses. Whether encountered in the community or admitted to an emergency department, these clients often present as a danger to themselves or others. These clients present with chaotic distress behaviors, which are not under the client's control. Many communities have trained first responders in methods of dealing with individuals experiencing psychiatric crisis and have crisis response teams.

The client who presents as a mental health emergency is generally unable to participate in his or her care. Although mental health emergencies share some similarities with other types of crisis, they usually require a higher, more immediate level of assessment and intervention to protect the client from harming himself or

others. Examples of a mental health emergency include suicidal, homicidal, or threatening behavior, self-injury, severe drug or alcohol impairment, and highly erratic or unusual behavior associated with serious mental disorders. Nurses can find it difficult to tolerate the intensity of the relationship associated with mental health emergencies.

Myer (2006) describes a triage assessment system (TAS) for mental health crises that can help nurses understand a client's responses across 3 domains: affective, behavioral, and cognitive. He suggests that clinicians identify the primary affective reaction, for example, anger, fear, or sadness. Next the client's behavioral reaction is assessed related to mobility, avoidance, or approach. The client's immediate perception of a transgression, threat, or loss in relation to the crisis event constitutes the cognitive domain. Treatment should focus on the most severe reaction.

This is where you should begin. Think about what the client sees. Remember that although defensive behaviors seem threatening, usually these clients feel vulnerable. Clients may feel they are in acute danger. They are not in control of their behavior or capable of logical reasoning. Keep communication short, compassionate and well defined. Do not be intimidated, but avoid intimidation. Find out where the fear is coming from. Go slow and avoid sudden movements. Box 21-2 provides de-escalation tips developed by Scott Davis of the Montgomery Police Department (2010) for use with clients presenting in the community with mental health emergencies.

Clinicians need to be respectful and avoid traumatizing individuals who are already experiencing a

BOX 21-2	De-escalation Tips for Mental Health Emergencies

- Use a nonthreatening stance—open, but not vulnerable. Have them "take a seat"
- Eye contact—not constant, brief to show concern
- Commands—brief, slow, with simple vocabulary, only as loud as needed, repeat as needed
- Movement—not sudden, announce actions when possible, keep hands where they can be seen
- Attitude—calm, interested, firm, patient, reassuring, respectful, truthful
- Acknowledge legitimacy of feelings, delusions, hallucinations as being real to the client "I understand you are seeing or feeling this, but I am not"
- Remove distractions, upsetting influences

- Keep the client talking/focused on the here and now
- Ignore rather than argue with provocative statements
- Allow verbal venting within reason
- Be sensitive to personal space/comfort zone
- Remove client to a quiet space; remove others from immediate area (avoid the "group spectators").
- Give some choices or options, if possible
- Set limits if necessary
- Limit interaction to just one professional and let that person do the talking.
- Avoid rushing—slow things down
- Give yourself an out; don't put the client between yourself and the door.

Adapted from Officer Scott A Davis, Crisis Intervention Team (CIT) Coordinator: De-escalation tips, Rockville, MD, February 10, 2010, Montgomery County Police Department.

chaotic, distressed state. Patient-centered care requires assessment and treatment approaches that are compassionate, and as acceptable to the client as is possible. Whenever possible, offer simple choices with structured coaching.

Psychiatric emergency clients usually require medication for stabilization of symptoms and close supervision. Whereas crisis intervention represents a short-term response, a mental health emergency requires an *immediate* coordinated response designed to alleviate the potential for harm and restore basic stability.

TYPES OF MENTAL HEALTH EMERGENCIES

Callahan (1998) identifies three types of mental health emergencies in health care: violence, suicide, and psychosis.

Violence

Violence is a mental health emergency that can create a critical challenge to the safety, well-being, and health of the clients and others in their environment. Officer Scott Davis, crisis intervention team coordinator with the Montgomery County Police Department shares a field expedient tool, using the acronym "DANGEROUS PERSON" (Box 21-3), to assess dangerousness to self or others in clients presenting as mental health emergency.

Nurses should assume an organic component (drugs, alcohol, psychosis, or delirium) underlying the aggression in clients presenting with disorganized impulsive or violent behaviors, until proven otherwise. Violent clients must be stabilized immediately for the protection of themselves and others. Perry and Jagger (2003) advise that at least two health care providers

BOX 21-3	Field Expedient Tool to Assess Dangerousness to Self or Others

Depression/suicidal
Anger/agitation, aggressive
Noncompliance with requests/taking medication
General appearance/inappropriate dress/poor hygiene
Evidence of self-inflicted injury
Responding/reacting to delusions or hallucinations
Owns/displays weapon(s)
Unorganized thoughts/appearance/behavior

Speech pattern/substance/rate (too fast, too slow, jumps all over)
Paranoid
Erratic or fearful behavior
Recent loss of job/loved one/home
Substance abuse
Orientation to date/time/location/situation/insight into illness
Number and type of previous contacts with police, social or crisis workers

From Officer Scott A Davis, Crisis Intervention Team (CIT) Coordinator: *Field expedient tool to assess dangerousness to self or others*, Rockville, MD, February 2010, Montgomery County Police Department.

should be present at the bedside for all procedures if the client is suicidal, delirious, or under the influence of drugs or alcohol.

The client's body language often offers the nurse clues to escalating anxiety, which can end in violent behavior if left unchecked. Table 21-3 presents characteristic indicators of increasing tension leading to violence. A history of violence, childhood abuse, substance abuse, mental retardation, problems with impulse control, and psychosis, particularly when accompanied by command hallucinations, are common contributing factors.

Treatment of violent clients consists of providing a safe, nonstimulating environment for the client.

TABLE 21-3	Behavioral Indicators of Potential Violence
Behavioral Categories	**Potential Indicators**
Mental status	Confused
	Paranoid ideation
	Disorganized
	Organic impairment
	Poor impulse control
Motor behavior	Agitated, pacing
	Exaggerated gestures
	Rapid breathing
Body language	Eyes darting
	Prolonged (staring) eye contact or lack of eye contact
	Spitting
	Pale, or red (flushed) face
	Menacing posture, throwing things
Speech patterns	Rapid, pressured
	Incoherent, mumbling, repeatedly making the same statements
	Menacing tones, raised voice, use of profanity
	Verbal threats
Affect	Belligerent
	Labile
	Angry

Data from: Keely B: Recognition and prevention of hospital violence. *Dimens Crit Care Nurs*, 21(6): 236-241, 2002; Luck L, Jackson D, Usher K. STAMP: components of observable behaviour that indicate potential for patient violence in emergency departments. *Journal of Advanced Nursing*. 59(1): 11-19, 2007.

Often clients calm down if taken to an area with less sensory input. The client should be checked thoroughly for potential weapons and physically disarmed, if necessary. Short-term medication is usually indicated to help defuse potentially harmful behaviors.

Communication strategies to defuse violent behaviors are useful adjuncts to treatment, and can prevent escalation of violent behavior. The nurse can use simple strategies such as calling the client by name; using a low, calm tone of voice; or presenting a show of force if necessary to help the client defuse tension. Encouraging the client to physically walk and to vent emotions verbally can be helpful.

Organically impaired clients may perceive necessary medical procedures as being intrusive and threatening. Perry and Jagger (2003) advise that, before you start any procedure, you should tell the client exactly what you are going to do and why the procedure is necessary, with a request to cooperate. If the client refuses, don't insist, but explain the reason for doing the procedure in a calm, quiet voice. If you help your client regain a sense of control, he or she will be more likely to cooperate with you. Your movements should be calm, firm, and respectful.

Suicide

Suicide is the ultimate personal crisis. People turn to suicide as an option in times of acute distress, when under the influence of drugs, or when they believe there are no other alternatives. A major goal in evaluating suicidal risk is to assess whether the client is in imminent danger of doing harm to self (Stellrecht, Gordon, Van Orden et al., 2006).

It is a myth that people who talk about harming themselves are at less risk. Every suicidal statement, however indirect, should be taken seriously. Even with clients who have indicated that they are "just kidding," the fact that they have verbalized the threat places them at greater risk. Verbal indicators of potential suicide include statements such as "I don't think I can go on without …" "I sometimes wish I wasn't here," or "People would be better off without me." Less direct indicators include statements like "I don't see anything good in my life." Any of these statements requires further clarification (e.g., "You say you can't go on any longer. Can you tell me more about what you mean?").

Nurses should ask directly:

* Are you thinking of hurting yourself? (include frequency and intensity of thoughts)
* Do you have a plan? (If the person indicates a plan, additional inquiry about the methods and availability of the method is needed.) Inquiring if the client has a plan is essential. Individuals with a detailed plan and the means to carry it out are at greatest risk for suicide, particularly if they do not have a reliable support system. In assessing the lethality of the plan, inquire about the method, and the client's knowledge and skills about its use (Roberts, Monferrari, & Yeager, 2008).
* What do you hope to accomplish with the suicide attempt? (look for hopelessness, including severity and duration)
* Have you thought about when you might do this? (immediate vs. chronic thinking)
* Who are you able to turn to when you are in trouble? (social support)

Behavioral indicators of escalating suicidal ideation include giving away possessions, apologizing for previous bad behaviors, writing letters to significant people, intense sharing of personal data from people who do not normally share with others, and frequent accidents.

Irrational behaviors, drug and alcohol abuse, previous suicide attempts, and verbal threats are matters of concern, as is a sudden mood change, especially if the client demonstrates much more energy. Clients with certain mental illnesses such as bipolar disorder or schizophrenia with command hallucinations are more at risk. Antisocial and borderline personality disorders are associated with increased suicide attempts. Suicide rates are greater for older adults, especially for white men, and among adolescents, particularly male African Americans. Men are more likely to complete suicide, whereas more women attempt suicide (American Psychiatric Association, 2003). Clients who verbalize or behaviorally demonstrate "a weight being lifted off the shoulders" should be watched carefully.

Other high-risk factors include:

* Previous attempts, or family history of suicide
* Major physical illness
* Social isolation
* Recent major loss
* History of trauma or abuse

Most clients are ambivalent about ending their life and experience relief that the decision has been taken out of their hands. Introduce the idea of psychiatric evaluation after disclosure of suicidal ideation in a calm, compassionate manner with a simple statement: "I'm worried that you might harm yourself because of how you say you are feeling right now. You have several of the factors that place you at high risk for suicide. I would like you to see Dr. Jones for an evaluation."

Stabilization and safety of the client is the most immediate concern with clients experiencing suicidal crisis. Clients exhibiting high-risk behaviors require one-to-one constant staff observation, and a potentially suicidal client should never be left alone. Possible weapons (e.g., mirrors, belts, knitting needles, scissors, razors, medications, clothes hangers) should be confiscated. When taking these items, explain in a calm, compassionate manner the general reason why the items should not be in the client's possession, and where they will be kept. The client needs to be compassionately informed of the reason unsafe items are being removed. They need to be assured that the items will be returned when the danger of self-harm resolves.

Documentation of the suicidal risk assessment, interventions, and client responses is essential. Included in the documentation should be any quotes made by the client, details of observed behavior, review of identified risk factors, and client responses to initial crisis intervention strategies. The names and times of anyone you notified and contacts with family should be incorporated in the narrative note. These data provide direction for future clinicians involved in the client's care. The Joint Commission requires that any death that is not consistent with a client's disease process or any permanent loss of function occurring as a consequence of an attempted suicide in a hospital be reported as a sentinel event (Captain, 2006).

Most inpatient settings have written suicide precaution protocols that must be followed with clients presenting with suicidal ideation. Observational monitoring of acutely suicidal clients ranges from constant 1:1 observation, to 15- or 30-minute observational checks. Less restrictive checks can include supervised bathroom, unit restriction or restriction to public areas, and supervised sharps (Jacobs, 2007). The frequency and type of observation is dependent on the suicidal assessment of the client.

After the initial focus of suicide intervention on stabilizing acute distress, helping the client identify triggers, and understand the reasons that led to suicidal ideation and/or suicide attempt becomes important. Helping people reestablish a reason for living and getting others involved as a support system are critical interventions.

Acceptance of the client is a critical element of rapport. Nurses need to explore their own feelings about suicide behaviors as the basis for understanding the client in danger of self-injury. Consistent with a high risk for suicidal behavior is a sense of hopelessness, lack of meaningful connection with others, and the feeling of being a burden to others (Stellrecht et al., 2006).

Speak slowly, gently, and clearly. Once the client's suicidal behaviors and feelings are brought under control, the crisis interventions presented earlier in the chapter can be instituted. Suicidal ideation waxes and wanes, so careful observation is critical even after the acute crisis has subsided. Captain (2006) suggests reassessing a client's suicidal intent every shift, using a 10-point scale and asking the client to "rate your level of suicidal intent on a 0-to-10 scale, with 0 meaning no thoughts of suicide and 10 meaning constant thoughts of suicide" (p. 47). Assessments should be repeated any time changes in behavior are noted and again before discharge.

Crisis Intervention with Psychotic Clients

A psychotic break in which a client is threatening harm to self or to others, is out of touch with reality, or is responding to hallucinations represents a serious mental health crisis. Acutely psychotic and delirious clients have disorganized thinking, reduced insight, and limited personal judgment. The individual is experiencing severe distress and is unable to manage himself or herself. Medication is usually indicated to manage psychotic symptoms.

The florid behavior symptoms associated with psychosis can be frightening for both nurse and client. Nurses should recognize the existence of the client's feelings and perceptions, even if the logic for their existence is not well understood. Psychotic clients do better in a quiet, softly lighted room, with no shadows, and out of the mainstream. One-to-one supervision usually is required for clients experiencing a psychotic break. Allow the client sufficient space to feel safe, and never try to subdue a client by yourself. Remain calm and positive. An open expression, eye contact, a calm voice, and simple concrete words invite trust. Do not use touch, as it can be misinterpreted.

CRISIS MANAGEMENT

DISASTER AND MASS TRAUMA SITUATIONS

A **disaster** is defined as "a calamitous event of slow or rapid onset that results in large-scale physical destruction of property, social infrastructure, and human life" (Deeny & McFetridge, 2005, p. 432). Recent years have borne witness to more unprecedented natural disasters, terrorism, and barbaric war than the world has seen in many decades. The September 11th terrorist attack on the World Trade Center in 2001, the Oklahoma City bombing, and the devastation of Hurricane Katrina, which demolished a thriving city in a matter of days, stimulated a fresh awareness of the need for community and national planned responses to mass trauma events that can happen anywhere, and at any time, to innocent masses of people. Webb (2004) identifies the components of mass trauma events in Table 21-4.

Myer and Moore (2006) note, "Crises do not happen in a vacuum, but are shaped by the cultural and social contexts in which they occur" (p. 139). From the perspective of its victims, terrorism is a random event, which reinforces insecurity, creates lingering anxiety, and increases avoidant behaviors around potential risks. The idea of a reciprocal relation between social forces and disaster crisis is supported by the Institute of Medicine (2003).

PLANNING FOR DISASTER MANAGEMENT

In the United States, The Federal Emergency Management Agency (FEMA) is responsible for setting forth recommendations related to creating an effective disaster plan (Hendriks & Bassi, (2009). FEMA recommendations provide guidelines for the creation of local disaster planning teams. Community-based governments and businesses, first responders, hospitals, and health providers are expected to be actively involved in community disaster planning. Around the globe, tsunamis in Indonesia, earthquakes occurring in rapid succession in China, Iceland, and South America, the threat of nations developing nuclear weapons, pandemic flu, and severe acute respiratory syndrome (SARS) remind us of a global approach to emergency preparedness.

Strategies for creating and sustaining community-wide emergency preparedness are published by the

TABLE 21-4	Assessing Elements of Mass Trauma Events
Element	**Example**
Single vs. recurring traumatic event	Type I (acute) trauma
	Type II (chronic or ongoing) trauma
Proximity to the traumatic event	On-site
	On the periphery
	Through the media
Exposure to violence/injury/pain	Witnessed and/or experienced
Nature of losses/death/destruction	Personal, community, and/or symbolic loss
	Danger, loss, and/or responsibility traumas
	Loved one "missing"/no physical evidence
	Death determined by retrieval of body or fragment
	Loss of status/employment/family income
	Loss of a predictable future
Attribution of causality	Random
	"Act of God" or deliberate
	Human-made

From Webb N: The impact of traumatic stress and loss on children and families (p. 6). In Webb N, editor: *Mass trauma and violence: helping families and children cope*, New York, 2004, The Guilford Press. Reprinted by permission.

Joint Commission (2003), which states, "It is no longer sufficient to develop disaster plans and dust them off if a threat appears imminent. Rather, a system of preparedness across communities must be in place everyday" (p. 5). Disaster planning can act as a deterrent to terrorist activity, as well as immediate resource in a disaster situation.

DISASTER INTERVENTION PROTOCOLS

Disaster intervention protocols focus on treating injury and acute illness, rather than chronic health conditions (Spurlock, Brown, & Rami, 2009). Crisis intervention responses to mass violence and disaster are quite distinct from treating individual traumas and crisis. Interventions must be embedded in community systems, and must be consistent with societal norms and available resources.

Disaster management requires providing immediate physical and emotional first aid. Instead of initially eliciting details of the experience, Everly and Flynn (2006) stress promotion of adaptive functioning and stabilization as a first response. They use the acronym BICEPS, which stands for brevity, immediacy, contact, expectancy, proximity, and simplicity to describe the type of psychological first aid needed in mass disaster situations.

Noji (2000) identifies four goals to guide disaster management:

- Assess the needs of disaster-affected populations.
- Match available resources to those needs.
- Prevent further adverse health effects; implement disease-control strategies for well-defined problems.
- Evaluate the effectiveness of disaster relief programs and improve contingency plans for various types of future disasters.

Any declared disaster situation affects individuals differently.

CRITICAL INCIDENT DEBRIEFING

Disasters, deliberate violence, and terrorist attacks are random events producing permanent changes in people's lives and shaking their perception of being in charge of their lives. Everly and Mitchell (2000) use the term **critical incident** to describe "an event, which is outside the usual range of experience and challenges one's ability to cope" (p. 212).

Critical incident debriefing is a type of crisis intervention used to help a group of people who have witnessed or experienced a mass trauma event process its meaning and talk about feelings that otherwise might not surface. The debriefing is designed to help the people directly involved in witnessing or caring for victims and survivors process first the facts and then the feelings associated with a traumatic or critical incident.

The process should allow for free expression of feelings, including guilt, anxiety, and anger. Guided mutual sharing of the crisis experience increases empathy and understanding of its meaning. The debriefing team teaches about the nature of distress reactions and offers helpful hints to mitigate their effects (Dietz, 2009).

The debriefing is conducted as a highly structured group intervention, which is held as soon as possible after the critical incident. The goal of critical incident debriefing is to lessen the symptoms of traumatic stress associated with a sudden crisis or trauma. The debriefing allows the people involved in a traumatic situation to achieve a sense of psychological closure. Although the critical incident will not be forgotten, people are better able to let go of its horror, which increases their potential for a return to normal life for individuals, communities, and organizations. Contact information for the group leader and possible referrals for further intervention should be provided.

Critical Incident Stress Debriefing Process

A specially trained professional generally leads the debriefing. Only those actively involved in the critical incident can attend the debriefing session.

The leader introduces the purpose of the group and assures the participants that everything said in the session will be kept confidential. People are asked to identify who they are and what happened from their perspective, including the role they played in the incident. After preliminary factual data are addressed, the next step is to explore feelings. The leader asks participants to recall the first thing they remember thinking or feeling about the incident. Participants are asked to discuss any stress symptoms they may have related to the incident. The final discussion focuses on the emotional reactions associated with the critical incident. This part of the session is followed by psycho-educational strategies to reduce stress. Any lingering questions are answered, and the leader summarizes the high points of the critical incident debriefing for the group (Rubin, 1990).

Critical incident debriefing is a useful strategy with families witnessing a tragedy involving one of their family members, for children and adolescents dealing with the death of a classmate, mass murders, or environmental disasters. A critical incident stress debriefing offers people an opportunity to externalize a traumatic experience through being able to vent feelings, discuss their role in the situation, develop a realistic sense of the big picture, and receive peer support in putting a crisis event in perspective (Curtis, 1995).

Critical Incident Debriefing for First Responders and Health Care Providers

Critical incidents in health care affect the personnel who respond to them. If there is no opportunity to process the meaning of a critical situation, an involved health care provider can become a psychological casualty. Research indicates that individuals, including health care providers who assist or witness critical incidents, are vulnerable to experiencing "secondary traumatization" similar to that experienced by direct survivors of the incident. Principles of critical incident debriefing can also be applied to strengthen the emotional coping skills of staff working in clinical settings on units with frequent or unexpected loss (Dietz, 2009).

Because of their magnitude, disasters present a more complicated coping process for family survivors and the community at large (Flannery, 1999). Survivors of disaster experience personal crisis response patterns similar to those described earlier in the chapter. In addition, they can experience what Lahad (2000) terms "breaks in continuity." He suggests that victims, their families, and those secondarily exposed to a disaster are subject to a sudden, serious break in their belief in the continuity of their personal lives that is difficult to ease. The break in continuity occurs in four spheres:

- I don't understand what is happening *(cognitive continuity)*.
- I don't know myself *(historical continuity)*.
- I don't know what to do, how to act here, what it is to be a bereaved person/an injured or wounded person *(role continuity)*.
- Where is everyone? I am so alone. Where are my loved ones? *(social continuity)*.

The experience of trauma from a disaster or terrorist event varies in intensity and impact for survivors. Each survivor brings to the experience a unique personal history, interpersonal strengths, and deficits. Each will interpret the meaning of the crisis differently. Individual, family, and community beliefs about a disaster's cause and meaning influence each person's response. Past experience with trauma makes a person more vulnerable to future impairment with traumatic situations (Maguen, Papa, & Litz, 2008). Having limited resources, lack of social support, or mental illness creates additional stress. The level of direct involvement, degree of uncertainty about outcome, nature of the loss, and personal resiliency of the individual and family also affects the impact of the trauma or disaster event, both short and long term. Client needs and individual service delivery requirements will also vary across the entire recovery period.

Another variable in crisis management is culture. Culture plays a role in how a crisis situation is interpreted, and the best means by which people and communities can be helped. Understanding and accepting cultural differences is an important dimension of helping to restore people to their precrisis level of functioning (Dykeman, 2005).

COMMUNITY RESPONSE PATTERNS

The Joint Commission (2003) explicitly portrays disaster management and emergency preparedness as a community responsibility. When disaster strikes, the existence and function of the community are significantly impaired, and even in danger of extinction. Initially people are confused and stunned. Emotions vary as the extent of the impact is realized. The closer the person is to the crisis event, the more intense is the impact (Myer & Moore, 2006). The immediate concern is protection of self and those closest to them. The community response to disaster characteristically consists of four phases:

- Heroic phase
- Honeymoon phase
- Disillusionment phase
- Reconstruction phase

The shock of the disaster pulls people together. Emergency medical teams, neighbors, and friends rally around the survivors, offering emotional support and tangible supplies needed for recovery. The *honeymoon phase* occurs when the "community pulls together and outside resources are brought in" after an initial search and recovery phase (Bowenkamp, 2000, p. 159). This phase typically lasts up to 6 months after disaster. The focus of intervention is to ensure the public health safety of the victims. Establishing an infrastructure to support the immediate needs of the population related to water, sanitation, food supplies, and insect and rodent control are essential services (Campos-Outcalt, 2006). Sharing the experience of the trauma with others and having tangible evidence of continuing support are crucial components of effective response.

The *disillusionment phase* usually appears as the initial emergency response starts to subside. The "shared community" feeling starts to leave as people begin to realize the extent of their losses and the limitations of external support. Survivors can experience anger, resentment, and bitterness at the loss of support, particularly if it is sudden and complete. Kaplan, Iancu, and Bodner (2000) suggest that opportunities for psychological debriefing sessions should continue for a period well beyond the initial disaster experience for victims of extreme stress.

The final *reconstruction phase* occurs when the survivors begin to take the primary responsibility for rebuilding their lives. This period can last for several years after a disaster. Ongoing support is required as survivors learn to cope with new roles and responsibilities, and to develop new alternatives to living a full life after trauma. Although the disaster experience recedes in memory, it is never lost, and the person may never again fully trust in the continuity of life and being in control of one's destiny. Kaminsky, McCabe, Langlieb, and Everly (2007) describe recovery from the clinical distress, impairment, and dysfunction associated with terrorism and mass disaster as evidenced in the ability to adaptively function psychologically and behaviorally.

DISASTER MANAGEMENT IN HEALTH CARE SETTINGS

In 2006, the Joint Commission added new standards for credentialing volunteer health care professionals in declared emergency situations. All hospitals are required to form disaster committees composed of key departments within the hospital, including nursing. That committee is charged with developing disaster plans and implementing practice with them at least twice a year. A rapid credentialing process must be in place. Nurses interested in emergency volunteer activities should become aware of credentialing requirements to ensure their participation as part of a national emergency volunteer system for health professionals.

The Uniform Emergency Volunteer Health Practitioners Act (UEVHPA) provides consistent standards designed to facilitate organized response efforts among volunteer health practitioners in declared emergencies, disaster relief, and public health crisis situations (National Conference of Commissioners on Uniform State Laws, 2006).

Hospital and community disaster planning must be coordinated so that all phases of the disaster cycle are covered. Designated hospital personnel must receive training to carry out triage at the emergency department entrance. Protocols should contain the capability to relocate staff and clients to another facility if necessary, and a plan must be in place detailing mechanisms for equipment resupply. Policies regarding notification, maintenance of accurate records, and establishment of a facility control center are required.

Citizen Responders

Unsolicited responders will play a large role in sudden onset, large scale disasters. Auf der Heide (2006) suggests that emergency plans should anticipate the presence of unsolicited responders and have an infrastructure for coordinating their efforts. Public education related to the citizen role in disaster management is essential.

Citizen Corps Programs, developed by FEMA, is a grassroots crisis intervention strategy that can provide community volunteers with a program to develop emergency preparedness and first-aid skills. The Web site (http://www.citizencorps.gov) provides training and tool kits to help improve the on-site care of disaster victims. It also provides links to information for families interested in developing emergency preparedness around the following issues:

- Providing children and family members with family work and cell phone numbers; name and number of neighbor, friend, or relative; emergency 911, fire, poison control, and police number (these should be posted in a conspicuous place).
- Choosing an out of town contact and instructions on how to make contact.
- Choosing a place to meet with other family members in case of emergency.
- Planning for pets, as they are not allowed in emergency shelters.

Family emergency preparedness plans should be updated annually.

HELPING CHILDREN COPE WITH TRAUMA

Children do not have the same resources when coping with traumatic events as adults do. Preexisting exposure to traumatic events and lack of social support increases vulnerability. It is not unusual for children to demonstrate regressive behaviors as a reaction to crisis. Knapp (2010) suggests that using rituals and memorials for children experiencing loss of peers at school is helpful in mitigating trauma impact. Having a place where children can bring flowers and other mementos commemorating their peer's death is important.

Children will look for cues from key adults in their lives and tend to mirror their adult caregivers, so it is essential to communicate calm and confidence. More than anything else, children need reassurance that they and the people who are important to them are safe. Encourage the family to maintain regular routines. Parents need to provide children with opportunities both to talk about crisis and to ask questions. Repetitive questions are to be expected. Often they reflect the child's need for reassurance. Offering factual information helps dispel misperceptions.

HELPING OLDER ADULTS COPE WITH TRAUMA

Functional limitations associated with compromised physical mobility, diminished sensory awareness, and preexisting health conditions can create special issues for older clients impacted by a disaster. Older adults have more injury and greater disaster-related deaths than adults in other age groups (Fernandez, Byard, Lin, Benson, & Barbera, 2002). Especially vulnerable are house bound and socially isolated individuals. Other population groups needing extra attention are those who require medical or nursing care, and those receiving services, care, or food from health, social, or volunteer agencies.

Disaster management for older adults needs to be proactive. The following core actions can make a difference in helping older adults weather a disaster event successfully. Proactive planning includes:

- Identify a support network that can be used in an emergency situation. Facilitate connections with social support systems and community support structures. Have this information readily available for use in an emergency situation.
- Older adults with a disability should wear tags or a bracelet to identify their disability. Keeping extra eyeglasses and hearing aid batteries on hand, and identifying any assistive devices is essential.
- Identify the closest special needs evacuation center.
- Develop a written list of all medications, with any special directions, for example, crushing pills, hours of administration, and dietary restrictions.
- Identify physicians and social support contacts, including someone apart from people in the local area who can be contacted.

Other actions, such as ensuring the safety, meeting mobility needs, and medication administration, will need careful attention during the course of actual disaster management. Even the most capable older adult can appear confused and vulnerable in a disaster situation. Reducing anxiety is especially important for the older adult disaster victim. Actions nurses can take include the following:

- Initiate contact and take the older adult to as safe a place as possible.
- Speak calmly and provide concrete information about what is happening, and what you need the older adult to do in simple terms.
- Assess for mobility and provide assistance where needed.
- Older adults may need warmer clothing because of compromised temperature regulation.

SUMMARY

Crisis is defined as an unexpected, sudden turn of events or set of circumstances requiring an immediate human response. People experience a crisis as overwhelming, traumatic, and personally intrusive. It is an unexpected life event challenging a person's sense of self and his or her place in the world. The most common types of crisis are situational and developmental crises. Most health crises are situational. Crisis can be private involving one person, or public involving large numbers of people. James (2008) describes two additional types of crisis: existential and ecosystem crisis.

Theoretical frameworks guiding crisis intervention include Lindemann's (1944) model of grieving, derived from his clinical work with survivors of a nightclub fire. Caplan's (1964) model is based on preventive psychiatry concepts. Aguilera's nursing model explores the role of balancing factors in defusing the impact of a crisis state. Erikson's (1982) model of psychosocial development forms the basis for developmental crisis.

Crisis intervention is a time-limited treatment that focuses only on the immediate problem and its resolution. Roberts' (2005) seven-stage model is used to guide nursing interventions: assessing lethality, establishing rapport, dealing with feelings, defining the problem, exploring alternative options, formulating a plan, and follow-up measures. The goal of crisis intervention is to return the client to his or her precrisis level of functioning.

Mental health emergencies require immediate assessment interventions and close supervision. The most common types are violence, suicide, and a psychotic break. Guidelines for communication with clients experiencing mental health emergencies (e.g.,

violence and suicide) focus on safety and rapid stabilization of the client's behavior.

As the world becomes more dynamically unstable, nurses will need to understand the dimensions of disaster management and develop the skills to respond effectively in disaster situations. Disaster management is a special kind of crisis intervention applied to large groups of people. The Joint Commission (2003) requires hospitals to develop and exercise disaster management plans at regular intervals. Critical incident debriefing is a crisis intervention strategy designed to help those closely involved with disasters process critical incidents in health care, thereby reducing the possibility of symptoms occurring.

ETHICAL DILEMMA   What Would You Do?

Sara Murdano was only 20 when she came to the mobile intensive care unit (MICU), but this is not her first hospital admission. She has been treated for depression previously. She states she is determined to kill herself because she has nothing to live for, and that is her right to do so because she is no longer a minor. As she describes her life to date, you can't help but think that she really doesn't have a lot to live for. How would you respond to this client from an ethical perspective?

REFERENCES

Aguilera D: *Crisis intervention: theory and methodology*, ed 7, St Louis, 1998, Mosby.

American Psychiatric Association: *Practice guidelines for the assessment and treatment of patients with suicidal behaviors*, Arlington, VA, 2003, American Psychiatric Association.

Artean C, Williams L: What we learned from the Oklahoma City bombing, *Nursing* 28(3):52–55, 1998.

Auf der Heide E: The importance of evidence-based disaster planning, *Ann Emerg Med* 47(1):34–49, 2006.

Bowenkamp C: Coordination of mental health and community agencies in disaster, *Int J Emerg Ment Health* 2:159–165, 2000.

Boyd MA: *Psychiatric nursing: contemporary practice*, ed 4, Philadelphia, 2008, Wolters Kluwer Health/Lippincott Williams & Wilkins.

Bluhm J: Helping families in crisis hold on, *Nursing* 17(10):44–46, 1987.

Callahan I: Crisis theory and crisis intervention in emergencies. In Kleespies PM, editor: *Emergencies in mental health: evaluation and management*, New York, 1998, Guilford Press.

Campos-Outcalt D: Disaster medical response: maximizing your effectiveness, *Fam Pract* 55(2):113–115, 2006.

Caplan G: *Principles of preventive psychiatry*, New York, 1964, Basic Books.

Caplan G: Recent developments in crisis intervention and the promotion of support service, *J Prim Prev* 10(1):3, 1989.

Captain C: Is your patient a suicide risk? *Nursing* 36(8):43–47, 2006.

Curtis J: Elements of critical incident debriefing, *Psychol Rep* 77 (1):91–96, 1995.

Dass-Brailsford P: *Crisis and disaster counseling: lessons learned from Hurricane Katrina and other disasters*, Thousand Oaks, CA, 2010, Sage Publications.

Davis S: *De-escalation tips in crisis situations,* Rockville, MD, 2010, Montgomery County, MD Police Department.

Davis S: *Field expedient tool to assess dangerousness in self and others,* Rockville, MD, 2010, Montgomery County, MD Police Department.

Deeny P, McFetridge B: The impact of disaster on culture, self, and identity: increased awareness by health care professionals is needed, *Nurs Clin North Am* 40(3):431–444, 2005.

Dietz D: Debriefing to help perinatal nurses cope with a maternal loss, *MCN* 34(4):243–248, 2009.

Dirkzwager A, Kerssens J, Yzermans C: Health problems in children and adolescents before and after a man-made disaster, *J Am Acad Child Adolesc Psychiatry* 45(1):94–103, 2006.

Dykeman BF: Cultural implications of crisis intervention, *J Instr Psychol* 32(1):45–48, 2005.

Erikson E: *The life cycle completed*, New York, 1982, Norton.

Everly G: Five principles of crisis intervention: Reducing the risk of premature crisis intervention, *Int J Emerg Ment Health* 2(1):1–4, 2000.

Everly G, Flynn B: Principles and practical procedures for acute first aid training for personnel without mental health experience, *Int J Emerg Ment Health* 8(2):93–100, 2006.

Everly G, Mitchell J: The debriefing "controversy" and crisis intervention: a review of lexical and substantive issues, *Int J Emerg Ment Health* 2(4):211–225, 2000.

Fernandez LS, Byard D, Lin CC, Benson S, Barbera JA: Frail elderly as disaster victims: Emergency management strategies, *Prehospital Disaster Med* 17(2):67–74, 2002.

Flannery R: Treating family survivors of mass casualties: a CISM family crisis intervention approach, *Int J Emerg Ment Health* 1(4):243–250, 1999.

Flannery RB Jr, Everly GS Jr: Crisis intervention: a review, *Int J Emerg Ment Health* 2(2):119–125, 2000.

Greene G, Lee M, Trask R, Rheinscheld J: How to work with strengths in crisis intervention: a solution focused approach. In Roberts AR, editor: *Crisis intervention handbook*, New York, 2005, Oxford University Press.

Hendriks L, Bassi S: Emergency preparedness from the ground floor up: a local agency perspective, *Home Health Care Manag Pract* 21 (5):346–352, 2009.

Hoff L: *People in crisis: cultural and diversity perspectives*, ed 6, New York, 2009, Routledge, Taylor & Francis Group.

Institute of Medicine, Butler AS, Panzer AM, Goldfrank LR: *Preparing for the psychological consequences of terrorism: a public health strategy*, Washington, DC, 2003, National Academies Press.

Jacobs D: *Screening for mental health: a resource guide for implementing the Joint Commission on Accreditation of Health Care Organizations (CAHO) 2007 patient safety goals on suicide*, Wellesley Hills, 2007, Screening for Mental Health Inc.

James R: *Crisis intervention strategies*, ed 6, Belmont, CA, 2008, Thomson Brooks/Cole.

Joint Commission: *Health care at the crossroads: strategies for creating and sustaining community-wide emergency preparedness systems*, Oakbrook Terrace, IL, 2003, Joint Commission on Accreditation of Health Care Organizations.

Kaminsky M, McCabe O, Langlieb A, Everly G: An evidence-informed model of human resistance, resilience, and recovery: the Johns Hopkins' outcome-driven paradigm for disaster mental health services, *Brief Treat Crisis Interv* 7(1):1–11, 2007.

Kaplan Z, Iancu I, Bodner E: A review of psychological debriefing after extreme stress, *Psychiatr Serv* 52(6):824–827, 2000.

Kavan M, Guck T, Barone E: A practical guide to crisis management, *Am Fam Physician* 74(7):1159–1164, 2006.

Keely B: Recognition and prevention of hospital violence, *Dimens Crit Care Nurs* 21(6):236–241, 2002.

Kleeman K: Families in crisis due to multiple trauma, *Crit Care Nurs Clin North Am* 1(1):25, 1989.

Knapp K: Children and crises. In Dass-Brailsford P, editor: *Crisis and disaster counseling: lessons learned from Hurricane Katrina and other disasters*, Thousand Oaks, CA, 2010, Sage Publications, pp 83–97.

Lahad M: Darkness over the abyss: supervising crisis intervention teams following disaster [online article],*Traumatology* 6(4):2000. Available online http://www.fsu.edu/~trauma/v6i4/v6i4a4.html.

Lindemann E: Symptomatology and management of acute grief, *Am J Psychiatry* 101:141–148, 1944.

Luck L, Jackson D, Usher K: STAMP: components of observable behaviour that indicate potential for patient violence in emergency departments, *J Adv Nurs* 59(1):11–19, 2007.

Maguen S, Papa A, Litz B: Coping with the threat of terrorism: a review, *Anxiety Stress Coping* 21(1):15–35, 2008.

Michalopoulos H, Micalopoulos A: Crisis counseling: be prepared to intervene, *Nursing* 39(9):47–50, 2009.

Myer R, Conte C: Assessment for crisis intervention, *J Clin Psychol* 62 (8):959–970, 2006.

Myer RA, Moore HB: Crisis in context theory: an ecological model, *J Couns Dev* 84(spring):139–147, 2006.

National Conference of Commissioners on Uniform State Laws: *Uniform Emergency Volunteer Health Practioners Act, 2006*. Available online http://www.uevhpa.org/DesktopDefault.aspx?tabindex=1&tabid=55. Accessed February 16, 2010.

Noji EK: The public health consequences of disasters, *Prehosp Disaster Med* 15(4):21–31, 2000.

Perry J, Jagger J: Reducing risks from combative patients, *Nursing* 33 (10):28, 2003.

Powley E: Reclaiming resilience and safety: resilience in the critical period of crisis, *Hum Relat* 62(9):1289–1326, 2009.

Roberts A: *Crisis intervention handbook: assessment, treatment and research*, New York, 2005, Oxford University Press.

Roberts A, Yeager K: *Pocket guide to crisis intervention*, New York, 2009, Oxford University Press.

Roberts A, Monferrari I, Yeager K: Avoiding malpractice lawsuits by following risk assessment and suicide prevention guidelines, *Brief Treat Crisis Interv* 8:5–14, 2008.

Rubin J: Critical incident stress debriefing: helping the helpers, *J Emerg Nurs* 16(4):255–258, 1990.

Spurlock W, Brown S, Rami J: Disaster care: delivering primary health care to hurricane evacuees, *Am J Nurs* 109(8):50–53, 2009.

Stellrecht N, Gordon K, Van Orden K, et al: Clinical applications of the interpersonal-psychological theory of attempted and completed suicide, *J Clin Psychol* 62(2)II:211–222, 2006.

Webb NB, editor: *Mass trauma and violence: helping families and children cope*, New York, 2004, Guilford Press.

CHAPTER 22

Communication for a Safe Environment

Kathleen Underman Boggs

OBJECTIVES

At the end of the chapter, the reader will be able to:

1. Identify client communication safety goals.
2. Identify how communication skills enhance client safety, as well as quality of care.
3. Describe why client safety is a complex system issue, as well as an individual function.
4. Describe how open communication and organizational error reporting contribute to a culture of safety.

5. Discuss how to advocate for safe, high-quality care as a team member.
6. Use simulations to demonstrate communication skills that affect client care; specifically apply standardized formats such as SBAR in a simulated conversation with a physician.

This chapter focuses on communication concepts designed to assist nurses and their health team colleagues in creating a safe environment for their clients. Although "safety" is recently getting increased attention, client safety is (and has always been) a priority in nursing care (Gore, Hunt, & Raines, 2008). Quality of care is dependent, in part, on communication (Joint Commission on Accreditation of Healthcare Organizations [JCAHO], 2008). Miscommunication is a dominant factor cited in error reports. The quality of communication and the quality of the client-provider relationship have long been used as indicators of quality of care (Agency for Healthcare Research and Quality [AHRQ,c]).

BASIC CONCEPTS

SAFETY DEFINITION

In healthcare organizations, safety is generally defined as freedom from accidental injury. Since the days of Hippocrates, the concept of "do no harm" has been incorporated into healthcare ethical practice. The nursing profession has always had safe practice as a major goal. It is the basic tenet of the American Nurses Association's Code of Ethics for Nurses. The National Patient Safety Foundation (NPSF; online, www.npsf.org/pdf/r/researchagenda. pdf) has a more specific definition: "avoidance, prevention, amelioration of adverse outcomes or injuries stemming from the process of healthcare itself." In a more comprehensive definition, the American Association of Colleges of Nursing (AACN, 2006a) defines safety as the minimalization of risk for harm to patients and to providers through both system effectiveness and individual performance. *Health care organizations* and *professional organizations* generally try to ensure safe care by establishing safety rules and procedures. This chapter restricts discussion to innovations in communication procedures designed to improve client safety.

RECENT OVERALL SAFETY ISSUES

In the early part of this century, the quality and safety of health care in the United States was mediocre or worse (Bates, 2009). In a British study comparing mortality data from the United States with 14 other Western countries between 1997 and 2003, the United States had only a 4% decrease in deaths from amenable causes, whereas the average decrease for other countries was 17% (Nolte & McKee, 2008). Much has changed in our practice since the landmark 1999 Institute of Medicine (IOM) study that found that preventable health care errors were responsible for almost 98,000 deaths each year in the United States. This IOM report, "To Err Is Human: Building a Safer Health System," made client safety a national American priority (Kohn, 1999).

Expense, resistance to change, and the lack of centralized data reporting slowed adoption of new practices. Worldwide, unsafe practice has compromised care for clients in many countries. Errors have a high financial cost in addition to the human cost, exceeding $29 billion dollars per year just in the United States (AHRQb). It is estimated that 70% of reported errors are preventable. "Preventable" means the error occurs through a medical intervention, not because of the client's illness. Fatigue is repeatedly cited as a factor contributing to errors. Risk doubled when nurses worked more than 12 consecutive hours (Scott, Rodgers, Hwang, & Zhang, 2006). Medical and Nursing organizations, as well as health care delivery organizations, have taken initiatives designed to foster "**best practice**" safer client care by designing protocols for care that are evidence based. At the same time, new technology tools are making care safer (refer to Chapters 25 and 26). This chapter limits discussion to only those practices relevant to communication.

Nurses are often the "last line of defense" against error. It is an ethical imperative (Lachman, 2008). Nurses are in a position to prevent, intercept, or correct errors. Individual nurses have many opportunities to prevent error, particularly by communicating clearly to others even when the hierarchy seems to discourage questioning authorities (Donaldson, 2008). The quality of your communication affects safety factors such as medication errors, client injuries from falls, clinical outcomes related to client adherence to his treatment plan, and rehospitalization rates. The Applications section of this chapter focuses on nursing communication practices to promote safer care.

POOR COMMUNICATION COMPROMISES CLIENT SAFETY

Multiple studies have pinpointed miscommunication as a major causative agent in sentinel events, that is, errors resulting in unnecessary death and serious injury (Leonard & Bonacum, 2008). Poor communication has been identified as the root cause of serious medical errors as much as 70% of the time in reported errors (Joint Commission, b,c). However, errors do not usually have one cause but result from a series of flaws in the care system. The problem is complex; therefore, solutions also will be complex.

MEDICATION ERRORS

According to the American Medical Association (AMA, eVoice, 2008), approximately 80% of medication errors are due to communication breakdown. Although some medication errors stem from lack of knowledge about the drug (its side effects, etc.), many other drug errors occur when a nurse fails to follow the rules for verification: right med, right client, right dose, and right time.

MISCOMMUNICATION DURING "HANDOFF" TRANSFERS OF CLIENT

Miscommunication errors most often occur during a handoff procedure, when one staff member transfers responsibility for care to another staff member. More than half of incidences of reported serious miscommunications occurred during *client handoff*, when those assuming responsibility for the client (coming on duty) are given a verbal, face-to-face synopsis of the client's current condition by those who had been caring for him and are now going off duty (Evans, Pereira, & Parker, 2008; Henkind & Sinnett, 2008).

CLIENT OUTCOMES

The literature suggests some progress in preventing sentinel events, but errors are still common, resulting in unnecessary harm to clients. In addition to errors, outcomes include increased costs, increased rates of hospitalization, longer recovery rates, and more medical complications. Beside risks to client safety, poor communication is also related to client dissatisfaction and risk for malpractice lawsuits. A survey of clients found that 34% experienced errors and 68% cited poor communication between nurses and physicians and others as a cause of errors (Kaiser Family Foundation, 2004). Annual current statistics about sentinel events are available on the Joint Commission Web site (TJC, c).

NEW INITIATIVES FOR SAFER CARE

We are redeveloping our health care system to make client care safer. There is consensus that this requires improving communication. Best nurse-physician collaborative communication has empirically been associated with lower risk for negative client outcomes and greater satisfaction. Research studies support this concept (DeVoe, Wallace, Pandhi, Solotaroff, & Fryer, 2008; Elder, Brungs, Nagy, Kudel, & Render, 2008). The current renewed focus on improving patient safety will cause standardization of many health care practices. "Standardization is among the best methods to improve quality and reduce costs of care…even if the standard is something as simple as a checklist" (Mathews & Pronovost, 2008, p. 2914). Changes in communication to reduce errors and increase safety need to be institutionalized at the system level and implemented consistently at the staff level. Safe communication about client care matters needs to be clear, unambiguous, timely, accurate, complete, open, and understood by the recipient to reduce errors (Amato-Vealey, Barba, & Vealey, 2008).

COMMUNICATION GOALS AND STANDARDS TO IMPROVE CLIENT SAFETY

Overall, medical goals are complex and have shifting priorities. Safe client care is always a priority, however. Measuring safety is problematic because not everyone uses the same definitions of "unsafe," nor do they use the same outcome measures. The number of surgeries done on the wrong site is a very specific outcome, even though most hospitals do not report to a national overseer in the United States, so data may not be readily accessible. When we focus on communication problems leading to adverse client outcomes, the data are much less specific. With the current increased focus on improving communication to promote a climate of client safety, we need communication that is open

and client centered. Safety goals to improve communication about clients among his or her various providers are aimed at reducing client mortality, decreasing medical errors, and promoting effective health care teamwork. These goals need to be mutually established by the health team in a climate of respect to assure maximum clarity among providers.

Communication health care safety goals from governing organizations include:

1. *IOM's 8 Goals.* A worldwide wake up occurred when IOM published their report, citing hospital errors as causing almost 100,000 deaths per year. Yet, 5 years later, Nolte and McKee's (2008) analysis showed more than 101,000 preventable deaths per year in clients younger than 75 years. The IOM specifically included improving accurate, complete communication as one of their eight goals. IOM has suggested that hospitals need to create structured handoff protocols, that is, a standardized format for reporting client status when care provider A goes off duty, turning care responsibility over to care provider B. This standardized communication format is needed to facilitate better communication for patient safety.

2. *AHRQ* in the Department of Health and Human Services, with a Congressional mandate, has taken a leading role in the United States to improve client safety. AHRQ's role is to prevent medical errors and promote client safety. They fund research and compile data to develop and publish "best practices" evidenced-based care protocols. Several other sites publish "best practice info" (online resources such as http://healthlinks.washington.edu/ebp).

3. The *World Health Organization* (WHO), a part of the United Nations, has actively sought to improve worldwide client safety. In 2005, WHO designated Joint Commission International as the WHO Collaborating Center for patient safety solutions. In 2007, WHO (Joint Commission International) published nine solutions; number 2 is "correctly identifying the patient," and number 3 is "better communication during patient hand-over" (from one caregiver to another).

Communication goals for healthcare safety from professional organizations include:

1. *Joint Commission Guidelines.* This organization regulates hospitals. They attribute more than

60% of sentinel events in hospitals to miscommunication. Many of their current National Patient Safety Goals are aimed at structuring and improving communication. Goal 2 is to improve the effectiveness of communication among caregivers. Section 2E addresses communication guidelines needed to manage handoff communication. When a client is transferred or "handed off" to another care provider, unit, or agency, hospitals are encouraged to develop a standard communication protocol to improve the effectiveness of communication. This should result in increased client safety (AHRQ,c).

2. *AACN*. Recommendations for nursing curriculums related to safety and communication include application of research-based/evidence-based knowledge as the basis for practice; recognition that safety is a complex issue that involves all providers; establishing and maintaining…open communication and cooperation within the interdisciplinary team; and using standardized "hand off" communications (AACN, 2006a).

CHANGES TOWARD BETTERING COMMUNICATIONS LEADING TO SAFER CARE

General communication problems identified by the AMA are listed in Box 22-1. Foremost recommendations include:

Use "best practices" by increasing use of evidenced-based "best practice" versus "usual practice." Agencies such as AHRQ (c) have begun to fund research to

BOX 22-1	Patient Communication Universal Precautions [Communication Problems]

1. Difficulty obtaining, processing, and understanding information
2. Health care system complexity
3. Practice pressures
4. Cultural and language issues
5. Lack of clinician training on effective communication strategies
6. Low health literacy

From AMA, Safe Communications Universal Precautions, Patient safety tip card. AMA Bookstore, 2008. Modified from AMA: American Medical Association eVoice, Best Practice Information, October 2, 2008. Only available on-line by subscription. Downloaded 5/2/09.

identify the most effective methods of promoting clear communication among health team members and agencies, as well as the most effective treatments. This information is used to develop and distribute protocols for best practice, including formats of standard communication techniques. We need more studies of interventions to promote best communication between nurse and physician with documented outcomes for clients.

Create a team culture of safety communication. Creating effective health teams means getting all team members to value teamwork more than individual autonomy. Team culture includes shared norms, values, beliefs, and staff expectations. In Canada, Sutter et al.'s 2009 study, as well as findings from the Canadian Health Services Research Foundation, identified effective team communication as a core competency. Team *collaborative communication strategies* involve shared responsibility for problem solving and decision making, as well as coordination of care. Teamwork failures including poor communication and failures in physician supervision have been implicated in two-thirds of harmful errors to clients (Singh, Thomas, Peterson, & Studdert, 2007). Creating a safe environment requires us to communicate openly, to be vigilant and accountable. Systems should create expectations of a work environment in which staff can speak up and express concerns, and alert team members to unsafe situations.

PROBLEMS OR BARRIERS FOR INDIVIDUAL HEALTH CARE WORKERS

Strategies for effective communication to promote client safety are listed in Box 22-2. They are discussed in the following subsections.

USUAL PRACTICE VERSUS EMPIRICALLY DERIVED BEST PRACTICES

There is a major lack of research utilization for best practice. Though you are exposed to the use of research findings in your practice, many staff nurses lack the time and skills to actively seek new study results that would improve their daily practice. Physicians are still likely to use their own experience rather than documented recommended best practice methods. Research-based

BOX 22-2	Strategies for Effective Communication to Promote Client Safety

1. Use standardized interdisciplinary communication tools/formats that promote collaboration, so everybody is "on the same page."
2. Use communication tools that promote clear, comprehensive communication when clients are moved between units or agencies, such as checklists.
3. Establish a psychological safe climate: identify opportunities for improving safety.
4. Participate in ongoing dialogue (via team meetings, periodic conference calls, etc.) to share successes.
5. Maintain awareness of potential situational safety concerns and planning standardized contingency responses (e.g., critical event training using simulation).
6. Restructure into teams that maintain a climate of open communication.

evidence is often absent or lacks high-quality consensus. Widespread adoption of best practices had not yet been accomplished in the decade after IOM's 1999 report. Best practice recommended therapies were found to have been received by only 55% of adult clients and 47% of child clients (Mangione-Smith et al., 2007).

COMMUNICATION DIFFERENCES AMONG PROFESSIONS

Each profession has its unique vocabulary and method of communicating. Physician's expectations may be "just the facts" briefly, whereas nurses have been educated to describe the broad picture. Medical communication is a goal-oriented, problem-solving behavior, which requires not only skill practicing but reflection on the process and outcome. Developing communication skills has now become a curriculum thread in nursing educational programs.

Hierarchical power differences exist between physicians and nurses. This difference in power intimidates some nurses communicating with physicians. Historic autonomy for physicians is being replaced by empowerment of teams for decision making. The concept of equity is integral to a functioning team. Historically, physicians and nurses are accustomed to working in a hierarchy where physicians make treatment decisions independently rather than though consultations with a team. This is sometimes termed medicine's "culture of individualism." Implementing measures specified by best practice evidence and sharing decision making about the client's care require that physicians correspondingly relinquish some autonomy (Mathews & Pronovost, 2008). Effective teamwork, including open communication, openness to new concepts, and honest error reporting, are basic components in establishing a new safety culture. This requires some readjustment in the way both physicians and nurses think about their roles.

RELUCTANCE TO REPORT ERRORS

According to IOM, only a tiny fraction of unsafe care incidents are submitted to reporting databases or agencies (Kohn, 1999). Some estimate that more than 90% of errors go unreported (Elder et al., 2008). A redesign is needed if we really want to create a culture of safety. The health care industry is looking at models created by other industries such as aviation or nuclear power, which have excellent safety records. Aviation's successful Crew Resource Management practice model has been used as a template for some in the health care industry. One needed step is to require the reporting of "near misses" so new safer protocols can be created. A centralized agency, such as the United Kingdom's Patient Safety Agency, with a database on instances of errors and near misses would provide a database for analyses that would be of great use in designing safer delivery systems. In the United States, error reporting is hidden, underreported, and local, rather than being nationally available. Accurate incident reporting and greater transparency are crucial if future errors are to be prevented.

Another step in creating a culture of safety is to overcome current fear of punitive outcomes involved in error reporting. Providers are concerned about negative consequences of disclosing errors, such as malpractice litigation, reputation damage, job security, personal feelings such as loss of self-esteem, among others. Elder et al.'s (2008) study reported that nurses remain strongly conflicted about disclosing their errors to peers and physicians. In their survey, less than half of the intensive care unit nurses witnessing a near-miss error were likely to report it. Creating a new safety climate would require retraining nurses in error disclosure to help prevent future errors. Meanwhile providers struggle with the current systems for reporting errors.

LOW LEVEL OF CLIENT HEALTH LITERACY VERSUS CLIENT EDUCATION

Multiple studies show that health-care–related communication occurs at a level far exceeding the understanding abilities of the majority of average persons (Denham, 2008). According to the AMA, 50% of adults are at increased risk for serious adverse health consequences because of their low level of understanding of medical terminology and their tendency to hide this problem from their doctors and nurses. Inadequate heath literacy leads clients to misunderstand information about their treatment, causing errors.

BARRIERS IN THE CURRENT HEALTH CARE SYSTEM

PROBLEMS WITH STRUCTURAL BARRIERS IN HEALTH CARE ORGANIZATIONS THAT IMPEDE COMMUNICATIONS

The greatest barrier to safer care is fragmentation of care systems. Evidenced-based practices have to be reinforced and implemented at a system-wide level. Although most hospitals and agencies have some form of error reporting, they lack a system-wide department for processing safety information. One model to be emulated is that of Kaiser Permanente, which implemented a national patient safety plan in 2000.

Developing an Evidenced-Based Practice

Messmer PR: Enhancing nurse-physician collaboration using pediatric simulation, *J Contin Educ Nurs* 39(7):319–327, 2008.

The purpose of this study was to describe levels of nurse-physician collaboration during simulation training. Videos of collaborative behaviors of 55 pediatric residents and 50 nurses during 3 mock codes using a pediatric human patient simulator depicting life-threatening scenarios were analyzed using standardized measures and observations.

Results: In the initial scenario, there was little collaborative discussion between nurses and residents, but overtime by the third scenario collaborative communication predominated. Scores showed high levels of group cohesion and collaboration, and participants expressed satisfaction with patient care decisions. Male respondents regardless of discipline had significantly greater cohesion scores than did female respondents. Competency scores increased over time.

Application to Your Practice: Interdisciplinary clinical simulation exercises can increase your ability to communicate and collaborate successfully with physicians, as well as increasing your care skill competency.

APPLICATIONS

Discussion in this section is limited to safety strategies that promote effective communication such as the mantra "Simplify, Clarify, Verify" (Fleischmann, 2008). A few general strategies are mentioned. (For a complete discussion, refer to IOM [2001, 2004].) Consider how you will apply evidence-based practice information such as that in the sample.

NEW TEACHING STRATEGIES TO HELP NURSES LEARN TO COMMUNICATE FOR SAFER CARE

Quality and Safety Education competencies for all Nurses (QSEN) have been developed by national leaders in nursing education (for full discussion, refer to Cronenwett et al. [2007]). Among these competencies are communicatión skills. Some new teaching strategies help students.

DEVELOP A SAFETY PRIORITY ATTITUDE

The IOM has urged organizations to create an environment in which safety is a top priority. For example, equipment can be standardized and simplified, and display a readout about the reason an alarm is ringing. One of our primary roles as nurses is to advocate for client safety. Beyea (2008a) recommends that nurses, as individuals, take active efforts to improve our safety understanding, beginning by assessing our own safety learning needs in our particular area of practice (online, NPSF: EdNeedsAsessment, www.npsf.org/pdf/r/researchagenda.pdf). Errors occur when you assume someone else has addressed a situation (Beyea, 2008b). A prime goal is to improve communication about client condition among all the people providing care to that client.

USE PRACTICE SIMULATIONS

Virtual client-nurse scenarios, whether using technologically enhanced dummies or active learning situations such as case studies provided in this textbook, allow practice without risk for potentially devastating outcomes with an actual client care situation. Nursing education programs are beginning to use "live models" to simulate clients. Actors are trained to portray clients with specific illnesses. Student nurses practice communicating with them to elicit histories, as well as practicing skills such as physical examinations. (For more ideas, read Gore et al. [2008] and Henneman [2009].)

DEVELOP AN EVIDENCE-BASED PRACTICE

Close the gap between best evidence and the way communication occurs in your current practice (Figure 22-1). Apply information from evidence-based best practice

databanks for safe practice. The process for development of practice guidelines, protocols, situation checklists, and so on is not transparent or easy. Solutions include gathering more evidence on which to base our practice. When is the "evidence" sufficiently strong to warrant adoption of a standardized form of communication about care? At the nurse-client level, Beauregard, nurse-administrator at Beaumont Hospital in Royal Oak, Michigan, has commented that "the nurse-patient relationship is a pivotal component of any patient safety program...(and) the number one driver of patient safety is communication" (Runy, 2008). We are beginning to compile best practice protocols for acute and preventative care; many are available on AHRQ's Web site (online, www.ahrq.gov) or in

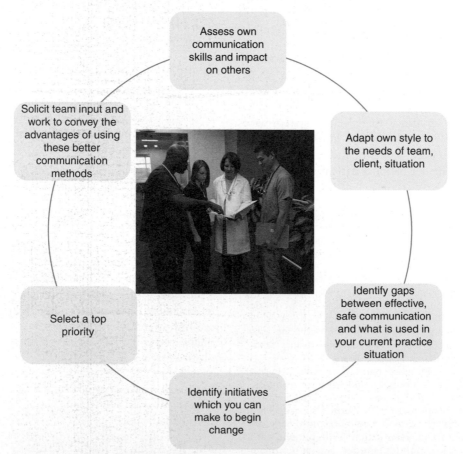

Figure 22-1 Communication competencies for creating safer care. *(Adapted from Carey M, Buchan H, Sanson-Fisher R: The cycle of change: implementing best-evidence clinical practice, Int J Qual Healthc 21(1):37–43, 2009; Cronenwett L, Sherwood G, Barnsteiner J, et al.: Quality and safety education for nurses, Nurs Outlook 55(3):122–131, 2007.)*

their *Patient Safety and Quality: An Evidence-Based Handbook for Nurses* (Hughes, 2008). Even though these are free and available to all, studies show that best care is delivered only half of the time (Mangione-Smith et al., 2007). In regard specifically to communication, so far there is relatively scant research to designate specific communication formats that will lead to safer care. Some of the clinical strategies that show promise are described in the following subsections.

Use Data from Analyses of Error Data Reporting to Improve Nursing Practices

A metaanalysis of results from error reporting demonstration grants found that as error reporting improves, error detection rates increase and severity decreases (AHRQ, b,d).

Use Standardized Communication Tools

Safety communication improvement solutions include using standardized communications tools, participating in team training communicating seminars, adopting technology-oriented tools, and empowering clients to be partners in safer care. Communication that promotes client safety needs to include both communication of concise critical information and active listening. Physicians, nurses, medical technologists, pharmacists, and other givers of care work in what Shortell and Singer (2008) call "functional silos"; that is, they are educated separately and for the most part work separately, which has caused them to have differing methods of communication. Educational programs impart very different communication expectations for nurses than those taught to medical students. Nurses are taught to communicate in detailed narrative form, to describe the broad picture when discussing a client with his physician. Physicians are taught to speak concisely, to diagnose and summarize. Or as Leonard and Bonacum (2008) say, "Physicians want bullet points," or just the headlines. Each group holds slightly different expectations about communication content and may have separate vocabularies. Nurses want their observations or assessments taken seriously. Solutions include team training and use of a standardized communication tool. Although currently there is no one universally accepted process, use of a shared format across disciplines can promote effective communication and client safety. The following are a sample of newer, more commonly used forms of team strategies designed to decrease or avoid errors of communication that lead to mistakes in health care.

Use of Checklists

Checklists serve as cognitive guides to accurate task completion. Checklists have been effectively used to improve client safety, especially in areas managing rapidly change, such as preoperative areas, emergency departments, and anesthesiology. Checklists have built-in redundancy. The floor nurse uses the preoperative checklist to verify that everything has been completed before sending the client to the surgical suite, but then this list is again checked when the client arrives but before the actual surgery. Such system redundancies are used to prevent errors. But they have limited and specific uses, and do not address underlying communication problems. No standardized protocol exists for checklist development, but use of expert panels with multiple pilot testing is recommended. One example found in most agency preoperative areas is a checklist where standard items are marked as having been done and available in the client's record/chart. For example, laboratory results are documented regarding blood type, clotting time, and so forth. In one cardiac area study, one common cause of adverse events was missing equipment; therefore, a checklist might be used before surgery to verify the presence of specific needed equipment (Wong et al., 2007). Adoption of assertion checklists empowers any team member to speak up when they become aware of missing information.

Use of SBAR

In 2002, at Kaiser Permanente's northern California regional risk management department's perinatal patient safety project, physicians and nurses training together expressed disappointment with their communication. In response, Bonacum, Leonard, and other Kaiser administrators developed and encouraged staff to begin implementing a standardized briefing format (known by its acronym **SBAR**) for use by all staff communicating with each other—nurses, physicians, and all other team members. Adapted by Bonacum (2009) from principles used in communication on nuclear submarines, the SBAR tool provides structured language and fosters active listening. SBAR is designed to convey only the most critical information by eliminating excessive language. SBAR eliminates the authority gradient, flattening the traditional physician-to-nurse hierarchy. This makes it possible for staff to say what they think is going on. This improves communication and creates collaboration. This concise format is gaining wide adoption in the United States and Great Britain (Bonacum, 2009; Fleishmann, 2008; Leonard, 2009; Leonard & Bonacum, 2008). Refer to Box 22-3.

SBAR is used as a situational briefing, so the team is "on the same page" (Bonacum, 2009). SBAR simplifies verbal communication between nurses and physicians because content is presented in an expected format. In addition to communications between two individuals, it is used in small groups, such as the obstetrical delivery team and the surgical team. Success soon spread this format to use in surgery, for telephone contacts and in other acute care settings. Velji et al. (2008) have shown SBAR use to also be effective in improving safe communication in other types of agencies, such as rehabilitation facilities. Some, including Kaiser Staff, have even informally adopted it for their e-mail communications (Bonacum, 2009). Some

hospitals use laminated SBAR guidelines at the telephones for nurses to use when calling physicians about changes in client status and requests for new orders (Leonard, 2009). Documenting the new order is the only part of SBAR that gets recorded. Refer to Table 22-1 for an example. Then practice your use of SBAR format in Exercise 22-1.

"Evidence-based reports show that [client] adverse events have decreased through use of SBAR" (Denham, 2008, p. 39). Practicing use of standardized communication formats by student nurses has been found to improve their ability to effectively communicate with physicians about emergent changes in client condition (Krautscheid, 2008). Use of a common communication tool with non-nurse members of the health team should also reduce risk (see Figure 22-1). This format sets expectation about what will be communicated to another member of the health care team. Practice using this format in Exercises 22-2 and 22-3.

TEAM TRAINING: MODELS OF COMMUNICATION STRATEGIES FOR COLLABORATIVE PRACTICE

HEALTH PROVIDER COLLABORATIONS

There is a close relationship between effective teamwork and client safety. Kramer and Schmalenberg developed a scale of five levels of collaboration based on their nursing research: collegial (equal in power but different); collaborative (mutual but not equal power); student-teacher (physicians have the power but are friendly and willing to inform nurses); neutral; and negative (physicians have total power and are disruptive to nurses, who then feel frustrated or hostile). The first three have good physician-nurse communication.

The majority of reported errors have been found to stem from poor teamwork and poor communication. An effective team has clear, accurate communication understood by all. All team members work together to promote a climate of client safety. To improve interdisciplinary health team collaboration, Boone and associates (2008) recommend that physicians and nurses jointly share communication training and team building sessions to develop an "us" rather than "them" work philosophy. When clashes occur, differences need to be settled. Specific conflict resolution techniques are discussed in Chapter 23.

BOX 22-3	SBAR Example

Clinical Example of Use of SBAR Format for Communicating with Client's Physician

S	Situation	"Dr. Preston, this is Wendy Obi, evening nurse on 4G at St. Simeon Hospital, calling about Mr. Lakewood, who's having trouble breathing."
B	Background	"Kyle Lakewood, DOB 7/1/60, a 53-year-old man with chronic lung disease, admitted 12/25, who has been sliding downhill × 2 hours. Now he's acutely worse: VS heart rate 92, reparatory rate 40 with gasping, B/P 138/94, oxygenation down to 72%."
A	Assessment	"I don't hear any breath sounds in his right chest. I think he has a pneumothorax."
R	Recommendation	"I need you to see him right now. I think he needs a chest tube."

Adapted from Leonard M, Graham S, Bonacum D: The human factor: the critical importance of effective teamwork and communication in providing safe care, *Qual Saf Health Care* 13(Suppl 1): i85–i90, 2004.

TABLE 22-1	SBAR Structured Communication Format	
S	Situation	Identify yourself; identify the client and the problem. In 10 seconds state what is going on. This may include client's date of birth, hospital ID number, verification that consent forms are present, etc.
B	Background	State relevant context and brief history. Review the chart if possible before speaking or telephoning to the physician. Relate the client's background, including client's diagnosis, problem list, allergies, as well as relevant vital signs, medications that have been administered, laboratory results, etc.
A	Assessment	State your conclusion, what you think is wrong. List your opinion about the client's current status. Examples would be client's level of pain, medical complications, level of consciousness, problem with intake and output, or your estimate of blood loss, etc.
R	Recommendation or request	State your informed suggestion for the continued care of this client. Propose an action. What do you need? In what time frame does it need to be completed? Always should include an opportunity for questions. Some sources recommend that any new verbal orders now be repeated for feedback clarity. If no decision is forthcoming, reassert your request.

Adapted from information during interviews with Leonard (2009), Bonacum (2009), and Fleishmann (2008).

EXERCISE 22-1	Using Standardized Communication Formats

Purpose: To practice the SBAR technique.

Case Study:
Mrs. Robin, date of birth 1/5/50, is a preoperative client of Dr. Hu's. She is scheduled for an abdominal hysterectomy at 9 a.m. She has been NPO [fasting] since last midnight. She is allergic to penicillin. The night nurse reported she got little sleep and expressed a great deal of anxiety about this surgery, immediately after her surgeon and anesthesiologist examined her at the time of admission. Preoperative medication consisting of atropine and were administered at 8:40 instead of 8:30 as per order. Abdominal skin was scrubbed with Betadine per order, and an IV of 1 L 0.45 saline was started at 7 a.m. in her left forearm. She has a history of chronic obstructive pulmonary disease, controlled with an albuterol inhaler, but has not used this since admission yesterday.

Directions:
In triads, organize this information into the SBAR format. Student #1 is giving report. Student #2 role-plays the nurse receiving report. Student #3 acts as observer and evaluates the accuracy of the report.

Adapted from Amato-Vealey EJ, Barba MP, Vealey RJ: Hand-off communication: a requisite for perioperative patient safety, *AORN J* 88(5): 763–770, 2008.

EXERCISE 22-2	Telephone Simulation: Conversation Between Nurse and Physician about a Critically Ill Client

Purpose: To increase your telephone communication technique using structured formats.

Procedure:
Read case and then simulate making a phone call to the physician on call. It is midnight.

Case:
Ms. Babs Pointer, date of birth 1/13/42, is 6 hours postop for knee reconstruction, complaining of pain and thirst. Her leg swelling has increased 4 cm in circumference, lower leg has notable ecchymosis spreading rapidly. Temp 99, R 20; pedal pulse absent.

Discussion/ written paper:
Record your conversation for later analysis. In your analysis, write up an evaluation of this communication for accurate use of SBAR format, effectiveness, and clarity.

| EXERCISE 22-3 | SBAR for Change of Shift Simulation |

Purpose: To practice use of SBAR.

Procedure:
In postconference have Student A be the day-shift nurse reporting to Student B, who is acting as the evening nurse. Practice reporting on their assigned client conditions or simulate four or five postoperative clients' status. Use the SBAR format.

Discussion:
Have the entire postconference group of students critique the advantages and disadvantages of using this type of communication.

VARIOUS MODELS OF TEAM TRAINING

Team training is a tool to increase collaboration between physicians and nurses. Use of teams is a concept that has been around for years within medical and nursing professions. For example, medicine has used medical rounds to share information among physicians. Nursing has end-of-shift reports, when responsibility is handed over to the next group of nurses. Team training programs are available such as "**TeamSTEPPS**," or Team Strategies and Tools to Enhance Performance and Patient Safety. This program emphasizes improving client outcomes by improving communication using evidence-based techniques.

Communication skills include briefing and debriefing, conveying respect, clarifying team leadership, cross-monitoring, situational monitoring feedback, assertion in a climate valuing everyone's input, and use of standard communication formats such as SBAR and CUS. Creating a team culture means each member is committed to:

- Open communication with frequent timely feedback
- Protecting others from work overload
- Asking for and offering assistance

NURSING TEAMWORK

The traditional client report from one nurse handing over care to another nurse needs to be accurate, specific, and clear, and allow time for questions to foster a culture of client safety. Using SBAR or any other standardized communication format for report would result in a safer environment for your clients (Amato-Vealey et al., 2008), as well as having staff work staggered shifts (Woods et al., 2008).

Regarding handoffs, AHRQ's TeamSTEPPS program (2008) recommends that all team members use the "I PASS the BATON" acronym during any transition by staff in client care. Table 22-2 explains this communication strategy.

INTERDISCIPLINARY ROUNDS

Contemporary health care teams use "interdisciplinary **rounds**" to increase communication among the whole team—physicians, pharmacists, therapists, nurses, and

TABLE 22-2		I PASS the BATON
I	Introduction	Introduce yourself and your role
P	Patient	State patient's name, identifiers, age, sex, location
A	Assessment	Present chief complaint, vital signs, symptoms, diagnosis
S	Situation	Current status, level of certainty, recent changes, response to treatment
S	Safety concerns	Critical laboratory reports, allergies, alerts (e.g., falls)
the		
B	Background	Comorbidities, previous episodes, current medications, family history
A	Actions	State what actions were taken and why
T	Timing	Level of urgency, explicit timing and priorities
O	Ownership	State who is responsible
N	Next	State the plan: what will happen next, any anticipated changes

Developed by the US Department of Defense. Department of Defense Patient Safety Program: Healthcare Communications Toolkit to Improve Transitions in Care. Falls Church, VA: TRICARE Management Activity; 2005.

dieticians (Woods et al., 2008). This strategy may increase communication and positively affect client outcome. For example, daily discharge multidisciplinary rounds have been correlated with decreased length of hospital stay.

Interdisciplinary "team" meetings can be used daily or weekly to explore common goals/concerns/options, smooth problems before they escalate into conflicts, or provide support. Lower on the scale are *clinical teaching rounds,* where a physician once weekly teaches nurses, which has the goal of encouraging physician communication with the nursing staff.

ESTABLISH OPEN COMMUNICATION ABOUT ERRORS

Most state Boards of Nursing require nurses to report unsafe practice by coworkers, but many nurses have mixed feelings about reporting a colleague, especially to a state agency (Elder et al., 2008). Physicians also have reservations about reporting problems (Zbar, Taylor, & Canady, 2009). One focus of team training can be creating an in-house agency system climate in which team members feel comfortable speaking out about their safety concerns. In this new nonpunitive reporting environment, staff are encouraged to report errors, mistakes, and near misses. In safety literature, compiling a database that includes near-miss situations that could have resulted in injury is important information in preventing future errors. They work in a climate in which they feel comfortable making such reports. A complete error reporting process should include feedback to the person reporting. Administrators should assume errors will occur and put in place a plan for "recovery" that has well-rehearsed procedures for responding to adverse events.

BRIEFINGS AND DEBRIEFINGS

In team situations, such as in the operating room, the team may use another sort of standardized format. The leader (the surgeon, in this case) presents to the team a brief overview of what procedure is about to happen, asking anyone who sees a potential problem to speak up. In this manner, the leader "gives permission" for every team member to speak up. This can include the client also, as many clients will not speak unless specifically invited to do so. A debriefing is usually led by someone other than the leader. It occurs toward the end of a procedure and is a "recap" or

summary as to what went well or what might be changed (Bonacum, 2009). This is similar to the feedback nurses ask clients to do after they have presented some educational health teaching, which verifies that the client understood the material.

TECHNOLOGY-ORIENTED SOLUTIONS CREATE A CLIMATE OF CLIENT SAFETY TO AVOID ERRORS

Prevention of misidentification of client is an obvious error prevention strategy. Before administering medication, the nurse needs to verify client allergies, use another nurse to verify accuracy for certain stock medications, and re-verify client's identity. **Joint Commission's** best practice recommendation is to check the client's name band and then ask him to verbally confirm his name and give a second identifier such as his date of birth. Use of technology such as *barcoded name bands* may offer protection against misidentification (AHRQ, d). Some name bands include the client's picture, as well as name, date of birth, and *bar code* for verification of client identity.

Many agencies including the Veterans Administration (VA) Hospital System have used bar codes for years. When a new medication is ordered by a physician, it is transmitted to the pharmacy, where it is labeled with the same bar code as is on the client's name band. The nurse administering that medication must first verify both codes by scanning with the battery-operated bar code reader, just as a

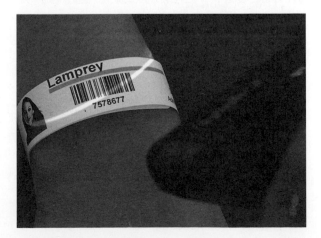

grocery store employee scans merchandise. In the VA, this resulted in a 24% decrease in medication administration errors (Wright & Katz, 2005). In a similar fashion, bar-coded labels on laboratory specimens prevent mixups.

OTHER TECHNOLOGY USED TO IMPROVE SAFE CARE

Health information technologies are said to be a key tool for increasing safety, as well as decreasing health care costs, and increasing quality of care (Bates, 2009). These are discussed in Chapters 25 and 26 and include electronic health records, clinical decision supports, and computerized registries or national databanks that monitor treatment. *Electronic transmission of prescriptions* to pharmacies in the community could help decrease errors caused by misinterpretation of handwritten scripts, yet by 2008 only 6% of American physicians had adopted electronic prescribing. *Radiofrequency identification* is an emerging technology allowing you to locate a certain nurse, identify a patient, or even locate an individual medication. Radiofrequency identification may be able to be incorporated into the nurse's handheld computer.

IMPROVE CARE EFFICIENCY

Measures to improve efficiency may also increase the time you have for communication with clients. Some changes such as equipment at bedside may increase client safety by decreasing possible infections.

TCAB (TRANSFORMING CARE AT THE BEDSIDE)

Begun in 2003, Transforming Care At the Bedside [**TCAB**; pronounced tee-cab] is an Institute for Healthcare Improvement Initiative funded by the Robert Wood Johnson Foundation to improve client safety and the quality of hospital bedside care by empowering nurses at the bedside to make system changes (online, TCAB;www.rwj.org/pr/product.jsp?id=31512; Runy, 2008; Stefancyk, 2008a, 2008b, 2009).

This program has four core concepts to improve care:
1. Create a climate of safe, reliable patient care. Uses practices such as brainstorming and retreats for staff nurses, to develop better practice and better communication ideas. One example is

nurses initiate presentation of the client's status to physicians at morning rounds, using a standard format. Another strategy is to empower staff nurses to make decisions.
2. Establish unit-based vital teams. Interdisciplinary, supportive care teams foster a sense of increased professionalism for bedside nurses. This together with better nurse-physician communication should positively affect client outcomes.
3. Develop client-centered care. This ensures continuity of care and respects family and client choices.
4. Provide value-added care. This eliminates inefficiencies, for example, by placing high-use supplies in drawers in each client's room

Evaluation in more 60 project hospitals showed that units using this method cut their mortality rate by 25% and reduced nosocomial infections significantly. Nurse-physician collaboration and communication was improved, with both physicians and nurses voicing increased satisfaction. Nurses said that overall they felt empowered (Stefancyk, 2008b).

CLIENT OUTCOMES OF TEAM TRAINING PROGRAMS

Multiple studies tend to demonstrate increased satisfaction, primarily from nurses, when team communication strategies are implemented. To date, little evidence exists about effects on client outcomes, although some literature indicates anesthesia team training has reduced errors. More research into the effects of communication interventions is needed. But what is really needed is an overhaul in the conception of what an interdisciplinary "team" is.

ADVANTAGES

Ideally, the health care team would provide the client with more resources, allow for greater flexibility, promote a "learning from each other" climate, and promote collective creativity to problem solving. Use of standardized communication tools would foster collaborative practice by creating shared communication expectations.

Obstacles to effective teamwork include lack of time, culture of autonomy, heavy workloads, and different terminologies and communication styles held by each discipline. Building in redundancy cuts errors but takes extra time, which can be irritating.

CLIENT-PROVIDER COLLABORATIONS

Communicating with clients about the need for them to participate in their care planning is a goal set in 2009 by Joint Commission (online, www. jcipatientsafety.org/). Goal 13 states, "Encourage patients' active involvement in their own care as a patient safety strategy," which includes having clients and families report their safety concerns. Clients and their families should be specifically invited to be an integral part of the care process. Another strategy is to provide more opportunities for communication.

Emphasize to each client that he is a valued member of the health team who is expected to actively participate in his care. Safe care is a top goal shared by client and care provider. Empowering your client to be a collaborator in his or her own care should enhance error prevention. Emphasizing this provider-client partnership is the second step in a communication model described by Fleischmann and Rabatin (2008). In building the relationship, to establish rapport, participants follow the acronym PEARLS: P = partnership; E = empathy; A = apology, such as "sorry you had to wait"; R = respect; L = legitimize or validate your client's feelings and concerns with comments such as "many people have similar concerns"; S = support. One outcome measured before and then 6 months after staff participated in a communications continuing education program was an increase in client satisfaction with care, up 16% in the emergency departments, up 17% in inpatient units, and up 28% in outpatient settings (Fleischmann, 2008). AHRQ advises clients to speak up if they have a question or concern, to ask about test results rather than to assume that "no news is good news."

DAILY CLIENT BRIEFINGS

Physicians have long used hospital rounds to briefly speak with each of their patients. Some supervising nurses have begun this practice.

USE OF WRITTEN MATERIALS

In one hospital system, written pamphlets are given to each client on admission instructing them to become a partner in their care. A nurse comes into the client's room at a certain time each day, sits, and makes eye contact. Together, nurse and client make a list of today's goals, which are written on a whiteboard in the client's room (Runy, 2008). As part of safety and communication, awareness of language barriers can be signaled to everyone entering the room by posting a logo on the chart, and room or bed. Use of interpreters and information materials written in the client's primary language may also reduce risk (AHRQ, 2004).

ASSESSMENT OF CLIENT'S LEVEL OF HEALTH LITERACY

The IOM has stressed that it is important to make verbal and written information as simple as possible (Denham, 2008). As a nurse, you need to assess the health literacy level of each client. Provide privacy to avoid embarrassment. Obtain feedback to determine client's understanding of teaching: Simplify, Clarify, Verify! In evaluating for literacy levels, some clues to low literacy or limited understanding are excuses such as "forgot my glasses," humor, or use of a family member to read written materials.

SUMMARY

There is a renewed effort to maximize client safety by minimizing errors made by all health care workers. Because miscommunication has been documented to be a most significant factor in occurrence of errors, this chapter focused on communication solutions. It described some individual and system solutions.

ETHICAL DILEMMA   What Would You Do?

You are a new nurse working for Hospice, providing in-home care for Ms. Wendy, a 34-year-old with recurrent spinal cancer. At a multidisciplinary care planning conference 2 months ago, Dr. Chi, oncologist, and Dr. Spenski, family physician, Hospice staff, and Ms. Wendy agreed to admit her when her condition deteriorated to the point that she would require ventilator assistance. Today, however, when you arrive at her home, she states a desire to forego further hospitalization. Her family physician is a personal friend and agrees to increase her morphine to handle her increased pain, even though you feel that such a large dose will further compromise her respiratory status.

1. What are the possibilities for miscommunication?
2. What steps would you take to get the health care team "on the same page"?

REFERENCES

Agency for Healthcare Research and Quality [AHRQ, a]: *National healthcare quality report*, Author. www.ahrq.gov/qual/nhqr05.htm.

Agency for Healthcare Research and Quality [AHRQ, b]: *Medical errors: the scope of the problem: an epidemic of errors*, Author. www.ahrq.gov/qual/errback.htm.

Agency for Healthcare Research and Quality[AHRQ, c]: Patient safety initiative: building foundations, reducing risk, 2009 Patient Safety Goals Available online: www.ahrq.gov/qual/pscongrpt/psinisum.htm. Accessed February 28, 2009.

Agency for Healthcare Research and Quality[AHRQ, d]: *Mistaken identity*, Author. http://cme.medscap.com/viewarticle/586256_2.

Agency for Healthcare Research and Quality [AHRQ, e]: *Literacy and health outcomes: summary, evidence report/technology assessment number 87*, 2004. Available online: http://www.ahrq.gov/clinic/epcsums/litsum.htm. Accessed March 1, 2009.

Agency for Healthcare Research and Quality: *TeamSTEPPS [trademark], pocket guide*, [Publication No. 06-0020-3], Rockville, MD, 2008, Author. Available online: http://teamsteps.ahrq.gov/index.htm.

Amato-Vealey EJ, Barba MP, Vealey RJ, et al: Hand-off communication: a requisite for perioperative patient safety, *AORN J* 88(5):763–770, 2008.

American Association of Colleges of Nursing: Hallmarks of quality and patient safety: recommended baccalaureate competencies and curricular guidelines to ensure high-quality and safe patient care, *J Prof Nurs* 22(6):329–330, 2006a. Available online: www.aacn.org or http://qsen.org/competencydomains/safety. Accessed June 1, 2009.

American Association of Colleges of Nursing: *Safety*, 2006b. Available online: http://www.qsen.org or www.pedsnurses.org/dmdocuments/BaccaliareateEssentials.pdf. Accessed June 6, 2009.

American Medical Association eVoice: *Best practice information*, 2008. Available online, http://co106w.col106.mail.live.com/. Accessed May 2, 2009.

American Medical Association: *Safe communications universal precautions. Patient safety tip card, AMA Bookstore*, Chicago, 2008b, Author.

Bates DW: The effects of Health Information Technology on inpatient care [editorial], *Arch Intern Med* 169(2):105–107, 2009.

Beyea SC: Learning more about the science of patient safety, *AORN J* 87(3):633–635, 2008a.

Beyea SC: Placing patient safety first, *AORN J* 87(4):829–831, 2008b.

Bonacum D: CSP, CPHQ, CPHRM, Vice President, Safety Management, Kaiser Foundation Health Plan, Inc. [Kaiser Permanente]: Personal interview, February 25, 2009.

Boone BN, King ML, Gresham LS, et al: Conflict management training and nurse-physician collaborative behaviors, *J Nurs Staff Dev* 24(4):168–175, 2008.

Cronenwett L, Sherwood G, Barnsteiner J, et al: Quality and safety education for nurses, *Nurs Outlook* 55(3):122–131, 2007.

Denham CR: SBAR for patients, *J Patient Saf* 4(1):38–48, 2008.

DeVoe JE, Wallace LS, Pandhi N, et al: Comprehending care in a medical home: a usual source of care and patient perceptions about health communication, *J Am Board Fam Med* 21(5):441–445, 2008.

Donaldson MS: An overview of 'To err in Human' reemphasizing the message of patient safety. In Hughes RG, editor: *Patient safety and quality: an evidence-based handbook for nurses*, [AHRQ pub no. 08-0043]. Rockville, MD, 2008, Agency for Healthcare Research and Quality.

Elder NC, Brungs SM, Nagy M, et al: Nurses' perceptions of error communication and reporting in the intensive care unit, *J Patient Saf* 4:162–168, 2008.

Evans AM, Pereira DA, Parker JM, et al: Discourses of anxiety in nursing practice: a psychoanalytic case study of the change-of-shift handover ritual, *Nurs Inq* 15(1):40–48, 2008.

Fleischman A, Rabatin J: "Provider-Patient Communication" conference materials supplied by Mayo Health Care System Medical Continuing Education Department, Rochester, MN, obtained May 27, 2008.

Fleischman JA: MD, Medical Vice President of Franciscan Skemp, Mayo HealthCare System, LaCrosse, WS: Personal interview, May 29, 2008.

Gore T, Hunt CW, Raines KH, et al: Mock hospital unit simulation: a teaching strategy to promote safe patient care, *Clin Simulation Nurs* 4(3):e57–e64, 2008. Available online: www.elsevier.com/locate/ecsn. Accessed February 13, 2009.

Henkind SJ, Sinnett JC: Patient care, square-rigger sailing, and safety, *JAMA* 300(14):1691–1693, 2008.

Henneman EA, Roche JP, Fisher DL, et al: Error identification and recovery by student nurses using human patient simulation: opportunity to improve patient safety, *Appl Nurs Res* 23(1):11–21, 2009.

Hughes RG, editor: *Patient safety and quality: an evidence-based handbook for nurses*, (vols 1–3), [AHRQ Publication No. 08-0043], Rockville, MD, April 2008, Agency for Healthcare Research and Quality.

Institute of Medicine: *Crossing the quality chasm: a new health system for the 21st century*, Washington, DC, 2001, National Academy Press.

Institute of Medicine: *Insuring America's health: principles and recommendations*, Washington, DC, 2004, National Academy Press.

Joint Commission on Accreditation of Healthcare Organizations [JCAHO,a]: Behaviors that undermine culture of safety, *Sentinel Event Alert* 40: 2008. Available online: http://www.jointcommission.org/SentinelEvents/SentinelEventAlert/sea_40.htm. Accessed July 9, 2008.

Joint Commission on Accreditation of Healthcare Organizations [JCAHO,b]: *Root causes of sentinel events*, 2006, Author, www.jointcommission.org/SentinelEvants/Statistics/.

Joint Commission on Accreditation of Healthcare Organizations [JCAHO,c]: Sentinel event statistics, www.jointcommissioninternational.org/24839/.

Joint Commission International: WHO Solutions, www.jointcommissioninternational.org/24839/.

Kaiser Family Foundation/AHRQ/Harvard School Family Foundation/AHRQ/Harvard School: *National survey on consumers' experiences with patient safety and quality information*, conducted 2004. Available online: http://www.kff.org/kaiserpolls/pomr111704pkg.cfm. Accessed February 20, 2009.

Kohn LT, Corrigan JM, Donaldson MS, editors: *To err is human: building a safer health system*, Washington, DC, 1999, Institute of Medicine, Committee on Quality in America, National Academy Press. Available online: http://www.guideline.gov/.

Kramer M, Schmalenberg C: Securing 'good' nurse-physician relationships, *Nurs Manag* 34:34–38, 2003.

Krautscheid LC: Improving communication among healthcare providers: preparing student nurses for practice, *Int J Nurs Educ Sch* 5(1), 2008, article 40. Available online: http://www.bepress.com/ijnes/vol5/iss1/art40/. Accessed October 21, 2008.

Lachman VD: Patient safety: the ethical imperative, *Dermotology Nursing* 20(2):134–136, 2008.

Leonard M: *SBAR,* personal communication [e-mail] February 20, 2009.

Leonard M, Bonacum D: SBAR application and critical success factors of implementation. Kaiser Permanente Health Care System presentation, May 2008, by Dr. Rabatin Jeff, Consultant, Pulmonary and Critical Care Medicine, Mayo Healthcare System, Rochester, MN.

Leonard M, Graham S, Bonacum D, et al: The human factor: the critical importance of effective teamwork and communication in providing safe care, *Qual Saf Health Care* 13(Suppl 1):i85–i90, 2004.

Mangione-Smith R, DeCristofara AH, Setodji CM, et al: The quality of ambulatory care delivered to children in the United States, *N Engl J Med* 357(15):1515–1523, 2007.

Mathews SC, Pronovost PJ: Physician autonomy and informed decision making, *JAMA* 300(24):2913–2915, 2008.

Nolte E, McKee CM: Measuring the health of nations: updating an earlier analysis, *Health Aff* 27(1):58–71, 2008.

Runy LA: The nurse and patient safety, *H&HN* 82(11):43–48, 2008. Available online: www.cinahl.com/cgi-bin/refsvc?jid=1774% accno=2010112696. Accessed January 6, 2009.

Scott LD, Rodgers AE, Hwang WT, et al: Effects of critical care nurses' work hours on vigilance and patients' safety, *Am J Crit Care* 15:30–37, 2006.

Shortell SM, Singer SJ: Improving patient safety by taking systems seriously, *JAMA* 299(4):445–447, 2008.

Singh H, Thomas E, Peterson L, et al: Medical errors involving trainees, *Arch Intern Med* 167(19):2030–2036, 2007.

Stefancyk AL: Transforming care at the bedside: transforming care at Mass General, *Am J Nurs* 108(9):71–72, 2008a.

Stefancyk AL: Transforming care at the bedside: nurses participate in presenting patients in morning rounds, *Am J Nurs* 108(11):70–72, 2008b.

Stefancyk AL: Transforming care at the bedside: high-use supplies at the bedside, *Am J Nurs* 109(2):33–35, 2009.

Sutter E, Arndt J, Arthur N, et al: Role understanding and effective communication as core competencies for collaborative practice, *J Interprof Care* 23(1):41–51, 2009.

Velji K, Baker GR, Fancott C, et al: Effectiveness of an adapted SBAR communication tool for a rehabilitation setting, *Healthc Q* 11(3 Spec No.):72–79, 2008.

Wong DR, Torchiana DF, Vander Salm TJ, et al: Impact of cardiac intraoperative precursor events on adverse outcomes, *Surgery* 141(6): 715–722, 2007.

Woods DM, Holl JL, Angst D, et al: Improving clinical communication and patient safety: clinician-recommended solutions, *J Healthc Qual* 30(5):4354, 2008. Available online: www.ahrq.gov/downloads/pub/advances2/vol3/Advances_woods_78.pdf. Accessed November 27, 2008.

Wright AA, Katz IT: Bar coding and patient safety, *N Engl J Med* 353(4):329–331, 2005.

Zbar RI, Taylor LD, Canady JW, et al: The disruptive physician: righteous Maverick or dangerous Pariah? *Plast Reconstr Surg* 123(1): 409–415, 2009.

CHAPTER 23

Communicating with Other Health Professionals

Kathleen Underman Boggs

OBJECTIVES

At the end of the chapter, the reader will be able to:

1. Identify standards for the healthcare work environment.
2. Identify communication barriers in professional relationships, including disruptive behaviors.
3. Describe methods to handle conflict through interpersonal negotiation when it occurs.
4. Discuss methods for communicating effectively in organizational settings.
5. Apply group communication principles to work groups.
6. Discuss application of research studies to clinical practice.

To be effective as a nursing professional, it is not enough to be deeply committed to the client. Ultimately, the workplace's corporate climate and work atmosphere will have an effect on the relationship that takes place between you and your client. **Disruptive behavior (workplace bullying)** creates conflicts on the job. The negative consequences of working in a dysfunctional atmosphere are adverse effects on client care and on the staff's physical and psychological health. This chapter focuses on principles of communication and strategies you can use to help deal with other professionals, promote more collaborative relationships, and function more effectively as an interdisciplinary team member and leader. Specific bridges to communication with other health professionals are described, together with strategies to remove communication barriers.

BASIC CONCEPTS
STANDARDS FOR A HEALTHY WORK ENVIRONMENT

A culture of collegiality is essential for a work environment that is to provide high-quality client care. Yet, when the Joint Commission surveyed nurses, more than 90% reported witnessing disruptive behavior; more than half reported they themselves had been subjected to verbal abuse (Joint Commission, 2008). As described in Chapter 22, failures in collaboration and communication among health care providers are among the most common factors contributing to increased errors and adverse client outcomes. Other outcomes include nurse dissatisfaction, job turnover, lost productivity, absenteeism, task avoidance, poor morale, impact on nurse's physical and mental health, and even legal action (Gerardi & Connell, 2007; Kerfoot, 2008; Olender-Russo, 2009; Rosenstein & O'Daniel, 2005; Spence-Laschinger, Leiter, Day, & Gilin, 2009).

The American Association of Critical Care Nurses (ACCN) in 2004 issued six standards characteristic of a healthy workplace (online, www.aacn.org):

- Nurses must be as efficient in communication skills as they are in clinical skills.
- Nurses must be relentless in pursuing and fostering true collaboration.
- Nurses must be valued and committed partners in making policy, directing and evaluating clinical care, and leading organizational operations.
- Staffing must ensure the effective match between patient needs and nurse competencies.
- Nurses must be recognized and recognize others for the value each brings to the work of the organization.
- Nurse leaders must fully embrace the imperative of a healthy work environment, authentically live it, and engage others in its achievement.

Professional Nursing organizations have identified eight elements of a healthy workplace environment:

- Collaborative culture with respectful communication and behavior
- Communication-rich culture that emphasizes trust and respect
- Clearly defined role expectations with accountability
- Adequate workforce
- Competent leadership
- Shared decision making
- Employee development
- Recognition of workers' contributions

CODE OF BEHAVIOR

The goal of collaboration is to communicate effectively with team members to provide best care. As part of creating a culture of teamwork where staff is valued, a standard across organizations should be zero tolerance for disruptive or bullying behaviors. To accomplish this, each organization needs one well-defined code of behavior applied consistently to all staff. The Joint Commission adopted standards originally scheduled to begin in 2009 that state each health care organization must create a code of conduct defining acceptable and unacceptable behaviors, as well as establishing an agency process for handling disruptive behaviors (Joint Commission line, www.jointcommission.org/SentinelEventAlert/Issue40, July 9, 2008).

INCIDENCE

Incivility is common in large organizations, especially hospitals. Although less than 3% of physicians and less than 3% of nurses exhibit disruptive behaviors, this is enough to effect client outcomes (Rosenstein & O'Daniel, 2005). Seventeen percent of professionals surveyed knew of a disruptive behavior that resulted in a specific adverse client outcome; 86% of nurses reported witnessing disrespect or harassment from physicians; and 72% reported receiving disrespectful behavior from other nurses (O'Daniel & Rosenstein, 2008). A number of authors have found that nurse-to-nurse destructive, disruptive behaviors occur more frequently than such physician-nurse interactions (Woelfle, 2007).

DEFINITIONS

Conflict was defined in Chapter 14 as a hostile encounter. The nursing literature uses a variety of terms to refer to persistent uncivil behaviors such as workplace bullying; verbal abuse; horizontal/lateral violence; "eating your young"; in-fighting; mobbing, harassment, or scapegoating. In this situation, the nurse victim is less powerful and is thus unable to bring an end to this behavior. For discussion in this textbook, we use the term *disruptive behavior* and use the original definition from Leymann in Sweden: at least two negative acts per week, occurring over more than 6 months in duration (Johnson, 2009).

Disruptive behaviors are prolonged and may include overt behaviors: rudeness, verbal abuse, intimidation, putdowns; angry outbursts, yelling, blaming, or criticizing team members in front of others; sexual harassment; or even threatening physical confrontations. Other disruptive behaviors are more covert and passive: withholding information, withholding help, giving unreasonable assignment loads, refusal to perform an assigned task, impatience or reluctance to answer questions, not returning telephone calls or pages, and speaking in a condescending tone (O'Reilly for Joint Commission, 2008, online). These behaviors threaten the well-being of nurses and the safety of clients (Wachs, 2009).

CREATING A CULTURE OF REGARD

Organizations have sometimes tolerated disruptive workplace behaviors (Olender-Russo, 2009). Australian nurses associated this with organizational restructuring or downsizing, or both (Hutchinson, Vickers, Jackson, & Wilkes, 2005). There are organizational pressures on nurses to increase their productivity and be more cost-effective. In Johnson's survey, 95% of emergency department nurses reported that disruptive bullying was done to two or more staff nurses by a supervisor in their department, leading us to speculate that agencies accept this as a useful management strategy (Johnson & Rea, 2009).

We need to become aware of how to discourage disruptive behaviors as we work to develop a healthy, collaborative workplace atmosphere. A climate that promotes collaboration and positive communication among caregivers contributes to satisfaction with one's work and better job retention. Most importantly, commitment to collaboration with other professionals helps sustain a high quality of client care (Joint Commission Resources, 2006). Building an organizational infrastructure that creates a climate that stresses our common mission and core values, and empowers nurses, starts with explicitly stated expectations of mutual respect. Administrators and nurse managers need to model behaviors that convey regard for staff and enforce policies of zero tolerance for disrespect.

RESPECT

Feeling respected or not respected is an integral part of how nurses rate the quality of their work environment (Bournes & Milton, 2009). Three key factors are a positive climate of professional practice, a supportive manager, and positive, respectful relationships with other staff.

ETIOLOGY

Nurses say they feel respected and appreciated if their opinions are listened to attentively and they receive feedback from authority figures as to the value of their work competence. When their opinions are discounted or ridiculed, they feel disrespected, angry, and frustrated (Parse, 2006). Feelings of powerlessness decrease self-esteem and increase anger. In an unhealthy atmosphere in which a staff member feels intimidated by authority and unable to change disruptive behaviors, they may direct their anger toward

peers (Gerardi & Connell, 2007). Respect is a natural extension of the practice of nursing, as identified in the American Nurses Association's Code of Ethics (2001). Typically, nurses describe behaviors indicating lack of respect to include demeaning verbal comments, nonverbal actions such as eye rolling, not paying attention to their opinions, interrupting, not responding to telephone or e-mail, and physical or sexual harassment.

Developing an Evidence-Based Practice

Bournes DA, Milton CL: Nurses' experience of feeling respected-not respected, *Nurs Sci Q* 22(1):47–56, 2009.

The purpose of this study was to gain understanding of nurses' experience in feeling respected or not respected. Participants were 37 staff or administrative nurses in a Canadian hospital. The Parse research method used involved analysis of content from small discussion groups.

Results: Concepts common to all the groups include respected nurses have their opinions listened to attentively, and they are given feedback as to the value of their work contributions (recognition). This made them feel good, empowered, and appreciated. Lack of respect was described as getting little appreciation, having your opinion discounted, and being patronized or belittled. This made them feel intimidated, demoralized, angry, or insecure.

Application to Your Clinical Practice: Each of us as nurses could make an effort to convey these positive behaviors to make our colleagues feel respected.

APPLICATIONS

CONFLICT RESOLUTION

Conflicts will inevitably arise in the work setting. Nurses have a responsibility to learn to work cooperatively. Refer to Box 23-1. Aside from the nurse-client conflicts described in Chapter 14, most workplace conflicts occur between the nurse and authority figures. In addition, conflict may arise from agency employee policies. Internal employee-management disputes detract from the agency's health care mission and from its financial bottom line.

Many of the same strategies for conflict resolution discussed for conflicts between client and nurse can be applied to conflicts between the nurse and other health care workers. Review the principles of conflict management in Figure 14-1 in Chapter 14. As mentioned,

BOX 23-1	Interpersonal Sources of Conflict in the Workplace: Barriers to Collaboration and Communication

1. Different expectations
   - Being asked to do something you know would be irresponsible or unsafe
   - Having your feelings or opinions ridiculed or discounted
   - Getting pressure to give more time or attention than you are able to give
   - Being asked to give more information than you feel comfortable sharing
   - Differences in language
2. Threats to self
   - Maintaining a sense of self in the face of hostility or sexual harassment
   - Being asked to do something to a client that is in conflict with your personal or professional moral values
3. Differences in role hierarchy
   - Differences in education or experience
   - Differences in responsibility and rewards (payment)
4. Clinical situation constraints
   - Emphasis on rapid decision making
   - Complexity of care interventions

conflict is not necessarily detrimental to productivity and job satisfaction. Successful resolution often has a positive effect on both outcomes.

IDENTIFY SOURCES OF CONFLICT

Conflict often stems from miscommunication. You need to think through the possible causes of the conflict. Conflict also stems from overly defensive responses to a situation. So you need to identify your own feelings about it and respond appropriately, even if the response is a deliberate choice not to respond verbally. Interpersonal conflicts that are not dealt with leave residual feelings that reappear in future interactions.

SET GOALS

Your primary goal in dealing with workplace conflict is to find a high-quality, mutually acceptable solution: a win-win strategy. In many instances, a better collaborative relationship can be developed through the use of conflict management communication techniques (Bacal, n.d.; Boone, King, Gresham, Wahl, & Suh, 2008). To reframe a clinical situation as a cooperative

process in which the health goals and not the status of the providers becomes the focus:

- *Identify your goal.* A clear idea of the outcome you wish to achieve is a necessary first step in the process. Remember the issue is the conflict, not your coworker.
- *Obtain factual data.* It is important to do your homework by obtaining all relevant information about the specific issues involved—and about the client's behavioral responses to a health care issue—before engaging in negotiation.
- *Intervene early.* Be assertive. The best time to resolve problems is before they escalate to a conflict. Create a forum for two-way communication, preferably meeting periodically. Structured formats have been developed for you to use in conflict resolution, especially in team meetings. Nielsen and Mann (2008) mention the format of **DESC**:
  - D = describe the behavior (the problem)
  - E = express your concern
  - S = specify a course of action
  - C = obtain consensus
- *Avoid negative comments that can affect the self-esteem of the receiver.* Even when the critical statements are valid (e.g., "You do . . ." or "You make me feel . . ."), they should be replaced with "I" statements that define the sender's position. Otherwise, needless hostility is created and the meaning of the communication is lost.
- *Consider the other's viewpoint.* Having some idea of what issues might be relevant from the other person's perspective provides important information about the best interpersonal approach to use. In addition to dealing with your own feeling, you need an ability to deal with the feelings of the others. Be cooperative, acknowledging the team's interdependence and mutual goals.

AVOIDING BARRIERS TO RESOLUTION

Refer to Box 23-2 for tips on how to turn conflict into collaboration. Much of the individual behavior was discussed in Chapter 14, such as avoiding the use of negative or inflammatory, anger-provoking words. Also avoid phrases that imply coercion or that are patronizing. Examples include: "We must insist that . . ." or "You claim that . . ." Most individuals react to anger directed at them with a fight-or-flight response. Anyone can have a moment of rudeness, but monitor your own communications to avoid any pattern of abusive

BOX 23-2	Strategies to Turn Conflict into Collaboration

1. Recognize and confront disruptive behaviors.
   - Use conflict-resolution strategies.
   - Take the initiative to discuss problems.
   - Use active listening skills (refrain from simultaneous activities that interrupt communication).
   - Present documented data relevant to the issue.
   - Propose resolutions.
   - Use a brief summary to provide feedback.
   - Record all decisions in writing.
2. Create a climate in which participants view negotiation as a collaborative effort.
   - Develop agency behavior policies with stated zero tolerance for disruptive or bullying behaviors.
   - Model communicating with staff in a respectful, courteous manner.
   - Participate in organizational interdisciplinary groups.
   - Solicit and give feedback on a regular, periodic basis.
   - Clarify role expectations.

behaviors, including blaming or criticizing staff to others. Katrinli et al.'s study (2008) showed that when nurse supervisors become aware of how their behavior affects their nurses, they can increase the nurses' performance, increase their job involvement, and increase organizational identification.

PHYSICIAN-NURSE CONFLICT RESOLUTION

The history of nurse-physician communication is described by Seago (2008) as a "game" in which nurses made treatment recommendations without appearing to do so, and physicians asked for recommendations without appearing to do so, with both parties striving to avoid open disagreements. She notes that the literature indicates that communication between doctor and nurse is still often contentious. Remarkable increases in safety in airline and space programs were achieved by creating a climate in which junior team members were free to question decisions of more senior, powerful team members. It is recommended that health care adopt a similar philosophy. The American Medical Association (AMA, 2008) has specifically stated that codes of conduct define appropriate behavior as including a right to appropriately express a concern you have

about client care and safety. While this is being set forth as a medical code of conduct for physicians, should it also apply to nurses?

Nurses influence physician-client communication. Nurses assess what physicians tell clients, encourage clients to seek clarification, encourage second opinions, and spend time defending the physician's competence. Better collaboration and better communication are associated with safer care and better client care outcomes. In a meta-analysis of existing research, Seago (2008) found these factors to be associated with reduced drug errors, reduced client mortality, improved client satisfaction, and somewhat with shorter hospital stays. Methods to improve safe communication are discussed in Chapter 22.

There will be occasions when you have collaboration difficulties. One major factor related to job satisfaction and job retention is *"disruptive" communication* between other professionals, especially physician-nurse interactions. Case law defines disruptive physician behavior as conduct that disrupts the operation of the hospital, affects the ability of others to get their jobs done, and creates a hostile work environment.

Gender and Historic Communication

The relationship between the doctor and the nurse remains an evolving process. Changes in the physician-nurse communication process are occurring as nurses become more empowered, more assertive, and better educated. Most nurses occasionally encounter problems in the physician-nurse relationship. The differences in power, perspective, education, pay, status, class, and sometimes gender are contributing factors. Contemporary society is redefining traditional gender role behavior, negating some of the traditional "nurse as subservient female" stereotypical behaviors. Reflect on content presented on gender differences in communication to determine whether your current situation might be related to gender differences in communication styles rather than a more serious problem. Some doctors are reluctant to be challenged; some nurses are quick to feel slighted. Some physician-nurse relationships are marked with conflict, mistrust, and disrespect. Although these feelings are changing, it is slow, and some physicians still regard themselves as the only legitimate authority in health care, seeing the professional nurse as an accessory. An attitude that excludes the nurse as a professional partner in health care promotion benefits no one and is increasingly challenged as being costly to professionals and clients alike.

It is important to remain flexible yet not to yield on important, essential dimensions of the issue. Sometimes it is difficult to listen carefully to the other person's position without automatically formulating your next point or response, but it is important to keep an open mind and to examine the issue from a number of perspectives before selecting alternative options. The communication process should not be prematurely concluded. You can apply the same principles of conflict resolution discussed in Chapter 14 when dealing with a physician-nurse conflict. Make a commitment to open dialogue. Listening should constitute at least half of a communication interaction. Foster a feeling of collegiality. Use strategies from that chapter to defuse anger. During your negotiation, discussion should begin with a statement of either the commonalities of purpose or the points of agreement about the issue (e.g., "I thoroughly agree Mr. Smith will do much better at home. However, we need to contact social services and make a home care referral before we actually discharge him; otherwise, he will be right back in the hospital again"). Points of disagreement should always follow rather than precede points of agreement. Empathy and a genuine desire to understand the issues from the other's perspective enhance communication and the likelihood of a successful resolution.

Nurses have a responsibility to foster good physician-client communication. This is especially true when it becomes obvious to you from content, tone, or body language that antagonism is developing. Do you think it is ever appropriate for a nurse to criticize a physician's actions to a client? A common underlying factor in at least 25% of all malpractice suits is an inadvertent or deliberate critical comment by another health care professional concerning a colleague's actions. So think before you speak!

Solutions that take into consideration the needs and human dignity of all parties are more likely to be considered as viable alternatives. Backing another health professional into a psychological corner by using intimidation, coercion, or blame is simply counterproductive. More often than not, solutions developed through such tactics never get implemented. Usually there are a number of reasons for this, but the basic issues have to do with how the problem was originally defined and the control issues that were never actually dealt

with in the problem-solving discussion. The final solution derived through fair negotiation is often better than the one arrived at alone.

NURSE-TO-NURSE CONFLICT RESOLUTION

Although it is inevitable that you will encounter some communication problems with nurse colleagues, remember that, if managed appropriately, these conflicts can lead to innovative solutions and improved relationships.

Negotiating with Nursing Authority Figures

Negotiating can be even more threatening with a nursing supervisor or an instructor who has direct authority, because these people have some control over your future as a staff nurse or student. Supervision implies a shared responsibility in the overall professional goal of providing high-quality nursing care to clients. The wise supervisor is able to promote a nonthreatening environment in which all of the aspects of professionalism are allowed to emerge and prosper. In a supervisor-nurse relationship, conflict may arise when expectations for performance are unclear or when the nurse is unable to perform at the desired level. Communication of expectations often occurs after the fact, within the context of an employee performance evaluation. To effectively manage requires that performance expectations are known from the beginning. The supervisor needs to advise you about the need for improvement as part of an ongoing, constructive, interpersonal relationship. When the supervisor gives constructive criticism, it is in a nonthreatening and genuinely caring manner. In studying approaches to authority figures, you are encouraged to analyze your overall personal responses to authority, as in Exercise 23-1.

Managing Nursing Staff Problems

Improving how nurses deal with conflict is an investment in coworkers, our organization, and ultimately in improved client outcomes. Nonaction has been identified as the most common repressive management strategy (Bacal, n.d.). Nurse managers have learned that ignoring conflict among staff does not solve problems. Avoidance perpetuates the status quo or leads to an escalation. When managed appropriately, you reduce time wasted by staff in griping, defending, and so on, as illustrated in the following case.

Purpose: To have students recognize their feelings about authority.

Procedure:

1. Lean back in your chair, close your eyes, and think of the word *authority*.
2. Who is the first person that comes to mind when thinking of that word?
3. Describe how this person signifies authority to you. Next, think of an incident in which this person exerted authority and how you reacted to it.
4. After you have visualized the memory, answer the following questions:
   a. What were your feelings about the incident after it was over?
   b. What changes of feelings occurred from the start of the incident until it was over?
   c. Was there anything about the authority figure that reminded you of yourself?
   d. Was there anything about the authority figure that reminded you of someone else with whom you once had a strong relationship (if the memory viewed is not mother or father)?
   e. How could you have handled the incident more assertively?
   f. Can you see any patterns in yourself that might help you handle interactions with authority figures?
   g. What about those patterns are not assertive?
   h. How could those patterns be improved to be more assertive?

Adapted from Levy R: *Self-revelation through relationships*, Englewood Cliffs, NJ, 1972, Prentice Hall.

Case Example

Two nursing teams work the day shift on a busy surgical unit. As nurse manager, Ms. Libby notices that both teams are arguing over use of the computer, have become unwilling to help cover the other team's client, and are taking longer to complete assigned work, and so on. To achieve a more harmonious work environment, she arranges a staff meeting to get the teams communicating. Rather than just issues about sharing the computer, these multiple problems suggest inadequate time management and overload. Ms. Libby listens actively, responds with empathy, and provides positive regard and feedback for solutions proposed by the group. She asks the group to decide on two prioritized solutions. Recognizing that her staff feel unappreciated and knowing that compromise is a strategy that produces behavior change, she resolves to offer more frequent performance feedback. She herself assumes responsibility for requesting an immediate second computer purchase under her unit budget's emergency funding allocation. A team member who is on the employee relations committee assumes responsibility for requesting that the Human Services Department schedule an inservice training on time management and stress reduction within the next month. The group agrees to meet in 6 weeks to evaluate.

COLLABORATING WITH PEERS

The nurse-client relationship occurs within the larger context of the professional relationship with other health disciplines. How the nurse relates to other members of the health team will affect the level and nature of the interactions that transpire between nurse and client. Interpersonal conflict between health team members periodically is concealed from awareness and projected onto client behaviors.

Case Example

On a psychiatric nursing unit, the nursing staff found Mr. Tomkins's behavior highly disruptive. At an interdisciplinary conference attended by representatives from all shifts, there was general agreement that Mr. Tomkins should spend 1 hour in the seclusion room each time his agitated behavior occurred. The order was written into his care plan. The plan was implemented for a week with a noticeable reduction in client symptoms. During the second week, however, Mr. Tomkins was be placed in the seclusion room for the reasons just mentioned, but the evening staff would release him after 5 or 10 minutes if he was quiet and well-behaved.

The client's agitated behavior began to escalate again, and another interdisciplinary conference was called. Although the stated focus of the dialogue was on constructive ways to help Mr. Tomkins cope with disruptive anxiety, the underlying issues related to the strong feelings of the day nursing staff that their interventions were being undermined. Equally strong was the conviction of the evening staff that they were acting in the client's best interest by letting him out of the seclusion room as soon as his behavior normalized. Until the underlying behaviors could be resolved satisfactorily at the staff level, the client continued to act out the staff's anxiety, as well as his own.

Similar types of issues arise now and again when there is no input from different work shifts in developing a comprehensive nursing care plan. The shift staff may not agree with specific interventions, but instead of talking the discrepancy through in regularly scheduled staff conferences, they may act it out, unconsciously undoing the work of the other shifts.

Occasionally you may have to work with a peer with whom you develop a "personality conflict." Stop and consider what led up to the current situation. Generally it is due to an accumulation of small annoyances that occurred over time. The best method to avoid such situations is to verbalize occurrences rather than ignoring them until they become a major problem. Avoid the "blame game" and discuss in a private, calm moment what you *both* can do to make things better.

Case Example

"Jane, we seem to disagree about the best way to teach Mr. Santos about his…He seems to be getting confused about our two different approaches. Let's talk about how we might be able to work more effectively together. What is the most important point you want to teach him?"

Use active listening skills to really pay attention to what Jane says. Do a self-inventory to eliminate any non-verbal behavior that is triggering Jane's reaction and eliminate it. Ask yourself, "Do I want to win, or do I want to fix this problem?" Then state your expectations in a calm tone.

Whenever there is covert conflict among nursing staff or between members of different health disciplines, it is the client who ultimately suffers the repercussions. The level of trust the client may have established in the professional relationship is compromised until the staff conflict can be resolved.

DELEGATION OR SUPERVISION OF UNLICENSED PERSONNEL

Delegation is defined as the transfer of responsibility for the performance of an activity from one individual to another while retaining accountability for the outcome. Whether delegating to a peer or unlicensed assistive personnel (UAP), the nurse is only transferring the responsibility for the performance of the activity, not the professional accountability for the overall care (American Nurses Association, 1994). In earlier times, delegating and trusting went hand in hand, because the nurse was transferring responsibility to a peer and had some assurance of the skills and knowledge of that peer. The present health care environment poses a

much different reality in which some UAPs possess minimal experience, skills, or knowledge.

The challenges of maintaining professional integrity and concurrently surviving in today's health care arena are felt by nurses in all settings. Effective and appropriate use of delegation can facilitate your ability to meet these challenges. But more often than not, novice nurses are inadequately prepared for the demands of delegating much of their nursing tasks to UAPs while retaining responsibility for interpreting patient outcomes.

Inherent in effective delegation is an adequate understanding of the skills and knowledge of UAPs, as well as of the Nurse Practice Act of the state in which you are practicing. Within each state's Nurse Practice Act are specific guidelines describing what nursing actions can and cannot be delegated, and to what type of personnel these actions can be delegated. In addition to knowing nurse practice guidelines and the skills and knowledge level of UAPs, the nurse must educate and reinforce the UAPs' knowledge base, assess the UAPs' readiness for delegation, delegate appropriately, oversee the task, and evaluate and record the outcomes. The appropriate implementation of these principles (e.g., educating, assessing, overseeing, and evaluating) is a costly process both in time and energy. Practice Exercise 23-2 to facilitate your understanding of the principles. The following case example highlights one particular principle.

Case Example

After receiving the report on her client assignments, Monica Lewis, RN, assigns a newly hired UAP to provide routine care (e.g., morning care, assistance with meals, vital signs, finger sticks for glucose, and reporting of any changes) to Mrs. Jones, who was recently admitted for exacerbation of her type 2 diabetes. While on routine rounds during lunch, Monica finds Mrs. Jones unresponsive, with cold, clammy skin, a heart rate of 110, and a finger stick reading of 60 mg/dL, which the UAP had obtained. Thinking Mrs. Jones was experiencing hypoglycemia, Monica requested the UAP to obtain another blood glucose reading. While administering high-glucose intravenous solutions to raise Mrs. Jones's blood sugar, Monica observed the UAP violate a number of basic principles in obtaining an accurate blood glucose level. On further questioning, the UAP admitted never having been taught the proper procedure and thought reading the directions was sufficient. Monica had wrongly assumed all UAPs underwent training on the principles of obtaining blood glucose finger sticks.

EXERCISE 23-2	Applying Principles of Delegation

Purpose: To help students differentiate between delegating nursing tasks and evaluating client outcomes.

Procedure:
Divide the class into two groups: A and B. The following case study is a typical day for a charge nurse in an extended-care facility. After reading the case study, Group A is to describe the nursing tasks they would delegate and instructions they would give the nursing assistants and certified medicine aides (CMAs). Group B is to describe the professional nursing responsibilities related to the delegated tasks. The two groups then share their reports.

Situation:
Anne Marie Roache is the day-shift charge nurse on one of the units at Shadyside Nursing and Rehabilitation Facility. On this particular day, her census is 24, and her staff includes four nursing assistants and two CMAs who are allowed to administer all oral and topical medications. Her nursing assistants are qualified to perform morning care: assist with feedings; obtain and record vital signs, fluid intake and output, and blood glucose finger sticks; turn and position residents; assist with ambulation; and perform decubitus dressing changes. Of the residents, 12 are bedridden, requiring complete bed baths and some degree of assistance with feeding. The remaining 12 require varying degrees of assistance with their morning baths and assistance to the dining rooms for their meals. Nine of the residents are diabetics requiring premeal blood glucose finger sticks; seven are recovering from cerebrovascular accidents and display varying degrees of right- or left-sided weakness; three require care of their sacral decubiti; and all of the residents are at risk for falling because of varying degrees of confusion, disorientation, or general weakness. The night shift reported that all the residents' conditions were stable and they had slept well. Ms. Roache is ready to assign her staff.

Discussion:
Entire class can identify client goals.

ADVOCACY

Nursing organizations have identified trends toward increased use of unlicensed workers in agencies wishing to reduce costs. Such organizations speak out about the burden this places on registered nurses. Becoming active in your state nurses' association or professional specialty organization allows you to add your voice to this debate. Obtain a copy of your state's Nurse Practice Act. Usually these can be downloaded from your state Board of Nursing's Web site. This document will spell out what you, as a registered nurse, can delegate and to whom.

Even as a beginning staff nurse you will be expected to delegate some client care duties to others. You are responsible for the completeness, quality, and accuracy of this care. To avoid conflicts in delegating client care, clearly state your expectations. It is your responsibility to ensure that care was given correctly.

STRATEGIES TO REMOVE BARRIERS TO COMMUNICATION WITH OTHER PROFESSIONALS

CONVEY RESPECT

Just as you treat clients with respect, you have an ethical responsibility to treat coworkers with respect. Nurses need to be appreciated, recognized, and respected as professionals for the work they do. Unsupportive and uncivil coworkers and workplace conflicts negatively influence retention of nursing staff. Communication can become distorted rather than open when you are concerned about offending a more powerful individual. Strategies for dealing with disrespectful or disruptive behaviors include establishing common communication expectations and skills (described in Chapter 22), teaching conflict resolution skills, and creating a culture of mutual respect within the health care system. Ideally, the system has ongoing education, leadership and team collaboration support, and policies to evaluate behavior violations.

CLARIFY COMMUNICATIONS

You can use skills taught in this textbook to improve both the clarity of message content and the emotional tone of interactions. Communication problems lead to a large percentage of disruptive behaviors, especially telephone communication. Message clarity is enhanced when standardized formats such as SBAR, discussed in Chapter 22, are used: The nurse identifies self by name, position, the client by name, diagnosis, the problem (include current problem, vital signs, new symptoms, etc.), and clearly states his or her request.

USE CONFLICT RESOLUTION STRATEGIES AND RESPOND TO PUTDOWNS AND DESTRUCTIVE CRITICISMS

The strategies for handling angry clients, as described in Chapter 14, can be applied to your relations with anger from colleagues. This chapter details a number of conflict resolution steps (see Box 23-3). In addition, you need to develop a strategy to respond to unwarranted putdowns and destructive criticisms. Generally, they have but one intent: to decrease your status and enhance the status of the person delivering the putdown. The putdown or criticism may be handed out because the speaker is feeling inadequate or threatened. Often it has little to do with the actual behavior of the nurse to whom it is delivered. Other times the criticism may be valid, but the time and place of delivery are grossly inappropriate (e.g., in the middle of the nurses'

station or in the client's presence). In either case, the automatic response of many nurses is to become defensive and embarrassed, and in some way actually begin to feel inadequate, thus allowing the speaker to project unwarranted feelings onto the nurse.

Recognizing a putdown or unwarranted criticism is the first step toward dealing effectively with it. If a comment from a coworker or authority figure generates defensiveness or embarrassment, it is likely that the comment represents more than just factual information about performance. If the comment made by the speaker contains legitimate information to help improve one's skill and is delivered in a private and constructive manner, it represents a learning response and cannot be considered a putdown. Learning to differentiate between the two types of communication helps the nurse to "separate the wheat from the chaff."

Case Example

You examine a crying child's inner ears and note that the tympanic membranes (eardrums) are red. You report to your supervisor that the child may have an ear infection.

A. *Response:* When a child is crying, the drums often swell and redden. How about checking again when the child is calm? *(Learning response)*

Or

B. *Response:* Of course they are red when the child is crying. Didn't you learn that in nursing school? I haven't got time to answer such basic questions! *(Putdown response)*

Which response would you prefer to receive? Why?

Whereas the first response allows the nurse to learn useful information to incorporate into practice, the second response serves to antagonize, and it is doubtful much learning takes place. What will happen is that the nurse will be more hesitant about approaching the supervisor again for clinical information. Again, it is the client who ultimately suffers.

Once a putdown is recognized as such, you need to respond verbally in an assertive manner as soon as possible after the incident has taken place. Waiting an appreciable length of time is likely to cause resentment and loss of self-respect. It may be more difficult later for the other person to remember the details of the incident. At the same time, if the nurse's own anger, not the problem behavior, is likely to dominate the response, it is better to wait for the anger to cool a little and then to present the message in a more reasoned manner.

BOX 23-3	Steps to Promote Conflict Resolution among Health Care Workers

1. Set the stage for collaborative communication.
   - Privacy: meet, bringing together all involved groups
   - Acknowledge the conflict problem
2. Maintain a respectful, nonpunative atmosphere.
   - Solicit the perspectives of each.
   - Define the problem issue clearly.
   - Respect the values and dignity of all parties.
   - Group members can be assertive but not manipulative.
   - Remember to criticize ideas, not people.
3. Discussion:
   - Identify the conflict's key points.
   - Have an objective or a goal clearly in mind.
   - Discuss solutions.
   - Identify the merits/drawbacks of each solution.
   - Be open to alternative solutions in which all parties can meet essential needs.
   - Depersonalize conflict situations.
   - Avoid emotion.
4. Decide to implement the best solution.
   - Specify persons responsible for implementation (role clarity).
   - Establish timeline.
   - Decide on the evaluation method.
   - Emphasize common goal is our shared value of quality client care.
   - Emphasize shared responsibility for team success.

PROCESS FOR RESPONDING TO PUTDOWNS

In responding to putdowns, the nature of the relationship should be considered. Attitudes are important. Respect for the value of each individual as a person should be evidenced throughout the interaction. Try to determine how to respond to this person in a productive way so that you are on speaking terms but still get your point across. Even if you do not fully succeed in your initial tries, you probably will have learned something valuable in the process.

Address the objectionable or disrespectful behaviors first. Briefly state the behavior and its impact on you. It is important to deliver a succinct verbal message without getting lost in detail and without sounding apologetic or defensive. Do not try to give a prolonged explanation of your behavior at this point in the interaction and do not suggest possible motivations.

Emphasize the specifics of the putdown behavior. Once the putdown has been dealt with, you can discuss any criticism of your behavior on its own merits. Refer only to the behaviors identified and do not encourage the other person to amplify the putdown.

Prepare a few standard responses. Because putdowns often catch one by surprise, it is useful to have a standard set of opening replies ready. Examples of openers might include the following:

"I think it was out of line for you to criticize me in front of the client."

"I found your comments very disturbing and insulting."

"I feel what you said as an attack. That wasn't called for by my actions."

"I thought that was an intolerable remark."

A reply that is specific to the putdown delivered is essential. The tone of voice needs to be even and firm. In the clinical example given previously, the nurse might have said to the head nurse: "My school is not an issue, and your criticism is unnecessary," or "It seems to me that the assessment of the child's ears, not my school, is the issue, and your superior tone is uncalled for."

An important aspect of putdowns is that they get in the way of the nurse's professional goal of providing high-quality nursing care to clients. The effect of the head nurse's second response is for both nurses to assume the reddened eardrums are from crying and not to reevaluate the child's eardrums. Feeling resentful

and less sure of her clinical skills, the staff nurse is less likely to risk stirring up such feelings again. If fewer questions are asked, important information goes unshared. In the clinical example just cited, a possible ear infection might not be detected.

CRITICIZE CONSTRUCTIVELY

Giving constructive criticism and receiving criticism is difficult for most people (Box 23-4). When a supervisor gives constructive criticism, some type of response from the person receiving it is indicated. Initially, it is crucial that the conflict problem be clearly defined and acknowledged. To help handle constructive criticism, nurses can do the following:

- Schedule a time when you are calm.
- Request that supervisory meetings be in a place that allows privacy.
- Defuse personal anxiety.

BOX 23-4   Constructive Criticism

Steps in Giving
1. Express sympathy.
   Sample statement: "I understand that things are difficult at home."
2. Describe the behavior.
   Sample statement: "But I see that you have been late coming to work three times during this pay period."
3. State expectations.
   Sample statement: "It is necessary for you to be here on time from now on."
4. List consequences.
   Sample statement: "If you get here on time, we'll all start off the shift better. If you are late again, I will have to report you to the personnel department."

Steps in Receiving
1. Listen and paraphrase. If unclear ask for specific examples.
   Sample reply: "You are saying being late is not acceptable."
2. Acknowledge you are taking suggestions seriously.
   Sample comment: "I hear what you are saying."
3. Give your side by stating supportive facts, without being defensive.
   Sample comment: "My car would not start."
4. Develop a plan for the future.
   Sample plan: "With this paycheck I will repair my car. Until then I'll ask Mary for a ride."

- Listen carefully to the criticism and then paraphrase it.
- Acknowledge that you take suggestions for improvement seriously.
- Discuss the facts of the situation but avoid becoming defensive.
- Develop a plan for dealing with similar situations; become proactive rather than reactive.

USE PEER NEGOTIATION

As students, you will encounter situations in which the behavior of a colleague causes a variety of unexpressed differences or disagreement because the colleague's interpretation of a situation or meaning of behavior is so different from yours. The conflict behaviors can occur as a result of age differences, differences in values, philosophical approaches to life, ways of handling problems, lifestyles, definitions of a problem, goals, or strategies to resolve a problem. These differences cause friction and turn relationships from collaborative to competitive.

Generally, conflict increases anxiety. When interaction with a certain peer or peer group stimulates anxious or angry feelings, the presence of conflict should be considered. Once it is determined that conflict is present, look for the basis of the conflict and label it as personal or professional. If it is personal in nature, it may not be appropriate to seek peer negotiation. It might be better to go back through the self-awareness exercises presented in previous chapters and locate the nature of the conflict through self-examination.

Sharing feelings about a conflict with others helps to reduce its intensity. It is confusing, for example, when nursing students first enter a nursing program or clinical rotation, but this confusion does not get discussed, and students commonly believe they should not feel confused or uncertain. As a nursing student, you face complex interpersonal situations. These situations may lead you to experience loneliness or self-doubt about your nursing skills compared with those of your peers. These feelings are universal at the beginning of any new experience. By sharing them with one or two peers, you usually find that others have had parallel experiences. In reviewing Exercise 23-3, think of a conflict or problem that has implications for your practice of nursing, one you would be willing to share with your peers.

Self-awareness is beneficial in assessing the meaning of a professional conflict. Now that you have had an opportunity to study different types of conflict, work on Exercise 23-4.

DEVELOP A SUPPORT SYSTEM

Collegial relationships are an important determinant of success as professional men and women entering

---

EXERCISE 23-3	Applying Principles of Confrontation

Purpose: To help students understand the importance of using specific principles of confrontation to resolve a conflict.

Procedure:
1. Divide the class into two groups: Group A is the day shift (7 a.m. to 7 p.m.) and Group B is the night shift (7 p.m. to 7 a.m.).
2. The following case study is an example of some problems between the night and day shifts resulting in mistrust and general tension between the two groups. After reading the case study, each group is to use three principles as identified in the text (i.e., identify concerns, clarify assumptions, and identify real issue). The two groups then share their concerns, assumptions, and what they believe to be the real issue. Finally, both groups are to apply the fourth principle, collaboratively identifying a solution or solutions that satisfy both groups.

Situation:
The night shift's (Group B) responsibilities include completing as many bed baths as possible and the taping report as close to the shift change (7 a.m.) as possible. The day shift (Group A) finds that few, if any, of the bed baths are completed and that the taped report is usually done at about 5 a.m., reflecting few of the client changes that occurred between 5 a.m. and 7 a.m. The day shift is angry with the night shift, feeling they are not assuming their fair share of the workload. The night shift feels the day shift does not understand their responsibilities; they believe they are contributing more than their fair share of work.

Discussion:
Instructor might role-play the part of the nurse manager who acts to facilitate resolution of this conflict.

Purpose: To help students understand the basic concepts of client advocacy, communication barriers, and peer negotiation in simulated nursing situations.

Procedure:

1. Here is an example of situations in which interprofessional communication barriers exist. Refamiliarize yourself with the concepts of professionalism, client advocacy, communication barriers, and peer negotiation.
2. Formulate a response.
3. Compare your responses with those of your classmates, and discuss the implications of common and disparate answers. Sometimes dissimilar answers provide another important dimension of a problem situation.

Dr. Tanlow interrupts Ms. Serf, RN, as she is preparing pain medication for 68-year-old Mrs. Gould.

It is already 15 minutes late. Dr. Tanlow says he needs Ms. Serf immediately in Room 20C to assist with a drainage and dressing change. Knowing that Mrs. Gould, a diabetic, will respond to prolonged pain with vomiting, Ms. Serf replies that she will be available to help Dr. Tanlow in 10 minutes (during which time she will have administered Mrs. Gould's pain medication). Dr. Tanlow, already on his way to Room 20C, whirls around, stating loudly, "When I say I need assistance, I mean now. I am a busy man, in case you hadn't noticed."

If you were Ms. Serf, what would be an appropriate response?

Discussion:

This situation could be discussed in class, assigned as a paper, or used as an essay exam.

---

nursing practice. Studies show the importance of mutual support (Woelfle & McCaffrey, 2007).

Although there is no substitute for outcomes that demonstrate professional competence, interpersonal strategies can facilitate the process. Integrity, respect for others, dependability, a good sense of humor, and an openness to sharing with others are communication qualities people look for in developing a support system.

Forming a reliable support system at work to share information, ideas, and strategies with colleagues adds a collective strength to personal efforts and minimizes the possibility of misunderstanding. With problem or conflict situations, getting ideas from trusted colleagues beforehand enhances the probability of accomplishing outcomes more effectively. An Australian study of 157 registered nurses working in a private hospital found that support lowered job-related stress and increased job satisfaction. Support was given to nurses by supervisors and other nurses (Bartram, Joiner, & Stanton, 2004).

Professional organizations do not usually have the primary purpose of providing emotional support; however, small subgroups within professional organizations may be used for personal support. A professional support group composed of individuals with similar work experience can be comforting. Often, family and friends have a limited understanding of the emotional impact of your experiences.

USE GROUP PROCESS

Creating opportunities for interdisciplinary groups to get together is a highly effective strategy for enhancing collaboration and communication. Ideas include collaborative rounds, team briefings, and committees to discuss problems. Some studies associate daily team rounds and joint decision making with shorter hospital stay and lower hospital charges.

TEAM BRIEFING MEETINGS

In addition to clarifying client information exchange and opening communication, some meetings could focus on opening up communication in a nonantagonistic fashion focusing on improving "people skills" such as conveying mutual respect and improving staff relations. Conflict situations among colleagues or among departments become negative when not dealt with. Recognition provides a potential opportunity for improvement. When effectively addressed, there is a tendency for the team to become stronger and to function more effectively.

ORGANIZATIONAL WORK GROUPS

Successful participation in work groups requires flexibility and good communication. This is especially true when the task is to implement some agency change. The Joint Commission also recommends violence audits and violence prevention inservice programs for all employees to address techniques for violence de-escalation (www.jointcommission.org/SentinelEvent Alert/Issue45, June 3, 2010).

WORK TOWARD AN ORGANIZATIONAL CLIMATE OF MUTUAL RESPECT

As mentioned earlier, the Joint Commission is requiring all health care organizations to have written codes of behavior and to establish internal processes to handle disruptive behaviors. Organizational strategies are discussed in Chapter 22; other strategies within the organization could include understanding the organizational system.

UNDERSTAND THE ORGANIZATIONAL SYSTEM

Whenever you work in an organization, you automatically become a part of a system that has norms for acceptable behavior. Each organizational system defines its own chain of command and rules about social processes in professional communication. Even though your idea may be excellent, failure to understand the chain of command or an unwillingness to form the positive alliances needed to accomplish your objective dilutes the impact. For example, if your instructor has been defined as your first line of contact, then it is not in your best interest to seek out staff personnel or other students without also checking with the instructor.

Although sidestepping the identified chain of command and going to a higher or more tangential resource in the hierarchy may appear less threatening initially, the benefits of such action may not resolve the difficulty. Furthermore, the trust needed for serious discussion becomes limited. Some of the reasons for avoiding positive interactions stem from an internal circular process of faulty thinking. Because communication is viewed as part of a process, the sender and receiver act on the information received, which may or may not represent the reality of the situation. Examples of the circular processes that block the development of cooperative and receptive influencing skills in organizational settings are presented in Table 23-1.

DOCUMENT AND USE THE COMPLAINT PROCEDURE TO REPORT INCIDENCES

In handling disruptive behavior occurrences, documentation is a key step. Some suggest beginning with a staff survey. Some agencies may hold "communication training sessions" after the offenses have been documented. Prevention strategies might include participation in assertiveness training inservices or the TeamSTEPPS program as cited in Chapter 22. Educational interventions that increase staff awareness are extremely effective, as are rehearsals similar to the exercises in this book (Bigony et al., 2009).

SUMMARY

In this chapter, the same principles of communication used in the nurse-client relationship are broadened to examine the nature of communication among health professionals. Most nurses will experience conflicts with coworkers at some time during their careers. The same elements of thoughtful purpose, authenticity, empathy, active listening, and respect for the dignity of others that underscore successful nurse-client relationships are needed in relations with other health professionals. Building bridges to professional communication with colleagues involves concepts of collaboration, coordination, and networking. Modification of barriers to professional communication includes negotiation and conflict resolution. Learning is a lifelong process, not only for nursing care skills but for communication skills. These will develop as you continue to gain experience working as part of an interdisciplinary group.

ETHICAL DILEMMA | What Would You Do?

You are working a 12-hour shift on a labor and delivery unit. Today, Mrs. Kalim is one of your assigned clients. She is fully dilated and effaced, but contractions are still 2 minutes apart after 10 hours of labor. Mrs. Kalim, her obstetrician Dr. Mary, and you have agreed on her plan to have a fully natural delivery without medication. However, her obstetrician's partner is handling day shift today, and Dr. Mary goes home. This new obstetrician orders you to administer several medications to Mrs. Kalim to strengthen contractions and speed up delivery, because he has another patient across town to deliver. Your unit adheres to an empowering model of practice that believes in client advocacy. How will you handle this potential physician conflict? Is this a true moral dilemma?

TABLE 23-1	Examples of Unclear Communication Processes That Block the Development of Cooperative and Receptive Influencing Skills	
Situation	**Cognitive Process**	**Reframed to Improve Communication**
Low self-disclosure	No one knows my real thoughts, feelings, and needs. *Consequently:* I think no one cares about me or recognizes my needs. Others see me as self-sufficient and are unaware that I have a problem. *Consequently:* Others are unable to respond to my needs.	I need to verbalize aloud my needs clearly so others can have an opportunity to respond.
Reluctance to delegate tasks	Other people think I do not believe that they can do the job as well as I can. *Consequently:* The others work at a minimum level. I do not expect or ask others to be involved. *Consequently:* Other people do not volunteer to help me. *Consequently:* I feel resentful, and others feel undervalued and dispensable.	I am part of a team. I need to assign team members to do the tasks they can complete competently.
Making unnecessary demands	I expect more from others than they think is reasonable. *Consequently:* I feel the others are lazy and uncommitted, and I must push harder. Others see me as manipulative and dehumanizing. *Consequently:* Others assume a low profile and do not contribute their ideas. *Consequently:* Work production is mediocre. Morale is low. Everyone, including me, feels disempowered.	I need to clearly define my expectations and capabilities, in a respectful manner. I need to set clear work goals and deadlines. I need to give feedback.

REFERENCES

American Association of Critical Care Nurses: *Zero tolerance for abuse position statement*, 2004.www.aacn.org/WD/Practice/Docs/Zero_Tolerance_for_Abuse.pdf.

American Medical Association: *Disruptive behavior: model medical staff code of conduct*, 2008. Available online: www.ama-assn.org/ama/pub/about-ama/our-people www.ama-assn.org/go/omss. Accessed March 14, 2009.

American Nurses Association: *Code of Ethics for nurses with interpretative statements*, Washington, DC, 2001, Author.

American Nurses Association: *Registered professional nurses and unlicensed assistive personnel*, Washington, DC, 1994, Author.

Bacal R: *Dealing with angry employees* [online article], n.d. Available online: http://work911.com/articles/angrye.htm.

Bacal R: *Organizational conflict: the good, the bad & the ugly* [online article], n.d. Available online:http://work911.com/articles/orgconflict.htm.

Bartram T, Joiner TA, Stanton P, et al: Factors affecting the job stress and job satisfaction of Australian nurses: implications for recruitment and retention, *Contemp Nurse* 17(3):293–304, 2004.

Bigony L, Lipke TG, Lundberg A, et al: Lateral violence in the perioperative setting, *AORN J* 89(4):688–696, 2009.

Boone BN, King ML, Gresham LS, et al: Conflict management training and nurse-physician behaviors, *J Nurses Staff Dev* 24(4): 168–175, 2008.

Bournes DA, Milton CL: Nurses' experiences of feeling respected-not respected, *Nurs Sci Q* 22(1):47–56, 2009.

Gerardi D, Connell MK: The emerging culture of health care: from horizontal violence to true collaboration, *Nebr Nurse* 40(3):16–18, 2007.

Hutchinson M, Vickers M, Jackson D, et al: I'm gonna do what I want to do: organizational change as a legitimized vehicle for bullies, *Health Care Manag Rev* 30(4):331–336, 2005.

Johnson SL: International perspectives on workplace bullying among nurses: a review, *Int Nurs Rev* 56:34–40, 2009.

Johnson SL, Rea RE: Workplace bullying: concern for nurse leaders, *J Nurs Admin* 39(2):84–90, 2009.

Joint Commission for the Accreditation of Healthcare Organizations: Behaviors that undermine a culture of safety, *Sentinel Event Alert* 40(July 9):1–3, 2008.www.jointcommission.org/SentinelEventAlert/.

Joint Commission for the Accreditation of Healthcare Organizations: Preventing Violence in the health care setting, *Sentinel Event Alert* 45 (June 3):1–3, 2010.www.jointcommission.org/SentinelEventAlert/.

Joint Commission Resources: *Civility in the health care workplace*, vol 6, pp. 1–8, 2006. Available online: http://www.jcipatientsafety.org/15419/ Accessed March 1, 2009.

Katrinli A, Atabay G, Gunay G, et al: Leader-member exchange: organizational identification and the mediating role of job involvement for nurses, *J Adv Nurs* 64(4):354–362, 2008.

Kerfoot K: Moving toward zero: the leader's mandate, *Nurs Econ* 26(5):331–332, 2008.

Nielsen P, Mann S: Team function in obstetrics to reduce errors and improve outcomes, *Obstet Gynecol Clin* 35(1):61–65, 2008.

O'Daniel M, Rosenstein AH: Professional communication and team collaboration. In Hughes RG, editor: *Patient safety and quality: an evidence-based handbook for nurses*, [AHRQ Pub no. 08-0043] Rockville, MD, 2008, Agency for Research and Quality.

Olender-Russo L: Creating a culture of regard: an antidote for workplace bullying, *Creat Nurs* 15(2):75–81, 2009.

O'Reilly KB: *AMA meeting: disruptive behavior standard draws fire.* Available online: www.ama-assn.org/amednews/2008/12/01/prse1201.htm.

Parse RR: Feeling respected: a Parse method study, *Nurs Sci Q* 19: 51–56, 2006.

Rosenstein AH, O'Daniel M: Disruptive behavior and clinical outcomes: perceptions of nurses and physicians, *Am J Nurs* 105(1): 54–64, 2005.

Seago JA: Professional communication. In Hughes RG, editor: *Patient safety and quality: an evidence-based handbook for nurses*, [AHRQ Publication no. 08-0043]Rockville, MD, 2008, Agency for Healthcare Research and Quality.

Spence-Laschinger HK, Leiter M, Day A, et al: Workplace empowerment, incivility and burnout: impact on staff nurse recruitment and retention outcomes, *J Nurs Manag* 17:302–311, 2009.

Wachs J: Workplace incivility, bullying, and mobbing, *AAOHN* 57(2):88, 2009.

Woelfle CY, McCaffrey R: Nurse on nurse, *Nurs Forum* 42(3):123–131, 2007.

CHAPTER 24

Communicating for Continuity of Care

Elizabeth C. Arnold

OBJECTIVES

At the end of the chapter, the reader will be able to:

1. Describe current challenges in health care delivery creating the need for continuity of care (COC).
2. Define COC and describe its relational, informational, and management dimensions.
3. Discuss the application of relational continuity concepts: client-centered care,

professional collaboration, and team communications.

4. Discuss the application of informational continuity concepts related to discharge planning and handoffs.
5. Discuss the application of management COC concepts related to case management and community advocacy.

Modern clinical practice requires new approaches to health care service delivery, with an emphasis on developing cost-saving coordination of health care delivery for individuals with chronic medical and mental disorders. This chapter provides a framework for exploring communication concepts and relationship strategies within and across health care systems. The chapter describes the concept of continuity of care (COC) and identifies its key components: relational, informational, and management continuity (Haggerty et al., 2003). Applications related to each dimension are discussed.

BASIC CONCEPTS

Continuity of Care COC provides a new model for describing the coordination and connections required across time, multiple clinical settings, and provider/agencies to effectively manage the health care of individuals with chronic conditions in the community (Sparbel & Anderson, 2000). Developing community-based collaborative models of care related to need

assessments, referral, and early intervention will be key to providing quality health care, particularly for youths and seniors as budgets tighten (Tractenberg, 2010).

The World Health Organization (WHO) calls for an emphasis on continuous care by skilled and primary care health teams, rather than on episodic hospital care of seriously ill clients to ensure quality care (Thomas, 2009). The Institute of Medicine (IOM, 2001a) identifies continuity of care (COC) as an essential component of quality primary care. At the core of COC is the therapeutic nurse-client relationship. This relationship serves as a critical communication bridge between clients and their health providers in developing and implementing comprehensive care plans.

CURRENT CHALLENGES IN HEALTH CARE DELIVERY

The nation's health care delivery system currently faces major challenges for complex interconnected reasons. The need for health care delivery systems organized around an acute, episodic medical model of care no longer suffices as a primary service model. Needed is a redesign of the health care system to include a prominent emphasis on chronic disease self-management (Thorne, 2008).

Clients today are discharged earlier, have complex medication and treatment regimens, and are seen by different health care providers in multiple care settings. Self-management, family involvement, and shared decision making have become an indispensable means of bridging the gap between diminishing financial support for chronic care and multifaceted health care demands that can last for years. To achieve quality health outcomes with chronic conditions, clients and families must have dependable relationships, accurate information, and ongoing collaborative support from coordinated health services.

Managed care is now the dominant form of health care financing in the United States. The goal of this new system of care reimbursement is to administratively lower costs, while providing quality health care delivery (Lein, Collins, Lyles, Hillman, & Smith, 2003). The bulk of health care is increasingly provided in primary care settings, with acute episodic care reserved for short-term hospital stays. People are better informed, more assertive, and more insistent on prompt access and value for their health care dollar (von Bultzingslowen, Eliasson, Sarvimaki, Mattson, & Hjortdah, 2006).

Other factors such as *Healthy People 2010* objectives, growing globalization, a sharp increase in migration of people without health insurance to the United States and Canada, and turbulent economic changes call sharp attention to widespread escalating public health issues and health care disparities. Provider shortages in the health care system, notably physicians and nurses, mandate a search for different and more effective, efficient ways of meeting client health care needs across multiple clinical settings.

CONTINUITY OF CARE FOR CHRONIC CONDITIONS

COC is recognized as an essential component of comprehensive care for individuals with chronic health conditions. WHO (2002) defines chronic health conditions as "health problems that require ongoing management over a period of years or decades" (p. 11). Examples include fibromyalgia, cancer, multiple sclerosis, and serious persistent mental disorders. What chronic conditions share in common is a requirement for ongoing health care management.

Kleinman (1988) describes chronic illness from the client perspective:

> The undercurrent of chronic illness is like the volcano: it does not go away, It menaces. It erupts. It is out of control...confronting crises is only one part of the total picture. The rest is coming to grips with the mundaneness of worries...Chronic illness also means the loss of confidence in one's health and normal bodily processes. (pp. 44–45)

CONTINUITY OF CARE

Sparbel and Anderson (2000) define **COC** as "a series of connected patient-care events both within a health care institution and among multiple settings" (p. 17). Nurses have an important role in implementing COC as a multidimensional concept, which according to Haggerty et al. (2003) is concerned with the following factors:

- Ensuring accessibility to coordinated health care services
- Personalization of care to meet a client's changing needs across delivery systems
- Informational data sharing of various elements of personal and medical data electronically over time and place, which contribute to appropriate care delivery
- Health services provided in an organized, logical, and timely manner, using a shared management plan

COC is described as a thread binding together episodes of care, and providing linkages across time, service providers and health care settings (Fletcher et al., 1984).

Dimensions of Continuity of Care

COC is an interdependent systems concept, consisting of three interlocking components: relational, informational, and management continuity. Each is dependent on the others (Schultz, 2009). Relational (interpersonal) continuity occurs through relationships with trusted care providers such that discrete health care events are experienced as being coherent and connected. Informational continuity is achieved through accurate record sharing and frequent team communication. Management continuity is accomplished through case management that can be flexibly adjusted to meet changing client needs in the community (Haggerty et al., 2003).

Relational Continuity. Haggerty et al. (2008) define relational continuity as "a therapeutic relationship with a practitioner that spans more than one episode of care and leads, in the practitioner, to a sense of clinical responsibility and an accumulated knowledge of the patient's personal and medical circumstances" (p. 118). A sustained relationship between health care providers and clients gives clients confidence that their providers know their circumstances well and are able to coordinate care between different providers and specialists.

Respect for client and family values, beliefs, knowledge, cultural background, and preferences are fundamental aspects of the relational continuity required for planning, delivery, and evaluation of comprehensive reliable care, particularly for chronic health conditions. Client participation offers health care providers unique insights into the context of an illness experience.

Providing health care for individuals with complex health care needs can exceed the energy and expertise of any one provider, even when highly talented. Current health care delivery systems emphasize team functioning in which professionals from different disciplines assume treatment responsibility for a common client population, develop common client-centered treatment goals, and function as a unified entity in providing client-centered care.

Professional team collaboration describes a communication process among health professionals required for promoting coordination of services and resolving complex treatment issues. Increasing the level of collaboration among health care professionals has been identified as one of the best strategies to improve the level of continuity in the health care system (San Martin-Rodriguez, D'Amour, & Leduc, 2008).

Informational Continuity. Communication of complete unbiased information is critical to ensuring safe, reliable care continuity (Kohn et al., 2000). Informational continuity refers to data exchanges among providers and provider systems, and between providers and clients related to care. Informational continuity is what "links provider to provider, and health care event to health care event" (Pontin & Lewis, 2008, p. 1199). As the client's condition changes, alterations are communicated quickly and accurately.

Sources of informational continuity include multidisciplinary team meetings, progress notes, handoff reporting, discharge plans, referral contacts, and client summaries. The SBAR is a new situational briefing format, which provides critical information about changes in a client's condition and is used in handoff or discharge/transfer of clients (Leonard, Graham, & Bonacum, 2004).

Management Continuity. Nazareth et al. (2008) define management continuity as "the delivery of health care by several providers in a complementary and timely manner through shared management plans that are consistent and flexible" (p. 570). The expectation is that health and complementary delivery services responsive to client needs will be provided to clients and families in a timely coordinated manner over an extended period. Management continuity represents a longitudinal pattern of health care utilization (Saultz & Albedaiwi, 2004), usually coordinated through case management.

Functionality of Continuity of Care

COC describes the communication bridge between discrete illness episodes and coordination of interventions by different providers to address changes in illness status (Mainous & Gill, 1998). When services are effectively coordinated, there is less potential for duplication of services, conflicting assessments, gaps in service, and decreased use of preventable acute care services. COC reduces medication and treatment errors, provides timely follow-up, and eases transitions between care settings for everyone concerned. Clients and families experience greater satisfaction.

Sharing of clinical activities makes for more holistic interventions (San Martin-Rodriguez, D'Amour, & Leduc, 2008). For chronically ill and elderly clients, COC means that they are more likely to have health care providers familiar with their overall history, who can notice subtle changes in the client's health status (von Bultzingslowen et al., 2006).

Developing an Evidence-Based Practice

Balaban M, Weissman J, Samuel P, Woolhandler S: Redefining and redesigning hospital discharge to enhance patient care: a randomized controlled study, *J Gen Intern Med* 23(8):1228–1233, 2008.

This randomized, controlled study was designed to evaluate a low-cost intervention for culturally and linguistically clients being discharged from a small community hospital. The intervention, designed to improve COC, involved a "user-friendly" patient discharge form, with electronic transmission to a primary care site, telephone contact from a nurse at the primary care site, and primary care review/modification of the discharge-transfer plan. The study sample of 122 patients was randomized to intervention and control groups (historical and concurrent). The outcome variable related to preventable negative clinical outcomes. Comparative differences between the control groups and the intervention group were statistically analyzed using chi-squared tests. *t* Tests were used to analyze continuous variables.

Results: Study results showed that among participants in the study sample, the intervention significantly increased outpatient follow-up and completion of outpatient workups recommended by the hospitalist. The intervention was especially effective with short hospital stays (1–2 days) and with study participants 60 years and older.

Application to Your Clinical Practice: The systematic transfer of client care from the hospital to a primary care "medical home" is needed to provide seamless medical care during the transition. This study proposes a new paradigm to formalize communication such that all parties involved in the client's care are well informed about postdischarge care. In what ways do you think studies of discharge-transfer interventions are important components of COC? How can you as a nurse facilitate compliance with follow-up treatment in a hospital setting? In a community or home setting?

APPLICATIONS

COC approaches are designed to provide a seamless continuum of care for clients through coordinated, acute, and community-based health services and relationships based on client needs and preferences. Multiple research studies have demonstrated improved clinical outcomes, satisfaction with care, and enhanced quality of life related to COC (van Servellen, Fongwa, & Mockus D'Errico, 2006).

CREATING RELATIONAL CONTINUITY

Relational stability is the interpersonal aspect of COC. It is a fundamental communication channel used to guarantee well-coordinated health care service delivery, free from errors and tailored to meet the individual client's health needs. Interdisciplinary collaboration within a health organization and professional communication across health care systems are essential characteristics of professional relationships.

In today's health care system, a person's health care is looked on as the joint responsibility of clients, their families, and professional care providers. Although the emphasis with each health care episode may differ depending on the type and setting of care, the client is always the central focus.

PATIENT (CLIENT)-CENTERED CARE

The IOM (2001a) defines **patient (client)-centered care** as "providing care that is respectful of and responsive to individual patient preferences, needs, and values, and ensuring that patient values guide all clinical decisions" (p. 40). Client-centered care is designed to recognize subtle differences among clients having the same diagnosis and cultural experiences, and to incorporate this knowledge into the care of the whole individual (Engebretson, Mahoney, & Carlson, 2008; Hasnain-Wynia, 2006).

Client-centered care requires individualizing nursing interventions based on a person's values, preferences, and beliefs as the basis for customized clinical decisions (Engebretson et al., 2008; Hasnain-Wynia, 2006). Being attuned to cultural cues about beliefs and values, including attitudes about illness, provider relationships, and the nature of healing helps nurses make better sense of the clinical reality of a client's illness from the client and family perspective.

Client-centered care supports client autonomy and helps people take control of their health care, to whatever extent is possible. Individual need for full disclosure can vary as the client's condition changes and is affected by cultural norms. Client-centered care respects the amount of information desired by clients and their families, and to whom it should be provided. Attending to the physical and emotional comfort of the client, providing sufficient information with plenty of time for questions, feedback, and time spent on reducing client or family anxiety about new information are significant aspects of patient-centered care. Box 24-1 identifies IOM guiding principles for providing client-centered care.

| **BOX 24-1** | Institute of Medicine Guiding Principles for Client-Centered Care |

- Care is based on continuous healing relationships and not just face-to-face visits, implying that the health care system must be responsive at all times and care should be provided by the most expedient means.
- Care should be designed to meet the most common types of needs but should have the capability to respond to individual patient choices, need, values, and preferences.
- The patient is the source of control by being given the necessary information and opportunity to exercise the degree of control they choose over health care decisions that affect them.

- Patients should have unfettered access to their own medical information and to clinical knowledge; clinicians and patients should communicate effectively and share information.
- Decision-making is research based, with care being consistent across clinicians and jurisdictions.
- Transparency is necessary, making available to patients and their families information that enables them to make informed decisions when selecting a health plan, hospital, or clinical practice, or when choosing among alternative treatments including information describing patient safety, research-based practice, outcomes, and patient satisfaction.

From Coleman EA, Fox PD: One patient, many places: managing health care transitions, Part 1: introduction, accountability, information for patients in transition, Annals of Long-Term Care, 12(9): 25-32, 2004.

BUILDING COLLABORATIVE PARTNERSHIPS WITH CLIENTS

Well-planned, competently executed, client-centered care results in improved practice efficiency and better client outcomes (Epstein, Fiscella, Lesser & Stange, 2010). . Client-centered care emphasizes partnerships between clients and providers, consisting of following factors:

- Mutual respect for the skills and knowledge of client consumers and the health care team
- Accessibility and respectful empathetic responsiveness to client and family needs
- Shared planning and development of mutually agreed-on goals that reflect the client's needs, beliefs, values, and preferences
- Frequent evaluation, based on a mutual exchange of information, constructive feedback, and negotiation of care strategies that are empowering and practical.

Family-centered care comes into play when the health needs of children are involved. Family-centered care is more complex. Parents may need help with parenting skills both in handling the needs of a chronically ill child and in providing support and direct care. Box 24-2 offers principles of family-centered care.

SHARED DECISION MAKING

A client-centered care views the client and family as equal partners with providers in negotiating treatment decisions and evaluating treatment outcomes (Engebretson et al., 2008; IOM, 2001b). To ensure that care decisions respect client values, needs, and

| **BOX 24-2** | Selected Principles of Family-Centered Care in Working with Parents |

- Families represent a central constant construct in children's lives.
- Each family is unique, with diverse clinical needs and strengths.
- Parents are ultimately responsible for the health and welfare of their children.
- Family-centered care should be based on family strengths and competencies.
- An important source of support for families is networking and family-to-family support.
- All family members should be encouraged to participate in the child's care.
- Family members should have the right to determine how much they will participate in decision making for their child.

Adapted from O'Neil M, Ideishi R, Nixon-Cave K, Kohrt A: Care coordination between medical and early intervention services: family and provider perspectives, *Fam Syst Health* 26(2):119–134, 2008.

preferences, health care providers need to: (1) observe and listen carefully; and (2) provide clients and families with the education and support they need to make reasoned decisions, and actively participate in their health care. Full disclosure of information is a prerequisite for effective shared decision making. Relevant information includes:

- Detailed information on diagnosis
- Options for treatment
- Anticipated clinical outcomes
- Treatment and care processes required to achieve desired clinical outcomes

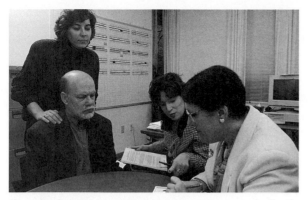

Shared decision making requires client and family involvement in all health care decisions.

RELATIONAL CONTINUITY: PROFESSIONAL PERSPECTIVES

Sheehan, Robertson, and Ormond (2007) differentiate between multidisciplinary and interdisciplinary teams. Professionals on multidisciplinary teams "each work within their particular scope of practice and interact formally. Interdisciplinary teams are characterized by greater overlapping of professional roles, formal and informal communication and shared problem solving for the good of the patient" (p. 18).

Although multidisciplinary teams share information with each other, and work in tandem with other disciplines, they function independently, with each being responsible for different care needs. By contrast, an interdisciplinary team develops a collective vision and common language to support a collaborative unified working approach to clinical problems. An interdisciplinary team actually integrates services, using teamwork principles, whereas on a multidisciplinary team, each profession maintains its own silo of expertise without much interaction (Margalit, Thompson, & Visovsky, 2009).

The interdisciplinary team consists of a core group of health professionals (commonly physician, nurse, social worker, pharmacist, and caseworker). Although each discipline has its central role, integrated client-centered care represents the team's core value. Decision making is nonhierarchal, with every professional being willing and ready to assume responsibility for achieving positive treatment outcomes (Jansen, 2008).

Interdisciplinary team function takes into account the diverse standards and behaviors associated with each clinical discipline, and emphasizes the common mission of working together to resolve complex clinical problems (Clark, Cott, & Drinka, 2007; D'Amour & Oandasan, 2005). Figure 24-1 presents the dimensions of patient centered care.

Each member of the team functions as both an individual and a health care professional representing a distinct discipline. Fundamental to effective participation on an interdisciplinary team is a clear understanding of one's own discipline, plus a knowledge and mutual respect for each other's discipline's roles, professional

Figure 24-1 Dimensions of client-centered care.

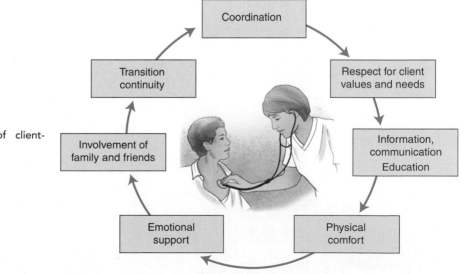

responsibilities, and expertise (Lidskog, Lofmark, & Ahlstrom, 2007).

Even when core personal and professional values, attitudes, and practices are not at odds with each other, professional training and interpretations of standards can shape how professional values are prioritized (D'Amour & Oandasan, 2005; Hall, 2005). Sparbel and Anderson (2000) identify team role confusion, fueled by professional rivalries, territoriality, and lack of clarification about job responsibilities, as a potential barrier to effective team communication. Exercise 24-1 explores the impact of discovering commonalities in people.

PROFESSIONAL COLLABORATION

The goal of interprofessional collaboration is to produce "a synthesis of the information such that the outcomes are more than additive" (Muir, 2008, p. 5). Interdisciplinary team collaboration enables practitioners to learn new skills and approaches, and encourages synergistic creativity among professionals. Collaboration decreases fragmentation and duplication of effort and promotes safe quality care (Figure 24-2) presents desired characteristics of professional collaboration.

Team collaboration includes the client as an essential collaborative partner. Within nurse-client relationships, nurses help clients interpret clinical findings, frame important questions about their diagnosis, treatment, or prognosis, and follow through with treatment recommendations.

TeamSTEPPS (Department of Defense, 2009) represents an accepted, evidence-based framework developed jointly by the Agency for Health Care Research and Quality and Department of Defense to guide development and implementation of interdisciplinary team collaboration in health care centers. Competency elements are identified in Box 24-3. Professional collaboration takes place through formally scheduled team meetings, informal huddles, and client comfort rounds.

Team Meetings

Interdisciplinary team collaboration differs from group communication in that team membership, focus of communication, and anticipated outcomes are consistently and solely focused on present moment client needs and solution planning. Team meetings serve the distinct purpose of concentrated discussion about targeted client and family needs, and meeting related treatment goals.

EXERCISE 24-1	Characteristics in Common

Purpose: To help students develop a sense of rapport with others as a basis for team understanding and communication.

Procedure:
1. Break up into teams of three students and appoint a scribe. Each group has 10 minutes.
2. In each group, answer this question: What is the most unexpected thing each group member holds in common with the other two group members?
3. Return to the larger group and share the answers with the larger class group.

Discussion:
1. How easy was it to share with others information about yourself that they didn't know previously?
2. What things made it easier or harder to share?
3. In what ways were you surprised to learn about something unexpected that you had in common with your teammates?
4. How could you use what you learned in this exercise to create better communication with other health care professionals?

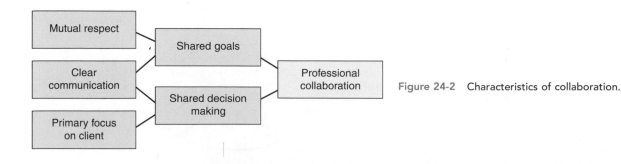

Figure 24-2   Characteristics of collaboration.

| BOX 24-3 | Competency Elements of TeamSTEPPS |

- Team leadership—the ability to direct and coordinate activities of team members, assess team performance, assign tasks, develop team knowledge and skills, motivate team members, plan and organize, and establish a positive team atmosphere
- Situation monitoring (or mutual performance monitoring)—the capacity to develop common understandings of the team environment and apply appropriate strategies to monitor teammate performance accurately
- Mutual support (or backup behavior)—the ability to anticipate other team members' needs and to shift workload among members to achieve balance
- Communication—including the efficient exchange of information and consultation with other team members

A smoothly run team meeting is one in which the team understands the mission of providing holistic care through defined membership, and where any problem related to client and family care can be worked through to the joint satisfaction of the team and client/family. Wise team leadership and careful attention to member relationships are essential.

The shared goals of client and health care team focus the discussion. Unrelated discussion or focus on routine details or on competing goals are discouraged because they distort or compromise the concentration of the team on key client/family needs and solutions. Time is a precious commodity for busy health care providers, so team meetings begin and end on time. Exercise 24-2 provides an opportunity for students to understand collaboration skills in team decision making.

Huddles

Sometimes an urgent problem arises that cannot wait until the team meets again. Huddles, defined as limited spontaneous or scheduled briefings, allow interdisciplinary team members to meet briefly with each other or with bedside caregivers for the purpose of staying

| EXERCISE 24-2 | Team Decision Making |

Purpose: To help students work together to discover how they work together to develop a consensus about an uncertain situation.

Procedure:
Break up the students into groups of four to six students. Each group should consider the scenario below and decide on which four people should be allowed to enter the life raft in a 15- to 20-minute time frame.
  The group should provide a rationale for selection.
Scenario:
A small aircraft crashes on a small island in the Pacific Ocean. There are six survivors, but the life raft can only hold four people.
  1. Bill is the pilot. He is a veteran pilot, with a good flying record. Recently, there has been a concern that he is depressed and showing signs of a drinking problem.
  2. Jack is a successful physician about to turn 60, and a bachelor. He is planning to retire next year and is looking forward to a life of leisure and travel, which he feels he deserves and has looked forward to all his life.
  3. Mary is a gifted musician in her early 30s. She is married, has three children, and recently received her first contract with a major orchestra.
  4. Maria is a 45-year-old diabetic. She has had a difficult life but is planning to marry the man of her dreams when she returns from this trip.
  5. Jeff is a broker with a major investment company. He recently resigned in the midst of a scandal involving insider trading, although he personally was never legally charged. He is married and has two teenage boys.
  6. John is a health director of an HIV treatment center. He was instrumental in acquiring properties and acceptance of HIV patients, which would not have been possible without his expertise. His treatment center is used as a model for treating HIV patients. Recently, John was diagnosed with HIV.

Discussion:
How did each group reach their decision?
What was it like to know you had to make a team decision about an issue for which there is no perfect answer?
What factors made the discussion easier or harder?
What did you learn about how people function as a team in making a difficult decision within a short time frame?

informed, making on-the-spot decisions, and being able to move ahead quickly in rapidly changing health circumstances. Huddles are held more frequently than team meetings, sometimes daily. They typically last no more than 7 to 10 minutes and are convened spontaneously in a convenient location with team members standing rather than sitting close to the site of action (Institute for Healthcare Improvement, 2007).

Sharing Critical information

Leonard et al. (2004) advocate the use of the SBAR format as a succinct way to share critical information with physicians and other team members about sudden changes in a client situation. The statements should contain a concise, convincing statement about the severity of the client's condition.

Case Example

- **Situation:** "Dr. Preston, I'm calling about Mr. Lakewood, who's having trouble breathing."
- **Background:** "He's a 54-year-old man with chronic lung disease who has been sliding downhill, and now he's acutely worse."
- **Assessment:** "I don't hear any breath sounds in his right chest. I think he has a pneumothorax."
- **Recommendation:** "I need you to see him right now. I think he needs a chest tube" (Leonard et al., 2004, p. i86).

Nursing Comfort Rounds

Studies have identified nursing rounds as a way to enhance client-centered care, improve client satisfaction, and enhance client safety (Bourgault et al., 2008; Meade, Bursell, & Ketelsen, 2006). Regular comfort rounds with professional nurses and/or clinical support staff provide opportunities to continuously meet client nonmedical needs and to share information with clients (Castledine, 2002). Common components include assessment of the environment to ensure that equipment is within easy reach of the client, adequate pain management, and attention to personal needs such as repositioning and toileting (Meade et al., 2006).

ROLE OF THE HOSPITALIST

A new professional role designed to improve COC in acute care settings is that of the "hospitalist" (Amin & Owen, 2006; Wachter & Goldman, 1996). The hospitalists may be a physician or nurse practitioner employed by the hospital to clinically manage inpatient medical care, with specialty physicians acting as consultants. The hospitalist assumes responsibility for coordinating care, integrating diagnostic test results, making decisions, presenting options to the client and family, and communicating with other professionals who may be or will become involved in the client's care after discharge. The specific dimensions of the hospitalist role are determined by the care site rather than clinical specialty (Schneller & Epstein, 2006).

Although hospitalists are often the client's main point of contact throughout the acute hospitalization phase, they may have limited knowledge of the client's health care patterns before hospitalization. The primary physician may have limited contact with the client during the hospitalization but will be expected to re-engage with the client on discharge.

Nurses have an important communication role with hospitalists. Clients cannot always easily interpret the events related to rapidly changing prognostic changes or treatment options. They are more likely to discuss their concerns regarding particular treatment issues with the nurse during the course of care provision than they are in formal meetings with the health care team. Nurses can and should be proactive in talking informally with physicians about their clients and in contributing data in huddles and team meetings.

Periodically, and or when the client's condition changes, the hospitalist or entire treatment team may meet with the family to discuss changes, treatment options, and family concerns. Even in the best of circumstances, client/family meetings with the health care team to discuss sensitive health issues such as discontinuing life support or transfer of clients to subacute or community settings with anxious clients and concerned family members can be highly intimidating. Nurses can help clients and families by continuing conversations after the health care team leaves, answering questions and providing support.

INFORMATIONAL CONTINUITY

Informational COC allows for an uninterrupted flow of data and clinical impressions between health care providers and agencies, with clients and their families, over time and space. Gaps in informational continuity can occur as a result of misplaced clinical records, inadequate discharge planning or referral data, deficient or delayed authorization for treatment, and lack of understanding by the client of their illness or treatment, or self-management guidelines. Lack of information at time of transfer can result in treatment delays, and can increase the client and/or family's anxiety unnecessarily. When clients get full information and a consistent message from their health care providers, regardless of where they are in the health care system, they become more relaxed and open to treatment recommendations.

Informational continuity requires sharing health and treatment information and changes with clients and families that are consistent, complete, accurate, value neutral, and delivered in an easily understandable and supportive manner. Notifying the family of changes in the client's condition or treatment recommendations is an essential part of ensuring informational continuity, particularly if the family is not in close contact with the client.

HANDOFF CARE TRANSITIONS

Communication at transition points in health care takes place in the form of handoffs. **Handoffs** refer to transfer processes taking place when clients are reassigned to another level of care, for example, from the intensive care unit to a step-down unit, or to a less intensive care facility for continued rehabilitation services. Carr (2008) advises, "Handoffs or care transitions shouldn't be an abrupt end of care previously provided, but rather considered to be a coordinated changeover for the patient to a new team of involved caregivers" (p. 26). The Joint Commission (2009)

mandates timely and accurate transfer of handoff information related to transfer of clients from one unit to another and from one clinical setting to another.

Transitions from one clinical unit to another, and discharge to a different clinical setting provide opportunities for unintentional information gaps (Coleman & Berenson, 2004; Greenwald, Denham, & Jack, 2007). Core functions for transitional sending and receiving teams designed to limit information gaps are presented in Box 24-4.

DOCUMENTING TRANSFER INFORMATION

SBAR is the most commonly used format for communicating pertinent information during handoff transfers and increasingly for shift reports. The format presents a clear, organized picture of a client's care during a shift or care episode to the different set of health professionals who will be assuming primary responsibility for client care. Mikos (2007) specifies the content information that nurses should include in Box 24-5. Exercise 24-3 provides practice with using the SBAR format.

DISCHARGE PLANNING AND REFERRALS

Han, Barnard, and Chapman (2009) use the American Hospital Association (AHA, 1983) definition of **discharge planning** "as a process of concentration, coordination and technology integration, through the cooperation of healthcare professionals, patients and their families, to ensure that all patients receive continuing care after being discharged" (p. 5).

BOX 24-4	SBAR Handoff Content Format in Inpatient Settings

Situation	Postoperative day (wounds/dressing/intravenous sites
Nurse name and unit	with date)
Reporting on (patient name and room number)	Mobility (number of staff and lifting device needed)
Background	Mental status
Admission diagnosis and date of admission	Pain assessment/reassessment (last time pain
Pertinent medical history	medication was given)
Brief synopsis of treatment to date	Physician orders (received, carried out, pending)
Patient code status (if applicable)	Oxygen (yes or no)
Family/significant other involvement	Changes from prior assessments (vital signs,
Isolation and type	neurologic changes, skin, pain)
Precautions (fall, suicide, seizure, restraints)	Recommendation
Medication reconciliation status	Items that require follow-up
Assessment	State of patient teaching needs
Vital signs	Discharge needs.
Abnormal laboratory results within 24 hours	

From Mikos K: Monitoring handoffs for standardization: 2008 guide to patient safety technology regulatory compliance, *Nurs Manag* 38(12): 16, 18, 20, 2007.

| BOX 24-5 | Nursing Components of a Comprehensive Discharge Process |

- Assessing the client's understanding of the discharge plan by asking them to explain it in their own words.
- Advising clients/family of any tests completed at the hospital with pending results at time of discharge, and notifying appropriate clinician of this contingency.
- Scheduling follow-up appointments or tests after discharge, if needed.
- Organizing home or health care services that needed to be initiated after discharge.

- Confirming the medication plan and ensuring that the client/family understands any changes (e.g., medication in the hospital not available or accessible in the community).
- Reviewing with the client/family what to do if a problem develops.
- Expediting transmission of the discharge summary to health care providers and case managers accepting responsibility.

| EXERCISE 24-3 | Using the SBAR Report Format |

Purpose: To provide an opportunity for students to use the SBAR format (found in Box 24-5) in a care transition report.

Procedure:
Using the following case study*, prepare a care transition report to accompany the client to his new unit.

Jeff O'Connor is a 66-year-old man originally admitted to the emergency department with severe chest pain, shortness of breath, dizziness, and intermittent palpitations. He was diagnosed with a myocardial infarction and admitted to the coronary care unit. He was placed on oxygen and remained there for several days because his serum markers continued to rise. He received morphine for pain and sedatives to keep him comfortable. He is currently stabilized with digoxin, demonstrates a normal sinus rhythm, and is being transferred to the step-down unit this afternoon. His wife and daughter have visited him several times each day. His wife states she is exhausted but is glad he is being transferred. Jeff has long-standing coronary artery disease, and a family history of cardiac events. This is his first heart attack.

Discussion:
If this is the only information you have on Jeff, what other data might you need to develop a full transitional report using the SBAR format?

*This exercise can be completed using a current client transfer.

Discharge planning begins with the client's admission to the hospital (Birmingham, 2004; Cotera-Perez, 2005). Nurses should educate clients and families about diagnosis and treatment throughout hospitalization, so that by the time the client is discharged, the client and family have a full understanding of the client's condition as a basis for follow-up care.

Assessment of Postdischarge Needs

Much of the care previously provided in acute care settings for clients has shifted to the home care environment (Cooke, Gemmill, & Grant, 2008). In the community, professional team care will involve interactions separated by both time and space.

Many clients/caregivers will require specific instruction in treatment-related tasks to successfully self-manage health problems at home. Arrangements and/or referrals for essential training needs should be implemented before discharge, if possible. Table 24-2

presents some of the key elements needed to plan for a successful transition from the hospital to the client's home.

Not all clients are discharged back to their home. Clients with complex disability or care needs may need to be discharged to a subacute or transitional skilled nursing facility for extended care. As soon as this is known, the client and the family need to be informed of the need for transfer and what parameters for discharge will be used for each client (Joint Commission, 2009). Recommendations for transfer should be thoroughly discussed with the family and included in the client's treatment plan. The goal of discharge planning is to provide clients and their families with the level and kind of information they will need to secure their recovery and/or maintain health status during the immediate posthospital period.

Clients may have multiple care transitions as part of their experience after discharge from a hospital setting (Boling, 2009). Frequent communication and careful coordination are keys to ensuring safe, effective care across settings. Successful transitioning involves consideration of the combined needs of the client and family, and the resources of the agency or health care provider to meet those needs. Table 24-1 provides guidelines for helping clients and families.

Clients admitted to emergency departments usually have limited information to prepare them for self-care after discharge. Nurses are responsible for communicating and coordinating postdischarge instructions with clients and families, quickly educating them about the client's condition and treatment-related tasks, and coordinating care with other health professionals as needed (Han et al., 2009).

Discharge Summary

The discharge summary is the most commonly used format for communicating diagnostic findings, hospital management, and plans for follow-up at the end of a client's hospitalization (Kripalani et al., 2007). Content mandated for each client's written discharge summary includes:

- Reason for hospitalization
- Significant findings
- Procedures and treatment provided
- The patient's condition at discharge
- Patient and family instructions (as appropriate)
- Attending physician's signature

TABLE 24-1	Collaborative Communication Protocol for Interdisciplinary Team Development

Name: Introduce yourself to other member(s) by name and discipline.

Role: Declare your professional role on the team, and describe it with respect to the target client under discussion.

Issue: Share with other team members your discipline-specific professional ideas regarding the treatment of the target client under discussion.

Feedback: As client issues are discussed, elicit interaction-specific feedback from other team participants in the interaction using prompts such as "Do you have any concerns?" or "Is there something else I should consider?"

Adapted from Zwarenstein M, Reeves S, Russell A, et al: Structuring communication relationships for interpersonal teamwork (SCRIPT): a cluster randomized controlled trial, *Trials* 8:23–36, 2007.

TABLE 24-2	Key Elements in Planning for Successful Transitions

Key Elements in Successful Transitions from Hospital to Home Health Care

Activity	Components
Assessment of need	Medical, functional, cognitive and behavioral, support system
Choose best next care setting	Nursing home Inpatient rehabilitation Assisted living Home with home health care Home with family or alone
Arrange services	Identify suitable agency(ies) and verify coverage
Clinical summary	Course (diagnosis and treatment) Key data (laboratory, radiographs, other) Care plan's main elements (how to care for the patient)
Medication reconciliation	Current medication list What was stopped and why What was started and why
Follow-up medical care	Appointments (names, times, dates, phone numbers)

Data from: Boling P: Care transitions and home health care, *Clin Geriatri Med* 25:135–148, 2009.

Clients should be encouraged to bring their discharge summary to initial follow-up appointments. The Joint Commission (2009) mandates that discharge summaries be completed within 30 days of hospital discharge.

Nurses are accountable for verbally reviewing discharge summaries with the client and/or caregiver as appropriate, providing written instructions, and completing discharge documentation in the chart. Although the physician is responsible for initiating and signing discharge summaries and orders, nurses play a critical role in the discharge of clients, as identified in Box 24-6.

Discharge instructions are not the same as discharge orders. Specific written discharge instructions should include a basic follow-up plan identifying diet, activity level, weight monitoring, what to do if symptoms develop or worsen, and the contact numbers of relevant hospital and primary care providers. Written instructions should be simple and concrete—for example, "Call the doctor if you gain more than 2 pounds in 1 week." A written list of all medications prescribed at discharge, including prescription, over-the-counter medications, and herbals, should be given to the client/caregiver.

| BOX 24-6 | Core Functions for Transitional Sending and Receiving Teams |

Both the sending and receiving care teams are expected to:

- Shift their perspective from the concept of a patient discharge to that of a patient transfer with continuous management.
- Begin planning for a transfer to the next care setting on or before a patient's admission.
- Elicit the preferences of patients and caregivers, and incorporate these preferences into the care plan, where appropriate.
- Identify a patient's system of social support and baseline level of function (i.e., How will this patient care for himself or herself after discharge?).
- Communicate and collaborate with practitioners across settings to formulate and execute a common care plan.
- Use the preferred mode of communication (i.e., telephone, fax, e-mail) of collaborators in other settings.

The sending health care team is expected to ensure that:

- The patient is stable enough to be transferred to the next care setting.
- The patient and caregiver understand the purpose of the transfer.
- The receiving institution is capable of and prepared to meet the patient's needs.
- All relevant sections of the transfer information form are complete.

- The care plan, orders, and a clinical summary precede the patient's arrival to the next care setting. The discharge summary should include the patient's baseline functional status (both physical and cognitive) and recommendations from other professionals involved with the patient's care, including social workers, occupational therapists, and physical therapists.
- The patient has a timely follow-up appointment with an appropriate health care professional.
- A member of the sending health care team is available to the patient, caregiver, and receiving health care team for 72 hours after the transfer to discuss any concerns regarding the care plan.
- The patient and family understand their health care benefits and coverage as they pertain to the transfer.

The receiving health care team is expected to ensure that:

- The transfer forms, clinical summary, discharge summary, and physician's orders are reviewed before or on the patient's arrival.
- The patient's goals and preferences are incorporated into the care plan.
- Discrepancies or confusion regarding the care plan, the patient's status, or the patient's medications are clarified with the sending health care team.

From HMO Work Group on Care Management: *One patient, many places: managing health care transitions* (p. 7), Washington, DC, 2004, AAHP-HIAA Foundation.

Discharge documentation in the client's chart should include the client's condition or functional status at time of discharge, followed by a summarization of the treatment and nursing care provided, discharge instructions given to the client/family and the client's responses. The place to which the client is charged (home, nursing home, rehabilitation center) should be identified. Subheadings help organize and highlight pertinent information for follow-up care (Kripalani et al., 2007). Nurses need to document that the client and/or caregiver was actually given a copy of the discharge instructions.

MANAGEMENT CONTINUITY

Management continuity represents a longitudinal approach to the clinical management of chronic disorders in the community. Care is delivered through coordinated referrals, case management, and community supports over a significant period.

THE MEDICAL HOME

A new concept in primary care service delivery designed to promote COC is the client/family-centered medical home. The **medical home** is defined as a community-based delivery process involving a primary care team, led by an identified personal physician for the client. The client's medical home accepts responsibility for coordinating health care across care settings, and providing accessible, comprehensive primary care services across time for designated clients and families.

The medical home serves as a central point of contact in primary care through which the majority of client health needs are met (Grumbach & Bodenheimer, 2002). Having a primary care home that coordinates care for all aspects of health care including acute and chronic care, preventive care, and palliative care is reassuring to clients and families. Over time, clients learn to depend on the medical home as a first-line treatment resource for all aspects of care. Physicians and other health care providers can provide better quality care because they have knowledge of the client's lifestyle and can better detect subtle changes in the client's situation or condition.

Using the medical home care delivery model provides an opportunity to effectively blend relational, informational, and management continuity into a holistic system of care for the client. A qualified provider consistent with the client's choice takes a clinical leadership role in coordinating care, with other care providers within and external to the medical home, providing skilled services when indicated. Medical homes provide quick access to health care and can facilitate connections to other providers or medical and mental health services when needed.

CASE MANAGEMENT

Whether one works in the hospital or primary care setting, all nurses should have knowledge of how case management works and how it fits into COC. Carter (2009) states, "Case management is a core component of what is needed to improve health care quality overall, while reducing costs" (p. 166). Knowledge of community resources needed to facilitate health care delivery in primary care settings allows nurse case managers to consistently deliver the right care at the right time to the right client/family.

The Case Management Society of America (2009) defines **case management** as "a collaborative process of assessment, planning, facilitation and advocacy for options and services to meet an individual's health needs through communication and available resources to promote quality cost-effective outcomes." Standards of practice for case management related to quality of care, collaboration, and resource utilization are consistent with National Patient Safety goals developed by the Joint Commission (Amin & Owen, 2006).

With the help of a case manager, clients with serious chronic conditions are able to stay in their homes and function in the community (Ploeg, Hayward, Woodward, & Johnston, 2008). Case managers help individuals and families identify providers and facilities in the community capable of providing an essential continuum of services. For example, the case manager might help the client and/or family locate rehabilitation facilities, make recommendations for placement, serve as a liaison with reimbursement sources, and/or help the family evaluate the care provided at the facility.

The goal of case management strategies is to help clients at their highest possible level in the least restrictive environment. Case management strategies are designed with the following purposes:

- To enhance the client's quality of life
- To decrease fragmentation and duplication of health delivery processes
- To contain unnecessary health care costs (Gallagher, Truglio-Londrigan, & Levin, 2009)

POPULATIONS SERVED BY CASE MANAGEMENT

Essentially, clients need a case manager when they are unable to establish or maintain self-management of a chronic health condition in a consistent manner without external support. Included in the population group served by case managers are frail elders and housebound adults or children, clients with minimal brain dysfunction, chronic mental illness, gait or balance problems, individuals with delirium or dementia and/or chronic physical disabilities affecting activities of daily living. Sometimes, the person requiring ongoing case management services is neither elderly nor mentally incapacitated. He or she can be overlooked as a potential recipient of case management services despite significant impairments that interfere with quality of life.

Case Example

Ray Bolton is a 48-year-old man with severe chronic Crohn's disease, which has gotten progressively worse since age 24. He has a permanent ileostomy and suffers from periodic exacerbations in his condition usually resulting in hospitalization. Because of the severity of his illness, he is on Social Security disability. Ray lives by himself with his cat. He has neurologic issues that affect his balance and gait, and cause him significant pain. In the past, he has had Meals-on-Wheels, but prefers to make his own food because he suffers less digestive disturbance. He can't sleep because of pain. Ray is socially isolated. Apart from his 80-year-old father and a brother, both of whom live some distance from him, Ray has no support system other than his physicians. He identifies them as his only friends. Ray's lack of a social support system, the seriousness of his medical condition, and his lack of knowledge about essential services warrant consideration of case management services.

In addition to symptom management, Ray's quality of life will require attention to the life skill domains needed to support Ray's independence. Exercise 24-4 provides an opportunity to assess and plan for client care using a case management approach.

EXERCISE 24-4	Planning Care for Ray Bolton: Case Management Approaches

Purpose: To provide practice with assessing and planning care for Ray Bolton using a case management approach.

Procedure:
(Initial consideration of Ray's issues can be completed as an out-of-class assignment.) In groups of four to five students, consider the case example of Ray Bolton on page 481.

Each group should identify:
- Relevant assessment data
- The best ways to address Ray's complex health needs and why

- What kinds of resources Ray will need to effectively self manage his multiple chronic health problems

After 15 to 20 minutes, have each student group share with the rest of the students what their plan would be, the resources they will need to accomplish the task, and why.

Discussion:
1. What was your experience of doing this exercise?
2. What were the commonalities and differences developed by different student teams?
3. Were you surprised by anything in doing this exercise?
4. What are the implications for your future practice?

CASE MANAGEMENT PRINCIPLES AND STRATEGIES

Case management strategies are designed to coordinate and manage client care across a wide continuum of health care services and community supports. With the help of a case manager, clients with serious chronic conditions are able to stay in their homes and function in the community (Ploeg et al., 2008). Case management frameworks follow the nursing process as a structural framework in service provision. Strategies incorporate COC concepts related to communication, team building, and data sharing with all members of the multidisciplinary care team, including the client and family caregivers.

Case Finding

Case management is a proactive form of care delivery. Case-finding activities, especially in areas of high prevalence, can identify individuals at high risk for potential health problems and provide opportunities for early intervention (Thomas, 2009). Networking and communication with other health professionals involved with the client helps prevent or minimize emergence of full-blown health problems.

Assessment

Comprehensive assessment forms the basis for case management care coordination. In addition to basic health and demographic information, assessment for case management purposes should include the names, addresses, and phone numbers of the client's health care providers, social service representatives, school or work contacts, if applicable, and health insurance

information. Availability of social supports and religious affiliations, previous hospitalizations, and history of treatment, current medications and allergies, advance directives and DNR (do not resuscitate) status, cognitive and mental status, mobility status, and functional assessment of activities of daily living is important case management assessment data. Identifying potential barriers to treatment adherence, including the impact that the client's diagnosis has on family members and coworkers can be helpful information. Baseline assessment data can be modified as the client's condition changes.

Treatment Planning

Case management treatment plans are designed to promote treatment compliance and continuity. Case management strategies are customized for each client, based on their needs, values, and preferences. The client/family has final power over decision making and control of a personal recovery process.

Because case management represents a longitudinal treatment management process, the plan will necessarily change over time to reflect changes in the client's situation and personnel/agency changes.

Implementation

Case managers meet with clients at regularly scheduled intervals. They assess client needs for changes in level of care, monitor client compliance with the plan of care, help clients procure needed supplies and medical equipment, and help clients obtain essential support services. Examples of non-nursing professional assistance clients may need to be linked with include legal aid, Social

Security benefits, safe affordable housing, social services, and/or mental health and addiction services.

Effective case managers have a strong understanding of community resources' strengths and weaknesses, including accessibility, availability, and affordability. They have an understanding of how health care systems work and can navigate the system.

Case managers need to be aware of the client's needs, values, and preferences, and they need to be able to express these data to the treatment team and agencies involved in the client's care in a clear, nonjudgmental, manner.

It is not enough to simply provide a referral. Additional follow-up may be necessary to assist clients with scheduling appointments, filling out required forms, getting transportation, or getting finances for participation in referral opportunities. Case managers may need to negotiate on the client's behalf with insurance companies and equipment suppliers. When single agency resources are insufficient to meet a client's complex health needs, case managers help clients and families identify and coordinate services with other agencies.

In the process of identifying and coordinating community-based resources, Hawranik and Strain (2007) note, "Nurses, as client advocates and agents of health promotion, can play an important role in modifying the focus of the system and of agency policies to include greater input by caregivers and clients" (p. 168).

Case managers are in a unique position to educate people in the community who work with disabled or chronically ill clients about the social aspects of disability to facilitate understanding and acceptance of the client's problems. They can be helpful in linking clients and families with faith or social support groups, in initiating contacts for housing or job training, and in coaching clients about seeking social acceptance.

Evaluation

Case management outcomes are described in terms of client satisfaction, clinical outcomes, and cost. Quality improvement variances related to achievement of actual clinical outcomes are analyzed with recommendations for treatment planning, related to observed changes in the client's situation, health condition, or in health care resources.

Documentation

The case manager is responsible for ensuring that all members of the multidisciplinary team accurately complete written documentation. Documentation from external providers and agencies needs to be included in the client's case management record, as do variances from the treatment plan, reasons for the variance, and plans for modification in care plans.

SUPPORTING INFORMAL FAMILY CAREGIVERS

COC involves supporting informal family caregivers. As health care delivery moves into the community, living with chronic illness increasingly becomes a home care responsibility, with family members as informal caregivers providing most of the care. Cott, Falter, Gignac, and Badley (2008) describe the home as "a unique clinical setting, different from acute care or institutional environments" (p. 19).

Family caregiving is neither a career choice nor a role for which one can prepare...and the caregiver has no "care map to lead the way," states Wright, Doherty, and Dumas (2009, p. 209). Exercise 24-5 offers insights into the role of family caregivers from the caregiver perspective. Although many variables cannot be controlled, research findings indicate that caregiver training and support reduces caregiver strain and results in better clinical outcomes for clients (Weinberg, Lusenhop, Gittell, & Kautz, 2007).

Caring for clients with significant disability at home has positive and negative aspects. Being cared for at home offers stronger COC management as home is associated with personal identity, security and relationships with people who genuinely care about the client. Variation exists in a family member's capacity to be supportive, especially if the caregiver's health is not optimal, the care is labor intensive and time consuming, or the relationship with the client is conflictual (Weinberg et al., 2007). The need for information and assistance by family caregivers is often unspoken, as demonstrated in this case example.

Case Example

A participant whose husband had urinary incontinence had been doing laundry every day, unaware that pads for incontinency were available free of charge through a publicly funded home-care program. A granddaughter expressed interest in attending a support group but did not know that there were support groups for family caregivers. These caregivers apparently assumed that no assistance was available and received no information about home care from acquaintances or family members (Hawranik & Strain, 2007, p. 166).

| EXERCISE 24-5 | Interview a Family Caregiver |

Purpose: To help students understand the caregiver role from the perspective of family caregivers.

Procedure:
1. Interview the family caregiver of a client with a long-standing chronic illness or mental disability, and write a summary of the caregiver's responses.
2. Use the following questions to obtain your data.
   a. Can you tell me why and how you assumed responsibility for caregiving?
   b. In what ways has your life changed since you became a caregiver for your parent, spouse, disabled child/adult, or mentally ill family member?
   c. What do you find most challenging about the caregiving role?
   d. What do you find rewarding about the caregiving role?
   e. How do you balance caring for your ill or disabled family member with caring for yourself?
   f. What advice would you give someone who is about to assume the caregiving role for a chronically ill or disabled family member?

Discussion:
What was it like to enter the life of the caregiver? Were you surprised by any of the responses? How can you incorporate what you learned doing this exercise in your clinical practice?

Case managers and home care nurses can fill in essential information gaps for family caregivers through careful questioning, observation, validation about feelings and observations, and consultation about emerging health issues.

CASE MANAGEMENT FOR CHRONICALLY MENTALLY ILL CLIENTS

Continuity of care is essential for effectively managing chronically mentally ill clients in the community (Wierdsma, Mulder, deVries, & Sytema, 2009). For clients with chronic mental illness, fulfilling even basic needs for shelter, food, clothing, and transportation can be issues, with the result that many of these clients are homeless and in poor physical health. Individuals with serious emotional and behavioral problems often function at a marginal level because of their symptoms. Many need consistent support to maintain themselves independently in the community. In addition to individualized treatment, COC for mentally ill and dually diagnosed clients includes formal wrap-around support services for mentally ill children and their families and case management for adults and children. Wrap-around services use a strengths based format and involve the family, community, school and service providers of the child's environment working together as a team with the family to prompt adaptive functioning (Walker & Schutte, 2004). Many of these clients will not avail themselves of the opportunity, even when available.

Case managers provide individual mentoring and coaching, and job training services. They help clients avert crisis relapses that precipitate rehospitalization. Case managers offer strength-based community interventions such as linking clients with counseling and alternative treatment services, social services, and community networks, based on recovery principles of care. Consumer advocacy groups such as the National Alliance for the Mentally Ill (NAMI) provide support and practical advice for clients and families.

ADVOCACY AT THE COMMUNITY LEVEL

Chinn (2009) challenges nurses as one of the largest professional groups in the health care system to become the leaders, movers, and shakers in bringing about essential and fundamental changes in health care delivery. Sustaining quality health programs and services costs money. Advocacy to influence policy change that promotes availability and adequacy of health services in the public sector becomes urgent as escalating financial constraints narrow availability of community services. The positive policy environment promoted by WHO (2002) and linking community and health organizational efforts to achieve better outcomes for chronic conditions is a useful framework (Figure 24-3) for achieving COC objectives.

Mason, Leavitt, and Chaffee (2007) define health policy as "the choices that a society, segment of society, or organization makes regarding its goals and priorities and the ways it allocates its resources to attain those goals" (p. 3). Advocacy at the system or community level tends to focus on adequate public health service

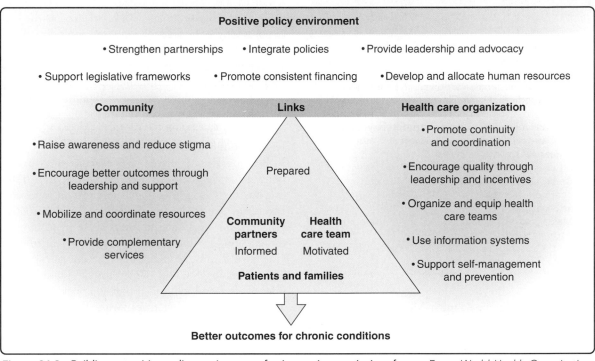

Figure 24-3 Building a positive policy environment for innovative continuity of care. *From: World Health Organization. Innovative Care for Chronic Conditions: Building Blocks for Action. Geneva, Switzerland, 2002, p. 65.*

provision, funding for essential health programs, and protecting the rights of vulnerable people to treatment.

Nursing practice in recent years has increasingly recognized political advocacy and involvement at the systems and policy level as a leadership responsibility of the professional nursing role (Francis-Baldesari & Williamson, 2008). Although nurses are on the front lines of the health care system as advocates of individual clients, they sometimes overlook their potential for helping to improve service delivery through advocacy at the community and national level. Clarke and Gottlieb (2008) declare that "keeping silent is no longer an option" (p. 7). Nurses must be willing to join together with other health professionals, their professional organizations, and community commissions and boards to argue for successful resolution of key quality-cost-access issues related to the financing and safe, effective delivery of health care (Spenceley, Reutter, & Allen, 2006).

Nurses can contribute to the development of effective health policy by writing e-mails to policy makers, becoming informed about public issues, sharing impressions with colleagues, testifying at public hearings, conducting and publishing research

with health policy implications, and joining professional organizations with advocacy missions (Taft & Nanna, 2008). Concrete suggestions for improving community advocacy are highlighted in Box 24-7.

To be effective, nurses must thoroughly understand the issues on current and proposed legislation, and the formal/informal processes involved in shaping policy and passing legislation. Social networking and interpersonal interaction between providers and policy makers is key to getting research and practice initiatives into policy (Taft & Nanna, 2008). If you testify at a public hearing, you will need to:

- Dress professionally.
- Keep your message simple and easy to understand; that is, What is your key message? Why is it important? What is the solution?
- Provide hard statistical data and support materials for your position. Produce one-page fact sheets.
- If there is time, add one powerful anecdote. Be descriptive, but concise.
- Know your audience; tailor your message and language accordingly.

BOX 24-7	Suggestions for Nurses Interested in Advocacy

1. Volunteer to serve on community advisory boards and commissions.
2. Join professional organizations and community groups with common interests in promoting advocacy (e.g., NAMI).
3. Encourage clients to provide personal testimonials related to program impact at public hearings.
4. Send e-mails (these are more effective than phone calls), with follow-up hard copy to public officials to support advocacy efforts.
5. Be an active participant. Show up at public hearings. Numbers and visibility count with advocacy efforts.
6. Make your voice heard in letters to the editor on important health issues.
7. Be persistent, cooperative, and solution focused; pay attention to timing.

- Keep within time limits. Memorize key points and practice your testimony. End with restating what you are advocating for.
- Acknowledge controversies and concerns, but do not dwell on them. Exercise 24-6 provides practice with effective advocacy efforts.

SUMMARY

COC is a dynamic, client-centered service delivery process characterized as much by attitude as by actions. It is a multidimensional concept, consisting of relational, informational, and management continuity, and focused on assisting individuals and families with the resources they need to manage chronic illness within and across clinical settings. Conceptualized as the joint responsibility of patient, family, and multidisciplinary health care provider teams, the goal of COC is to ensure a seamless continuum of care for clients, provided through coordinated, community-based health services.

COC in clinical practice means building integrated delivery systems that focus on what really matters to a patient and family, and have the capacity to provide services to meet the patient's needs.

Relational continuity embraces collaborative relationships and shared decision making between health care providers and clients to whatever extent is possible. Successful outcomes also depend on interdisciplinary collaboration and interprofessional team communication caring for the client, who can be defined as an individual, family, or community in need of care.

Informational COC allows for an uninterrupted flow of data and clinical impressions between health care providers and agencies, with clients and their families, in a care experience that is connected and coherent over time.

Discharge planning and handoff reporting represent important linkages between changes in clinical settings and between nurses at change of shift. The SBAR format for communicating important information offers a standardized comprehensive methodology for transmitting information.

Management continuity is achieved through case management strategies preparation and support of family caregivers in the home, and advocacy to ensure access and adequate funding for high-quality community-based care across health care systems.

EXERCISE 24-6	Nurse Advocacy

Purpose: To help students think through on a relevant health issue.

Procedure:
1. As an out-of-class assignment, each student should develop a one-page advocacy letter on a relevant health care issue in his or her community, using the chapter suggestions. Check your local government Web sites, newspapers, or state legislative Web sites for ideas.
2. Bring your advocacy letter to class. Break the group into three to five students, depending on the size of the group. Each group should pick one advocacy topic and develop a 5-minute public testimony script highlighting important elements (allow 20 minutes to develop the testimony).
3. One student will present the testimony, followed by a 5-minute period for questions or public comment from the group.

Discussion:
1. How difficult was it to condense the material into a 5-minute segment?
2. Were you surprised at any of the comments or questions?
3. How could you use what you learned in this exercise in your practice?

Paul is ready to be discharged from the hospital, but it is clear that he can no longer live independently by himself. He has had several heart attacks in the past with significant heart damage and currently suffers from chronic obstructive pulmonary disease (COPD). His recent hospitalization was for uncontrolled diabetes. Paul has difficulty complying with diet restrictions and his need to take daily insulin. He is not an easy person to live with, but Paul is sure that his daughter will welcome him into her home because he is family.

Although his daughter agrees to assume care for her father, she does so reluctantly as she has her own life and has never had a positive relationship with her father. Without her support, however, Paul cannot live independently in the community. What would you do as the nurse in this situation to promote quality of life for both individuals involved in the discharge process?

REFERENCES

American Hospital Association: *Introduction to discharge planning for hospital,* Washington DC, 1983, American Hospital Association.

Amin A, Owen M: Productive interdisciplinary team relationships: the hospitalist and the case manager, *Lippincott Case Manag* 11(3):160–164, 2006.

Birmingham J: Discharge planning: a collaboration between provider and payer case managers using Medicare's Condition of Participation, *Lippincott Case Manag* 9(3):147–151, 2004.

Boling P: Care transitions and home health care, *Clin Geriatr Med* 25:135–148, 2009.

Bourgault A, King M, Hart P, et al: Circle of excellence: does regular rounding by nursing associates boost patient satisfaction? *Nurs Manag* 39(11):18–24, 2008.

Carr D: On the case: effective care transitions, *Nurs Manag* 32(1):25–31, 2008.

Carter J: Finding our place at the discussion table: case management and heath care reform, *Prof Case Manag* 14(4):165–166, 2009.

Case Management Society of America: *What is a case manager,* 2009. Available online: http://www.cmsa.org/Home/CMSA/WhatisaCaseManager/tabid/224/Default.aspx Accessed August 6, 2009.

Castledine G: Patient comfort rounds: a new initiative in nursing, *Br J Nurs* 11(6):407, 2002.

Chinn P: History in the making, *Adv Nurs Sci* 32(1):1, 2009.

Clark P, Cott C, Drinka T, et al: Theory and practice in interprofessional ethics: a framework for understanding ethical issues in health care teams, *J Interprof Care* 21(6):591–603, 2007.

Clarke S, Gottlieb L: Editorial: influencing health policy for the imminent health-care crisis: a task for informed citizens, proactive nurses, and committed researchers, *Can J Nurs Res* 40(4):5–9, 2008.

Coleman E, Berenson R: Lost in transition: challenges and opportunities for improving the quality of transitional care, *Ann Intern Med* 140:533–536, 2004.

Cooke L, Gemmill R, Grant M, et al: Advance practice nurses core competencies: a framework for developing and testing an advanced practice nurse discharge intervention, *Clin Nurse Spec* 22(5):218–225, 2008.

Cotera-Perez O: Discharge planning in acute care and long-term facilities, *J Legal Med* 26(1):85–94, 2005.

Cott C, Falter L, Gignac M, et al: Helping networks in community home care for the elderly: types of team, *Can J Nurs Res* 40(1):18–37, 2008.

D'Amour D, Oandasan I: Interprofessionality as the field of interprofessional practice and interprofessional education: an emerging concept, *J Interprof Care* 19(Suppl 1):8–20, 2005.

Department of Defense (DoD) Patient Safety Program, in collaboration with the Agency for Healthcare Research and Quality (AHRQ): The TeamSTEPPS™ Teamwork System. Available online: http://dodpatientsafety.usuhs.mil/index.php?name=News&file=article&sid=31. Accessed August 13, 2009.

Engebretson J, Mahoney J, Carlson E, et al: Cultural competence in the era of evidence based practice, *J Prof Nurs* 24:172–178, 2008.

Epstein R, Fiscella K, Lesser CS, et al: Why the nation needs a policy push on patient-centered health care, *Health Aff (Millwood)* 29(8):1489–1495, 2010.

Fletcher RH, O'Malley MS, Fletcher SW, et al: Measuring continuity and coordination of medical care in a system involving multiple providers, *Med Care* 22:403–411, 1984.

Francis-Baldesari C, Williamson D: Integration of nursing education, practice and research through community partnerships, *Adv Nurs Sci* 31(4):E1–E10, 2008.

Gallagher L, Truglio-Londrigan M, Levin R, et al: Partnership for healthy living: an action research project, *Nurse Res* 16(2):7–29, 2009.

Greenwald JL, Denham CR, Jack BW, et al: The hospital discharge: a review of high risk care transition with highlights of a reengineered discharge process, *J Patient Saf* 3(2):97–106, 2007.

Grumbach K, Bodenheimer T: A primary care home for Americans: putting the house in order, *J Am Med Assoc* 288(7):889–893, 2002.

Haggerty JL, Reid RJ, Freeman GK, et al: Continuity of care: a multidisciplinary review, *Br Med J* 327:1219–1221, 2003.

Haggerty JL, Pineault R, Beaulieu M, et al: Practice features associated with patient reported accessibility, continuity, and coordination of primary health care, *Ann Fam Med* 6(2):116–123, 2008.

Hall P: Interprofessional teamwork: professional cultures as barriers, *J Interprof Care* 19(Suppl 1):188–196, 2005.

Han CY, Barnard A, Chapman H, et al: Emergency department nurses' understanding and experiences of implementing discharge planning, *J Adv Nurs* 65(6):1283–1292, 2009.

Hasnain-Wynia R: Is evidence-based medicine patient-centered, and is patient-centered care evidence-based? *Health Serv Res* 41:1–8, 2006.

Hawranik P, Strain L: Giving voice to informal caregivers of older adults, *Can J Nurs Res* 39(1):156–172, 2007.

Institute for Healthcare Improvement: *Use regular huddles and staff meetings to plan production and to optimize team communication.* Available online: http://www.ihi.org/IHI/Topics/OfficePractices/Access/Changes/IndividualChanges/UseRegularHuddlesandStaffMeetingstoPlanProductionandtoOptimizeTeamCommunication.htm. Accessed April 30, 2007.

Institute of Medicine (U.S.). Committee on Quality of Health Care in America: *Crossing the quality chasm: a new health system for the 21st century,* Washington, DC, 2001a, National Academies Press. Available online: http://www.nap.edu.proxy-hs.researchport.umd.edu/books/0309072808/html.

Institute of Medicine: *Envisioning the National Health Care Quality Report*, Washington, DC, 2001b, National Academies Press.

Jansen L: Collaborative and interdisciplinary health care teams: ready or not? *J Prof Nurs* 24:218–227, 2008.

Joint Commission: *2010 Portable comprehensive accreditation manual for hospitals (CAMH): The official handbook*, Oakbrook Terrace, IL, 2009, Joint Commission on Accreditation of Healthcare Organizations.

Kleinman A: *The illness narratives: suffering, healing, and the human condition*, New York, NY, 1988, Basic Books.

Kohn LT, et al, editor: *To err is human: building a safer health system*, Washington, DC, 2000, National Academies Press. Available online: http://www.nap.edu.proxy-hs.researchport.umd.edu/books/0309068371/html.

Kripalani S, LeFevre F, Phillips C, et al: Deficits in communication and information transfer between hospital-based and primary care physicians: implications for patient safety and continuity of care, *J Am Med Assoc* 297(8):831–841, 2007.

Lein C, Collins C, Lyles J, et al: Building research relationships with managed care organizations: issues and strategies, *Fam Syst Health* 21(2):205–214, 2003.

Leonard M, Graham S, Bonacum D, et al: The human factor: the critical importance of effective teamwork and communication in providing safe care, *Qual Saf Health Care* 13(Suppl 1):i85–i90, 2004.

Lidskog M, Lofmark A, Ahlstrom G, et al: Interprofessional education on a training ward for older people: students conceptions of nurses, occupational therapists and social workers, *J Interprof Care* 21(4):387–399, 2007.

Mainous AG, Gill JM: The importance of continuity of care in the likelihood of future hospitalization: is site of care equivalent to a primary clinician? *Am J Public Health* 88:1539–1541, 1998.

Margalit R, Thompson S, Visovsky C, et al: From professional silos to interprofessional education: campuswide focus on quality of care, *Qual Manag Health Care* 18(3):165–173, 2009.

Mason DJ, Leavitt JK, Chaffee MW, editors: *Policy & politics in nursing and health care*, ed 5, St. Louis, MO, 2007, Elsevier.

Meade C, Bursell A, Ketelsen L, et al: Effects of nursing rounds on patients call light use, satisfaction, and safety, *Am J Nurs* 106(9):58–70, 2006.

Mikos K: Monitoring handoffs for standardization. 2008 Guide to Patient Safety Technology regulatory compliance, *Nurs Manag* 16–20, 2007.

Muir JC: Team, diversity and building communities, *J Palliat Med* 11(1):5–7, 2008.

Nazareth I, Jones L, Irving A, et al: Perceived concepts of care in people with colorectal and breast cancer—a qualitative case study analysis, *Eur J Cancer Care* 17:569–577, 2008.

Ploeg J, Hayward L, Woodward C, et al: A case study of a Canadian homelessness intervention programme for elderly people, *Health Soc Care Community* 16(6):593–605, 2008.

Pontin D, Lewis M: Maintaining the continuity of care in community children's nursing caseloads in a service for children with life-limiting, life-threatening or chronic health conditions: a qualitative analysis, *J Clin Nurs* 18:1199–1206, 2008.

San Martin-Rodriguez L, D'Amour D, Leduc N, et al: Outcomes of interprofessional collaboration of hospitalized cancer patient, *Cancer Nurs* 31(2):E18–E27, 2008.

Saultz J, Albedaiwi W: Interpersonal continuity of care and patient satisfaction: a critical review, *Ann Fam Med* 2(5):445–451, 2004.

Schneller E, Epstein K: The hospitalist movement in the United States; agency and common agency issues, *Health Care Manag Rev* 31(4):308–316, 2006.

Schultz K: Strategies to enhance teaching about continuity of care, *Can Fam Physician* 56:666–668, 2009.

Sheehan D, Robertson L, Ormond T, et al: Comparison of language used and pattern of communication in interprofessional and multidisciplinary teams, *J Interprof Care* 21(1):17–30, 2007.

Sparbel K, Anderson MA: Integrated literature review of continuity of care: part 1, conceptual issues, *J Nurs Sch* 32(1):17–24, 2000.

Spenceley S, Reutter L, Allen M, et al: The road less traveled; nursing advocacy at the policy level, *Policy Polit Nurs Pract* 7(3):180–194, 2006.

Taft S, Nanna K: What are the sources of health policy that influence nursing practice, *Policy Polit Nurs Pract* 9(4):274–287, 2008.

Thomas D: Case management for chronic conditions, *Nurs Manag* 15(10):22–27, 2009.

Thorne S: Chronic disease management: what is the concept? *Can J Nurs Res* 40(3):7–14, 2008.

Tractenberg D: County Council Member, Montgomery County Member, Rockville, MD, January 7, 2010, *Montgomery County Mental Health Advisory Committee Presentation.*

van Servellen G, Fongwa M, Mockus D'Errico E, et al: Continuity of care and quality care outcomes for people experiencing chronic conditions: a literature review, *Nurs Health Sci* 8:185–195, 2006.

Von Bultzingslowen I, Eliasson G, Sarvimaki A, et al: Patients' views on interpersonal continuity based on four core foundations, *Fam Pract* 23(2):210–219, 2006.

Wachter RM, Goldman L: The emerging role of "hospitalists" in the American health care system, *N Engl J Med* 335:514–517, 1996.

Weinberg D, Lusenhop RW, Gittell J, et al: Coordination between formal providers and informal caregivers, *Health Care Manag Rev* 32(2):140–149, 2007.

Wierdsma A, Mulder C, de Vries S, et al: Reconstructing continuity of care in mental health services: a multilevel conceptual framework, *J Health Serv Res Policy* 14:52–57, 2009.

World Health Organization: *Innovative care for chronic conditions: building blocks for action*, Geneva, Switzerland, 2002, Author.

Wright J, Doherty M, Dumas L, et al: Caregiver burden: three voices-three realities, *Nurs Clin North Am* 44:209–221, 2009.

Zwarenstein M, Reeves S, Russell A, et al: Structuring communication relationships for interpersonal teamwork (SCRIPT): a cluster randomized controlled trial, *Trials* 8:23–36, 2007.

CHAPTER 25

Documentation in the Age of the Electronic Health Record

Kathleen Underman Boggs

OBJECTIVES

At the end of the chapter, the reader will be able to:

1. Identify five purposes for documentation.
2. Discuss electronic health records (EHRs) as part of a larger electronic Health Information Technology (HIT) system.
3. Discuss the need for coding and nursing taxonomy in the use of EHRs.
4. Identify how use of clinical pathways and electronic HIT systems improves client outcomes.
5. Identify legal aspects of documenting in client records.
6. Discuss how evidence-based clinical practice may change the way nursing is practiced and documented.
7. Discuss why "use of technologies to assist in effective communication in a variety of healthcare settings" is listed as an expected nurse competency by nursing organizations

The process of obtaining, organizing, and conveying client health information to others in print or electronic format is referred to as **documentation**. As illustrated in Figure 25-1, documentation serves five purposes: communicates to others care received or not received; conveys pertinent information about the client's condition and response to treatment interventions; substantiates the quality of care by showing adherence to care standards; provides evidence for reimbursement; and serves as source of data, which can be aggregated and analyzed for client care research to establish "best practice" interventions. Documentation should show evidence of effective care and client outcomes during accreditation reviews.

This chapter focuses on electronic health records (EHRs) and documenting client care. In recent years, computerization of records in hospitals has gone from a leading-edge experiment to mainstream management. Regulatory and ethical implications of documentation, use of coding and of nursing

taxonomies, as well as use of clinical pathways are also discussed in this chapter. The newest technology devices for medical communication at the point of care, including clinical decision support, remote monitoring, secure messaging, and telehealth, are discussed in Chapter 26.

BASIC CONCEPTS
DOCUMENTING CLIENT INFORMATION

Documentation of client care must be complete and accurate. Standards of documentation must meet the requirements of government, health care agency, professional standards of practice, accreditation standards, third-party payers, and the legal system. Every health care agency has its own version of clinical documentation, but in the United States, Medicare has published guidelines for primary providers affecting advanced

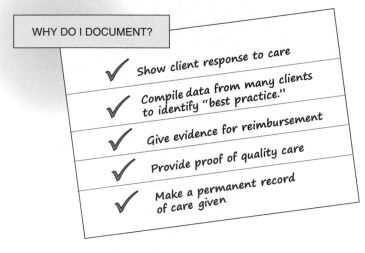

WHY DO I DOCUMENT?

✓ Show client response to care

✓ Compile data from many clients to identify "best practice."

✓ Give evidence for reimbursement

✓ Provide proof of quality care

✓ Make a permanent record of care given

Figure 25-1   Why do I document?

nurse practitioners. This documentation includes a client history (a database that often includes a summary list of health problems and needs); physical examination findings; a description of the presenting problem; and rationales for decision making, counseling, and coordination of care in a client-centered care plan. These guidelines specify what is to be examined in each body system. Nursing documentation also includes a Nursing Care Plan, daily records of client progress, and evaluation of outcomes. These daily records may include flow sheets, nursing notes, intake and output forms, and medication records.

COMPUTERIZED HEALTH INFORMATION TECHNOLOGY SYSTEMS

A major communication revolution in health care is under way internationally, made possible by the increased use of computers. The U.S. Health Information Technology for Economic and Clinical Health Act of 2009 provides major resources to care providers to assist them in computerization of client care information. Computers make information more accessible to all who are involved, including your client. The U.S. Federal Government, the American Nurses Association, and the Institute of Medicine, among

others, believe computerization offers opportunities to improve the quality of health care and to reduce its cost. This use of **Health Information Technology (HIT)** involves creation of a whole new electronic interactive system. It is far more than just putting existing documentation, as in paper charting, on a computer. HIT is designed to support the multiple information needs required by today's complex client care by providing you with assistance such as clinical decision support. Refer to Table 25-1 for a list of EHR components. Despite the federal government mandate that every American's health records be electronic by 2014, hospitals in the United States have been amazingly slow to adopt fully integrated computerized health systems. By 2008, less than 11% of hospitals and 20% of physician offices had even basic EHR systems, in contrast with 98% in the Netherlands and 89% in Great Britain (Carter, 2008; Silva, 2009).

ADVANTAGES OF COMPUTERIZED CLIENT ELECTRONIC HEALTH RECORDS

EHRs, as one part of the overall computerized HIT system, are now the accepted process for documenting care. The authors use the term *EHR* in this book, although electronic records are also known as electronic clinical records, electronic patient records, person-centered health records, or electronic medical records (Figure 25-2).

TABLE 25-1	Components of a Health Information Technology System

- An integrated, accessible electronic repository of client data with easy access by a variety of health care providers and agencies
- Client health record history, physical examination findings, medications, laboratory tests, imaging files with real-time access at the point of care
- Electronic clinical documentation of care available to nurses, physicians, other providers
- Computerized provider (or physician) order entry (CPOE)
- Clinical decision support alerts and reminders, standard "best practice" protocols that monitor your care and send you prompts if care is not recorded
- Ease of access to allow aggregation of data from many clients

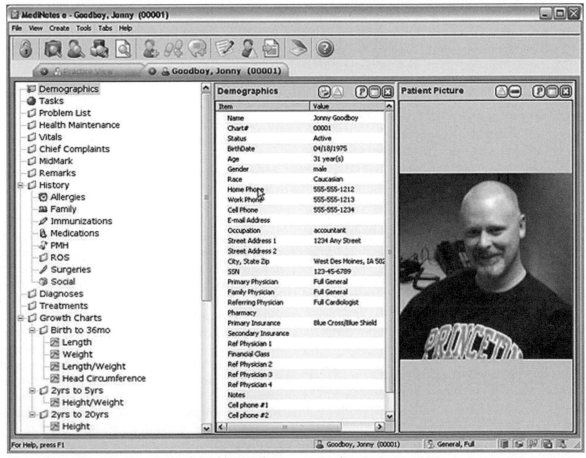

Figure 25-2 **Example of an electronic health record.** (Courtesy MediNotes Corporation.)

Interagency Accessibility

Electronic records are more durable than paper charting and easily transferable. For example, during Hurricane Katrina in 2005, the New Orleans Veterans Administration (VA) was able to send their 50,000 client health records to a secure site, while untold thousands of paper records at other New Orleans hospitals were destroyed by flood waters. The VA record system is fully integrated with the Department of Defense. Therefore, if a soldier is wounded abroad, diagnosed and treated, shipped home, and eventually discharged, his record including computed axial tomography (CAT) scans are seamlessly available to his VA doctor. Another example might be a client who travels across the country on vacation. His records are potentially available if he is admitted to an emergency department in another state.

Cost Savings

Initial transition from paper records is expensive, but cost reduction is expected to occur in the long run. Administrators estimate that the cost of using paper records in an agency is 25% of total health care costs. In addition to the actual paper and printing costs, there are costs involved in record transcription, filing, storage, and retrieval of information. Under Medicare and Medicaid reimbursement, hospitals maximized reimbursement through use of the computer-driven MS-DRG system.

Increased Access to Client Information

A client's EHR may be stored so that it is accessible to all of a client's care providers. Electronic records support telehealth, for example, in the case of a fully computerized medical record that includes graphic files (e.g., sonograms, x-ray scans, and other diagnostic imaging) that can be sent and analyzed by specialists hundreds of miles away. Information is instantly available to a variety of users. Results of your client's laboratory tests, posted in the laboratory, can be accessed by you from the client's inpatient unit, by the community health nurse, and by the primary physician's office as soon as the laboratory technician enters them into the hospital computer system. Your clients also can have access to some areas of their EHR. For example, Kaiser Permanente's nearly 9 million members can access their immunization records at any time from anywhere. When seeking care outside their own health system, clients can carry their entire health record on a flash drive until we achieve universal interoperatibility.

Efficiency and Ease of Use

The potential impact of EHRs on nursing efficiency is measured by a reduction in the amount of time you spend doing activities other than direct care of your client (Thompson, Johnston, & Spurr, 2009). Computer-assisted charting can reduce the time you spend charting. This allows you to spend more time with your client, possibly increasing client satisfaction. In a meta-analysis by Poissant et al. (2005), nurses

reduced their time documenting by 24%, an average of almost an hour of their time in an 8-hour workday. Though there are some study results showing that computer charting takes a nurse more time, the Agency for Healthcare Research and Quality reports that there is up to a 50% decrease in time spent charting.

EHR also improves the quality of charting (Moody et al., 2004). Duplication is eliminated, increasing efficiency. This includes eliminating duplication in questioning your client about his history, as his answers about his medical history are available to you from admission. A greater impact on nursing efficiency is the elimination of duplication when charting.

Efficiency is increased because providers across all agencies have immediate access to client information. Some Canadian provinces and states such as Minnesota are examples of regions with integrated electronic health infrastructures, attained by legislating and financing a region-wide system. Thompson and colleagues (2009) list HIT benefits that improve nursing efficiency in other "downstream" ways beyond what is apparent in documentation activities, such as medication record resolution, automatic medication calculations, automatic downloading of bedside monitoring records, automated nursing discharge summaries, and so forth.

Computers should be easy to use. Your terminal may be located at the nurses' station, in your client's room, or it may be portable wherever you go, including to a client's home or a community clinic. When charting, you type in your password/identification number, scan your identity card, or scan your fingerprint. Then you enter data into the client's computer file. Some systems use a mouse or light pen to select from a menu of standard groupings or categories in documenting client care information. Many systems have template outlines to prompt you, for example, when you are doing your intake interview. Capability to document your care from your client's bedside or home is known as "point of care" and is described in Chapter 26.

Enhanced Quality of Care and Communication

A comprehensive computer information system changes the way information flows through the health care delivery system. Communication is more rapid. For example, after the client's admission to an acute care hospital, a physician's orders entered into the computer are transmitted simultaneously to the pharmacy, the laboratory, and the nursing unit. HIT can be used to communicate quickly among doctors, nurses, client, families, and across agency departments.

Quality of care can be maximized with clinical decision-making electronic "prompts" that remind you to do complete care or to chart comprehensively. This prompt function also enhances the quality of care by reminding you about the specific standards of care that may apply to your client. Most electronic client monitors, such as those recording blood pressure, pulse, and oxygenation, record this information directly into the client's EHR. This saves charting time and eliminates transcription errors. The computer sends you an "alert" to notify you about increases in your client blood pressure or other abnormalities. Records over time can be examined to determine the percentage of time you delivered care that was "best practice." In another example, your diabetic client's insurance company may be able to monitor whether his physician is appropriately checking his HbA1c levels routinely. Your client may also have limited access to his own health record, for example, to check results of his laboratory tests, his immunization records, and so on. Participation in Centralized Disease Registries can give real-time feedback to providers of care. For example, participants in the National Cancer Data System can receive electronic "alerts" if "best practice" care is not started within a certain time frame. So if the standard of care for your postoperative lumpectomy client for diagnosed early-stage breast cancer is to begin radiation within a week, the registry notifies the hospital and the physician if this fails to happen.

Communication among health professionals coordinating client care can also be improved with HIT use. For example, Nemeth's study (2007) showed that point-of-care access to current laboratory tests allowed providers to discuss changes in care at the time of the visit. An example might be instant access to laboratory results on blood clotting time, allowing you to contact the physician for a change in medication levels while you are still at your client's home.

Safety

As discussed in Chapter 22, one of the most important reasons for computerizing is to reduce errors. HITs force standardization of nursing terminology, eliminate use of inappropriate abbreviations, and avoid problems of illegibility. Errors are prevented because assistance is given with drug calculations, and in assisting with decision support such as checking drug incompatibility, allergies, and so on.

Aggregated Data

Computerized systems offer ease of access to aggregate (combine together) information from many clients for reports, disease surveillance, and to research best practice nursing care. An audit trail promotes greater accountability. Aggregated information from a number of records can be analyzed to determine outcomes, for example, the number of postoperative infections that have occurred on your unit. Access time to records is also enhanced. For example, when using paper files, it took a lengthy time to do audits for agency quality assurance or by insurance companies verifying reimbursement.

In addition to documentation, nurses use HIT systems to identify contributions nurses make to attain better client outcomes. By combining data, nurses identify better treatment methods and transfer this new knowledge to colleagues (Gruber, Cummings, Leblanc, & Smith, 2009). It is crucial to nursing that nursing terminologies become embedded into EHRs, both to improve communication between nurses, such as at change of shift, and to allow data to be extracted to describe nursing care. In the past, EHRs did not contain nursing terminologies (Westra, Delaney, Konicek, & Keenan, 2008). Thus, no data could be aggregated to identify best practice nursing care.

Keepnews, Capitman, and Rosati (2004) demonstrated that one computer charting system could be used to obtain reports about predictors of client outcomes in home health care. For example, you can easily get information identifying the most effective specific nursing interventions to establish best practice and identify other interventions that need to be changed. Combining data from many clients quickly can speed identification of adverse outcomes. For example, public health agencies analyze information about illness to generate epidemiologic information such as the spread of influenza across the world. In another example, Kaiser Permanente was able to analyze information from 1.3 million clients receiving Vioxx to identify potential harm from this medication, which led to its removal from the market.

DISADVANTAGES OF COMPUTERIZED PATIENT ELECTRONIC HEALTH RECORDS

In 2009, the American Health Information Management Association published a citizen's Health Information Bill of Rights, which states that all clients have the right to secure and accurate electronic records which they can access free of charge. Other professional organizations and governments advocate protection and privacy of client information, including electronic records.

Initial Cost

Barriers to adoption of the EHR include high start-up costs. In the United States, several government statutes provide financial incentives for adopting EHR, but beginning in 2014, there are penalties for not e-prescribing. Future changes in technologies associated with your client care will necessitate expensive software periodic revisions. These may be offset by the increased efficiency and the improved ability to capture billing levels.

Lack of Legal Guidelines

Your client's record is a legal document. Few nations have adequate laws governing information misuse of EHRs. In the United States, government Health Insurance Portability and Accountability Act of 1996 (HIPAA) regulations provide some privacy guidelines for your client's records, limiting with whom you can share this information, and these will be expanded to include associated businesses. More rigorous penalties will be imposed. When computers are located at the bedside, the screen displays information to anyone who stops by the bedside. You need to be alert to this potential violation of your client's privacy.

Lack of Uniform Standards and Universal Client Identifier Numbers

Although many countries use the same universal number to identify the client in all their agencies, in the United States, our clients often have multiple identity numbers across agencies. Proposals for using one's Social Security number have received criticism, with some favoring a separate national identification number. During the transitional phase-in stage, some information is still in paper charts whereas other data are in a computer.

Problems with System Function

Vendors created systems that were incompatible with competing software. The Office of the National Coordinator for HIT created a certification process to harmonize EHR products for better interoperability. Not only must EHRs be integrated in multiple departments such as pharmacy, radiology, physical therapy, and nursing, they must be accessible across agencies. A number of companies are now marketing software applications to maximize interoperability.

User Frustration

Incompatibility of software would make it difficult to follow care from acute treatment to rehabilitation to home care. The lack of standardized data terminology and classification in the past was a key barrier to EHR information sharing. As with the medical profession, the nursing profession has been intensely engaged in developing standardized languages for their practice.

Insurance companies, banks, and others have been doing business electronically for years. But initially, health care providers complained that software was difficult to use. Staff do have a challenge, particularly those who work in multiple agencies having different computer systems, such as nurses who float to several hospitals. New users complain HIT is time consuming, but once use is mastered, their efficiency increases. Periodic system upgrades also require readjustment.

A staff nurse on a busy unit might not have a computer terminal immediately available. Client files are routinely backed up usually once a day. If there is a dysfunction or glitch and your computer crashes, you get frustrated. Computer systems require "downtime" for storing records on backup software or while technicians service system hardware. Any time the computer is unavailable for entering your documentation, you need alternative documentation forms.

Misuse of Technology

Several articles have addressed the potential possibility of abusing the unique capabilities of computer entry, such as a temptation to "cut and paste" an old client care entry when documenting today's care (Siegler & Adelman, 2009).

Confidentiality Issues

Confidentiality and legal issues are by far the biggest areas of concern. Whenever there are multiple users, there are risks that others not involved in a client's care may access confidential information. This is particularly true for computerized data, but it is also a concern with any data transmitted electronically (e.g., information sent by fax or through telehealth networks). Ensuring privacy and developing security safeguards have become a requirement for electronic records. Procedures requiring passwords, preset log-on time limitations, and internal computer system safeguards to prevent tampering with or unauthorized access to client data are now routine expectations of nursing documentation.

CLASSIFICATION OF CARE: USE OF STANDARDIZED TERMINOLOGIES

The nursing profession has been very active in developing **coding systems** for the classification of nursing care. If nursing cannot categorically classify the care provided and the outcomes of that care, there is little hope that the profession will be able to effectively communicate, document nursing care electronically, or get reimbursed for its essential role in the health care of the individual, family, and community.

GOAL FOR THE CLASSIFICATION OF NURSING CARE

Problem statements, interventions, and outcomes recorded using a standard language communicate a commonly understood message across a variety of health care settings. These terms, consistent with the scope of nursing practice, are necessary to electronically document our care. When standardized language is used to document practice, we can compare and evaluate effectiveness of our care, regardless of which nurse in which setting is delivering this care. In the past, nursing has been unable to describe the units of care, its effect on client outcome, or to establish a cost for its contributions to client care. Nowhere on a client's hospital bill does the cost of our nursing care appear. It traditionally has been part of the "room charge." The goals of developing standardized terminology and classification codes are to improve communication, to make nursing practice visible within (computerized) health information systems, and to assist in establishing evidenced-based nursing practices.

DEVELOPING CLASSIFICATIONS FOR CODING

Use of a standardized nursing classification language can save time by clearly describing clients' needs, interventions used, and the outcomes of care; by improving communication among staff members, in writing nursing care plans and nursing notes; and in conferring with health team members across the continuum of primary care, acute care, and home care practices. Use of standard language is instrumental in describing nursing

practice. The time spent teaching, providing support, and assisting in grieving are the types of nursing activities that nurses spend considerable time doing, yet they rarely show up in the medical record. In home health records, nurses most often document nursing problems or diagnoses related to the medical diagnosis, but some report they spend most of their care in client teaching.

Taxonomies: Standardized Language Terminology in Nursing

The challenge for nursing is to communicate clearly. For decades, efforts have been made to improve communication among nurses caring for the same clients, as well as those working across different health care settings and different cultures. Our profession is building a scientific knowledge base so we can identify, teach, and give "best care" that creates the best possible outcome for our clients. With the shift to electronic records, terms must also be codable. Utilization of standardized nursing terms to describe nursing practices and their outcomes accomplishes this (Rutherford, 2008). The American Nurses Association recognizes a number of different taxonomies for describing nursing care, based on specific criteria. In 1998, McCormick and Jones predicted that because no one system could meet the needs of nurses in all areas of practice, technologic applications would be developed that would communicate across classification systems.

Taxonomy is defined as a hierarchical method of classifying a vocabulary of terms according to certain rules. Various taxonomies have been developed to be used in communication and comparisons across health care settings and providers, insurers/payers, and policy makers who set priorities and allocate resources. So far, the international nursing community has not agreed on one common terminology. Research by Muller-Staub and colleagues (2007) found North American Nursing Diagnosis Association International (NANDA-I) to be the best researched and most widely implemented nursing classification internationally.

Four of the most commonly used nursing taxonomies are briefly discussed: NANDA-I, the Nursing Interventions Classification system (NIC), the Nursing Outcomes Classification system (NOC), and the Omaha system.

The first three terminologies (NANDA-I, NIC, and NOC), are used together to plan and document nursing care, sometimes referred to as **NNN**. NNN use creates a systematic schema for implementing

TABLE 25-2	Example of Linkages of North American Nursing Diagnosis Association, Nursing Interventions Classification, and Nursing Outcomes Classification

Nursing Diagnosis	Nursing Outcome (rate each indicator on 1–5 scale)	Nursing Intervention
Chronic Pain [Domain: Perceived Health V] **Defining Characteristics:** • Sudden or slow onset • Consistent or reoccurring • Duration > 6 months	Pain Control -1605 *Indicators:* • Recognizes pain onset -160502 • Uses analgesics as recommended -160505 • Uses diary to monitor symptoms over time -160510 • Reports symptom changes to provider -160513 • Reports pain controlled -160511	Pain Management *Nursing Activities:* • Determine impact of pain on quality of life. • Evaluate effectiveness of past pain-control measures. • Administer analgesics as prescribed. • Administer or teach client nonpharmacology measures of pain control (such as massage, biofeedback, heat/cold, guided imagery, music therapy, therapeutic touch). • Use pain-control measures before pain increases. • Promote adequate rest. • Teach client to monitor own pain levels.
	Pain: Disruptive Effects -2101 *Indicators:* • Impaired role performance -210102 • Impaired concentration -210108 • Interrupted sleep -210112 • Loss of appetite -210115 • Impaired mood -210110 • Lack of patience -210111	
	Pain Level -2102 *Indicators:* • Length of pain episode -210204 • Reported pain -210201 • Facial expressions of pain -210206 • Rubbing affected area -210221	

Modified from Bulechek GM, Butcher HK, Dochterman J [McCloskey]: *Nursing classification (NIC)*, ed 5, St. Louis, 2008, Mosby/Elsevier; Johnson M, Bulechek G, Dochterman JM et al: *Nursing diagnosis, outcomes, and interventions: NANDA, NOC, and NIC linkages*, St. Louis, 2001, Mosby; and Moorhead M, Johnson M, Maas M, Swanson E: *Nursing outcomes classification (NOC)*, ed 4, St. Louis, 2008, Mosby/Elsevier.

the nursing process. Table 25-2 presents an example of the linkages for the nursing diagnosis of chronic pain, linking nursing diagnosis, intervention, and outcome aids in developing electronic records so that for each diagnosis there are specific interventions and outcomes that can be selected and saved into a client database.

North American Nursing Diagnosis Association International. NANDA uses domains based on Gordon's Functional Health Patterns with diagnoses of actual problems, at-risk for diagnoses, potential problems

or syndromes in illness, as well as wellness diagnoses. A nursing diagnosis is a clinical judgment and is the basis for your selection of nursing interventions. Diagnosis domains are health promotion, nutrition, elimination, rest/activity, perception/cognition, self-perception, role relationships, sexuality, coping-stress tolerance, life principles, safety/protection, comfort, and growth and development. NANDA has approved for clinical testing and refinement more than 150 standardized terms to describe nursing diagnoses. Initially designed to classify the problems of hospitalized ill clients, nursing diagnoses have been expanded to include community nursing, especially in areas used by home health nurses

A nursing diagnosis is not another name for a medical diagnosis; rather, it delineates areas for independent nursing actions. When a physician orders a primary intervention, the nursing actions are collaborative, secondary interventions that include monitoring and managing physician-prescribed interventions. A sample list of NANDA-I diagnoses is provided in Box 25-1, with the intent of generating enough material for application in the accompanying learning exercises. Refer to books on nursing diagnoses for complete information. Writing nursing diagnoses takes practice.

Nursing Interventions Classification. This classification of nursing interventions was developed as a standardized language that names and defines an intervention you will use to give direct and indirect care.

BOX 25-1	Sample North American Nursing Diagnosis Association Nursing Diagnoses

Nursing Diagnosis Problem Statement Relevant to Interpersonal Relationships
Directions: When writing a diagnostic statement for an actual nursing diagnosis (which describes a human response the nurse can treat), the nurse should use the PES formula, stating the *Problem*, the *Etiology*, and the *Symptoms* or signs of risk factors that validate the diagnosis. Take any of the case studies in this textbook and practice writing a diagnosis.

Example: *Impaired verbal communication* related to inability to speak English as evidenced by inability to follow instructions in English and verbalizing requests in Spanish

Sample Diagnosis (updated 1/2/2010):
1. Regarding ROLE (interpersonal) relationships:
   Impaired parenting (associated with...)
   Risk for impaired parenting...
   Sexual dysfunction
   Social isolation (related to...)
   Interrupted family processes (related to...)
   Readiness for enhanced family processes...
   Ineffective role performance (related to...)
2. Regarding PERCEIVING:
   Disturbed sensory perception: visual (associated with...)
   Chronic low self-esteem
   See North American Nursing Diagnosis Association (NANDA): *Nursing diagnoses: definitions and classifications 2009-2011*, Philadelphia, 2009, Wiley-Blackwell.

The interventions are actions that nurses perform in settings relevant to illness prevention, illness treatment, and health promotion. The NIC is used to communicate a common meaning across settings. Its focus is on describing nursing behaviors in the logical order you use to improve client outcomes. There are 542 recognized nursing interventions that are classified in 7 domains. The domains are physiologic basic, physiologic complex, behavioral, safety, family, health systems, and community. Under each domain are classes, and under the classes are the specific interventions. For example, in the domain of physiologic basic there is a class called "immobility management." Specific intervention activities include bedrest care, cast care maintenance, physical restraint, positioning, splinting, traction, and transport. You can use or modify these interventions to meet your client's need. Each nursing intervention has a unique code number, and thus can be computerized and potentially could be used to reimburse the nurse. In one example relevant to mobility, the code for "Body mechanics promotion" is 0140, under Class A "Activity and exercise management" (Park, Lu, Konicek, & Delaney, 2007). More than half of the most common nursing interventions are in the physiologic domain. The following case example demonstrates how NIC is used.

Case Example

Barbara, a 64-year-old woman, is 1 day after surgery for heart valve replacement. Using NIC with a diagnosis in the Physiologic Domain, Class: 1 (Respiratory management: ventilation adequate to maintain arterial blood gases within normal limits), our NIC Intervention is Labeled: Airway management with a code [#3140] and Definition: Facilitation of patency of air passages. Thus, our standardized activities include maintaining our client in a position that maximizes ventilation potential; monitoring rate, rhythm, depth, and effort of respirations q4h; removing secretions by teaching client how to cough effectively and assess ability; and auscultating breath sounds, noting changes in SaO_2 and arterial blood gases.

(Case example is based on content in Bulechek, Butcher, & Dochterman [2008].)

NIC experts identify core nursing interventions. A partial list is presented in Box 25-2 (refer to the Elsevier Evolve Web site for complete information). Identification of core interventions provides nurse educators and clinicians with a focus for developing entry-level competencies for nursing practice.

BOX 25-2   Nursing Intervention Classification Core Nursing Interventions

Example Core NIC Interventions, codes, and definitions, with two samples of the many nursing intervention activities listed for each intervention:

- Active Listening (4920): attending closely to and attaching significance to a client's verbal and nonverbal messages, using activities such as using nonverbal behaviors to facilitate communication; verifying understanding of messages by use of questions or feedback
- Anxiety Reduction (5820): minimizing apprehension, dread, foreboding, or uneasiness related to an unidentified source of anticipated danger using activities such as using a calm, reassuring approach; explaining all procedures
- Coping Enhancement (5230): assisting a client to adapt to perceived stressors...using activities

such as appraising client's understanding of his disease process; encouraging verbalization of concerns

- Documentation (7920): recording all pertinent client data in a clinical record using activities such as recording complete assessment findings in initial record; charting baseline assessments and care activities using agency-specific forms/flow sheets
- Emotional Support (5270): provision of reassurance, acceptance, and encouragement during times of stress using activities such as making supportive or empathetic statements; encouraging client to express feelings of anxiety, anger, or sadness

For a complete listing of interventions, definitions, and specific nursing activities, see Bulechek GM, Butcher HK, Dochterman JM: *Nursing interventions classification (NIC)*, St. Louis, 2008, Mosby/Elsevier.

Nursing Outcomes Classification. NOC provides a standard language to name and define client outcomes attained through nursing actions to communicate among nurses and across settings. NOC complements NANDA-I and NIC, and provides a language and coding numbers for evaluating the nursing process. NOC experts identified 385 nursing-sensitive outcomes. An outcome assesses the client's actual status on specific behaviors (indicators) using a five-point scale, ranging from 1 (severely compromised function) to 5 (function not compromised). The following case example demonstrates how NOC is used.

Case Example

Mr. Lee, 46 years old, is admitted with right-sided paralysis. In the physiologic Health Domain, neurocognitive class, we use the nursing diagnosis of impaired verbal communication related to a left hemisphere bleed as evidenced by expressive aphasia. Using NOC, we get a code number (0903), Communication: Expressive, and rate him as 1 (severely compromised) on seven indicators listed. A student is assigned to his care. Her interventions to increase his expressive communication ability as listed in NOC include naming things aloud as she gives care, encouraging speech, encouraging nonverbal gestures, introducing a board displaying the pictures and words for several common needs for him to point at. After 2 days of care, Mr. Lee is assessed on the seven indicators. His use of spoken language is still rated as 1 (severely compromised). But the nurse assesses two of the other listed indicators (his use of nonverbal language and ability to point to the picture board to

communicate) as having progressed to 4, mildly compromised. This shows a specific change in Mr. Lee's status after specific nursing interventions. It is numerical and thus can be coded.

(Updated based on Moorhead, Johnson, Maas, & Swanson [2008].)

The Omaha System. In the 1970s, Omaha System research was initiated to address the needs of community health nurses, managers, and administrators. The **Omaha System** is a comprehensive practice, documentation, and information management tool used by nurses and other health providers (Martin, 2005). Studies show it can also be used in acute care situations. Categories cover common transitional care problems as clients move from hospitalized care to long-term or home care. Transitional care problems include categories such as nutrition, communication, pain, physical activity, and medication administration.

The Omaha System includes an assessment, or Problem Classification Scheme. This consists of four levels: (a) the major domains (environmental, psychosocial, physiologic, and health-related behaviors), (b) specific problems, (c) modifiers, and (d) signs and symptoms. The Intervention Scheme is similarly organized into categories: (a) teaching guidance and counseling, (b) treatments and procedures, (c) case management, and (d) surveillance. Each domain has targets of the intervention. Lastly, it has an outcome component, the Problem Rating Scale for Outcomes. This consists of a five-point ordinal scale assessing the client's knowledge, behavior, and condition (the status or symptoms of the identified problem). The outcomes rating scale can be applied as a baseline and then reevaluated after the intervention to measure change in knowledge, related behaviors, and symptoms of the originally identified problem (Martin, 2005).

ADVANTAGES OF NURSING CLASSIFICATION SYSTEMS

Nursing classification systems provide a standard and common language for nursing care so that nursing contributions to client care become visible and define professional practice. The ANA has issued a position statement stating that standards for terminology are an essential requirement for a computer-based patient record (ANA, 1995b). A standardized language of nursing can help develop realistic standards of care. Groups of client records can be analyzed to describe the client population (e.g., to discover the most common interventions used for a specific nursing diagnosis). Analyzing client records in this way can lead to developing benchmarks that set the desired outcomes for a condition or diagnosis and then measure the client's actual level of achievement. Agencies could use a nursing classification system to bill for specific nursing care and build further accountability into the care and its documentation. Figure 25-3 shows how coding allows a client's data to be easily aggregated

Coding Nursing Practice Provides Information:

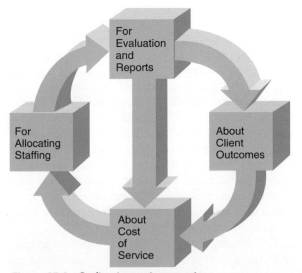

Figure 25-3 Coding in nursing practice.

with other cases to produce a larger picture describing health care delivered by the agency.

DISADVANTAGES OF NURSING CLASSIFICATION SYSTEMS

Standardized nursing languages need to convince the business and medical interests managing health care agencies of the need to incorporate nursing classification codes as part of their information technology systems. The greatest problem has been that nursing classifications have not yet been thoroughly incorporated into many agency clinical records. Other difficulties include awkward syntax, lack of completeness, and problems with portability to other cultures. As is true of medical classification systems, nursing classification systems continue to evolve and develop as they are used in practice.

OTHER CODING SYSTEMS IN HEALTH CARE

The National Library of Medicine maintains a metathesaurus for a unified medical language. Because of the complexity of health care and the variety of providers involved, multiple medical classification systems have emerged. Often providers use several in combination. A major drawback for nursing is that use of computerized documentation systems based on medical code numbers often forces nurses to use classification systems designed to describe medical practice instead of describing nursing assessment and care of clients. In doing so, the richness of the nursing care provided often goes undocumented. Four common medical classification and coding systems are described here.

INTERNATIONAL CLASSIFICATION OF DISEASES

One of the most common medical coding systems is the ICD codes. Classifications in use include ICD-9-CM, ICD-10-CM (codes for inpatient and outpatient diagnoses), and ICD-10-PCS (codes for procedures). The World Health Organization (WHO) published a revised 10th edition in 1994, but the United States did not mandate use until 2013.

Generally, diseases are classified according to body system. ICD-10 uses three to seven digits in an alphanumeric code that begins with a letter to record diagnosis and care interventions, and has 3,000 more categories than ICD-9, which used a 4-digit numeric code. The first digit is always alpha. For example, fractures are coded beginning with S, so a displaced fracture of the neck of the right radius in an initial treatment for closed fracture is S52.131a. In another example, respiratory diseases are all classified beginning with the letter J. Pneumonia is listed in this grouping. Death from pneumonia and influenza is classified under ICD-9 as 480, but under ICD-10 code, it is J10, while to the right of this decimal, the coder can enter codes that identify very specific information, such as the type of pneumonia, which lung was affected, and so on. It is crucial when documenting care to provide enough specificity so that information management workers can correctly and accurately code. Data management and reimbursement depend on the accuracy of this coding.

ICD-10-PCS (CODES FOR PROCEDURES)

These new codes replace CPT codes, which were originally developed by the American Medical Society to provide coding for diagnostic procedures. The client's record must provide sufficient information about a diagnosis so that the insurance company computer accepts the diagnostic test as relevant and necessary for reaching a correct diagnosis. For example, the ordering of a digoxin level by a provider would be appropriate related to a diagnosis with a code for hypertension with congestive failure, but would not be appropriate or reimbursable for a diagnosis code for epilepsy.

DIAGNOSIS-RELATED GROUPS

Diagnosis-related groups [DRGs] were originally developed for use in prospective payment for the Medicare program. Diagnosis-related group coding provided a small number of codes for classifying client hospitalizations based on diagnosis and severity of illness.

DIAGNOSTIC AND STATISTICAL MANUAL OF MENTAL DISORDERS, FOURTH EDITION, TEXT REVISION

The *Diagnostic and Statistical Manual of Mental Disorders,* Fourth Edition, Text Revision (DSM-IV-TR) is the standardized diagnostic classification for mental illness. The *DSM-IV-TR* is organized using five axes describing psychiatric diagnosis and functional status. It provides a comprehensive assessment and labeling of psychiatric and mental health–related conditions. The five axes are clinical disorders, personality disorders, general medical conditions, psychosocial and environmental problems, and global assessment of functioning (American Psychiatric Association, 2000).

JOINT COMMISSION COMPUTERIZED DOCUMENTATION GUIDELINES

Electronic Clinical Information Systems promote entry, storage, and linkage of *all* information about a client's health care. Ideally, any Clinical Information System allows ease of access to one client's information as inputted by any of the client's health care providers, including the hospital and community. The Joint Commission on Accreditation of Healthcare Organizations has developed standards for uniform data for agencies it accredits. In the past, the Joint Commission required that nurses repeat information recorded by the physician. Now, nursing documentation may consist merely of updating.

OUTCOME AND ASSESSMENT INFORMATION SET

Beginning in 1998, home care agencies phased in a new requirement to complete a functional health assessment on all Medicare clients before they begin care. The results of the assessment feed into a standardized database. The Health Care Financing Administration (HCFA) developed the Outcome and Assessment Information Set (OASIS) assessment for the purpose of describing home care clients, developing outcome benchmarks, and providing feedback regarding quality of care to home health agencies.

The OASIS assessment is required for home health agencies to receive reimbursement for the care provided to Medicare recipients. Home health care agencies are sent reports comparing their client populations and functions with benchmarks established through analysis of multiple home health agency clients. OASIS can be used to establish standards of quality. The report can also be used by individual home health agencies to monitor and improve outcomes of care. The components of OASIS are essential items for documenting a comprehensive assessment of functional health status of adult home care clients. The assessment documentation is used by HCFA to analyze the health status and needs of Medicare recipients.

OASIS data items include the sociodemographic, environmental, support system, health status, and functional status attributes of nonmaternity adult clients, as well as the attributes of health service utilization. OASIS was not developed as a comprehensive health assessment tool, and home care agencies need to supplement the assessment items. The items of OASIS have evolved over time.

Home health agencies are required to submit OASIS data to a designated state site. The state agency then has the responsibility of collecting OASIS data that can be retrieved from a central repository. These data provide a national picture of health status, outcome, and cost of Medicare enrollees who require home health care. To learn more, visit HCFA's Medicare Web site (www.HCFA.gov).

REFERENCE TERMINOLOGY SYSTEMS THAT EXCHANGE DATA BETWEEN CLASSIFICATION SYSTEMS

The American Nurses Association recognizes two reference terminologies that can translate the terms between the various classification systems. These allow us to retrieve data even when agencies use several different classification systems.

SYSTEMATIZED NOMENCLATURE OF MEDICAL-CLINICAL TERMS

Systematized nomenclature of medical-clinical terms (SNOMED-CT) is the most comprehensive reference of medical terminology from many health care languages. Originally developed by American pathologists and the U.K. Department of Health (National Health Service), its goal is to accurately record health care encounters to avoid the injuries or deaths arising from poor communication between health care practitioners. It is endorsed by the American Nurses Association and is used in several other countries including Australia (www.ihtsdo.org/snomed-ct/).

LOGICAL OBSERVATION IDENTIFIERS NAMES AND CODES

Logical Observation Identifiers Names and Codes (LOINC) was developed originally to provide electronic exchange of laboratory data but evolved to include data from lots of classification systems. For example, it includes terms from the Omaha System and the Nursing Management Minimum Data Set (Westra et al., 2008).

CHARTING FORMATS FOR DOCUMENTING NURSING CARE

Use of structured documentation has been found to be associated with more complete nursing records, better continuity of care, more meaningful nursing data, and perhaps with better client outcomes. Use of EHRs has made written charting formats, such as the narrative **Problem-Oriented Record** (POR), the SOAP format, and so on, obsolete. Still, the focus of the POR on the client's identified list of health problems can be adapted for electronic charting. A problem list typically consists of medical diagnoses. In POR, nurses refer to the problem list and chart their observations by referring to the listed problem. Information about the client's progress in each problem area is documented when some measurable change occurs.

In charting electronically, the nurse can call up a preformulated template to record today's data. There is some evidence that use of EHRs that provide reminders or "prompts" results in more complete documentation (Gunningberg, Fogelberg-Dahm, & Ehrenberg, 2009).

Electronic charting can use **flow sheets** with predefined client progress parameters based on written standards with preprinted categories of information. They contain daily assessments of normal findings. For example, in assessing lung sounds, the nurse needs to merely check "clear" if that information is normal. Deviations from norm must be completely documented. By marking a flow sheet, you are saying all care was performed according to existing agency protocols. The best example of this format is known as critical pathways or clinical pathways.

Clinical pathways are a documentation system based on standardized plans of care. They are derived by aggregating computerized assessment and outcome data from client records. Locally developed by consensus, they incorporate national evidence-based best practice recommendations. A "pathway" is created, with benchmark milestones clients are expected to achieve within an identified time frame. Each specific disease or procedure has a standard path developed by an interdisciplinary team. The path describes expected care for each day and also permits the nurse to record care given. This improves communication and reduces unnecessary variations in care.

The trend toward more streamlined yet comprehensive and meaningful charting is exemplified in clinical pathways. The goals are to provide a structured tool for planning the highest quality of care; encourage interdisciplinary communication; decrease the time spent charting, because you are **charting by exception**; focus care on expected client outcomes; and facilitate quality assurance evaluations. Most agencies give the client a copy of the pathway at the time of admission, so that he understands what is expected each day (Figure 25-4). Thus, the pathway becomes a teaching tool for client education and a tool to measure quality.

The clinical pathway is truly an *interdisciplinary tool*. It allows the entire health team to monitor the client's progress compared with a standard time frame for progress. A variance or exception occurs when a client does not progress as anticipated or an expected outcome does not occur. A variance is a red flag, alerting staff of a need for further action to assist the client.

ADVANTAGES

Use of clinical pathways provides a concise method for documenting routine care. Nurses direct attention to abnormal or significant findings, rather than spending time detailing normal findings. This documentation method is efficient and cost-effective. Multiple studies show it takes less nursing time. Use of pathways is associated with fewer complications and reduced length of hospital stays (Barbieri et al., 2009). Loeb et al.'s 2006 study in nursing home clients showed use of pathways was associated with fewer admissions to hospital, again showing pathways to be cost-effective.

DISADVANTAGES

Charting by exception does not allow for qualitative information. If you fail to perform even one step of the protocol, you are guilty of falsifying the client's record.

Patient Name _____   Date _____

DRG# _____   Expected LOS ___<23 hours___

	Preprocedure	Preoperative	Intraoperative	Postoperative Phase I PACU	Postoperative PHASE II PACU	Discharge	Postoperative PHASE II PACU
Medication	Review medical history	Start IV	Administer meperidine	Administer naloxone, flumazenil pm	Pain med prn	Start on Rx omeprazole	Continue medications
Diagnostic tests	H & P chest x-ray, ECG, blood work	Review tests	Endoscopy procedure	None, unless complications	None	None	None
Diet	Regular	NPO	NPO	NPO	Clear liquids & progress	Regular	Regular
Activity	Not restricted	Ambulate	None	Turn, cough, and deep breathe	Increase activity to ambulation	Normal ambulation	Not restricted
Nursing action	Assessment	Vital signs	Vital signs, O$_2$ saturation	Vital signs, level of consciousness, O$_2$ saturation	Monitor as before	Prepare for discharge	Follow-up evaluation via phone
Teaching/ discharge planning	Phone call	Patient education about procedure	Transport to PACU	Discharge when Aldrete criteria I met	Discharge when Aldrete criteria II met	Instructions reviewed	Phone call for follow-up

Figure 25-4 Clinical pathway for endoscopy. *DRG*, Diagnosis-related group; *ECG*, electrocardiogram; *H&P*, history and physical; *IV*, intravenous; *LOS*, length of stay; *NPO*, nothing by mouth; *O₂*, oxygen; *PACU*, postanesthesia care unit; *prn*, as needed. *(From Monahan FD: Phipps' Medical-Surgical Nursing: Health and Illness Perspectives, ed 8, 2007, Mosby.)*

Legal decisions in the early 1990s found that certain nurses charting by exception were negligent by virtue of items not charted. Clinical pathways are labor-intensive to develop, and they require "buy-in" by both physicians and nursing staff.

ETHICAL, REGULATORY, AND PROFESSIONAL STANDARDS

The use of electronic medical records and storage of personal health information in computer databases has refocused attention on issues of ethics, security, privacy, and confidentiality. For example, a nurse in one unit of a hospital who accesses the electronic medical record of a client who is in another unit and for whom the nurse has no responsibilities for care is violating confidentiality. Ethical professional practice requires that you do not allow others to use your access log-on. Other ethical issues with electronically generated care plans and standard orders center on how to determine who is responsible for the computer-generated care decisions.

CONFIDENTIALITY AND PRIVACY

The Institute of Medicine defines **confidentiality** as the act of limiting disclosure of private matters appropriately, maintaining the trust that an individual has placed in an agent entrusted with private matters. In the United States, most states have laws that grant the client ownership rights to the information contained in the client's health record. Electronic storage and transmission of medical records have sparked intense scrutiny over privacy protection. More than two thirds of consumers express concerns that their personal health records stored in an EHR with Internet connections will not remain private. Violations of confidentiality because of unauthorized access or distribution of sensitive health information can have severe consequences for clients. It may lead to discrimination at the workplace, loss of job opportunities, or disqualification for health insurance. Issues of privacy will dominate how nurses and other health care providers address clinical documentation in the years ahead. Currently, a **personal medical identification number** is used on client records. Hardware safeguards such as workstation security, keyed lock hard drives, and automatic log-offs are used in addition to user identification and passwords to prevent unauthorized access. Some advocate that clients be able to choose how much of their information is shared and be notified when their information is accessed. In the United States, federal law now requires clients be notified in the event of a breach of their EHR. Authorization is not needed in situations concerning the public's health, criminal, or legal matters. Refer to Chapter 2 for Federal Medical Record Privacy Regulations (HIPAA).

OTHER LEGAL ASPECTS OF CHARTING

Management literature emphasizes the need for quicker documentation that still reflects the nursing process. At the same time, documentation must be legally sound. The legal assumption is that the care was not given unless it is documented in the client's record. Malpractice settlements have approached the multimillion-dollar mark for individuals whose charts failed to document safe, effective care.

"If it was not charted, it was not done." This statement stems from a legal case *(Kolesar v. Jeffries)* heard before Canada's Supreme Court, in which a nurse failed to document the care of a client on a Stryker frame before he died. Because the purpose of the medical record is to list care given and client outcomes, any information that is clinically significant must be included. Legally, all care must be documented. Aside from issues of legal liability, third-party reimbursement depends on accurate recording of care given. Major insurance companies audit client records and contest any charges that are not documented. Every nurse should anticipate having their clients' records subpoenaed at some time during their nursing career (refer to Box 25-3 for recommendations).

Any method of documentation that provides comprehensive, factual information is legally acceptable. This includes graphs and checklists. By signing a protocol, check sheet, pathway, and so forth, you are documenting that every step was performed. If a protocol exists in a health care agency, you are legally responsible for carrying it out.

COMMUNICATING MEDICAL ORDERS

WRITTEN ORDERS

Nurses are required to question orders that they do not understand or those that seem to them to be unsafe. Failure to do so puts the nurse at *legal risk*. "Just following orders" is not an acceptable excuse. On the other

| BOX 25-3 | Documentation Suggestions |

Content
- Chart promptly, but never ahead of time. Do not wait until end of shift.
- Document complete care reflecting the nursing process.
- Document all noncooperative or bizarre behavior.
- Document all refusals of ordered treatments.
- Document teaching (information you gave the client and/or family).
- When care or medicine is omitted, document action and rationale (who was notified and what was said).
- Document all significant changes in the client's condition and who was notified, as well as your nursing interventions.

Mistakes to Avoid
- Failing to record complete, pertinent health information
- Making "untimely" entries (e.g., charting after the fact, passed the day)
- Failing to record drug administration, route, outcome
- Not recording all nursing actions
- Recording on the wrong chart
- Failing to document a discontinued medication
- Failing to record outcome of an intervention such as a medicine
- Writing about mistakes or incident reports in the client record; incident reports are stored separately.

hand, nurses can be held liable if they arbitrarily decide not to follow a legitimate order, such as choosing to withhold ordered pain medication. Reasons for such a decision would have to be explicitly documented. With computerization, it is possible to have standing orders, such as for administering vaccines. The computer is programmed to recognize the absence of a vaccination and then to automatically write an order for a nurse to administer. What might the legal implications be?

Persons licensed or certified by appropriate government agencies to conduct medical treatment acts include physicians, advance practice nurses, and physician assistants. These providers have their own state prescribing numbers and must abide by government rules and restrictions. To prescribe controlled substances they must also have a Drug Enforcement Agency (DEA) number. Nurse practitioners may choose not to apply for a DEA number. Consult your agency policy regarding who is allowed to write client orders for the nurse to carry out.

FAXED ORDERS

The physician or nurse practitioner may choose to send a faxed order. Because this is a form of written order, it has been shown to decrease the number of errors that occur when transcripting verbal or telephone orders. However, there is the risk for violating client confidentiality when faxing health-related information. See the American Health Information Management Association's general guidelines for faxing medical orders (Hughes, 2001).

VERBAL ORDERS

Often, a change in client condition requires the nurse to telephone the primary physician or hospital staff resident to obtain new orders. Most primary providers work in group practices, so it is necessary to determine who is "on call" or who is covering your client when the primary provider is unavailable. It may be necessary to call for new orders if there is a significant change in the client's physical or mental condition as noted by vital signs, laboratory value reports, treatment or medication reactions, or response failure. Before calling for verbal orders, obtain the chart and familiarize yourself with current vital signs, medications, infusions, and other relevant data. Read Chapter 22 on using the SBAR format to communicate with doctors.

With the growth of unlicensed personnel, there is greater likelihood that a verbal order will be relayed through someone with this status. The legality is vague, but basically, if harm comes to the client through miscommunication of a verbal order, you (the licensed nurse) will be held responsible. The following case examples demonstrate typical scenarios you may encounter:

Case Example

Tracy, the secretary on your unit, answers the telephone. Dr. Uganda gives her an order for a medication for a client. Tracy asks him to repeat the order as soon as she gets a registered nurse to take the call. If you cannot answer the telephone immediately, have her tell him you will call back in 5 minutes to verify the order.

CHARTING FOR OTHERS

It is not acceptable to chart for others.

Case Example

Juanita Diaz worked day shift. At 6 p.m. she calls you and says she forgot to chart Mr. Reft's preoperative enema. She asks you to chart the procedure and his response to it. Can you just add it to your notes? In court this would be portrayed as an inaccuracy. The correct solution is to chart "1800: Nurse Diaz called and reported..."

Developing an Evidence-Based Practice

Banner L, Olney CM: Automated clinical documentation: does it allow nurses more time for patient care? *CIN Comput Inform Nurs* 27(2):75–81, 2009.

The purpose of this study was to compare time spent in nursing activities before and then 1 year after implementation of an electronic information system. The research question was whether automation would mean more time for direct patient care and less time spent on documentation. In this time-motion study, raters observed six categories of nurse work behavior on a progressive cardiac unit using a pretest and post-test design. The six categories were direct care, indirect care, documentation, administrative tasks, housekeeping, and personal.

Results: There was a statistically significant 6% *increase* in the amount of time nurses spent in direct care ($P \leq 0.05$), work such as assessing and teaching.

There was a decrease in time spent in indirect activities ($P = 0.008$).

There was an increase in time spent documenting ($P = 0.000$).

There was a 12% decrease in time nurses spent on administrative tasks ($P = 0.000$), such as searching for charts, verifying all paper forms were completely filed in, and so on.

No change in time spent on housekeeping or personal tasks was noted.

Application to Your Clinical Practice: Many studies support these results indicating EHR gives the nurse more time at the bedside interacting with his or her client. You can use this time to make more complete assessments, to reassure ill clients, but most importantly to educate them to promote maximal health. One Canadian study found HIT also improved communication-related activities such as time spent on the telephone, paging staff, or searching for a staff member, as well as improving work flow.

Vandenkerkhof EG, Wilson R, Gay A, Duhn L: Evaluation of an innovative communication technology in an acute care setting, *CIN Comput Inform Nurs* 27(4):254–262, 2009.

APPLICATIONS

COMPUTER LITERACY

To practice nursing in coming years, you will need to continually upgrade your technology skills. As students, you learn skills such as data entry, data transmission, word processing, Internet accessing, spreadsheet entry, and use of standard language and codes describing practice. Voice recognition software may eventually revolutionize clinical documentation, making documentation easier for nurses.

DOCUMENTING ON A CLIENT'S HEALTH RECORD

Documenting electronically requires learning the specific system at your agency. There is a learning curve; that is, initially it may take longer, but as you become familiar with the system, EHRs should increase your nursing efficiency. Use Exercise 25-1 to stimulate discussion of appropriate documentation.

CONFIDENTIALITY

Ethical and legal dilemmas inherent in use of computerized systems require continued vigilance, especially regarding the concern of protecting client privacy. As cases come to court, a body of case law will provide some guidance. HIPAA regulations mandating clients' right to privacy are the current guidelines. You need to become aware of threats to privacy and your obligation to protect your clients' privacy where possible. Discuss the ethical dilemma provided.

USE OF UNIVERSAL NURSING LANGUAGES AND CODES

The need to identify and analyze outcomes of nursing practice requires computer-compatible frameworks. Adoption allows us to gather and analyze large amounts of information to identify which nursing interventions produce positive client outcomes. Interoperable computer coding applications help do this across health settings. Think about this "bigger picture" as you learn use of nursing terminology in your clinical practice.

Dochterman and colleagues (2005) were among the first to demonstrate that NIC-coded patterns of

---

EXERCISE 25-1   Documenting Nursing Diagnoses

Purpose: To clarify diagnoses.

Procedure:
Discuss in small groups which of the following examples help provide a direction for independent nursing interventions.
Example 1
Incorrect: Inability to communicate related to deafness
   Suggested: Impaired social interaction (00052) related to anatomical (auditory), as evidenced by refusal to interact with others

Discussion:
What additional information is provided in the correct diagnosis? Why would the first statement be

incorrect? Are all people who are deaf unable to communicate?
Example 2
Incorrect: Acute lymphocytic leukemia
   Suggested: Acute pain (00132) during ambulation related to leukemia disease process, as evidenced by limping, grimacing, and increased pulse

Discussion:
Could a nurse make any independent intervention based on the information provided by the diagnosis "acute lymphocytic leukemia"?

---

nursing interventions can be analyzed. They examined three types of interventions for older adults in 13,758 acute care hospitalizations. Data were obtained for interventions for clients with diagnoses of heart failure and hip fracture, and for fall prevention interventions. Results demonstrated that interventions occurred throughout the hospitalization period, were individualized, and could be classified into daily patterns (and potentially could produce better health outcomes). Information describing the type and amount of nursing care delivered could also potentially help staff managers plan for amount and type of staff needed on a unit.

Standardization work is ongoing internationally, as evidenced by groups such as the Association for

Common European Nursing Diagnoses, Interventions, and Outcomes. Try Exercise 25-2 to explore how you might apply information.

SUMMARY

This chapter focuses on electronic documentation of care in the nurse-client relationship. Documentation refers to the process of obtaining, organizing, and conveying information to others in the client record. Discussion of new HIT including the nurse's role in using EHRs emphasized their role in reducing redundancy, improving efficiency, reducing cost, decreasing errors, and improving compliance with standards of practice. Chapter 26 discusses technology that can

---

EXERCISE 25-2   Application of Nursing Intervention Classification Finding

Purpose: To make use of NIC meaningful.

Procedure:
Consider the following finding from Dochterman's 2005 study, then answer the questions.
   On Day 3 of hospitalization, nurses averaged four intravenous therapy interventions for clients with a diagnosis of hip fracture but averaged only two interventions for (oral) fluid management.
   1. How could you use this information to justify the need for skilled nursing care?
   2. Suppose data showed that by Day 6, skilled care activities had been cut in half. How might the

nurse manager readjust the client assignment for her nurse aides?
   On Day 3, clients with hip fractures received three times as many nursing interventions encouraging proper coughing as were made for clients with congestive heart failure.
   1. Speculate about why there was this difference.
   2. Suppose hospital units with more nursing interventions to encourage coughing were shown to have greatly decreased rates of clients with pneumonia complications. Could this information be used to justify a better nurse-to-client ratio?

From Dochterman J, Titler M, Wang J, et al: Describing use of nursing interventions for three groups of patients, *J Nurs Scholarsh* 37(1): 57–66, 2005.

facilitate communication among health care workers, increase client education, and assist the providers of health care with decision making.

ETHICAL DILEMMA What Would You Do?

You work in an organization with a computerized clinical documentation system. A coworker mentions that Alice Jarvis, RN, has been admitted to the medical floor for some strange symptoms and that her laboratory results have just been posted, showing she is positive for hepatitis C, among other things.
1. Identify at least two alternative ways to deal with this ethical dilemma. (What response would you make to your coworker who retrieved information from the computerized system? What else might you do?)
2. What ethical principle can you cite to support each answer?

From Sonya R. Hardin, RN, PhD, CCRN.

REFERENCES

American Nurses Association: ANA Position Statement No.12.22, On access to patient data, 1995a. http://nursingworld.org/readroom/position/joint/jtdata.htm.

American Nurses Association: ANA Position Statement No. 12.20, Position paper on computer-based patient record standards, 1995b. http://nursingworld.org/readroom/position/joint/jtcpri1.htm.

American Psychiatric Association: *Diagnostic and statistical manual of mental disorders*, ed 4, text revision, Washington, DC, 2000, Author.

Barbieri A, Vanhaecht K, Van Herck P, et al: Effects of clinical pathways in the joint replacement: a meta-analysis, *BMC Med* 7:32, 2009.

Bulechek GM, Butcher HK, Dochterman J [McCloskey]: *Nursing classification (NIC)*, ed 5, St. Louis, 2008, Mosby/Elsevier.

Carter JH, editor: *Electronic health records*, ed 2, Philadelphia, 2008, ACP Press.

Dochterman JM, Bulechek GM, editors: *Nursing interventions classification (NIC)*, ed 4, St. Louis, 2004, Mosby.

Dochterman J, Titler M, Wang J, et al: Describing use of nursing interventions for three groups of patients, *J Nurs Scholarsh* 37(1): 57–66, 2005.

Gruber D, Cummings GG, Leblanc L, et al: Factors influencing outcomes of clinical information systems implementation, CIN, *Comput Inform Nurs* 27(3):151–163, 2009.

Gunningberg L, Fogelberg-Dahm M, Ehrenberg A, et al: Improved quality and comprehensiveness in nursing documentation of pressure ulcers after implementing an electronic health record in hospital care, *J Clin Nurs* 18:1557–1564, 2009.

Hughes G: Practice brief: facsimile transmission of health information (updated), AHIMA Practice Brief, *J AHIMA* 72(6):64E–64F, 2001.

Available online: http://library.ahima.org/ xpedio/groups/public/documents/ahima/bok2_000116.hcsp?dDocName=bok2_000116.

Johnson M, Bulechek G, Dochterman JM, et al: *Nursing diagnosis, outcomes, and interventions: NANDA, NOC, and NIC linkages*, St. Louis, 2001, Mosby.

Keepnews D, Capitman JA, Rosati RJ, et al: Measuring patient-level clinical outcomes of home health care, *J Nurs Scholarsh* 35(1):79–85, 2004.

Loeb M, Carusone SC, Goeree R, et al: Effect of a clinical pathway to reduce hospitalizations in nursing home residents with pneumonia, *JAMA* 295(21):2503–2510, 2006.

Martin KS: *The Omaha System: a key to practice, documentation and information management*, ed 2, St Louis, 2005, Elsevier.

McCormick KA, Jones CB: Is one taxonomy needed for health care vocabularies and classifications? *Online J Issues Nurs* 3(2): manuscript 2, 1998. Available online: www.nursingworld.org/MainMenueCategories/ANAMarketplace/ANAPeriodicals/OJIN/TableofContents/Vol31998/No2Sept1998/Isonetaxonomyneeded.aspx. Accessed December 6, 2009.

Moody LE, Slocumb E, Berg B, et al: Electronic health records documentation in nursing: nurses' perceptions, attitudes and preferences, *Comput Inform Nurs* 22(6):337–344, 2004.

Moorhead M, Johnson M, Maas M, et al: *Nursing outcomes classification (NOC)*, ed 4, St. Louis, 2008, Mosby/Elsevier.

Muller-Staub M, Lavin MA, Needham I, et al: Meeting the criteria of a nursing diagnosis classification: evaluation of ICNP, ICF, NANDA, and ZEFP, *Int J Nurs Stud* 44(5):702–713, 2007.

Nemeth LS, Wessell AM, Jenkins RG, et al: Strategies to accelerate translation of research into primary care with practices using electronic medical records, *J Nurs Care Qual* 22(4):343–349, 2007.

North American Nursing Diagnosis Association (NANDA): *Nursing diagnoses: definitions and classifications 2009–2011*, Philadelphia, 2009, Wiley-Blackwell.

Park H, Lu D, Konicek D, et al: Nursing interventions classification in systematized nomenclature of medical terms: a cross-mapping validation, *CIN Comput Inform Nurs* 25(4):198–208, 2007.

Poissant L, Pereira J, Tamblyn R, et al: The impact of electronic health records on time efficiency of physicians and nurses: a systematic review, *J Am Med Inform Assoc* 12(5):505–516, 2005.

Rutherford MA: Standardized nursing language: what does it mean for Nursing Practice? *OJIN* 13(1), 2008. Available online: www.nursingworld.org/MainMenuCategories/ANAMarketplace/ANAPeriodicals/OJIN/Table ofContents/vol132008/No1Jan08/ArticlePreviousTopic/StandardizedNursingLanguage.aspx.

Siegler EL, Adelman R: Copy and paste: a remediable hazard of electronic health records, *Am J Med* 122(6):493–494, 2009.

Silva C: Only 1.5% of non-Federal hospitals report having full EHRs, *Am Med News* April 6, 2009. Available online: www.ama-assn.org/amednews/2009/04/06/gvsc0406.htm. Accessed April 6, 2009.

Thompson D, Johnston P, Spurr C, et al: The impact of electronic medical records on nursing efficiency, *J Nurs Admin* 39(10):444–451, 2009.

Westra BL, Delaney CW, Konicek D, et al: Nursing standards to support the electronic health record, *Nurs Outlook* 56(5):258–266, 2008.

CHAPTER 26

Communicating at the Point of Care: Application of eHealth Information Technology

Kathleen Underman Boggs

OBJECTIVES

At the end of the chapter, the reader will be able to:

1. Identify types of wireless technologies of use in decentralized "point of care" nursing.
2. Discuss the advantages and disadvantages of various assistive technologies for continual communication.
3. Describe advantages to staff nurses for using clinical decision support systems software, especially with regard to potential to increase communication in health care.
4. Discuss application of technology at the point of care.

Three major transformations are occurring in use of Health Information Technology [HIT] that will greatly change traditional patterns of nursing communication:

- Electronic health record (EHR) and accompanying ordering and taxonomy (discussed in Chapter 25)
- *Decentralized access* to client information at the point of care
- Handheld wireless devices allowing continual real-time exchange of information

According to Dr. David Blumenthal, National coordinator for HIT in the United States, no healthcare provider can practice effectively without use of eHealth technology (2009). Nurses are expected to be competent in HIT use and keep abreast as innovations are introduced to help us meet professional standards (Fetter, 2009). Broad use of HIT can improve our communication, the quality and safety of our care, and our efficiency. At the same time, HIT can decrease costs of health care in the long term.

This chapter focuses on using electronic HIT to enhance communication between nurse and client or between nurse and other professional health care providers. Communication is the cornerstone for teamwork, safety, and support. New emerging technologies facilitate our communication. Portable electronic devices with Internet access small enough to be easily carried are referred to in this textbook as "handheld" devices. Decentralized access to information and ability to document at your client's location are referred to as "point of care" capability. You can use your handheld device to access nursing information databases or to document care while at your client's bedside and in his or her home. Content in this chapter also covers other HIT tools such as computerized clinical decision support programs (CDS), secure messaging, telehealth, remote monitoring, Internet client education and support, and Internet professional education. Discussion of these emerging technologies is limited to a focus on their relation to communication.

BASIC CONCEPTS

DECENTRALIZED ACCESS TECHNOLOGY FOR COMMUNICATION AT THE POINT OF CARE

Available electronic technology is revolutionizing our nursing care communication (Figure 26-1). In addition to the EHR discussed in Chapter 25, new hand-held devices with Internet capability allow nurses decentralized access to client records. Nursing practice now incorporates Point of Care Information and Documentation, allowing continual use of updated client information and reference material at any client location via the Internet. Communication in a timely manner is one of four standards of effective communication (Table 26-1). Communication in "real time" is the new hallmark of bedside nursing in the age of new technology. With fiscal cutbacks, fewer nurses per client, and increased acuity of client situations, use of technology can enhance our critical thinking, clinical decision making, and delivery of safe, efficient

TABLE 26-1	TeamSTEPPS: Standards of Effective Communication
Complete	• Communicate all relevant information.
Clear	• Convey info in a plainly understood manner.
Brief	• Be concise.
Timely	• Offer and request info in an appropriate time frame. • Verify authenticity. • Validate or acknowledge info.

Online: www.ahrq.gov/teamsteppstools/instructor/fundamentals/module6/

care (Carter & Rukholm, 2008; HIT, http://healthit.hhs.gov/portal/server.pt, accessed 1/2/10).

Development of technology is advancing hundreds of times faster than at any previous time in history. This chapter describes a few of the current choices. The goal is to improve health care outcomes and in the long range to decrease the cost of health care. Governmental agencies in many countries have been funding use of eHealth technology and giving incentives to providers. Government programs mandate use of aspects of HIT. For example, in the United States, the Medicare Modernization Act [MMA] requires that e-prescribing be done for Part D–covered clients. EHRs must be in use before 2014. Statutes address the delivery of information to the point of care to enable more informed decisions about appropriate, more cost-effective medications. Active electronic participation by clients is seen as a way to alleviate demands on staff. Among others, the American Academy of Family Physicians supports the concept of a "medical home" embodying active client participation via e-mail, client use of Internet portals, and remote monitoring.

WIRELESS DEVICES IN HEALTH CARE: ACCESS TO INFORMATION AT THE POINT OF CARE

Unlike other industries such as banking, health care was slow to adopt new technology. But now that wireless handheld devices with Internet access are commonly used, the transition to HIT is making rapid progress. Box 26-1 presents a summary of advantages and disadvantages for use of wireless technology by nurses. As a new generation of wireless technology comes into common use, nurses have continual access

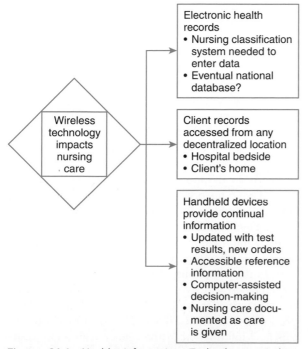

Figure 26-1 Health Information Technology: wireless technology has an impact on nursing care.

BOX 26-1	Use of Wireless Handheld Computers

Advantages
- Easily portable; can be used at the point of care (client's bedside, in the home, etc.)
- Quick charting when nurse enters information by tapping menu selections
- Can contain reference resources about treatment, for medication dosage, and so forth, if uploaded
- May provide dictionary, and reminders about standards of care
- When accompanied by Internet access, provides quick communication (e.g., nurse is signaled by beep regarding receipt of new orders)
- Provides quick access to client records

Disadvantages
- Possible threats to client's legal privacy rights
- Long learning curve; may take a while to become familiar with how to use
- Nurse does not have a printed copy of information (until downloaded to agency printer)
- Small screen does not allow you to view entire page of information
- Technical problem may result in dysfunction/ downtime

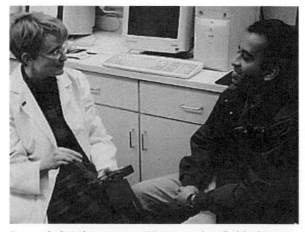

Personal digital assistants (PDAs) are handheld electronic devices that may contain multiple databases, possibly including a language translator for use when interviewing a patient from another culture. With these devices, data can be entered at the point of care, whether it is in a clinic or a patient's home, then transmitted wirelessly to a central agency computer or printer. *(Photo courtesy Adam Boggs.)*

to client records. HIT will transform our nursing care, enhancing our ability to give quality care, reduce risk for making errors, and improve our communication competency.

Personal Digital Assistant

Personal digital assistant (PDA) is a generic term for any of several brands of small, handheld computerized electronic devices that fit in the palm of the nurse's hand. First introduced in the mid-1990s as the U.S. Robotics Pilot (Palm Pilot), PDAs organize and retrieve information. PDAs store assessment and diagnostic tools, best practice guidelines, and references for nursing and drug information. They reduce paperwork and help the nurse save time tracking client information, leaving more time to focus on client care (Stroud, Smith, & Erkel, 2009). PDA applications can check for drug interactions, calculate dosages, analyze laboratory results, schedule procedures, order prescriptions, serve as a dictionary, or provide language translation, among other functions. It is easy to upload reference sources, such as the latest medication information or disease treatment protocols, making them akin to a portable medical and nursing library. PDAs can be taken to wherever the client is located.

PDA operating systems incorporate various types of handwriting recognition, allowing the user to tap, draw, or write on the screen using a stylus. The great advantage of PDAs over laptop computers is they are small, lightweight, and easy to carry. Because they are wireless, they can be used in the client's hospital room, in an outpatient clinic, or in the community—even in the client's home. Most PDAs can send stored information to another PDA, to the agency computer, or directly to a printer.

PDAs are used to record client data. You can enter your client's history, your assessment of this client, compile a problem list, update data, and write nursing notes. Your wireless handheld device can also be used to track information such as client's medications and dosages or laboratory test results in a flow sheet format. In the community, PDAs with Internet capability can be used to access client records. For example, a nurse practitioner using a PDA can call up a client's previous prescriptions, renew them at a touch, record this new information in the agency mainframe computer, correctly calculate the dosage of a new medication, write the order, and send this prescription to the client's pharmacy instantly—all without writing any-thing on paper.

Nursing programs and agencies worldwide are beginning to require use of portable devices such as PDAs. For example, a survey of emergency department nurses in Australia showed they find PDAs a useful tool in their practice (Gururajan, 2004). Some study findings indicate that providers using PDAs make more accurate judgments and write more complete reports than do control groups without access to a PDA (Skeate, Wahi, Jessurum, & Connelly, 2007).

A number of brands of hardware are available to run operating systems like Palm OS or Windows CE Pocket PC. Downloadable health care information programs are available, as well as programs that support the documentation of client care data. Limited battery life and incompatibility of software uploadable pro-grams are limitations that need to be considered before adoption.

Cellular (Mobile) Telephones or Pagers

Some staff nurses use tools of convenience such as cell phones or pagers in their daily work. Ordinary cell phones can be used to locate clinicians, or verify and clarify information. Some hospitals are issuing mobile phones to staff nurses to use at work so they can directly contact physicians or other hospital departments from the client's bedside, give condition updates, or obtain verbal orders. The major cost is not the actual phone device but the monthly service provider cost. Nurses working in the community use cellular phones to con-tact clients on the way to give home care. Phones pro-vide easy access from the field back to the agency, to the client's primary physician, and to other resources.

In the United Kingdom, nurses making home visits use mobile phones to improve communication with agencies and community services and to trans-mit client data (Blakc, 2008a, b). Some community nurses prefer pagers, which notify them of telephone messages so they can return calls. Cellular phones equipped with cameras and picture transmission cap-abilities have potential for long distance diagnosis, a "snapshot" version of telemedicine/telehealth inter-active video and vocal transmissions.

Smartphones

Smartphones represent the convergence of cellular mobile phones and mobile computers. These devices, such as the Blackberry Storm, have three functions:

They enable you to download and access PDA-type information resources, provide Internet access to client information (new laboratory results or physician orders), and make and receive telephone calls or instant messages. Some downloaded applications provide "alerts" by beeping when there are new orders or newly available test results. In addition to housing down-loaded reference programs such as those described for the PDA, smartphones with large enough memory may even house computer-assisted decision support systems. Downloadable programs such as Epocrates, a free drug information program, not only provide drug information, but when you type in client information such as age, weight, and diagnosis, they provide you with guidelines for correct dosage, contraindications, and side effects. New information "alerts" are sent to your device in a timely manner. National guidelines for best practice can also be downloaded. Smartphones are now outselling PDAs by a wide margin. Busis (2010) suggests a barcode reader as an add-on applica-tion for a smartphone.

Phones may also increase direct access to health care for the client. Companies such as TelaDoc, pro-vide access to a physician's advice or treatment by telephone to its members for a nominal annual fee.

Laptop Computers

Laptop computers are more powerful than PDAs, yet are still small and portable enough to be taken into the client's home. They are used to chart and transmit your client's care. If a laptop with a networking card is near a wireless Internet transmitter, information can be sent in a wireless fashion. Another option is to use a telephone to transmit your nursing documentation.

COMPUTERIZED CLINICAL DECISION SUPPORT SYSTEMS

A most important asset of HIT adoption is the provi-sion of computerized clinical decision support sys-tems, which the authors refer to as CDS. A CDS is defined as an electronic information technology–based system designed to improve clinical decision making to enhance client care and safety. More sophisticated CDS systems give interactive advice, after comparing entries of your client data with a computerized knowledge base. The information offered to you is personalized to your client's condition (filtered) and is offered at appropriate times in your workday.

Multiple research studies indicate that integrated decision support systems offer timely information, improve provider performance, and result in better outcomes for clients (Poissant, Taylor, Huang, & Tamblyn, 2010). Computerized physician order entry systems have been heavily promoted as assets in prescribing medications because they reduce the incidence of adverse outcomes. In addition to helping you provide safer care, outcomes include reduced costs, increased adoption of best-practice care, and improved treatment responses (Bertsche, 2009).

Since the Institute of Medicine and the Canadian Institutes of Health Research began advocating CDS programs or supporting research into CDS effect on client care, suggested types of data in the CDS system have come to include:

- Diagnosis and care information displays with care management priorities listed
- A method for communication, that is, for order entry and for entering client data (system offers prompts so you enter complete data; offers "smart" or model forms)
- Automatic checks for drug-drug, drug-allergy, and drug-formulary interactions
- Ability to send reminders to clients according to their stated preference
- Medication reconciliations and client summary of care at transitions of client care
- Ability to send you electronic "alerts" or prompts if problem occurs or you haven't acknowledged receipt of information, such as client's laboratory test results

The hardware can be a computer terminal on your hospital unit or wireless handheld device, such as a PDA or smartphone. A software database can be information residing in the agency server, or a central repository such as a disease registry or government database (Berner, 2009).

For the nurse, CDS software generates specific information for your client care including assessment guidelines and forms, analyses of their laboratory test results, and use of best practice protocols to make specific recommendations for safe care (Hayes & Wilczynski, 2010). Ideally, this is integrated into the EHR system you are using. Based on input about the current condition of your client (coded data), the system is programmed to provide you with appropriate reminders. For example, after you complete care for your first assigned client, specific information is presented to you if you have not yet documented a needed intervention. This assists you in preventing treatment errors or omissions and helps improve your documentation. Blaser and colleagues (2007) demonstrated that their computerized decision support system based on clinical pathways could also speed up the time to intervention. More timely interventions should lead to fewer client complications.

CDS technology is slowly being adopted. Early systems were "stand-alone"; but technology is rapidly advancing, leading to more user-friendly, integrated systems that provide timely, relevant content. Because the system stores your information about your activity, you can obtain reports about your overall compliance with standards of care or provide data for research. More studies on CDS effects on client health outcomes and client provider communication are needed. Current research results show better client outcomes and more accurate, complete documentation (Eslami, Abu-Hanna, de Jonge, & de Keizer, 2009; Gerard et al., 2008). Key CDS issues are speed and ease of access.

SEARCHABLE REFERENCES FOR NURSING INFORMATION

Nurses have the opportunity to search databases when they need information, using computers or smartphones. There are many free, downloadable guides to care. One example is "The Guide to Clinical Preventive Services," which has care recommendations. You can search by age, sex, and risk factors (U.S. Preventive Services Task Force: www.epss.ahrq.gov). Many regional nurse associations have or soon will have such databases. Most hospitals and larger agencies have resident experts such as medical librarians or clinical nurse specialists to help staff nurses access information about evidenced-based care guidelines.

REMOTE CLIENT HEALTH MONITORING

Rapid upgrades in electronic applications are changing the way we deal with our clients. A few examples are described here.

"SMART ROOM" TECHNOLOGY

"Telecare" programs have been implemented that communicate client vital signs, monitor whether nurses wash hands, or signal you if a client falls and does not get up via sensors embedded in the hospital room or client's house. Families in America and England are using such sensors placed throughout the client's home to monitor for potential problems such as stove burners left on, doors left open, a too cold house, or a client crisis, such as an epileptic seizure. In the literature, this is referred to as "Smart Rooms" a form of automated medical technology.

REMOTE MONITORING

Wireless technology extends decision support into the client's home. Use allows for self-monitoring, reduces time client spends in physician offices, reduces demands on staff time, and promotes efficient monitoring of your client's status (Blake, 2008a,b). A variety of monitors worn by clients can periodically transmit data directly to a primary provider or nurse in a health agency via ground telephone lines or even using wireless technology (Yao, Schmitz, & Warren, 2005). Such devices include 24-hour heart monitors, pacemakers, uterine contraction monitors, and respiratory function peak flow readings, among others. Nurses are assuming increased responsibilities for interpretation of these data and for instituting interventions.

ELECTRONIC COMMUNICATION

E-MAIL

According to the American Medical Association (AMA, 2004), e-mail can be a convenient, inexpensive method of communicating follow-up instructions, test results, and educational information to the client in his or her home. Almost all clients express a desire to communicate with their health care providers via e-mail, but only a small percentage of physicians actually use e-mail for scheduling appointments, providing prescription refills, and other routine tasks. Physicians express concern about lack of income generation, confidentiality, malpractice, and the belief that it would be too time-consuming (Gerstle & AAP Task Force on Medical Informatics, 2004). Yet, studies show e-mail access to physicians improves communication, is desirable, decreases phone calls, may improve health outcomes, and does not impede client satisfaction (Goldman, 2005; Stalberg et al., 2008). Nurses also use e-mail as a way to communicate with clients, for example, in tracking the response of clients who are on new medication, instead of waiting until their next office appointment. AMA guidelines (2004) suggest that electronic or paper copies be made of e-mail messages sent to clients.

SECURE MESSAGING

Text instant messaging (IM) is commonly used in daily life, but IM can also be used to improve communications between clients and providers as a part of eHealth. IM can be used by clients to communicate self-monitored information to their care provider. The provider can also text message reminders to the client. Nurses provide personalized IM to clients as one intervention in preventive or chronic care, such as weight management, smoking cessation, or drug rehabilitation. IMs are also used as interventions with clients managing their cancer, asthma, diabetes, or other chronic diseases (Blake, 2008a,b).

ELECTRONIC REFERRALS AND CONSULTATIONS

With computerization and Internet, making eReferrals is easy. The Internet provides a common platform among agencies, even those that do not have integrated systems. Technology offers great potential for nurses, nurse-practitioners, and physician assistants, especially those who comprise a significant portion of the rural health care labor force. Rural populations comprise 20% in the United States, and tend to be poorer and medically underserved. Use of HIT discussed in this chapter can increase resources available to rural providers (Effken & Abbott, 2009). This form of communication needs guaranteed privacy protection and reimbursement provisions for the professionals for time spent to become successful (Bodenheimer, 2008).

TELEHEALTH

Telehealth is also called telemedicine, or occasionally, telenursing (eHealth in England). Telehealth is a broader term encompassing any use of the Internet for health purposes. Telecommunication technology is used for exchanging information across geographic distances with professional health care providers. It can be used to diagnose and treat illness, provide preventive health care, or provide medical consultation. It initially was used to provide care to clients in rural areas but is now also used in urban areas. The goal is to increase care to the underserved, while eliminating long trips to providers, especially to emergency departments. Many studies show use of this technology reduces hospitalizations, emergency department visits, and health care costs (Dansky, Vasey, & Bowles, 2008; McConnochie, Wood, Harendeen, Noyes, & Roghman, 2009).

Telehealth provides live, real-time audio and visual transmissions from one care provider to another or to a client. This technology is hailed as a boon to rural practitioners, facilitating long-distance consultations by expert specialists. Telehealth nursing communicates monitoring data to the nurse from the client (Prinz, 2008). There is some evidence that communication devices can improve client health outcomes, but more research is needed. It requires expensive hardware equipment at both ends of the transmission, as well as the infrastructure to support its use, but has the potential to reduce the cost of conventional health services (Wang, 2009). Privacy and information secuirty are concerns expressed by potential users (George, Hamilton, & Baker, 2009).

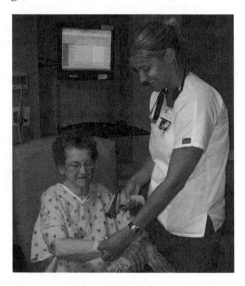

CLIENT HEALTH EDUCATION AND SUPPORT

CONSUMER HEALTH INFORMATION

People are willing to access the Internet for self-education to meet their health care needs. The Pew Internet and American Life Project (2005) found that about 80% of Internet users search for health information, especially on specific medical problems, wellness information, or treatment procedures. Many Web sites provide consumer health information. There is strong potential for improved health learning associated with interactive computer teaching programs.

LIFESTYLE MANAGEMENT

Not only do these educational programs increase client knowledge about their disease and their role in health promotion and disease management, but computers have been shown to positively impact client outcomes. Support and reminders about health self-management have already been described. Many Web sites provide interactive management. Others provide access to client support groups, such as the National Institute of Health. Nurses frequently recommend Internet sites to clients.

Agency for Healthcare Research and Quality's analysis of 146 studies of the impact of computer health modules on client outcomes found that these programs succeeded in engaging client attention, but more significantly they improved client clinical health (AHRQ, a). Just as studies have documented positive health outcomes after telephone support from nurses, contact with providers using interactive computer programs for Client Health Education using Webcam technology real-time (synchronous) communication between nurse and client can deliver health maintenance information, provide answers to illness-related questions, and lead to positive health outcomes.

PROVIDER AND CLIENT COMMUNICATION

WEB PORTALS FOR CLIENT EDUCATION

Many health care systems use portals to allow their clients access to communicate both with physicians and nurses. Most major pharmaceutical companies have portals that provide consumer and health care provider access to drug information.

ALERTS

Using the Internet, you can send electronic "alerts" to your clients who need medication renewals, screening examinations or other health services. A 2009 Kaiser Permanente study showed a marked decrease in primary care office visits after implementation of an electronic system with intensive provider-client communication via a secure Web site. They cite a separate Kaiser survey showing that 85% of users reported that being able to communicate electronically with their physicians improved their ability to manage their own health (Kaiser, 2004). A personalized Web site can be used by an agency for far broader functions than providing business hours or travel directions. In an American

Hospital Association study report, O'Dell (2005) says that nearly all health care organizations now have their own Web sites. Such sites can include health assessment tools and allow clients to schedule appointments. Another primary function is to provide health information. Web sites can have hyperlinks embedded that clients can use to access general information about their condition, medications, or treatment. They can also contain an e-mail link so that clients can directly contact the nurse responsible for patient education.

GROUP COMMUNICATION AS SUPPORT

Computers are used to mediate support groups for families and clients with various health problems. These formal Internet groups provide information, but they also importantly have been shown to provide improved social support for the ill client. Rains and Young's 2009 analysis of 28 research studies showed Internet group participants report less depression, increases in quality of life, as well as improved ability to manage their disease condition. Technologies associated with providing support include e-mail, instant (text) messaging, chat rooms, and discussion forums. The chat rooms are usually synchronous, in real time, providing immediate feedback. Usually discussion forums are asynchronous with time delays between postings and responses, allowing for more reflection before posting. Communication with group members over the Internet has been shown to be associated with lower levels of reported stress, especially in older adults. More studies are needed before we can specify the needed frequency, duration, or quality of content for optimal client support.

PROFESSIONAL EDUCATION

In addition to the portals used by clients, most professional organizations and government agencies offer free access to health care information dealing with protocols, standards of practice, and medication information. The American Nurses Association provides a popular, useful resource (www.nursingworld.org).

Developing an Evidence-Based Practice

Vandenkerhof EG, Hall S, Wilson R, Gay A, Duhn L: Evaluation of an innovative communication technology in an acute care setting, *CIN Comput Inform Nurs* 27(4):254–262, 2009.

Purpose: To assess staff attitude toward use of wireless communications device (Vocera) and compare communication patterns before and after implementation.

This quasi-experimental prestudy and poststudy was conducted to measure nurses' use of a wireless communication system, called Vocera, at Kingston General Hospital in Canada. Vocera is a personal communication tool that uses voice-over-Internet protocol. Each nurse wears a communication badge the size of a small cell phone clipped to his or her uniform or on a lanyard around the neck. Except when initiating a call by pressing a button of this badge, all the rest of the communication is hands-free. You can designate the recipient of your communication by name, title, or function—eliminating the need to know a phone number. The badge can call within the hospital or outside.

Results: Use of Vocera reduced the time for key communications, such as looking for the medication keys, looking for others, paging doctors, or walking to the telephone, by 25% overall. The distance each nurse walked to communicate was also reduced.

On average, each nurse reduced the time they spent attempting to communicate from 16.2 times per shift to 11.6 times. The most significant time savings were related to looking for other staff. There was a 45% reduction in the time spent looking for others ($P \leq 0.01$). Attitudes were compared before and after implementation. The increase in efficiency after implementation alleviated most concerns, except those involving confidentiality issues.

Application to Your Clinical Practice: Adoption of any innovative communication system needs to take into account nurses attitudes before implementation. Could your personal cell phone be used perhaps in its "texting" function for similar within-hospital communication? Should your employing agency provide such a device for all staff? These researchers believe their findings indicate that this communication system has the potential to improve client safety, as well as improve the general acute care work environment by improving work flow or eliminating some distractions. If further research should bear this out, employers might consider purchase of communications devices as economically prudent.

APPLICATIONS

In 2004, the U.S. National Coordinator for HIT set several goals, including the need to use new technology to improve health by facilitating quality of care monitoring and quickly disseminating research findings into practice. Competency in HIT use has broadly been cited by national nursing and policy organizations as an essential of basic nursing practice (Fetter, 2009). In addition to employers, regulatory agencies, professional agencies, and academic agencies, individual nurses themselves are responsible for attaining competency (ANA: role competency statement issued 3/12/09; accessed 1/11/10).

POINT OF CARE

Wireless entry of data at the point of care can increase your access to and use of evidence-based resources in your practice. If smartphones are used for personal business, as well as in work situations, separate e-mail/messaging accounts would be needed. Study results suggest that after an initial learning period, you will save time spent documenting care. Handheld devices at point of care provide timely access to client information, are convenient, and are cost-effective in the long run. Their prompts should help you provide safer, more comprehensive care.

WIRELESS HANDHELD COMPUTER USE
Electronic Mail

Guidelines are available for physician use of e-mail to communicate with clients (AMA, 2004); these guidelines are also appropriate for nurses. No one knows how many nurses are accustomed to using wireless technology devices in their care of clients. Guidelines for their use in giving client care still need to be developed.

Personal Digital Assistants and Smartphones

Although just about every nursing student has seen or used a wireless or cellular telephone, not everyone has used them as an aid to giving client care. These devices can save time, decrease errors, and simplify information retrieval at the point of care. Nursing is just beginning to deal with guidelines. Ethically, you do not send personal, non-professional messages.

Electronic Messaging

Electronic provider-client IM can be used to communicate simple data. This may promote better quality care and improved client utilization. Multiple articles in the literature describe the efficacy of using personalized IM for helping clients manage their conditions. In one example, your hypertensive client taking a new medication could text message his blood pressures to you today after self-monitoring, or your diabetic client could send today's glucose results after testing his or her blood sugar. Potentially, this could lead to better control, as in Harris et al.'s 2009 study in which clients who sent electronic messages to providers had better glycemic control. In addition, you can use IM to send personalized reminders to your client to schedule an appointment or take a medication.

CLINICAL DECISION SUPPORT SYSTEMS

CDS systems were introduced in the 1970s but have not yet matured into widespread use. Various CDS systems include knowledge management, triage systems, assessment forms, prescribing systems, or systems for test ordering and analysis. Multiple studies show that CDS provision of information based on evidence-based best practice improves quality of care (Damiani et al., 2010). This is most likely to occur when the CDS system is integrated into existing EHR systems and automatically provides care recommendations. The "active" or automatic provision of suggestions or prompts to the nurse to support his or her decisions is more effective than "passive" systems, which wait for the user to request data. Access to CDS programs by staff nurses is improving but still limited in most countries, including the NHS agencies in England surveyed by Mitchell and colleagues (2009).

For staff nurses, suggestions about care are offered as "pop-ups" or "alerts" when you access the client's record. For example, when you access a medication order on your client's EHR, you can use the CDS system to verify the five rights before administering the drug (Table 26-2). This reveals whether there would be any possible harmful interactions with other medications your client is already taking. CDS "reminders" integrated with your work flow gives you suggestions about interventions that are based on researched best practice. Perhaps the CDS offers you a suggested alternative to the intervention you plan. In another example, nurses working with pediatric cancer clients have long used calculators to determine correct fractional dosage based on the child's weight. Now instead, they can use this automated support system because it automatically predetermines the correct doses.

Case Example

The following case is an example of how this technology is designed to assist us to deliver better and safer nursing care more efficiently.

Gail Myer, RN, is assigned to Mrs. Sanchez as one of her eight clients on an obstetrical unit. Mrs. Sanchez is

TABLE 26-2	Five Rights of Medication Administration as Communicated by Clinical Decision Support	
1	Right information	• Use of this medication is evidence based, pertinent, and suitable for my client's current condition or circumstance, as well as cost-effective.
2	Right person	• Was ordered by the appropriate provider. (Nurse will verify right client via coded ID bracelet on client, preferably with his or her picture attached; CDS matches this with bar code on the medication container.)
3	Right format	• CDS does automatic check for contraindications, allergies, etc. Matches drug with laboratory data. Checks correct dose/amount, correct form for ordered route (oral, injection, rectal suppository, etc.), and verifies that there are no harmful interactions with other drugs client is receiving.
4	Right channel	• Communicated to all via electronic health record disseminated through computer terminal, laptop, or handheld wireless device.
5	At the Right time	• Order and drug received by nurse at the right time in her work flow; before administration, nurse is prompted to assess any needed information, such as the client's blood glucose level. (Nurse will document as administered at the approximate time specified in the order.)

CDS, Clinical decision support programs.

in preterm labor. Gail's CDS automatically lists desired client outcomes based on her work assignment, lists "best practice" interventions, and then gives real-time feedback about client outcomes. Her handheld device receives electronic prompts to assist in clinical decision making. For example, the hospital's CDS program calculates expected delivery date for Mrs. Sanchez and supplies the correct dose of the prescribed medication based on her weight. It alerts Gail if the prescribed dose she intends to administer exceeds maximum standard safety margins, and also cross-checks this new drug for potential drug interactions with the drugs Mrs. Sanchez is already taking. It pops up a screening tool for Gail to use to assess Mrs. Sanchez's current status and then alerts Gail if she should forget to document today's results.

BARRIERS

Current handheld devices and CDS software programs are somewhat cumbersome to use. It may take too much time to input the data the program needs to make recommendations to you. Another problem is that the CSD system might send you clinically irrelevant information or it might send you so many alerts that you ignore them. Studies suggest that customizing alerts to your client assignment is more effective (Tamblyn et al., 2008). A number of studies show positive results, especially in areas of drug-dosing alerts or reminders about preventive care. More studies are needed to examine effects of CDSs on communication, but data

suggest a positive effect. In a Canadian study, nurses used PDAs to access the Registered Nurses Association of Ontario best-practice guidelines specific to their assigned clients' outcome assessments. Overall study results indicated communication was improved and nurses were more likely to receive information in a timely manner when their client's condition changed (Doran & Mylopoulos, 2008). Interestingly, the majority of participating nurses had not accessed the best practice resource in the month before the Doran study when they began using PDAs.

Cost and usability are the main issues in adopting CDS technology. Of course, a nurse needs the hardware, as well as easy access to the CDS software program. Access needs to be user friendly, integrated into your work flow, relevant to your care, and provide information quickly at times that really fit into your existing work flow. Some current CDS systems are cumbersome to use, provide information that is irrelevant or in too much detail to be visualized on small handheld device screens. If your CDS requires separate access from your client EHRs, provides details you did not seek or want, or repeatedly sends you alerts that are not useful, you would probably not find it helpful. On the other hand, if CDS use improves your work environment and client care, you would probably support its use. Bakken and colleagues (2008) suggest that effective use begins when this technology is integrated into the student learning experience.

INTERNET USE

We are just beginning to realize the positive impact that Internet use can have on client health.

CYBER HEALTH CARE FOR HEALTH PROMOTION

There is considerable evidence about the efficacy of providing health care education and information online. The Internet can be used to remind clients of appointments, replacing telephone calls. Limited areas of the client's EHR can be accessed for information. Clients could sign on and obtain results of laboratory tests. One advantage is that this information would be available at all times, rather than just during office hours. Appointments can be made and reminders given via the Internet.

CYBER EDUCATION FOR CLIENT DISEASE MANAGEMENT

Disease self-management using computers will greatly change the way nurses deliver health education. Health information about preventive health or about controlling their chronic disease conditions can be provided to clients effectively, quickly, and inexpensively via the Internet. Van der Meer and colleagues (2009) studied outcomes of an Internet-based education program for asthma self-management and found that the Internet group had better quality-of-life scores and, more importantly, maintained better asthma control than did the traditional care group. Consider other conditions that might have similar outcomes.

Client education programs via the Internet are so popular that entire companies have sprung up to provide for this need. Commercial companies produce many software packages that nurses could use to supplement their own teaching. Client learning would need to be evaluated. Outcome studies show some clients learn more from computer-based programs than from traditional teaching. One example is the HIV/AIDS program described by Marsch and Bickel (2004). PDAs can be used to play videos to educate clients about their health care. In Brock and Smith's 2007 study, clients reported PDAs were an appropriate medium for learning, regardless of their literacy skills. They demonstrated increased knowledge after watching. One problem for clients accessing health information using general Web search engines is that not all online information is accurate or easy for the user to verify. Refer to Chapter 16 for in-depth discussion of health education.

CYBER SUPPORT FOR CLIENTS

Caregivers or clients with chronic conditions can use Internet support groups, chat rooms, or direct communication with care providers to gain support. Also, nurses can gain insight and better understand the "lived experiences" of their clients by participating in these Internet opportunities. Clients are accustomed to accessing support from friends when they use Facebook, Twitter, and so on. Because support via telephone has been shown to be a cost-effective method for improving functioning and quality of life for diabetic clients, the same effects need to be documented for cyber support. For example, use of cyber support opportunities has been shown to empower asthma caregivers (Sullivan, 2008). Client use of CDS programs that provide information about treatment options and the benefits and risks for each option can help them clarify their choice and can improve nurse-client communication (O'Connor et al., 2009).

CAUTIONS OR BARRIERS TO APPLICATION OF NEW TECHNOLOGIES

USER RESISTANCE

The transition to use of eHealth technology in nursing implies a learning curve. Some providers cite problems such as the time involved in use, equipment design limitations, access issues, and fears about losing handheld devices. Australian and Swedish studies suggest that administrators need to educate and support nurses while addressing the impact of computerization on nursing work flow (Dahm & Wadensten, 2008; Eley et al., 2008).

OUTCOMES

Is the cost involved in adopting new technology worth it? Measurable effects such as work efficiency and effects on client health need to be carefully evaluated to determine the effectiveness of use of these new communication technologies.

ILLITERACY

Illiteracy could be a barrier to consumer use. For example, in some developed countries, one-fifth of the population may be reading below fifth-grade level. Although the number of citizens who have no access to the Internet is shrinking, there are those who have yet to learn use. Experts suggest that availability of technology will have a significant, widespread, positive impact on citizen health in Third World countries. In all cases, our communication needs to be tailored to the needs and literacy level of our client (Neuhauser & Kreps, 2008).

LIABILITY ISSUES

Use of the Internet presents many questions about how to maximize its communication potential with an increasingly diverse population. Liability and regulatory issues are outmoded, relevant to the century gone by. For example, if transmission (and treatment) crosses state lines, in which region does the provider need to be licensed? If malpractice occurs, in which region or state would legal action occur?

PRIVACY

As with any computer use, we are also concerned about *security*. Today, concerns about maintaining privacy are linked in people's minds with the ability of agencies to maintain secure records. Many surveys of consumer concerns cite breach of privacy as their biggest concern. See the Ethical Dilemma box at the end of this chapter for an exercise that explores this problem.

PROFESSIONAL ONLINE NURSING PRACTICE GUIDELINES

A number of nursing organizations provide policy and procedure information to nurse users. One

example is the Visiting Nurse Association (VNA) which offers telecare protocols used by more than 900 agencies.

PROFESSIONAL ONLINE NURSING EDUCATION

Some nursing programs are offered entirely online, but most have incorporated at least some computer-enhanced courses in response to student demand. Students say they prefer asynchronous (not in real time) courses that they can access at their convenience. After graduation, would you prefer this method to earn continuing education credits as required for your relicensure or recertification? How about for work-related meetings? Gross and Gross (2005) have suggested using the asynchronous format for meetings, especially when content is controversial or has emotional aspects. This format may increase participation. Try Exercise 26-1 as practice.

SUMMARY

HIT is an emerging new technology transforming the way nurses communicate with other professionals, with clients, and with data. HIT provides nurses with new tools to deliver nursing at the client's point of care. Moreover, it is anticipated that use of HIT will improve the quality of care. Tools discussed in this chapter include CDS programs, messaging, telehealth, and remote monitoring. HIT gives clients new ways to educate themselves, to manage their health, and to communicate with health care professionals.

EXERCISE 26-1	Critique of an Internet Nursing Resource Database

Purpose: To encourage students to gain familiarity with Internet resources.

Procedure:
As an out-of-class assignment, access any nursing resource database, preferably using a handheld wireless device. Many sites are listed in the online references.

    Write a one-paragraph critique; rate the Web site from 0 = useless to 10 = excellent.

1. How quickly were you able to find a specific piece of information?
2. How applicable to your clinical practice?
3. To what degree was the information evidenced based?

Discussion:
Use results as a basis for a general in-class discussion.

ETHICAL DILEMMA   What Would You Do?

A large insurance company's medication service routinely fills 20 million prescriptions on the client's request transmitted over the Internet. The system contains client identification numbers, names, addresses, and diagnoses. After rebooting their system after a temporary shutdown to upgrade, a technician begins to reply to accumulated e-mails. Unfortunately, he sends these e-mail responses to the wrong recipients. Clients complain that they had been promised confidentiality of medical records as long as they did not give out their password, yet they were receiving e-mails containing other members' medical information.

In another case, a pharmacy chain replaced their computers, donating old computers to a local school system. However, they neglected to wipe out customer medical information from the hard drives. Users were able to access confidential information, such as which customers were taking AIDS-suppression medications.

1. What safeguards could have prevented these violations of confidentiality?
2. If you were the nurse sending the "e-mails gone astray," what would you do?
3. Are you responsible or is only the agency responsible?

REFERENCES

AHRQ, a: Evidence Report, Publication No.10-E019. www.ahrq.gov/clinic/tp/chiapptp.htm. Accessed December 23, 2009.

AHRQ, b: TeamSTEPPS. www.ahrq.gov/teamsteppstools/instructor/fundamentals/module6/. Accessed March 11, 2010.

American Medical Association: *Guidelines for physician-patient electronic communications* [online], 2004. Available online: http://www.ama-assn.org/ama/pub/category/2386.html. [type title into the search box]. Accessed August 18, 2010.

ANA: *American Nurses Association statement on nursing practice*, www.nursingworld.org/NursingPractice. Accessed January 11, 2010.

Bakken S, John R, Currie LM, et al: Advancing evidence-based practice and patient safety through integration of personal digital assistants into clinical nursing education, *Nurs Outlook* 56(1):3840, 2008.

Berner ES: *Clinical decision support systems: state of the art*, AHRQ Publication No. 09-0069-EF, Rockville, MD, 2009, Agency for Healthcare Research and Quality.

Bertsche T, Askoxylakis V, Habl G, et al: Multidisciplinary pain management based on a computerized clinical decision support system in cancer pain patients, *Int Assoc Study Pain* 147:20–28, 2009.

Blake H: Innovation in practice: mobile phone technology in patient care, *Br J Community Nurs* 13(4):160, 162–165, 2008a.

Blake H: Mobile phone technology in chronic disease management, *Nurs Stand* 23(12):43–46, 2008b.

Blaser R, Schnabel M, Biber C, et al: Improving pathway compliance and clinician performance by using information technology, *Int J Med Inform* 76:151–156, 2007.

Blumenthal D: Speech at the 2009 National Conference of Health Information Management Association, Dallas, TX, October 6, 2009.

Bodenheimer T: Coordinating care—a perilous journey through the health care system, *N Eng J Med* 358(10):1064–1071, 2008.

Brock TP, Smith SR: Using digital videos displayed on personal digital assistants [PDAs] to enhance patient education in clinical settings, *Int J Med Inform* 76:829–835, 2007.

Busis N: Mobile phones to improve the practice of neurology, *Neurol Clin* 28:395–410, 2010.

Carter LM, Rukholm E: A study of critical thinking, teacher-student interaction, and discipline-specific writing in an online educational setting for registered nurses, *J Contin Educ Nurs* 39(3):133–138, 2008.

Dahm MF, Wadensten B: Nurses' experiences of and opinions about using standardized care plans in electronic health records—a questionnaire study, *J Clin Nurs* 18:2137–2145, 2008.

Damiani G, Pinnarelli L, Colosimo SC, et al: The effectiveness of computerized clinical guidelines in the process of care: a systematic review, *BMC Health Serv Res* 10:2, 2010.

Dansky KH, Vasey J, Bowles K, et al: Impact of Telehealth on clinical outcomes in patients with heart failure, *Clin Nurs Res* 17(3):182–199, 2008.

Doran DM, Mylopoulos J: *Outcomes in the palm of your hand: improving the quality and continuity of patient care*, Ottawa, 2008, Canadian Health Services Research Foundation. Available online: www.chsrf.ca/final_research/ogc/documents/DoranReport1_3_25_FINAL.pdf. Accessed September 13, 2009.

Effken JA, Abbott P: Health IT-enabled care for underserved rural populations: the role of nursing, *J Am Med Inform Assoc* 16(4):439–445, 2009.

Eley R, Fallon T, Soar J, et al: Barriers to use of information and computer technology by Australia's nurses: a national survey, *J Clin Nurs* 18:1151–1158, 2008.

Eslami S, Abu-Hanna A, de Jonge E, et al: Tight glycemic control and computerized decision-support systems: a systematic review, *Intensive Care Med* 35:1505–1517, 2009.

Fetter MS: Improving information technology competencies: implications for psychiatric mental health nursing, *Issues Ment Health Nurs* 30:3–13, 2009.

George SM, Hamilton A, Baker R, et al: Pre-experience perceptions about Telemedicine among African-Americans and Latinos in South Central Los Angeles, *Telemed J E Health* 15(6):525–530, 2009.

Gerard MN, Trick WE, Das K, et al: Use of clinical decision support to increase influenza vaccination: multi-year evolution of the system, *J Am Med Inform Assoc* 15:776–779, 2008.

Gerstle RS: AAP Task Force on Medical Informatics: E-mail communication between pediatricians and their patients, *Pediatrics* 114(1):317–321, 2004.

Goldman RD: Community physicians' attitudes toward electronic follow-up after an emergency department visit, *Clin Pediatr (Phila)* 44(4):305–309, 2005.

Gross D, Gross C: Impact of an electronic meeting system on the group decision-making process, *Comput Inform Nurs* 23(1):46–51, 2005.

Gururajan R: A study of the use of hand-held devices in an emergency department, *J Telemed Telecare* 10(Suppl 1):33–35, 2004.

Harris LT, Haneuse SJ, Martin DP, et al: Diabetes quality of care and outpatient utilization associated with electronic patient-provider messaging: a cross-sectional analysis, *Diabetes Care* 32(7):1182–1187, 2009.

Hayes RB, Wilczynski NL: Effects of computerized clinical decision support systems on practitioner performance and patient outcomes: methods of a decision-maker-researcher partnership systematic review, *Implement Sci* 5(12), 2010. Available online: www.implementationscience.com/content/5/1/12 Accessed March 9, 2010.

Kaiser Family Foundation/AHRQ/Harvard School of Public Health: *National survey on consumers experiences with patient safety and quality info*, 2004. www.kff.org/kaiserpolls/pomr111704pkg.cfm.

Marsch LA, Bickel WK: Efficacy of computer-based HIV/AIDS education for injection drug users, *Am J Health Behav* 28(4):316–327, 2004.

McConnochie KM, Wood NE, Harendeen NE, et al: Acute illness patterns change with use of Telemedicine, *Pediatrics* 123(6): e989–e995, 2009.

Mitchell N, Randekk R, Foster R, et al: A national survey of computerized decision support systems available to nurses in England, *J Nurs Manag* 17:772–780, 2009.

Neuhauser L, Kreps GL: Online cancer communication: meeting the literacy, cultural and linguistic needs of diverse audiences, *Patient Educ Couns* 71:365–377, 2008.

O'Connor AM, Bennett CL, Stacey D, et al: Decision aids for people facing health treatment of screening decisions, *The Cochrane Library* (3), 2009.

O'Dell GJ: American Hospital Association environmental assessment, *Hosp Health Netw* 79(10):69–71, 2005.

Pew Internet and American Life Project Report: Doctor, doctor give me the Web, *Smart Comput Plain English* 16(8):6, 2005.

Poissant L, Taylor L, Huang A, et al: Assessing the accuracy of an inter-institutional automated patient-specific health problem list, *BCM Med Inform Decis Mak* 10:10, 2010. Available online: www.biomedcentral.com/1472-6947/10/10/abstract.

Prinz L, Cramer M, Englund A, et al: Telehealth: A policy analysis for quality, impact on patient outcomes, and political feasibility, *Nurs Outlook* 56(4):152–158, 2008.

Rains SA, Young V: A meta-analysis of research on formal computer-mediated support groups: examining group characteristics and health outcomes, *Hum Commun Res* 35:309–336, 2009.

Skeate RC, Wahi MM, Jessurum J, et al: Personal digital-enabled report content knowledgebase results in more complete pathology reports and enhances resident learning, *Hum Pathol* 38:1727–1735, 2007.

Stalberg P, Yeh M, Ketterridge G, et al: E-mail access and improved communication between patient and surgeon, *Arch Surg* 143(2): 165–169, 2008.

Stroud SD, Smith CA, Erkel EA, et al: Personal Digital Assistants use by nurse practitioners: a descriptive study, *J Am Acad Nurse Pract* 21:31–38, 2009.

Sullivan CF: Cybersupport: empowering asthma caregivers, *Pediatr Nurs* 34(3):217–224, 2008.

Tamblyn R, Huang A, Taylor L, et al: A randomized trial of effectiveness of on-demand verses computer triggered drug decision support in primary care, *J Am Med Inform Assoc* 15(4):430–438, 2008.

Van der Meer V, Bakker MJ, van der Hout WB, et al: Internet-based self-management plus education compared with usual care in asthma, *Ann Intern Med* 151(2):110–120, 2009.

Wang F: The role of cost in Telemedicine, *Telemed J E Health* 15(10): 1–7, 2009.

Yao J, Schmitz R, Warren S, et al: A wearable point-of-care system for home use that incorporates plug-and-play and wireless standards, *IEEE Trans Inf Technol Biomed* 9(3):363–371, 2005.

GLOSSARY

Accommodation A desire to smooth over a conflict through cooperative but nonassertive responses. (ch. 14)

Acculturation Describes how a person from a different culture initially learns the behavior norms and values of the dominant culture, and begins to adopt its behaviors and language patterns. (ch. 11)

Active listening A dynamic process in which a nurse hears a client's message, decodes its meaning, and provides feedback to the client. (ch. 10)

Acute grief Somatic distress that occurs in waves with feelings of tightness in the throat, shortness of breath, an empty feeling in the abdomen, a sense of heaviness and lack of muscular power, and intense mental pain. (ch. 8)

Advance directive A legal document, executed by a competent client or legal proxy, specifically identifying individual preferences for level of treatment at end of life, should the client become unable to make valid decisions at that time. (chs. 2, 8)

Advanced practice nurses Registered nurses with a baccalaureate degree in nursing, and an advanced degree in a selected clinical specialty with relevant clinical experience. (ch. 7)

Advocacy Interceding or acting on behalf of the clients to provide the highest quality of care obtainable. (chs. 7, 19, 24)

Affective domain Domain concerned with emotional attitudes related to acceptance, compliance, and taking personal responsibility for health care. (ch. 16)

Aggregated Data Compilation of multiple bits of factual information into large groupings allowing analysis. (ch. 25)

Aggressive behavior A response in which the individual acts to defend the self and to deflect the emotional impact of the perceived threat to the self through personal attack, blaming, or an extreme reaction to a tangential issue. (ch. 14)

Aging A lifelong process, advancing through the life cycle, beginning at birth and ending at death. (ch. 19)

Andragogy Art and science of helping adults learn. (ch. 16)

Anticipatory grief An emotional response that occurs before the actual death around a family member with a degenerative, or terminal disorder. (ch. 8)

Anticipatory guidance Education which helps the client foresee health outcomes. (ch. 20)

Anxiety A vague, persistent feeling of impending doom. (ch. 6, 20)

Aphasia A neurological linguistic deficit that is most commonly associated with neurological trauma to the brain. (ch. 17)

Apraxia The loss of ability or the inability to take purposeful action even when the muscles, senses, and vocabulary seem intact. (ch. 19)

Art of nursing Nurse's mode of being knowing and responding; represents an attunement rather than an activity. It is the element of care that nurses and clients tend to remember best. (ch. 1)

Assertive behavior Setting goals, acting on those goals in a clear, consistent manner, and taking responsibility for the consequences of those actions. (ch. 14)

Assimilation A person's full adoption of the behaviors, customs, values, and language of the mainstream culture. (ch. 11)

Authenticity The capacity to be true to one's personality, spirit, and character in interacting with clients and others in the nurse-client relationship. (ch. 5)

Authoritarian leadership A leadership style in which leaders take full responsibility for group direction and control group interaction. (ch. 12)

Autonomy The client's right to self-determination. (chs. 3, 19)

Avoidance A withdrawal from conflict. (ch. 14)

Beneficence Ethical principle guiding decisions, based on doing the greatest good for the greatest number and avoiding malfeasance. (ch. 3)

Best practice Nursing interventions derived from research evidence demonstrating successful outcome for client. (ch. 22)

Biofeedback Immediate and continuous information about a person's physiological responses; auditory and visual signals that increase one's response to external events. (ch. 20)

Boards of nursing State governmental agencies that are responsible for the regulation of nursing practice in each respective state. Boards of Nursing are authorized to enforce the Nurse Practice Act, develop administrative rules/regulations and other responsibilities per state statutes. (ch. 2)

Body image The physical dimension of self-concept. (ch. 4)

Body language also kinesics Involving the conscious or unconscious body positioning or actions of the communicator. (ch. 9, 10)

Boundaries Invisible limits surrounding the family unit, protect the integrity of the family system. (chs. 2, 5, 12, 13)

Boundary crossings Boundary crossings are less serious infractions. They give the appearance of impropriety but do not actually violate prevailing ethical standards. (ch. 5)

Boundary violations Boundary violations take advantage of the client's vulnerability and represent a conflict of interest that usually is harmful to the goals of the therapeutic relationship. (ch. 5)

Burnout A state of fatigue or frustration brought about by devotion to a cause, way of life, or relationship that failed to produce an expected reward. (ch. 20)

Caring An intentional human action characterized by commitment and a sufficient level of knowledge and skill to allow the nurse to support the basic integrity of the client. (chs. 1, 6)

Case management A collaborative process of assessment, planning, facilitation and advocacy for options and services to meet an individual's health needs through communication and available resources to promote quality cost-effective outcomes. (ch. 24)

Catastrophic reactions Older adult tantrums that represent a completely disorganized set of responses. (ch. 19)

Chaining Linking single behaviors together in a series of steps leading to the targeted desired behavior. (ch. 16)

Channels Channels of communication through which a person receives messages are the five senses:sight, hearing, taste, touch, and smell. (ch. 1)

Charting by exception A type of charting in which normal data are charted using check marks on flow sheets, with only abnormal/significant findings, called exceptions, being charted in a descriptive format. (ch. 25)

Chronic sorrow An ill-defined form of grief, occurring while a person is still alive, in relation to a limiting disease, or as an ongoing loss of potential in a loved one. (ch. 8)

Circular questions Questions that focus on family interrelationships and the impact of a serious health alteration has on individual family members and the equilibrium of the family system. (chs. 10, 13)

Civil laws Developed through court decisions, which are created through precedents, rather than written statutes. (ch. 2)

Clarification A therapeutic active listening strategy designed to aid in understanding the message of the client by asking for more information or for elaboration on a point. (ch. 10)

Client education also patient education A set of planned educational activities, resulting in changes in health related behaviors and attitudes as well as knowledge. (ch. 16)

Clinical pathways (also critical pathway) A documentation tool based on standardized plans of care for a specific health condition, usually demonstrating predefined progress toward recovery. (chs. 2, 25)

Clinical preceptor An experienced nurse, chosen for clinical competence, and charged with supporting, guiding and participating in the evaluation of student clinical competence. (ch. 7)

Closed-ended questions A question that can be answered with yes, no, or another one-word syllable. (ch. 10)

Closed groups Groups that have a pre-defined selected membership with an expectation of regular attendance for an extended time period, usually at least 12 sessions. (ch. 12)

Coding systems Alphanumerics assigned to label each type of healthcare intervention, making computerization possible. (ch. 25)

Cognitive dissonance The holding of two or more conflicting values at the same time. (ch. 3)

Cognitive distortions Faulty or negative thinking that causes a person to interpret neutral situations in an unrealistic, exaggerated, or negative way. (ch. 1)

Cognitive domain The focus when the client has a knowledge deficit. (ch. 16)

Cognitive learning Knowledge obtained from information a person did not have before. (ch. 16)

Cohesion The value a group holds for its members and their investment in being a part of the group. (ch. 12)

Collaboration A solution-oriented response in which we work together cooperatively to problem solve. (chs. 7, 14)

Collaborative nursing interventions Interventions that are those performed by the nurse and other health care team members with the mutual goal of providing the most appropriate and effective care to clients (ch. 2)

Commendations The practice of noticing, drawing forth, and highlighting previously unobserved, forgotten, or unspoken family strengths, competencies or resources. (ch. 13)

Communication A combination of verbal and nonverbal behaviors integrated for the purpose of sharing information. (ch. 9)

Communication disability Includes any client who has any impairment in body structure or function that interferes with communication. (ch. 17)

Compassion fatigue A syndrome associated with serious spiritual, physical and emotional depletion related to caring for clients that can affect the nurse's ability to care for other clients. (ch. 8)

Competition A response style characterized by domination. (ch. 14)

Complicated grieving Represents a form of grief, distinguished by being unusually intense, significantly longer in duration, or incapacitating. (ch. 8)

Computerized Clinical Decision Support programs Software programs which input specific information about your client, analyze it, and make care recommendations based on standardized care practices to promote best care outcomes as derived from research evidence. (ch. 26)

Concrete operations period Piaget's developmental stage in which a child can play cooperatively and employ complex rules. (ch. 18)

Confidentiality The respect for another's privacy that involves holding and not divulging information given in confidence except in case of suspected abuse, commission of a crime, or threat of harm to self or others. (chs. 2, 6, 25)

Conflict A mental struggle, either conscious or unconscious, resulting from the simultaneous presence of opposing or incompatible thoughts, ideas, goals, or emotional forces, such as impulses, desires, or drives. (ch. 14)

Connotation A more personalized meaning of the word or phrase. (ch. 9)

Coping Any response to external life strains that serves to prevent, avoid, or control emotional distress (ch. 20)

Countertransference Feelings represent unconscious attitudes or exaggerated feelings a nurse may develop toward a client. (ch. 1)

Criminal laws Reserved for cases in which there was intentional misconduct, and/or the action taken by the health care provider represents a serious violation of professional standards of care. (ch. 2)

Crisis A crisis occurs when a stressful life event overwhelms an individual's ability to cope effectively in the face of a perceived challenge or threat. (ch. 21)

Crisis incident An event, which is outside the usual range of experience and challenges one's ability to cope. (ch. 21)

Crisis intervention The systematic application of problem-solving techniques, based on crisis theory, designed to help the client move through the crisis process as swiftly and painlessly as possible and thereby achieve at least the same level of pre-crisis functioning. (ch. 21)

Crisis state An acute normal human response to severely abnormal circumstances; it is not a mental illness. (ch. 21)

Critical incident stress debriefing (CISD) A type of crisis intervention, used to help a group of people who have witnessed or experienced a mass trauma event process its meaning and talk about feelings that otherwise might not surface. (ch. 21)

Critical thinking An analytical process in which you purposefully use specific thinking skills to make complex clinical decisions. (ch. 3)

Cultural competence A set of cultural behaviors and attitudes integrated into the practice methods of a system, agency, or its professionals, that enables them to work effectively in cross cultural situations. (ch. 11)

Cultural diversity Variations among cultural groups. (ch. 11)

Cultural relativism The belief that each culture is unique, and should be judged only on the basis of its own values, and standards. (ch. 11)

Cultural sensitivity The ability to be appropriately responsive to the attitudes, feelings, or circumstances of groups of people that share a common and distinctive racial, national, religious, linguistic, or cultural heritage. (ch. 11)

Culture A complex social concept that encompasses the entirety of socially transmitted communication styles, family customs, political systems, and ethnic identity held by a particular group of people. (ch. 11)

Decentralized access A nurse can use internet devices to view or document client information even when in the community or in the client's home. (ch. 26)

Delegation The transfer of responsibility for the performance of an activity from one individual to another while retaining accountability for the outcome. (ch. 23)

Democratic leadership The leadership style in which the leader involves members in active discussion and decision making, encouraging open expression of feelings and ideas. (ch. 12)

Denial An unconscious refusal to allow painful facts, feelings, and perceptions into conscious awareness. (ch. 8)

Denotation The generalized meaning assigned to a word. (ch. 9)

Deontological model (also duty-based model) A duty based model for making ethical decisions. (ch. 3)

Dependent nursing interventions Interventions that require an oral or a written order from a physician to implement. (ch. 2)

Disaster A calamitous event of slow or rapid onset that results in large-scale physical destruction of property, social infrastructure, and human life. (ch. 21)

Discharge planning A process of concentration, coordination and technology integration, through the cooperation of healthcare professionals, clients and their families, to ensure that all patients receive continuing care after being discharged. (ch. 24)

Discipline A community of interest that is organized around the accumulated knowledge of an academic or professional group. (ch. 1)

Discrimination A legal statute refers to actions in which a person is denied a legitimate opportunity offered to others because of prejudice. (ch. 6)

Disease prevention A concept concerned with identifying modifiable risk and protective factors associated with diseases and disorders. (ch. 15)

Disenfranchised grieving The grief nurses can experience following the death of a client with whom they have had an important relationship. (ch. 8)

Distress A negative stress causes a higher level of anxiety, and is perceived as exceeding the person's coping abilities. (ch. 20)

Documentation The process of obtaining, organizing, and conveying client health information to others in print or electronic format. (ch. 25)

Dysfunctional conflict Conflict in which information is withheld, feelings are expressed too strongly, the problem is obscured by a double message, or feelings are denied or projected onto others. (ch. 14)

Ecomap A sociogram, illustrating the shared relationships between family members and the external environment. (ch. 13)

Ego defense mechanisms The conscious and unconscious coping methods used by people to change the meaning of a situation in their minds. (chs. 1, 20)

Ego despair The failure of a person to accept one's life as appropriate and meaningful. (ch. 19)

Ego integrity The capacity of older adults to look back on their lives with satisfaction and few regrets, coupled with a willingness to let the next generation carry on their legacy. (ch. 19)

Electronic health record (EHR): Various types of computerized client health records. (ch. 25)

Emancipated minors Mentally competent adolescents under the age of 18, who petition the courts for adult status. (ch. 2)

Emotional Cutoff A person's withdrawal from other family members as a means of avoiding family issues that create anxiety. (ch. 13)

Emotion-focused coping (ch. 20)

Empathy The ability to be sensitive to and communicate understanding of the client's feelings. (chs. 5, 6)

Empowerment Helping a person become a self-advocate; an interpersonal process of providing the appropriate tools, resources, and environment to build, develop, and increase the ability of others to set and reach goals. (ch. 6)

End-of-life decision making The process that healthcare providers, patients and patients' families go through when considering what treatments will or will not be used to treat a life threatening illness. (ch. 8)

Environment The internal and external context of the client, as it shapes, and is affected by a client's health care situation. (ch. 1)

Ethical dilemma (also moral dilemma): The conflict of two or more moral issues; a situation in which there are two or more conflicting ways of looking at a situation. (ch. 3)

E-prescribing Prescriptions typed into the health record and transmitted as hardcopy, and electronically. (ch. 26)

Ethnicity A chosen awareness that reflects a person's commitment to a cultural identity; a personal awareness of certain symbolic elements that bind people together in a social context. (ch. 11)

Ethnic group A social grouping of people who share a common racial, geographical, religious, or historical culture. (ch. 11)

Ethnocentrism A belief that one's own culture should be the norm, because it is considered better or more enlightened than others. (ch. 11)

Eustress A short term mild level of stress. (ch. 20)

Facial expression Facial configurations convey feelings without words. Facial expression either reinforces or modifies the message the listener hears. (ch. 9, 10)

Familismo A strong value in the Hispanic community. The family is the center of Hispanic life, and serves as a primary source of emotional support. (ch. 11)

Family A self-identified group of two more or individuals whose association is characterized by special terms, who may or may not be related by bloodlines or law, but who function in such a way that they consider themselves to be a family. (ch. 13)

Family Projection Process An unconscious casting of unresolved family emotional issues, or attributes people in the past from the past onto a child. (ch. 13)

Feedback A message given by the nurse to the client in response to a message or observed behavior. (chs. 1, 10)

Flow sheets Charting on sheets with client's progress in preprinted in categories of information. (ch. 25)

Formal operations period Piaget's developmental stage in which abstract reality and logical thought processes emerge and independent decisions can be made. (ch. 18)

Functional similarity Choosing group members who have enough common intellectually, emotionally, and experientially to interact with each other in a meaningful way. (ch. 12)

Functional status A broad range of purposeful abilities related to physical health maintenance, role performance, cognitive or intellectual abilities, social activities, and level of emotional functioning. (ch. 19)

Genogram A standardized set of connections to graphically record basic information about family members and their relationships over three generations. (ch. 13)

Goals (ch. 17)

Good death One that is free from unavoidable distress and suffering for patients, families and caregivers; in general accord with patients and families' wishes; and reasonably consistent with clinical, cultural, and ethical standards. (ch. 8)

Grand theories Addresses the key concepts and principles of the discipline as a whole. (ch. 1)

Grief Describes the personal emotions, and adaptive process a person goes through in recovering from loss. (ch. 8)

Group A gathering of two or more individuals who share a common purpose and meet over time in face-to-face interaction to achieve an identifiable goal. (ch. 12)

Group dynamics A term used to describe the communication processes and behaviors occurring during the life of the group. (ch. 12)

Group norms The behavioral rules of conduct expected of group members. (ch. 12)

Group process The identifiable structural development of the group that is needed for a group to mature. (ch. 12)

Group think A phenomena that occurs when loyalty and approval by other group members becomes so important that members are afraid to express conflicting ideas and opinions for fear of being excluded from the group. (ch. 12)

Handheld wireless communication devices Any small portable computer which uses the Internet to transmit client information. (ch. 26)

Handoffs Transfer process taking place when clients are reassigned to another team of health care providers. (chs. 22, 24)

Health A broad concept that is used to describe an individual's state of well-being and level of functioning. (chs. 1, 15)

Health disparities A chain of events signified by a difference in the environment, access to, utilization of, and quality of care, health status, or a particular health outcome that deserves scrutiny. (ch. 11)

Health Insurance Portability and Accountability Act (HIPAA) Federal privacy standards enacted in 2003, designed to protect client records and other health information provided to health plans and other health care providers. (chs. 2, 25)

Health Information Technology (HIT) Creation of a whole new electronic interactive system designed to support the multiple information needs required by today's complex client care. (ch. 25)

Health literacy The degree to which people have the capacity to obtain, process, and understand basic health information and services needed to make appropriate health decisions. (ch. 15, 16)

Health promotion An interactive educational support process that enables people to reach their highest health potential by taking control of, and improving the circumstances pertaining to their health and well-being. (ch. 15)

Health teaching A specialized form of teaching, defined as a focused, creative, interpersonal nursing intervention in which the nurse provides information, emotional support, and health-related skill training. (ch. 16)

Hearing screening Includes testing for receptive acuity, pitch, and tone perception via use of whisper, tuning fork or an audiometry machine. (ch. 17)

Heterogeneous groups Groups that represent a wider diversity of human experience and problems. (ch. 12)

Homeostasis (also dynamic equilibrium): A person's sense of personal security and balance. (ch. 20)

Homogeneous groups Groups that share common characteristics, for example, diagnosis (e.g., breast cancer support group) or a personal attribute (e.g., gender or age). (ch. 12)

Human rights-based model Based on the belief that each client has basic rights. (ch. 3)

Independent nursing interventions Interventions that nurses can provide without a physician's order or direction from another health professional. (ch. 2)

Inference An educated guess about the meaning of a behavior or statement. (ch. 2)

Informed consent A focused communication process in which the professional nurse or physician discloses all relevant information related to a procedure or treatment, with full opportunity for dialogue, questions, and expressions of concern, prior to asking for the client's signed permission. (chs. 2, 16)

Interactive videodiscs Contain onscreen figures that sign words preprogrammed into bar codes that you select or that you speak into a microphone. (ch. 17)

Interagency Accessibility Transmission and availability of client information across departments in a healthcare agency. (ch. 25)

Intercultural communication Conversations between people from different cultures that embrace differences in perceptions, language and non-verbal behaviors, and recognition of dissimilar contexts for interpretations. (ch. 11)

Interpersonal communication A cyclic, reciprocal, interactive and dynamic process, with value, cultural, and cognitive variables influencing its transmission and reception. (ch. 1)

Interpersonal competence The ability to interpret the content of a message from the point of view of each of the participants and the ability to use language and non-verbal behaviors strategically to achieve the goals of the interaction. (ch. 9)

Interprofessional education Occasions when two or more professions learn from and about each other to improve collaboration and the quality of care. (ch. 7)

Intrapersonal communication Takes place within the self in the form of inner thoughts; beliefs are colored by feelings and influence behavior. (ch. 1)

Justice Ethical principle guiding decision making. Justice is actually a legal term; however, in ethics it refers to being fair or impartial. (ch. 3)

Laissez-faire A hands-off approach. (ch. 12)

Leadership Interpersonal influence that is exercised in situations and directed through the communication process toward attainment of a specified goal or goals. (ch. 12)

Learning readiness A person's mind-set and openness to engage in a learning or counseling process for the purpose of adopting new behaviors.

Lifestyle Patterns of choices made from the alternatives that are available to people according to their socioeconomic circumstances and the ease with which they are able to choose certain ones over others. (ch. 15)

Loss A generic term that signifies absence of an object, position, ability or attribute. (ch. 8)

Magnet Recognition Program ANA national program that recognizes quality patient care and nursing excellence in health care institutions and agencies and identifies them as work environments that act as a "magnet" for professional nurses desiring to work there because of their excellence. (ch. 7)

Maintenance functions Group role functions that foster the emotional life of the group. (ch. 12)

Medical home A community based delivery process involving a primary care team, led by an identified personal physician for the client. (ch. 24)

Mentoring A special type of professional relationship in which an experienced nurse or clinician (mentor) assumes a role responsibility for guiding the professional growth and advancement of a less-experienced person (protégé). (ch. 7)

Message Consists of the transmitted verbal or nonverbal expression of thoughts and feelings. (ch. 1)

Message competency The ability to use language and non-verbal behaviors strategically in the intervention phase of the nursing process to achieve the goals of the interaction. (ch. 9)

Metacommunication A broad term used to describe all of the verbal and nonverbal factors that influence how the message is perceived. (chs. 9, 10)

Mid-range theories Cover more discrete aspects of a phenomenon specific to professional nursing, exploring them in depth rather than exploring the full phenomena of nursing. (ch. 1)

Minimal cues The simple, encouraging phrases, body actions, or words that communicate interest and encourage clients to continue with their story. (ch. 10)

Modeling A behavioral strategy that describes learning by observing another person performing a behavior. (ch. 16)

Moral distress A feeling that occurs when one knows what is "right" but feels bound to do otherwise because of legal or institutional constraints. (ch. 3)

Moral uncertainty A difficulty in deciding which moral rules (e.g. values or beliefs) apply to a given situation. (ch. 3)

Motivation The forces that activate behavior and direct it toward one goal instead of another. (ch. 15)

Multiculturalism A term to describe a heterogeneous society in which diverse cultural world views can coexist with some general characteristics shared by all cultural groups and some perspectives that are unique to each group. (ch. 11)

Multigenerational transmission The emotional transmission of behavioral patterns, roles, and communication response styles from generation to generation. (ch. 13)

Mutuality An agreement on problems and the means for resolving them; a commitment by both parties to enhance well-being. (ch. 6)

NNN Abbreviation designating the combination of NANDA, NIC, and NOC. (ch. 25)

Nonmaleficence Avoiding actions that bring harm to another person. (ch. 3)

Nonverbal gesture A body movement that conveys a message without words. (ch. 9)

North American Nursing Diagnosis Association International (NANDA-I) A professional organization of registered nurses that promotes accepted nursing diagnoses. (chs. 25)

Nuclear Family Emotional System The way family members relate to one another within their immediate family, when stressed. (ch. 13)

Nurse Practice Acts Legal documents that communicate professional nursing's scope of practice, and outline nurses' rights, responsibilities, and licensing requirements in providing care to individual clients, families, and communities. (ch. 2)

Nursing Encompassing autonomous and collaborative care of individuals of all ages, families, groups and communities, sick or well and in all settings. (ch. 1)

Nursing Interventions Classification (NIC) A standardized language describing direct and indirect care that nurses perform. NIC and Nursing Outcomes Classification (NOC) attempt to quantify nursing care so that it becomes visible and defines professional practice. (chs. 2, 25)

Nursing outcomes classification (NOC) The measure of how nursing care affects client outcomes. NOC and Nursing Interventions Classifications (NIC) attempt to quantify nursing care so that it becomes visible and defines professional practice. (ch. 25)

Nursing's Social Policy Statement the discipline's covenant with society and contractual obligations for care (ch. 2)

Objective data Data that are directly observable or verifiable through physical examination or tests. (ch. 2)

Omaha System A comprehensive computerized information management system for documentation at the point of care (i.e., the client's location). (ch. 25)

Open-ended questions A question that is open to interpretation and that cannot be answered by yes, no, or another one-word response. (ch. 10)

Open groups Groups that do not have a defined membership. Individuals come and go depending on their needs. (ch. 12)

Optacon A reading device that converts printed letters into a vibration that can be felt by the client who is both deaf and blind. (ch. 17)

Orientation phase The period in the nurse-client relationship when the nurse and client first meet and set the tone for the rest of their relationship, assessing the client's situation and setting goals. (ch. 5)

Pager Converts voice mail into e-mail that can be read. (ch. 17)

Palliative care A clinical approach designed to improve the quality of life for clients and families coping with a life threatening illness. (ch. 8)

Paralanguage The oral delivery of a verbal message expressed through tone of voice and inflection, sighing, or crying. (ch. 9)

Paraphrasing Transforming the client's words into the nurse's words, keeping the meaning intact. (ch. 10)

Patterns of Knowing A unified form of knowledge embedded in nursing practice and grounded in empirical principles, intuitive personal responses, creative aesthetics used to connect with a client, and ethics, which the nurse uses to address the individualized needs of clients (ch. 1)

Pedagogy The processes used to help children learn. (ch. 16)

Perception A personal identity construct by which a person transforms external sensory data into personalized images of reality. (ch. 4)

Person A unitary concept that includes physiological, psychological, spiritual, and social elements. (ch. 1)

Personal digital assistant (PDA) A wireless electronic device containing databases that may also have the potential for electronic message transfer. (ch. 26)

Personal identity An intrapersonal psychological process consisting of a person's perceptions or images of personal abilities, characteristics and potential growth potential. (ch. 4)

Personal space The invisible and changing boundary around an individual that provides a sense of comfort and protection to a person and that is defined by past experiences and culture. (ch. 6)

Point of care Whatever location the nurse is in to provide care to the client, whether at the bedside in his hospital room, in an outpatient clinic, or even in the client's own home. (ch. 26)

Point of care information Client information and reference material that is updated via wireless Internet devices at any location. (ch. 26)

Possible selves Used to explain the future oriented component of self concept. (ch. 4)

Practice theories The most limited form of nursing theory. (ch. 1)

Prejudices Stereotypes based on strong emotions. (ch. 6)

Premack principle The choice of reinforcer should always be something of value to the individual learner. (ch. 16)

Preoperational period Piaget's developmental stage in which learning by the toddler is developed through concrete experiences and devices and the child is markedly egocentric. (ch. 18)

Primary prevention Actions taken to preclude illness or to prevent the natural course of illness from occurring; focus is on teaching people how to establish and maintain lifestyles conducive to optimal health. (ch. 15)

Privacy A client's right to have control over personal information whereas confidentiality refers to the obligation not to divulge anything said in a nurse-client relationship. (ch. 2)

Problem-oriented record (POR) A chart containing four basic sections:(1) a database, (2) a list of the client's identified problems, (3) a treatment plan, and (4) progress notes. (ch. 25)

Professional boundaries The invisible structures imposed by legal, ethical, and professional standards of nursing that respect nurse and client rights and protect the functional integrity of the alliance between nurse and client. (ch. 5)

Professional networking Establishing and using contacts for information, support, and other assistance in order to achieve career goals. (ch. 7)

Professional performance standards A competent level of professional role behavior related to quality of care, practice evaluation, continuing education, collegiality, collaboration, ethics, research, resource utilization and leadership. (ch. 2)

Professional standards of practice The knowledge and clinical skills required of nurses to practice competently and safely. (ch. 2)

Proxemics The study of an individual's use of space. (ch. 6, 9)

Psychomotor domain Learning a skill through hands-on practice. (ch. 16)

Quality of life A personal experience of subjective well-being, and general satisfaction with life that includes, but is not limited to, physical health. (ch. 1)

Real-time captioning devices Allow spoken words to be typed simultaneously onto a screen. (ch. 17)

Receiver The recipient of the message. (ch. 1)

Reflective appraisals The personalized messages received from others that help shape self-concepts, and contribute to self evaluations. (ch. 4)

Reframing Changing the frame in which a person perceives events in order to change the meaning. (ch. 10)

Reinforcement (also conditioning) The consequences of performing identified behaviors; positive reinforcement increases the probability of a response, and negative reinforcement decreases the probability of a response. (ch. 16)

Resilience Strength in the midst of change and stressful life events; the power of springing back or recovering readily from adversity. (ch. 15)

Safety The minimalization of risk of harm to clients and to providers; the avoidance of adverse outcomes or injuries stemming from the healthcare process. (chs. 14, 22)

SBAR A standardized communication format, used in handoffs and discharge/transfer of clients to communicate critical information about a client. (Ch. 2, 22, 24)

Scope of practice A broad term referring to the legal and ethical boundaries of practice for professional nurses established by each state; it is defined in written state statutes. (ch. 2)

Secondary prevention Interventions designed to promote early diagnosis of symptoms through health screening, or timely treatment after the onset of the disease, thus minimizing their effects on a person's life. (ch. 15)

Self-concept An acquired constellation of thoughts, feelings, attitudes and beliefs that individuals have about the nature and organization of their personality. (ch. 4)

Self-differentiation A person's capacity to define him/herself within the family system as an individual having legitimate needs and wants. (ch. 13)

Self-disclosure Intentional revealing of personal experiences or feelings that are similar to, or different from those of the client. (ch. 5)

Self-efficacy A term originally developed by Albert Bandura referring to a personal perceptual belief that a person has the capability to perform general or specific life tasks successfully. (ch. 4, 15)

Self-esteem The emotional value a person places on his or her personal self worth in relation to others and the environment. (ch. 4)

Self-talk A cognitive process people can use to lessen cognitive distortions. (ch. 4)

Sender The source or initiator of the message. (ch. 1)

Sensorimotor period Piaget's developmental stage in which the infant explores its own body as a source of information about the world. (ch. 18)

Shaping The reinforcement of successive approximations of the target behavior. (ch. 16)

Sibling Position A belief that sibling positions shape relationships and influence a person's expression of behavioral characteristics. (ch. 13)

Social cognitive competency The ability to interpret message content within interactions from the point of view of each of the participants. (ch. 9)

Social support The emotional comfort, advice, and instrumental assistance that a person receives from other people in their social network. (ch. 20)

Societal Emotional Process Parallels that Bowen found between the family system and the emotional system operating at the institutional level in society. (ch. 13)

Speech amplifiers Devices to assist hearing. (ch. 17)

Speech-generating devices Laptop computers, fax machines, and PDAs (ch. 17)

Spirituality A unified concept, closely linked to a person's worldview, providing a foundation for a personal belief system about the nature of God or a Higher Power, moral-ethical conduct, and reality. (chs. 4, 8, 11, 20)

Standard communication tools Uniformly used formats for communication of client information among all care providers, such as SBAR. (ch. 22)

Statutory laws Legislated laws, drafted and enacted at federal or state levels. (ch. 2)

Stereotyping The process of attributing characteristics to a group of people as though all persons in the identified group possessed them. (ch. 6)

Stress A natural physiologic, psychological, and spiritual response to the presence of a stressor. (ch. 20)

Stressor A demand, situation, internal stimulus, or circumstance that threatens a person's personal security or self-integrity. (ch. 20)

Subculture A smaller group of people living within the dominant culture who have adopted a cultural lifestyle distinct from that of the mainstream population. (ch. 11)

Subsystems Member unit relationships within the family such as spousal, sibling, and child-parent subsystems. (ch. 13)

Sundowning Episodic agitated behavior occurring in the late afternoon, or early evening with clients in the middle stages of dementia. (ch. 19)

Task functions The group role functions that facilitate goal achievement. (ch. 12)

TCAB An acronym for the program 'Transforming Care at the Bedside' which empowers nurses to make changes which improve client safety. (ch. 22)

TeamSTEPPS A program which emphasizes improving client outcomes by improving communication. (ch. 22)

Telehealth Any use of Internet transmitted visualization for health care diagnosis or treatment. Also known as Telemedicine, Telenursing, eHealth. (chs. 1, 26)

Tellatouch A portable machine into which the nurse types a message that emerges in Braille on a punched-out paper in Braille format. (ch. 17)

Termination phase (also resolution) A period in the nurse-client relationship when the nurse and client examine and evaluate their relationship and its goals and results; the time when they deal with the emotional content (if any) involved in saying good-bye. (ch. 5)

Tertiary prevention Rehabilitation strategies designed to minimize the handicapping effects of a disease or injury, once it occurs. (ch. 15)

Theme The underlying feeling associated with concrete facts a client presents (e.g. feelings of powerlessness, fear, abandonment, and helplessness). (ch. 10)

Theory A theorist's thoughtful examination of a phenomenon, defined as a concrete situation, event, circumstance, or condition of interest. (ch. 1)

Therapeutic communication An interactive active dynamic process entered into by nurse and client for the purpose of achieving identified health related goals. (ch. 10)

Therapeutic relationship A professional interpersonal alliance in which the nurse and client join together for a defined period of time to achieve health-related treatment goals. (ch. 5)

Touch Providing comfort and communication through purposeful contact. (ch. 9)

Transference Projecting irrational attitudes and feelings from the past onto people in the present. (ch. 1)

Triangles A defensive way of reducing, neutralizing or defusing heightened anxiety between two family members by drawing a third person, or object into the relationship. (ch. 13)

Trust A relational process, one that is dynamic and fragile, yet involving the deepest needs and vulnerabilities of individuals. (chs. 5, 6)

Uniform standards Guidelines of accepted practice. (ch. 25)

Universal client identifier numbers A unique series of digits assigned to each client, used by every health agent/agency. (This would replace use of identifying numbers such as social security number, which were not intended to be used for health care.) (ch. 25)

Utilitarian/goal-based model A framework for making ethical decisions in which the rights of the client and the duties of the nurse are determined by what will achieve maximum welfare. (ch. 3)

Validation A form of feedback involving verbal and non-verbal confirmation that both participants have the same basic understanding of the message. (chs. 1, 10)

Values A set of personal beliefs and attitudes about truth, beauty, and the worth of any thought, object, or behavior. Attitudes, beliefs, feelings, worries, or convictions that have not been clearly established are called value indicators. (ch. 3)

Values acquisitions The conscious assumption of a new value. (ch. 3)

Values clarification A process that encourages one to clarify one's own values by sorting them through, analyzing them, and setting priorities. (ch. 3)

Verbal responses The spoken words people use to communicate with each other. (ch. 10)

Violence A mental health emergency, which can create a critical challenge to the safety, well-being and health of the clients and others in their environment. (ch. 21)

Web portal An agency website that provides opportunities for consumers to use hyperlinks to access a variety of information, receive cyber support, or even make appointments. (ch. 26)

Well-being A person's subjective experience of satisfaction about his/her life related to six personal dimensions: intellectual, physical, emotional, social, occupational, and spiritual. (ch. 15)

Wireless text communication text messaging (ch. 17)

Wisdom The virtue associated with Erikson's 8th, and final stage of ego development, represents an integrated system of 'knowing' about the meaning and conduct of life. (ch. 19)

Working phase The period in the nurse-client relationship when the focus is on communication strategies, interventions for problem resolution, and enhancement of self-concept. (ch. 5)

World view The way people tend to look out upon their world or their universe to form a picture or value stance about life or the world around them. (ch. 11)

PHOTOGRAPH CREDITS

Chapter 1

Lowdermilk D, Perry S: Maternity and Women's Health Care, ed. 9, St. Louis, 2007, Mosby

Marriner Tomey A: Guide to nursing management and leadership, ed 8, Mosby, 2009.

Yoder-Wise PS:, Leading and Managing in Nursing, ed. 5, St. Louis, 2011, Mosby

Chapter 2

Sorrentino SA: Mosby's Textbook for Nursing Assistants, ed. 7, St. Louis, 2008, Mosby

Chapter 3

©2010, PhotoDisc, *Medicine Today*

Chapter 4

Courtesy Elizabeth Arnold

Chapter 5

Potter PA, Perry AG: Basic Nursing, ed. 7, St. Louis, 2011, Mosby

©1996, Digital Stock, *Medicine and Health Care 2*

Chapter 6

Courtesy Adam Boggs

Chapter 7

©1996, Digital Stock, *Medicine and Health Care 2*

©2010, Comstock, *Medical 3*

Chapter 9

Sorrentino SA: Mosby's Textbook for Nursing Assistants, ed. 7, St. Louis, 2008, Mosby

Chapter 10

Potter PA, Perry AG: Basic Nursing, ed. 7, St. Louis, 2011, Mosby

Potter PA, Perry AG: Basic Nursing, ed. 7, St. Louis, 2011, Mosby

Potter PA, Perry AG: Fundamentals of Nursing, ed. 7, St. Louis, 2009, Mosby

Chapter 11

©2010, PhotoDisc, *Medicine Today*

Sorrentino SA: Mosby's Textbook for Nursing Assistants, ed. 7, St. Louis, 2008, Mosby

Chapter 12

Yoder-Wise PS:, Leading and Managing in Nursing, ed. 5, St. Louis, 2011, Mosby

Chapter 14

Yoder-Wise PS:, Leading and Managing in Nursing, ed. 5, St. Louis, 2011, Mosby

Chapter 16

©2010, Comstock, *Medical 3*

©2010, PhotoDisc, *Medicine Today*

©2010, Comstock, *Medical 3*

Potter PA, Perry AG: Basic Nursing, ed. 7, St. Louis, 2011, Mosby

Chapter 17

Potter PA, Perry AG: Basic Nursing, ed. 7, St. Louis, 2011, Mosby

Potter PA, Perry AG: Fundamentals of Nursing, ed. 7, St. Louis, 2009, Mosby

Chapter 19

Leake P: Community/Public Health Nursing Online for Stanhope and Lancaster Foundations of Nursing in the Community, ed. 3, St. Louis, 2010, Mosby.

Chapter 20

Potter PA, Perry AG: Fundamentals of Nursing, ed. 7, St. Louis, 2009, Mosby

Chapter 22

Yoder-Wise PS: Leading and Managing in Nursing, ed. 5, St. Louis, 2011, Mosby

Courtesy Endur ID Incorporated, Hampton, NH

Chapter 24

Potter PA, Perry AG: Basic Nursing, ed. 7, St. Louis, 2011, Mosby

Chapter 26

Potter PA, Perry AG: Basic Nursing, ed. 7, St. Louis, 2011, Mosby

INDEX

Note: Page numbers followed by *b* indicate boxes, *f* indicate figures and *t* indicate tables.

A

Abuse, elder, 381
Acceptance stage, of dying, 143
Accommodation, 273
Accountability, 17, 25, 26
Acculturation, 200
Acting-out behaviors, 361–362
Active listening
  to child, 363
  conflict resolution using, 282
  definition of, 176, 179–180
  language used in, 190–191
  responses, 184–188
    clarification, 185–186, 186*b*
    feedback, 191–192
    minimal cues and leads, 184–185, 185*b*
    paraphrasing, 186, 187*b*
    reflection, 186, 187*b*
    restatement, 186
    silence, 187–188, 188*b*
    summarization, 186–187, 187*b*
    validation, 192
Activities of daily living, 376
Acupressure, 215
Acute grief, 146–147
Adaptive functioning, 69
Adolescents
  communication with, 356, 360–361
  teaching strategies for, 318*t*
Advance directives, 28–30, 29*t*, 30*b*, 150
Advance organizers, 328
Advance practice roles, 122–123, 123*b*
Adventitious crisis, 416
Advocacy
  children, 367
  community, 484–486
  description of, 134–136, 135*b*, 137*b*, 166, 347
  legal protections, 382
  methods of, 486*b*
  older adults, 381–382
  safety, 441
Aesthetic way of knowing, 6
Affect, 178
Affective domain of learning, 314–315
African American clients, cultural considerations, 212–213
Agency for Healthcare Research and Quality, 438
Aggression
  behavior associated with, 275
  clients showing, 287–288
  by dementia patients, 388*t*
Aging. *See also* Older adults
  attitudes toward, 370
  communication affected by, 370
  concepts of, 369–371
  definition of, 369
  health affected by, 370–371
  successful, 369, 371
  wisdom of, 372, 372*b*
Agitation, 388*t*
Aguilera, Donna, 418
Alerts, 514–515
Allostasis model of stress, 394, 395*f*
Altruism, 126*t*
Alzheimer's disease, 382
  professional education models of, 124
  safety and, 436, 439
American Association of Critical Care Nurses, 453
American Health Information Management Association, 493–494
American Nurses Association
  Bill of Rights for Registered Nurses, 131*b*
  Code of Ethics for Nurses, 24, 28, 28*b*, 38, 54, 134, 436
  nursing standards, 314
  Social Policy Statement, 25
American Nurses Credentialing Center, 24
  Magnet Recognition Program, 131–132, 132*f*
American Sign Language, 164, 341–343
Americans with Disabilities Act, 338
Andragogy, 316, 317*f*
Anger, 273*b*, 279–280, 401, 402*b*, 424
Anger stage, of dying, 143
Angry clients, 285–287
Anticipatory grief, 146
Anticipatory guidance, 364, 366, 405–406
Anxiety
  anger and, 402*b*
  behaviors associated with, 400
  in children, 356, 361
  conflict effects on, 463
  crisis-related, 424
  description of, 279–280
  family, 403*t*
  health teaching affected by, 322
  nurse-client relationship affected by, 108–110, 109*b*, 109*t*, 110*b*
  separation, 355
Aphasia, 339, 344
Apraxia, 383–385
Art of nursing, 5–7
Art therapy groups, 238
Articles, 5*b*
Asian American clients, cultural considerations, 69, 207, 208, 213–216
Assertive behavior, 275, 275*b*
Assertive skills, 283–285
Assertiveness, 275, 276*b*

Assessment
  case management, 482
  client needs, 32
  cognition, 71–72, 375
  communication deficits and disabilities, 341
  conflict, 277–278
  cultural. *See* Cultural assessment
  family. *See* Family assessment
  nursing process, 31*t*, 32–33
  older adults, 373–377
  pain, 150, 376–377
  self-esteem, 74–76
  social support, 401–402
  spirituality, 78–80
  stress, 399–404
Assessment summary, 33
Assimilation, 200–201
Attending behaviors, 115
Audiovisual aids, 359–360
Authenticity, 88
Authoritarian leadership, 240–241
Authority, 457, 458*b*
Autonomy, 46–47, 53*b*, 126*t*, 208–209, 331, 379, 471
Avoidance, 273
"Awfulizing," 73
Ayurveda, 215

B

Baby boomers, 371, 371*b*
Bar-coded name bands, 447–448
Bargaining stage, of dying, 143
Beck, Aaron, 12–13
Behavioral cues, 178*b*
Behavioral models, 316–319
Behavioral strategies
  modeling, 315
  premack principle, 315
  reinforcement, 315, 317*t*
  shaping, 315, 316
  chaining, 316
Beneficence, 47–48, 53*b*
Benner's stages of clinical competence, 128*t*
Best practices
  description of, 437, 439–440
  evidence-based, 442–444
Bias
  description of, 110–111
  self-awareness of, 203
Bioethical principles, 46–47
  autonomy, 46–47, 53*b*
  beneficence, 47–48, 53*b*
  justice, 48, 53*b*
  nonmaleficence, 47–48
  paternalism, 46–47

Biofeedback, 408
Blaming, 281
Blended family, 247–248, 248*t*
Blind self, 64
Bloom, Benjamin, 314
Body cues, 168
Body image
  definition of, 68
  disturbances of, 68–69
  meaning of, 69
Body language, 167
Boundaries, 250
Boundary crossings, 86
Boundary violations, 86
Bowen's systems theory, 249–250
Brainstorming, 94, 243*b*
Briefings, 447
Bullying, 452
Burnout, 409–412, 411*f*, 411*t*, 412*b*

C

Canadian Nurses Association Code of Ethics
    for Registered Nurses, 28
Capacity building, 305–306
Caplan, Gerald, 417–418
Caregiver
  family as, 267–268, 483–484
  role as, 122*t*
Caregiving skills, 329–332
Caring
  communication improvement through,
    104–105
  description of, 8, 8*b*
  steps involved in, 113–114
Case finding, 482
Case management, 481–484
  chronically medically ill clients, 484
  definition of, 481
  description of, 481
  goal of, 481
  implementation, 482–483
  informal family caregivers, 483–484
  populations served by, 481
  principles and strategies for, 482–483
  treatment planning, 482
Case manager, 122*t*, 481, 482–483, 484
Catastrophic reactions, 387–388
Cellular telephones, 511
Center for the Advancement of Health,
    330–331
Centers for Disease Control and Prevention,
    294
Certified nurse-midwives, 123
Certified registered nurse anesthetists, 123
Charting by exception, 501–503
Children. *See also* Pediatric care
  acting-out behaviors by, 361–362
  active listening with, 363
  adolescents
    communication with, 356, 360–361
    teaching strategies for, 318*t*

advocacy for, 367
anticipatory guidance for, 364, 366
anxiety in, 361
autonomy in, 355
cognition in
  communication considerations,
    350–351
  developmental stages of, 350*t*
  impairments in, 339
communication by
  hobbies used for, 360–361
  play as, 353–357, 358
  regression as form of, 352
communication with
  active listening, 363
  adolescents, 356, 360–361
  age-appropriate considerations, 352–353,
    354*b*
  assessments, 352–353, 353*f*
  authenticity in, 363–364
  developmentally appropriate levels of,
    350–351, 350*t*
  gender differences, 351
  infants, 354–355, 357
  interpersonal, 351–352
  location for, 349
  1- to 3-year-olds, 355
  overview of, 349
  physically ill child, 353–357, 354*b*
  preschoolers, 355–356, 357–364
  respect in, 364
  school-age children, 356, 358–360
  3- to 5-year-olds, 355–356
  toddlers, 357
  veracity in, 363–364
disaster management for, 433–434
end-of-life care for, 155–158
family-centered care of, 351–352
hearing loss in, 338
hospitalization of, 351–352
infants, 354–355, 357
medical terminology usage with, 359*b*
nurse as advocate for, 367
obesity in, 367
1- to 3-year old, 355
pain in, 361
physically ill
  assessment of child's reaction, 352–353
  communication with, 353–357, 354*b*
  needs of, 351
  parents of, communication with, 349,
    364–366
  peers of, 352–353
preschoolers
  communication with, 355–356,
    357–364
  teaching strategies for, 318*t*
regressive behavior by, 352
school-age
  communication with, 356, 358–360
  teaching strategies for, 318*t*

with special health care needs, 351, 366
  stress in, 404
  supportive care for, 155–158, 157*t*
  teaching strategies for, 318*t*
  3- to 5-year old, 355–356
  toddlers, 357
  vision loss in, 338
Chronic conditions, 469–471
Chronic sorrow, 146–147
Circular questions, 183, 262
Circular transactional model of
    communication, 14–15, 14*f*, 15*b*
Citizen Corps Program, 433
Citizen responders, 433
Civil laws, 26–27
Clarification, 185–186, 186*b*
Clarifying feelings, 75*f*
Client
  advocacy. *See* Advocacy
  aggressive, 287–288
  angry, 285–287
  coaching of, 331–332, 332*b*, 332*f*
  culturally diverse. *See* Culturally diverse
    clients
  definition of, 83–84
  health literacy assessments, 449
  medication administration rights for, 517*t*
  nurse and, relationship between.
    See Nurse-client relationship
  physician communication with, 456, 457
  rights and responsibilities, 134, 135*b*
  violent, 287–288
Client advocate role, 122*t*
Client education
  client health literacy vs, 441
  definition of, 312
  Internet programs for, 518
  Web portals for, 514
Client handoff, 437. *See also* Handoffs
Client needs
  assessment of, 32
  identifying of, 92–93
  therapeutic relationships, 92–93
Client-centered care, 471–472, 473*f*
Client-centered communication, 179–180
  active listening in, 179–180
  asking questions, 181–183
  characteristics of, 179
  description of, 177
  goal of, 180
  introductions, 180
  nonverbal, 181
  observation, 181
  patterns of, 184
  rapport building, 180–181
  role-play exercise for, 181*b*
  themes, 183, 184*b*
Client-centered health teaching, 315–316
Client-centered interactions, 89*b*
Client-centered outcomes, 34–35
Client-centered partnership, 85

Clinical competence, 128*t*
Clinical decision support systems, computerized, 511–512, 516–517
Clinical incompetence, 382
Clinical judgments, 52, 56
Clinical nurse leader, 124
Clinical nurse specialists, 123
Clinical pathways, 501, 502, 502*f*
Clinical practice, 7–8
Clinical research, 52
Clock drawing test, 375
Closed groups, 231
Closed-ended questions, 183
Clustering of information, 57
Coaching, 331–332, 332*b*, 332*f*
Code of Ethics for Nurses, 24, 28, 28*b*, 38, 54, 134, 436
Coding systems, 499–501
    diagnosis-related groups, 500
    Diagnostic and Statistical Manual of Mental Disorders, Fourth Edition, Text Revision, 500
    International Classification of Diseases, 499–500
    Joint Commission computerized documentation guidelines, 500
    Outcome and Assessment Information Set, 500–501
Cognition, 71–74
    assessment of, 71–72, 375
    definition of, 71
    dementia-related changes in, 385*b*
    in older adults, 375
    personal identity affected by, 70, 71–74
Cognitive behavioral communication strategies, 194, 194*b*
Cognitive behavioral therapy, 12–13, 73
Cognitive dissonance, 50
Cognitive distortions, 13, 73, 73*b*
Cognitive domain of learning, 314
Cognitive impairments
    delirium, 384*t*
    dementia. *See* Dementia
    description of, 339, 345
    older adults, 383–389
Co-leadership, 230–231
Collaboration, 130, 138–139, 274
Collaborative nursing interventions, 36
Colleagues. *See also* Peers
    professional nursing roles with, 129–130
    verbal communication with, 130
Collegiality culture, 452–453
Commendations, 264, 265*b*
Commune, 247
Communication. *See also* Therapeutic communication
    aging effects on, 370
    barriers to, 103
    channels of, 14
    with children. *See* Children, communication with

circular transactional model of, 14–15, 14*f*, 15*b*
client involvement in, 165
cognitive behavioral strategies, 194, 194*b*
colleagues, 130
concepts to improve, 104
    caring, 104–105
    empathy, 106–107
    empowerment, 105–106, 114
    mutuality, 107
    respect, 104
    trust, 106, 106*b*, 107*b*
    veracity, 107–108
cross-cultural, 112
cultural influences on, 165
culturally competent, 112
culturally diverse clients, 208–209
definition of, 163
dementia patients, 385–387, 386*b*
description of, 13
distortion in, 75*f*
electronic health records benefits for, 492–493
electronic methods of, 513–514
end-of-life care, 151–154, 152*b*
environment for, 173
group, 231, 515
humor, 193–194
intercultural. *See* Intercultural communication
interpersonal, 13
interprofessional, 464*b*
intrapersonal, 13
linear model of, 14, 15*b*
malpractice claims prevented through, 27
metaphors, 193
negligence claims prevented through, 27
nonverbal, 166–169
    behaviors used in, 166, 167, 168
    body cues, 168
    body language, 167, 177
    congruent, 281
    cultural differences, 202
    description of, 91, 93*b*, 166
    function of, 166
    silence, 166
    styles of, 165*t*, 166–169
    touch, 167, 192–193
in nursing process, 30–31
with parents, 349, 364–366, 366*b*
participant responsiveness, 172–173
personality characteristics that affect, 170
profession-specific differences in, 440
real-time, 509
reciprocity in, 172–173
reframing, 194
role relationships in, 15
safety. *See* Safety communication
self-esteem affected by, 76
sociocultural factors that affect, 169–170
    culture, 169–170, 170*b*

    gender, 169
    location, 170
    specialized strategies for, 193–194
    styles of, 165–166, 170–171
    technology used in, 195
    theories of, 13–15, 14*b*
    therapeutic. *See* Therapeutic communication
    tips for improving, 172*b*
    touch as form of, 167, 192–193
    unclear, 466*t*
    verbal, 164–166, 165*t*, 281
    violence defusing through, 427
    voice inflection in, 165
Communication deficits and disabilities
    assessment of, 341
    cognitive impairments as cause of, 339, 345
    concepts associated with, 337–338
    early recognition of, 341
    environmental deprivation caused by illness, 340–341
    hearing loss, 338, 341–343, 343*b*
    language deficits as cause of, 339, 344–345, 345*b*
    legal mandates, 338
    mental disorders, 339–340, 345–346
    nursing goals for, 341
    speech deficits as cause of, 339, 344–345, 345*b*
    strategies for, 341–347
    treatment-related, 346–347
    types of, 338–341
    vision loss, 338–339, 343–344
Community
    advocacy in, 484–486
    crisis interventions resources, 422
    definition of, 302
    disaster management response patterns, 432
    empowerment in, 302, 305–306
    family-centered relationships in, 267–268
    health promotion, 301–303
    stress management resources, 402, 403*b*
Community education, 302–303, 303*t*
Community engagement, 306*b*
Community health agencies, 239
Compact state recognition model, 26
Compassion, 106–107
Compassion fatigue, 160
Competition, 273
Complaint procedures, 465
Complicated grieving, 147
Computer literacy, 505
Computerized clinical decision support systems, 511–512, 516–517
Concrete operations stage, 350*t*
Confidentiality, 40
    adolescent issues with, 356
    definition of, 40, 503
    electronic health records, 494–495, 503, 505
    Health Insurance Portability and Accountability Act provisions for, 38–39, 39*b*, 419

Confidentiality (*Continued*)
limits to, 233
mandatory reporting, 40
professional sharing of information, 40
violations of, 116–117
Conflict
anxiety affected by, 463
assessment of, 277–278
causes of, 272
covert, 277
cultural effects on, 274
de-escalation of, 278–279
definition of, 271–272, 453
dysfunctional, 275
escalation of, 286–287
features of, 272
functional uses of, 274
gender effects on, 274
in home health care settings, 288
interpersonal, 272, 274
intrapersonal, 274, 282, 283
lack of communication as cause of, 272
management of, 272–274
nature of, 272
in nurse-client relationship, 277–278
personal responses to, 272–274, 273*b*
personal rights and responsibilities, 274*b*
prevention of, 277
sources of, 455, 455*b*
staff, 457–458
Conflict resolution
angry clients, 285–287
behavior change for, 281
cultural considerations, 281–282
demanding, difficult clients, 285
evaluation of, 282
health professionals, 461*b*
"I" statements for, 283
nursing strategies to enhance, 278–283
options for, 281
principles of, 275–277
reasons for working toward, 272
tension-reducing actions for, 282–283
therapeutic communication for, 280
timing of, 280
in work environment, 454–459
barriers to, 455–456, 456*b*
conflict sources, 455, 455*b*
goal setting, 455
nurse-nurse, 457–458
physician-nurse, 456–457
Confrontation, 463*b*
Connotation, 164–165, 325
Consent, informed, 40–41
Constructive criticism, 465*b*
Constructive feedback, 96
Consultant role, 122*t*
Consultations, electronic, 513
Consumer(s)
expectations of, 16
health information sources for, 514

roles of, 16–17
Consumer advocacy groups, 484
Continuity of care
case management. *See* Case management
for chronic conditions, 469–471
chronically medically ill clients, 484
community advocacy, 484–486
definition of, 469
description of, 19, 173, 468
dimensions of, 469–470
discharge planning, 477–480, 478*b*
functionality of, 470–471
handoffs, 477–481
hospitalist's role in, 476
informational, 470, 476–481
interdisciplinary teams for.
See Interdisciplinary teams
management, 470, 480–481
medical home, 480–481
policy environment for, 485*f*
relational, 469
transitions. *See* Transitions
Coping, 395–399
stress
adaptive strategies for, 396*b*
assessment of, 401
defensive strategies for, 397–398, 397*t*
definition of, 395–396
ego defense mechanisms for, 9, 64–65,
397–398, 397*t*
emotion-focused, 396
maladaptive strategies for, 396*b*
previously used strategies, 422
problem-focused strategies for, 396
purposes of, 395–396
strategies for, 396–398, 396*b*
trauma, 433–434
Counseling role, 89
Countertransference, 8–9, 21, 87
Criminal law, 27
Crisis
adventitious, 416
Burgess and Roberts continuum of, 416,
417*t*
definition of, 415–416
developmental, 416
environmental, 416
existential, 416
feelings associated with, 421
mental health. *See* Mental health
emergencies
powerlessness feelings, 422
private, 416
situational, 416
theoretical frameworks for, 417–418
types of, 416
Crisis intervention, 416–417
action plan for, 422, 423
client's perception of, 420
community resources for, 422
critical incident debriefing as, 430–432

cultural influences, 431–432
definition of, 416–417
disaster and mass trauma crisis management,
428–432
family support in, 423, 424*b*
follow-up protocol for, 423–425
goal setting for, 423
mental health emergencies. *See* Mental
health emergencies
personal support systems, 421, 421*b*
Robert's Stage Model for crisis intervention,
418–424
social support systems, 422
strategies for, 419–425
task selection for, 423
termination protocol for, 423–425
theoretical frameworks of, 416–418
Crisis state, 415–416
Critical incident, 430
Critical incident debriefing, 430–432
Critical thinkers, 49–50, 50*t*
Critical thinking, 49–52
applications of, 52, 55–61
barriers to, 50–51
characteristics of, 56
clinical decision-making applications of,
55–61
in clinical judgments, 52, 56
data integration, 57–58
definition of, 49
description of, 44
learning about, 60
summary of, 60–61
Criticisms, 461
Critiquing of nursing theory article, 5*b*
Cross-cultural communication, 112
Cross-cultural dissonance, 117
Cultural assessment
client preferences, 206*t*
guides to, 205, 206*t*
Purnell's model, 205, 206*t*
sample questions for, 205, 206*t*
Cultural brokering, 210
Cultural care theory, 8
Cultural competence, 112, 202–204, 205, 206*t*
Cultural diversity, 199–200
definition of, 199
in health care, 198*b*
health teaching accommodations for,
328–329
in nursing, 201*b*
Cultural identity, 69
Cultural relativism, 199
Cultural sensitivity, 203, 209*b*
Culturally diverse clients
care of, 204–207
communication issues, 207, 208–209
family involvement, 208
health teaching principles, 209
interpreters for, 209–210, 210*b*
rapport building with, 204–205

role relations, 207–208
time orientation, 208
Culture, 197–199 *See also specific cultural group*
  acculturation, 200
  assimilation, 200–201
  communication affected by, 169–170, 170*b*
  conflict resolution affected by, 281–282
  conflict responses affected by, 274
  crisis management affected by, 431–432
  decision making affected by, 208
  definition of, 197
  diagnoses affected by, 205–207
  end-of-life care affected by, 154–155, 208–209
  ethnicity, 199
  ethnocentrism, 199
  family experiences, 198*b*
  gender roles based on, 208
  health promotion strategies affected by, 308–309
  perceptions associated with, 200*b*
  poverty, 217–218
  role relations affected by, 207–208
  self-awareness assessments, 203*b*
  social behavior affected by, 197
  stereotypes based on, 200*b*
  stress responses affected by, 399
  subculture, 198
  time orientation based on, 208
  touch and, 167
  values associated with, 200*b*
  verbal communication affected by, 165
  worldview vs, 197
Curanderos, 211
Curative care, 151*f*

D

Data cues, 32–33
Death. *See also* Dying; End-of-life care
  children and, 156–158
  client care after, 159
  good, 158–159
  lifestyle factors, 292
  as loss, 142
  Muslims' beliefs about, 215
  self-awareness about, 149*b*
  signs of approaching death, 158–159
  stages of dying, 142–143
Debriefing
  critical incident, 430–432
  safety uses of, 447
Decision making
  bioethical principles for, 46–48, 46*f*
  client-centered care, 472
  computerized systems for, 511–512, 516–517
  cultural differences, 208
  end-of-life, 148
  ethical, 48–49
  models of, 45–48
  mutuality in, 360

shared, 472, 473*f*
Delegation of unlicensed personnel, 459, 460*b*
Delusions, 345–346
Demanding, difficult clients, 285
Dementia
  advanced, 388–389
  aggression associated with, 388*t*
  agitation associated with, 388*t*
  catastrophic reactions by clients with, 387–388
  characteristics of, 384*t*
  cognitive changes associated with, 385*b*
  communication difficulties associated with, 385–387, 386*b*
  description of, 375, 383
  neuropsychiatric symptoms associated with, 388, 388*t*
  sundowning, 388
  touch considerations, 387
  validation therapy for, 387
Democratic leadership, 240–241
Denial, 397*t*
Denial stage, of dying, 142
Denotation, 164–165
Deontologic model, 46
Dependent nursing interventions, 36
Depression, 3–4, 71, 377, 384*t*, 424
Depression stage, of dying, 143
Descriptive theory, 2
Development level
  empowerment, 308
  teaching strategies based on, 318*t*
Developmental crisis, 416
Developmental family theory, 251
Diagnosis-related groups, 500
Diagnostic and Statistical Manual of Mental Disorders, Fourth Edition, Text Revision, 500
Disaster management, 429
  for children, 433–434
  citizen responders in, 433
  community response patterns, 432
  critical incident debriefing, 430–432
  in health care settings, 432–433
  intervention protocols for, 430
  for older adults, 433–434
  planning for, 429–430
Discharge instructions, 479
Discharge planning, 477–480, 478*b*
Discharge summary, 479–480
Discipline
  characteristics of, 5
  definition of, 1–2
  Flexner's criteria of, 120*b*
  of nursing, 1–2
Disease prevention, 291–293
  application of, 299–301
  definition of, 291
  goal of, 291
  levels of, 291–292
  lifestyle, 292–293

national agendas for, 293–294
  well-being, 292, 292*f*
Disenfranchised grieving, 159–160
Disengagement, 87
Displacement, 397*t*
Disruptive behaviors, 452, 453
Distraction, 357
Distress
  behavioral observations associated with, 400
  definition of, 393
  moral, 54
  spiritual, 78, 80*b*, 155
Distributive justice, 48
Do not resuscitate order, 29*t*, 154
Doctor of nursing practice, 124
Doctor-assisted suicide, 46
Documentation
  charting formats, 501–503
  client information, 489–490
  definition of, 489
  electronic health record. *See* Electronic health records
  guidelines for, 504*b*
  health care outcome, 35
  health teaching, 334–335
  legal aspects of, 503
  nursing process, 36–37
  purposes of, 489, 490*f*
  tips for, 504*b*
Domestic violence, 217
Drug Enforcement Agency, 504
DSM-IV-TR. *See* Diagnostic and Statistical Manual of Mental Disorders, Fourth Edition, Text Revision
Durable mental health power of attorney, 29*t*
Durable power of attorney, 29*t*
Duty-based model, 46
Duvall's developmental framework, 251, 252*t*
Dying. *See also* Death; End-of-life care
  caring environment during, 159
  comfort care during, 158–159
  communication during, 152*b*
  loss of appetite during, 159
  as narrative, 151–152
  presence during, 159
Dysfunctional conflict, 275

E

Ecomaps, 258, 259*b*, 259*f*
Education
  client
    client health literacy vs, 441
    definition of, 312
    Internet programs for, 518
    Web portals for, 514
  nursing, 123–124
    interdisciplinary collaboration, 125
    interprofessional, 124–125
    models in, 124–125
    online, 519
Effective groups, 233*t*

Ego defense mechanisms, 9, 64–65, 397–398, 397*t*
Ego despair, 372
Ego integrity, 372
Egocentrism, 355, 357–358
Elder abuse, 381
Electronic communication, 513–514
Electronic consultations, 513
Electronic health records
    access benefits of, 492
    advantages of, 490–493
    aggregated data, 493
    charting formats, 501–503
    charting quality improved with, 492
    client's rights, 493–494
    communication benefits, 492–493
    components of, 490, 491*t*
    confidentiality issues for, 494–495, 503, 505
    costs of, 492, 494
    description of, 489
    disadvantages of, 493–495
    ease of use, 492
    efficiency of, 492
    error reduction using, 493
    ethical considerations, 503
    example of, 491*f*
    interagency accessibility to, 491–492
    legal considerations, 494, 503
    misuse of, 494
    nursing classification systems, 495–499
        advantages of, 499
        development of, 495–499
        disadvantages of, 499
        goal for, 495
        Nursing Interventions Classification, 37, 496*t*, 497, 498*b*, 506*b*
        Nursing Outcomes Classification, 37, 496*t*, 498
        Omaha System, 498–499
        taxonomies, 495–499, 496*t*, 497*b*
    nursing terminologies embedded in, 493
    personal medical identification number, 503
    privacy issues, 503
    professional standards, 503
    quality of care benefits, 492–493
    regulatory considerations, 503
    safety benefits of, 493
    system function issues, 494
    uniform standards lacking for, 494
    universal client identifier numbers, 494
    user frustration with, 494
Electronic records, 1–2
Electronic referrals, 513
E-mail, 130, 513, 516
Emancipated minors, 41
Emblems, 178
Emergent informal leaders, 230
Emotional cutoff, 250
Emotional objectivity, 183
Emotion-focused coping, 396
Empathetic objectivity, 180

Empathy, 83–84, 84*b*, 99, 106–107, 114–115, 286
Empirical way of knowing, 6
Empowerment
    communication affected by, 105–106, 114
    community, 305–306
    description of, 47
    developmental level effects, 308
    health literacy for, 306–308, 307*b*, 308*t*
    health promotion, 302, 305–309
    learner involvement and, 305
    strategies for, 305–309, 315–316
End-of-life care
    advance directives, 28–30, 29*t*, 30*b*, 150
    children, 155–158
    communication in, 151–154, 152*b*
    cultural differences, 154–155, 208–209
    decision making in, 148
    family conversations about, 150*b*, 152*b*
    guiding principles for, 153*b*
    pain control and management, 150–151
    quality measures for, 144*t*
    spiritual needs, 154–155
    transparent decision making in, 148–150
End-of-Life Nursing Education Consortium (ELNEC), 144
Engel, George, 145
Environment
    concept of, 3
    definition of, 3
    illness-related deprivation of, 340–341
    influence on relationship, 91
    person and, 3
    self-concept and, relationship between, 63–64
    therapeutic communication affected by, 178–179
    work. *See* Work environment
Environmental crisis, 416
Environmental hazards, 344
Equifinality, 248–249
Erikson, Erik
    description of, 9
    psychosocial development model, 65–67, 66*t*, 67*b*, 350, 371–372, 416
Essential values, 125–127, 126*t*
Ethical decision making, 48–49
Ethical dilemmas
    causes of, 54
    definition of, 54
    description of, 46
    solving of, in nursing, 53–54, 53*b*
Ethical reasoning, 45–49, 52
Ethical standards and issues, 28–30
    advance directives, 28–30, 29*t*
    code of Ethics, 24, 28, 28*b*
Ethical theories, 45–48
Ethnicity, 199
Ethnocentrism, 199
Eustress, 393
Euthanasia, 46

Evaluation phase of nursing process
    description of, 31*t*, 36
    family application of, 268
    health teaching application of, 334
Evidence-based practice, 17–18
    best practices, 442–444
    definition of, 17–18
    elements of, 17
    nursing theory and, 17
Existential crisis, 416
Explanatory theory, 2
Expressive aphasia, 339
Extended family, 247
Eye contact, 167, 168

F
FACES Pain Rating Scale, 148*f*, 376
Facial expressions, 167, 168
Faith, 412
False inferences, 188*t*
False reassurance, 188*t*
Familismo, 211
Family
    assessment of
        data collection in
            tools used in, 255
                ecomaps, 258, 259*b*, 259*f*
                genograms, 255–258, 256*f*, 257*b*, 257*f*
                time lines, 258–259, 260*f*
    in African American culture, 212
    anxiety in, 403*t*
    in Asian American culture, 214
    biological and blended, 247–248, 248*t*
    of chronically ill children, 268
    common law, 247
    composition of, 247–248, 247*b*
    conferences with, 153–154
    crisis intervention support, 423, 424*b*
    of critically ill clients, 265–266, 265*b*
    culture experiences of, 198*b*
    definition of, 246–247, 255
    dynamics of, 247
    evaluation of, 268
    extended, 247
    health teaching participation by, 323
    in Hispanic culture, 211
    illness effects on, 252, 253
    informational needs of, 267
    informational support for, 265
    intervention skills with, 268*b*
    in Native American culture, 216
    in palliative care, need of, 152
        strategies for, 143–144
    psychosocial support for, 254–255
    stress effects on, 403, 407
    theoretical frameworks of, 248–254
        Bowen's family systems theory, 249–250
        Duvall's developmental framework, 251, 252*t*
        general systems theory, 248–249, 248*f*

McCubbin's Resiliency Model of Family Coping, 251–254
  Munchin's structural model, 250–251
types of, 247*b*
Family assessment, 255
  data collection, 260–262
  framework for, 260–261, 261*b*
  interventive questioning, 262–263, 262*b*
  nursing process applied to, 260–266
Family assets, 252
Family boundaries, 250
Family caregiver, 267–268, 483–484
Family nursing care plan, 263*b*
Family resilience, 253–254
Family strengths, 264
Family-centered care, 255–259
  principles of, 472, 472*b*
  purpose of, 255
Faxed medical orders, 504
Feedback
  active listening and, 191–192
  constructive, 96
  description of, 74
  group leader, 242*b*
  health teaching, 329, 330*b*
Feedback loops, 248–249
Feelings
  crises and, 421
  loss and, 141
  stress and, 405
"Fight or flight" response, 393–394
First responders, 431–432
Flat affect, 340
Flow sheets, 501
Focus groups, 239–240
Focused questions, 182–183
Formal operations stage, 350*t*
Freud, Sigmund
  psychoanalytic theories of, 8, 9
  psychosexual stages of personality development, 10*t*
Functional similarity, 224
Functional status
  assessments of, 375–376
  definition of, 375–376

G

Gaze aversion, 168
Gender
  communication affected by, 169, 351
  conflict responses affected by, 274
  nurse-client relationship affected by, 113
  stress response differences based on, 393
Gender bias, 171*b*
Gender roles
  cultural influences on, 208
Gendergram, 258*b*
General adaptation syndrome, 394
General systems theory, 248–249, 248*f*
Generativity vs. stagnation stage, 66*t*
Genograms, 255–258, 256*f*, 257*b*, 257*f*

Gestures, 167, 168
Gift giving, 98, 99*b*
Global aphasia, 339
Goals
  client-centered communication, 180
  conflict resolution, 455
  crisis intervention, 423
  disease prevention, 291
  group, 232
  professional, 90
  therapeutic relationships, 94
Good death, 158–159
Gordon's Functional Health Patterns, 33, 33*b*
Grand theories, 5
Grass roots health promotion, 302
Grief, 145–146, 424
  acute, 146–147
  anticipatory, 146
  definition of, 145
  Lindemann's work on, 145
Grieving, 145–146
  complicated, 147
  contemporary models of, 146
  disenfranchised, 159–160
  patterns of, 146–147
  personal inventory of, 146*b*
  reflections on, 147*b*
  theory-based frameworks of, 145
Group(s). *See also* Therapeutic groups
  adjourning phase of, 227–228, 235, 244
  closed, 231
  cohesion of, 234, 234*b*
  definition of, 222–226
  discussion groups, 240, 240*t*
  educational groups, 239
  focus groups, 239–240
  dynamics, 223
  effective, 233*t*
  forming stage of, 226–227, 232–233, 242
  functional roles of, 228
  goals
    heterogeneous, 232
    homogeneous, 232
  leader tasks applied to stage development of, 232–235
  phases of, 226–228, 227*f*
  norming phase of, 227, 233–235, 242
  open, 231
  performing phase of, 227, 234–235, 235*t*, 242–243
  primary and secondary, 222
  size of, 231–232
  storming phase of, 227, 233
  structure and format of, 231
  themes, 183, 184*b*
  therapeutic, *see* therapeutic groups
  work, *see* professional work groups
Group communication characteristics, 231, 515
Group dynamics, 223–226
  definition of, 223–224
  factors that affect, 224*f*

functional similarity, 224
maintenance functions in, 228, 228*b*, 229*b*
monopolizing, 234–235
norms, 225, 225*b*
task functions in, 228, 228*b*, 229*b*
Group family, 247
Group leader
  feedback, 242*b*
  responsibilities of, 241–242
  stage development-based tasks of, 242–244
Group leadership, 228–231
Group presentations, 332–334
Group process, 226
Group purpose, 225
Group think, 242–243, 243*b*
Guided imagery, 409
Guilt, 424

H

Hallucinations, 345–346
Handbooks, 327–328
Handoffs, 437, 477–481
Hands-on training, 315
Health, 290–291
  aging effects on, 370–371
  definition of, 3, 290–291
  as nursing concept, 3–4, 4*b*
Health care
  barriers to safety in, 441
  cultural diversity in, 198*b*
  demographic changes in, 17
  focus of, in 21st century, 18–19
  reforms in, 17
Health care delivery
  challenges in, 468–469
  changes in, 15–17, 16*f*, 313
  community-based model of, 313
  consumer roles, 16–17
  continuity of care in, 19
  hospital-based model of, 313
  professional roles, 16–17
  technological advances in, 19–20
Health care laws, 26–27
Health care outcome
  definition of, 34
  documentation of, 35
Health communication, 103
Health disparities, 203–204
Health information technology
  advances in, 508
  applications of, 515–517
  barriers to, 517, 518–519
  client communication using, 514–515
  communication benefits of, 493
  computerized clinical decision support systems, 511–512, 516–517
  definition of, 490
  description of, 448
  electronic communication, 513–514
  electronic health record. *See* Electronic health record

Health information technology (*Continued*)
 misuse of, 494
 point of care uses of, 516–517
 professional education uses of, 515
 provider communication using, 514–515
 remote client health monitoring, 512–513
 searchable databases, 512
 "Smart Rooms,", 512–513
 wireless devices, 509–511, 509*f*, 510*b*, 510*f*,
  516
Health Insurance Portability and
  Accountability Act
 confidentiality protections, 39*b*, 419
 privacy protections of, 38–39, 39*b*, 494
Health literacy, 306–308, 307*b*, 308*t*, 441, 449
Health policy, 484–485
Health professionals
 barriers to communication with, strategies
  for removing, 460–463
  clarifying of communications, 460
  constructive criticism, 465*b*
  destructive criticisms, 461
  peer negotiation, 463
  putdowns, 461, 462
  respect, 460
 client and, collaboration between, 449
 collaborations among, 444–445, 446
 conflict resolution among, 461*b*
 interdisciplinary rounds, 446–447
Health profile, 300*b*
Health promotion, 290–291
 application of, 299–301
 Centers for Disease Control and Prevention
  agenda for, 294
 at community level, 301–303
 counseling for, 305
 cultural factors, 308–309
 definition of, 291
 education for, 305
 empowerment strategies, 305–309
 grass roots, 302
 for individuals, 300–301
 learner variables in education for, 304–309
 national agendas for, 293–294
 older adults, 382–383, 382*b*
 organized strategies for, 291
 as population concept, 291
 self-awareness, 309
 theoretical frameworks for, 295–299
  motivational interviewing, 297–298
  Pender's model, 295–296, 295*f*, 296*b*, 304
  social learning theory, 298–299
  transtheoretical model of change,
   296–297, 298*b*
Health teaching, 209. *See also* Learning
 accommodations for special learning needs,
  328–329
 advance organizers for, 328
 anxiety effects on, 322
 behavioral models of, 316–319
 caregiving skills, 329–332

categories of, 320*f*
client-centered, 315–316
coaching clients, 331–332, 332*b*, 332*f*
comorbid conditions that affect, 322
contexts of, 313
cultural diversity accommodations, 328–329
definition of, 312
documentation of, 334–335
ethical mandates for, 313–314
family support for, 323
feedback, 329, 330*b*
format of, 313, 326
group presentations, 332–334
handouts used in, 333
in home, 333–334
language used in, 326–327
learning domains, 314–315
legal mandates for, 313–314
medications, 330*b*
nursing diagnoses amendable to, 323, 323*b*
nursing process applied to, 319–332
 assessment, 320–323
 evaluation, 334
 implementation, 326–329
 planning, 323–326
older adults, 383
problem-solving approach used in, 330–331
self-management skills, 329–332
special learning needs accommodations,
 328–329
teach-back method, 331
theoretical frameworks of, 315–319
 andragogy, 316, 317*f*
 behavioral models, 316–319
 client-centered health teaching, 315–316
 pedagogy, 316
timing of, 325–326, 325*b*
transitional cues, 332
visual aids used in, 327, 328*f*
written handbooks used in, 327–328
Healthy lifestyle, 407
Healthy People 2010, 3–4, 17, 136–137, 203–204,
 293–294, 293*b*, 364, 367, 380, 469
Healthy People 2020, 293–294
Hearing
 loss of, 338, 341–343, 343*b*, 374–375
 screening of, 338
Helping relationships, 84*t*
Henderson, Virginia, 2–3
Heterogeneous groups, 232
Hidden self, 64
Hispanic clients, cultural considerations,
 210–212
Hobbies, 360–361
Holistic nursing theories, 7
Home care
 conflict in, 288
 health teaching, 333–334
Home health agencies, 501
Homeostasis, 248–249, 393
Homogeneous groups, 232

Hope, 424
Hopefulness, 79
Hospice, 144
Hospital
 disaster planning for, 432
 health care delivery in, 313
Hospitalist, 476
Hospitalization
 of children, 351–352
 stress caused by, 399–400
Hostility, 286, 401, 424
Hot-cold balance, 211
Huddles, 475–476
Human dignity, 126*t*
Human rights-based model, 46
Humor, 193–194, 282–283
Hypothalamic-pituitary-adrenal axis, 394

I

"I" statements, 283
ICD-9-CM, 499
ICD-10-PCS, 500
Identity, 63–64. *See also* Personal identity
Ignoring, 318*t*
Illiteracy, 306–307, 518–519
Illness-related environmental deprivation,
 340–341
Illustrators, 178
Implementation phase of nursing process
 description of, 31*t*, 36
 family assessment application of, 263–265
Independent nursing interventions, 36
Individualized education plan, 366
Infants, 354–355, 357
Inference, 32
Informal family caregivers, 483–484
Informational continuity, 470, 476–481
Informed consent, 40–41, 208–209
Inquiry, 44
Instant messaging, 513, 516
Institute of Medicine, 17, 124, 199–200, 294,
 294*t*, 438, 441, 449, 471, 472*b*, 503
Instrumental activities of daily living, 376
Intake assessment, 32
Integrity, 126*t*
Intellectualization, 397*t*
Intensive care unit
 communication with clients in, 346*b*
 environmental deprivation associated with,
  340–341
 family needs in, 265–266, 265*b*
Interactive videodiscs, 343
Intercultural communication, 201–202
 definition of, 201
 planning and intervention considerations,
  207
 principles of, 208–209
 rapport building, 204–205
 role relations, 207–208
Interdisciplinary collaboration, 125, 138–139
Interdisciplinary rounds, 446–447

Interdisciplinary teams
  collaborative communication protocol, 479*t*
  description of, 473
  meeting of, 474–475
  sharing of critical information in, 476
International Classification of Diseases coding, 499–500
Internet
  consumer health information on, 514
  educational uses of, 518
  health promotion uses of, 518
  liability issues, 519
  privacy issues, 519
  support groups on, 518
Interpersonal communication
  with children, 351–352
  description of, 13, 176
Interpersonal competence, 171
Interpersonal conflict
  assertive skills, 283–285
  description of, 272, 274
  escalation of, 286–287
  interventions for, 283–288
Interpersonal relationships
  Peplau's mid-range theory of, 7
  trust and respect in, 171–172
Interpreters, 209–210, 210*b*
Interprofessional collaboration, 474, 474*f*
Interprofessional communication, 464*b*
Interprofessional education, 124–125
Interventive questioning, 262–263, 262*b*
Interview, assessment, 32, 373*b*
Intrapersonal communication, 13
Intrapersonal conflict, 274, 282, 283
Intuitive feelings, 184
Irrational beliefs, 13*t*

J

James, William, 64
Jargon, 172, 190–191
Job maturity, 241
Johnson, Dorothy, 2–3
Joint Commission on Accreditation of Health Care Organizations
  best practice guidelines, 447
  computerized documentation guidelines, 500
  nursing care plan requirements, 31*b*
  professional standards, 25
  violence recommendations, 464–465
Jung, Carl, 9
Justice, 48, 53*b*

K

Kinesics, 167
Kinesthetic communication, 354, 355
Knowing, patterns of, 6, 7
  aesthetic way of, 6
  empirical way of, 6
  ethical way of, 6
  personal way of, 6

L

Laissez-faire leadership, 240–241
Language deficits, 339, 344–345, 345*b*
Language proficiency, limited, 202, 202*b*, 207
Laptop computers, 511
Laughter, 193–194
Laws, 26–27
Leadership
  authoritarian, 240–241
  democratic, 240–241
  group, 228–231
  laissez-faire, 240–241
  situational, 241
  styles of, 240–242
Leadership role, 89
LEARN mnemonic, 209
Learning. *See also* Health teaching
  domains of, 314–315
  factors that affect ability for, 322–323
  goal setting for, 324, 324*b*, 325*b*
  physical barriers that affect, 322
  styles of, 315*b*
Learning delay, 345
Learning needs
  at discharge, 333*b*
  questions for assessing, 320, 320*b*
  special, 328–329
Learning readiness, 306*b*, 321–322
Legal advocacy, 382
Legal standards, 26–27
Leininger, Madeleine, 8, 205
Licensure, 26
Lidocaine, 361
Life review, 155, 378
Lifestyle, 292–293, 407, 514
Limit setting, 286, 362, 362*b*
Lindemann, Eric, 145, 417
Linear model of communication, 14, 15*b*
Listening. *See* Active listening
Literacy
  computer, 505
  health, 306–308, 307*b*, 308*t*, 441, 449
Living will, 29*t*
Logical Observation Identifiers Names and Codes, 501
LOINC. *See* Logical Observation Identifiers Names and Codes
Lose–lose situation, 273–274
Lose–win situation, 273
Loss
  concept of, 141–142
  death as, 142–143
  definition of, 141
  feelings associated with, 141
  meaning of, 142*b*
  multiple, 142

M

Magnet Recognition Program, 131–132, 132*f*
Malpractice, 26–27
Managed care, 469

Management continuity, 470, 480–481
Manager role, 122*t*
Mandatory reporting, 40
Maslow's hierarchy of needs, 10–11, 11*b*, 11*f*, 12*b*, 34, 34*t*, 306*b*, 372–373
Mass trauma, 429, 430*t*
McCubbin's Resiliency Model of Family Coping, 251–254
Mead, George, 64
Mead, Margaret, 4
Medical home, 480–481
Medical jargon, 172
Medical orders
  communication of, 503–505
  faxed, 504
  verbal, 504
  written, 503–504
Medical power of attorney, 29*t*
Medical terminology, 359*b*
Medicare, 489
Medicare Modernization Act, 509
Medication administration rights, 517*t*
Medication errors, 437, 440, 447–448, 493
Medication groups, 239
Medication support, for older adults, 380–381, 381*b*
Meditation, 81, 408, 408*b*
Mental disorders, 339–340, 345–346, 353
Mental health emergencies, 425–429
  challenges associated with, 425
  de-escalation tips for, 426*b*
  examples of, 425
  psychotic clients, 429
  suicide, 427–429
  triage assessment system for, 425
  types of, 426–429
  violence, 426–427, 426*b*, 427*t*
Mental status
  assessment of, 419
  testing of, 376*b*
  mini-mental Status Examination, 286, 374
Mentoring, 128–129
Message, 14
Message competency, 171
Metacommunication, 163–164, 164*f*, 176
Metaparadigm, 3–4
  nursing description of, 3
  concept of environment, 3
  concept of health, 3–4, 4*b*
  concept of person, 3
  concept of nursing, 4
Metaphors, 193
Mid-range theories, 5, 7
Mind reading, 73
Mind/body therapies, 407–409, 408*b*, 409*b*
Mindfulness, 408
Minorities, 204
Minors, 41
Mistrust, 106
Mnemonics, 328
Modeling, 316

Moral distress, 54
Moral uncertainty, 53–54
Moralizing, 188*t*
Morphostasis, 248–249
Motivation, 298
Motivational interviewing, 297–298, 300
Multiculturalism, 197
Multidisciplinary teams, 473
Mutuality, 107, 360

N

National Cancer Institute, 157
National Council of State Boards of Nursing, 25, 26
National Library of Medicine, 499
Native American clients, cultural considerations, 216–217, 309
Negative feedback, 288
Negative reinforcement, 318*t*
Negative stereotypes, 110
Negligence, 26–27, 27*t*
Networking, 129
Newman, Margaret, 7
Nightingale, Florence, 2, 88
Nonmaleficence, 47–48
Nonverbal communication, 166–169
    of anger, 285
    behaviors used in, 166, 167, 168
    body cues, 168, 181
    body language, 167, 177
    congruent, 281
    cultural differences, 202
    description of, 91, 93*b*, 166
    function of, 166
    silence, 166
    styles of, 165*t*, 166–169
    touch, 167
Nonverbal feedback, 192
Norms, 225, 225*b*
North American Nursing Diagnosis Association, 33–34, 68, 495–497, 496*t*, 497*b*
Nurse. *See also* Registered nurse
    accountability of, 17, 25
    core competencies, 121*f*
    legal liability of, 27
    professional role of, 121–122.
        See also Professional nursing roles
Nurse Practice Acts, 25–26, 36
Nurse practitioners, 123
Nurse-client relationship
    advocacy roles in, 134–136
    barriers to, 108–113
        anxiety, 108–110, 109*b*, 109*t*, 110*b*
        bias, 110–111
        cultural, 112
        gender differences, 113
        level of involvement, 87, 111
    caring as element of, 8
    confidentiality in, 40
    conflict in, 277–278

context of, 17
description of, 1
emotional integrity in, 85–86
interdependent nature of, 84
legal liability in, 27
limit setting in, 362, 362*b*
nursing process application to, 30–41, 31*t*
older adults, 377–383
professional role behaviors in, 133–134
termination of, 98
therapeutic. *See* Therapeutic relationships
Nurse-parent partnership, 366
Nursing
    advocacy for, 460
    art of, 5–7
    core competencies, 121*f*
    concept of, 4
    contemporary roles associated with, 4
    core values of, 51*b*
    criteria for survival of, 20*t*
    discipline characteristics of, 1–7
    definition of, 1
    goal of, 4
    knowledge base necessary for, 2
    metaparadigm of. *See* Metaparadigm
    professional standards of, 313
    performance standards of, 25
    role behaviors in, 121
    roles of, 89*b*
    social policy statement of, 25
    teamwork in, 446
    themes of, 120
    theoretical perspective of other disciplines in, 8–13
Nursing actions, 115*t*
Nursing classification systems, 495–499
    advantages of, 499
    development of, 495–499
    disadvantages of, 499
    goal for, 495
    Nursing Interventions Classification, 37, 496*t*, 497, 498*b*, 506*b*
    Nursing Outcomes Classification, 37, 496*t*, 498
    Omaha System, 498–499
    taxonomies, 495–499, 496*t*, 497*b*
Nursing diagnoses, 33–34
    definition of, 497
    health teaching, 323, 323*b*
    role performance as, 136–138
    self-concept as, 68–76
Nursing education, 123–124
    interdisciplinary collaboration, 125
    interprofessional, 124–125
    models in, 124–125
    online, 519
Nursing intervention
    classification of, 36
    collaborative, 36
    definition of, 36
    selection considerations for, 36*b*

Nursing Interventions Classification, 37, 496*t*, 497, 498*b*, 506*b*
Nursing licensure, 26
Nursing outcomes, 35
Nursing Outcomes Classification, 37, 496*t*, 498
Nursing practice
    online guidelines for, 519
    political factors that affect, 15
Nursing process, 30–41
    assessment. *See* Assessment
    communication's role in, 30–31
    definition of, 30
    diagnosis, 31*t*
    documentation of, 36–37
    evaluation. *See* Evaluation
    family assessment use of, 260–266
    health teaching application of. *See* Health teaching, nursing process applied to
    implementation. *See* Implementation
    nurse-client relationship application of, 30–41, 31*t*
    outcome identification, 31*t*, 34–35
    phases of, 30–31
    planning. *See* Planning
    values clarification and, 51–52
Nursing research, 5
Nursing rounds, 476
Nursing theory, 2–5
    definition of, 2
    development of, 2–3
    evidence-based practice and, 17
    frameworks of
        clinical practice application of, 7–8
        description of, 5, 7–8
    grand, 5
    as guide to practice, 5–7
    historical development of, 2–3
    holistic, 7
    levels of, 4–5
    mid-range, 5
    practice, 5
    types of, 2

O

OASIS. *See* Outcome and Assessment Information Set
Occupational stress, 409–412
Older adults. *See also* Aging
    abuse of, 381
    activities of daily living in, 376
    advocacy support for, 381–382
    assessment of, 373–377
    autonomy of, 379
    baby boomers, 371, 371*b*
    categories of, 369
    cognitive assessments, 375
    cognitive impairments, 339, 383–389
        assessment and support interventions, 383–389
        catastrophic reactions, 387–388
        reality orientation groups, 387

comorbidities in, 376
contemporary, 371
delirium in, 384*t*
dementia in. *See* Dementia
depression in, 377, 384*t*
disaster management for, 433–434
discrimination against, 371
environmental supports for, 379
functional status assessments, 375–376
health promotion for, 382–383, 382*b*
health teaching for, 383
hearing loss in, 338, 374–375
independence of, 379, 380
individual differences among, 370–371
instrumental activities of daily living in, 376
interviews with, 373*b*
legal advocacy for, 382
life review by, 378
medication support for, 380–381, 381*b*
mental status testing in, 376*b*
nurse-client relationships, 377–383
pain assessments in, 376–377
polypharmacy in, 380
population growth, 370
psychosocial assessments in, 377
psychosocial communication supports for, 377–378
reminiscence groups, 378, 378*b*
rights of, 381, 381*b*
safety supports for, 380–381
sensory changes in, 374–375
sensory function loss in, 342*b*
social supports for, 378–379
spiritual supports for, 378–379
stress issues for, 404
teaching strategies for, 318*t*
theoretical frameworks used in care of, 371–373
vision loss in, 338–339, 375
Omaha System, 498–499
Online nursing education, 519
Online nursing practice guidelines, 519
Open groups, 231
Open self, 64
Open-ended questions, 181–182, 182*b*, 300, 321
Opioids, 151
Optacon, 342
Organizational work groups, 464–465
Ottawa Charter for Health Promotion, 291
Outcome and Assessment Information Set, 500–501
Outcome identification, 31*t*, 34–35
Overgeneralizing, 73

P

Pagers, 342, 511
Pain
    assessment of, 150, 376–377
    behavioral indicators of, 150–151
    in children, 361

in older adults, 376–377
Wong-Baker FACES Pain Rating Scale, 148*f*, 376
Pain management
    end-of-life care, 150–151
    Joint Commission standards, 150
    opioids for, 151
Palliative care, 143–144
    definition of, 143
    dimensions of, 143*b*
    hospice vs, 144
    indications for, 143–144
    model of, 151*f*
    nursing initiatives, 144
    nursing roles in, 148
    palliative care team, 148
    principles of, 144
    quality measures for, 144*t*
    stress issues for nurses in, 159–160
Paralanguage, 165
Paraphrasing, 186, 187*b*
Parents of physically ill child
    communication with, 349, 364–366, 366*b*
    nurse-parent partnership, 366
    nurse's interactions with, 365–366
    stress in, 366
    support groups for, 367
Parse, Rosemarie, 7
Participant observation, 93
Paternalism, 46–47, 135–136
Patient education. *See also* Client education
    definition of, 312
    elements of, 319–320
Patient Protection and Affordable Care Act, 17
Patient Self-Determination Act, 28–30
Patient-centered care, 3, 471–472
Patterns of knowing, 6
PDAs. *See* Personal digital assistants
Pedagogy, 316
Pediatric care. *See also* Children
    child's participation in, 350
    location for, 349
Pediatric intensive care unit, 266
Peers. *See also* Colleagues
    collaborations with, 458–459
    delegation to, 459
    negotiation with, 463
Pender's health promotion model, 295–296, 295*f*, 296*b*, 304
Peplau, Hildegard, 7, 9, 21, 89
Perception, 70–71, 72*b*
Person
    client as, 3
    concept of, 3
    environment and, 3
Person centered models, 12–13
Personal digital assistants, 510–511, 510*f*, 516
Personal identity, 69–70
    body image and, 68
    cognition effects on, 70, 71–74
    definition of, 69

health status changes that affect, 70
interventions to enhance, 72, 72*b*
perception effects on, 70–71
serious injury or illness effects on, 71–72
spiritual aspects of, 77–80
supportive nursing strategies for, 72–74
Personal medical identification number, 503
Personal space
    respect for, 115–116
    therapeutic conversation, 178–179
    violation of, 111–112, 112*b*
Personal support systems, 421, 421*b*
Personal values, 50–51
Personality, 10*t*, 65
Personalizing, 73
Person-centered care, 18–19
Person-centered models, 12–13
Pew Commission, 18*b*
Pew Health Professions Commission, 125
Physician
    client communication with, 456, 457
    disruptive behavior by, 456
    nurse conflicts with, 456–457
Physiologic needs, 11
Piaget, Jean, 350, 350*t*
Pictographs, 342
Planning phase of nursing process
    description of, 31*t*, 33–38
    family assessment application of, 262–266
    health teaching application of, 323–326
Play, 353–357, 358
Point of care
    decentralized access technology for communication at, 509–511
    health information technology applications, 516–517
Polypharmacy, 380
Positive reinforcement, 318*t*
Possible selves, 63
Posture, 167, 168, 177*f*
Poverty, 217–218
Powerlessness, 422, 454
Practical wisdom, 372
Practice simulations, 441–442
Practice theories, 5
Prayer, 81
PRECEDE-PROCEED model, 302–303, 303*t*
Preceptor, 127
Predictive theory, 2
Pregroup interview, 232
Pregroup tasks, 242
Premack principle, 316
Preoperational stage, 350*t*
Presbycusis, 338
Preschoolers
    communication with, 355–356, 357–364
    play by, 358
    storytelling, 358, 359*b*
    teaching strategies for, 318*t*

Presence
  during dying, 159
  nursing, 88
Primary appraisal, 395, 396f
Primary group, 222
Primary prevention, 291, 299
Priority setting, 406
Privacy
  confidentiality, 40
  definition of, 38
  Health Insurance Portability and
    Accountability Act protections for,
    38–39, 39b, 494
  Internet, 519
  protection of, 38–41
  respect for, 116
  for spiritual activities, 80
  strategies for protecting, 39–40
Private crisis, 416
Problem-focused coping, 396
Problem-oriented record, 501
Prochaska's transtheoretical model of change,
  296–297, 297t, 298b
Professional behaviors, 125–127
Professional boundaries, 85–86
Professional education, 515
Professional goals, 90
Professional licensure, 26
Professional nursing roles
  advanced practice, 122–123, 123b
  behaviors, 129–130
  with colleagues, 129–130
  development of, 120
  registered nurse, 127–129
  types of, 121–122, 122t
Professional performance standards, 25
Professional rights, 130
Professional role behaviors
  with colleagues, 129–130
  in nurse-client relationships, 133–134
Professional self-awareness, 177–178
Professional standards of care, 25–26
Professional values, 50–51, 54–55, 55b
Professional work groups, 240–244
  group maturity, 241
  group think, 242–243
  leadership styles, 240–241
  leader and member responsibilities, 241
  leader stage appropriate applications,
    242–244
Professionalism, 126t
Progressive relaxation, 408, 409b
Projection, 397t
Proxemics, 111, 168, 171–172.
  See also Personal space
PSDA. See Patient Self-Determination Act
Psychiatric advance directives, 30
Psychodynamic models, 8–9
Psychological job maturity, 241
Psychomotor domain of learning, 315
Psychosexual development, 9

Psychosocial assessments, 377
Psychosocial development theories
  description of, 9–11, 10t
  Erikson's, 65–67, 66t, 67b, 371–372, 416
Psychotherapy, 236
Psychotic clients, 236–237, 429
Punishment, 318t
Purnell, Larry, 205, 206t
Putdowns, 461, 462

Q
Qi, 215
Quality of life, 3–4

R
Rapport
  building of, 180–181, 204–205, 419–420,
    429
  humor and, 194
Rationalization, 397t
Reaction formation, 397t
Readiness to learn, 306b, 321–322
Real-time captioning, 343
Real-time communication, 509
Reasoning, 55t
Receiver, 14
Receptive aphasia, 339
Reciprocity, 172–173
Recognition role, 229t
Reference terminologies, 501
Referrals, electronic, 513
Reflection, as listening response, 186, 187b
Reflective appraisals, 63
Reframing, 194
Registered nurse. See also Nurse
  American Nurses Association Bill of Rights
    for, 131b
  professional role development of, 127–129
Regression
  by children, 352
  as defense mechanism, 397t
Regulatory bodies
  nurse practice acts, 25–26
  state boards of nursing, 25
Reinforcement, 316, 318t
Relational continuity, 470
  creation of, 471
  definition of, 470
  interprofessional collaboration, 474, 474f
  professional perspectives on, 473–477
  team meetings, 474–475
Relationships. See Nurse-client relationship;
    Therapeutic relationships
Religion
  spirituality vs., 77. See also Spirituality
Reminiscence groups, 237, 378, 378b
Remorse, 424
Remote client health monitoring, 512–513
Remotivation groups, 237, 237b
Repression, 397t
Researcher role, 122t

Resilience, 253–254, 293
Resiliency Model of Family Coping, 251–254
Resocialization groups, 237
Resource role, 89
Respect
  in communication with children, 364
  for coworkers, 460
  description of, 104
  interpersonal conflict resolution and, 283
  in interpersonal relationships, 171–172
  organizational climate of, 465
  for personal space, 115–116
  for privacy, 116
  in work environment, 454, 465
Restatement, 186
Rightness, 45–46
Rogers, Carl, 12–13, 65, 315
Role
  definition of, 119
  performance dimension of, 119
  professional. See Professional nursing roles
Role disruption, 138
Role modeling, 381–382
Role performance
  disturbance of, 139
  as nursing diagnosis, 136–138
Role relationships, 119–129, 134, 138b, 173
Role socialization
  definition of, 125–126
  nursing values, 125
  professional, 125–129

S
Safety
  advocacy for, 441
  barriers to, in current health care system, 441
  best practices for, 437, 439–440
  checklists for improving, 443
  client outcomes, 437–438
  culture of
    creation of, 439
    error reporting and, 440
  definition of, 436
  electronic health record benefits for, 493
  evidence-based best practices for, 442–444
  initiatives to improve, 438
  issues associated with, 437–438
  medication errors, 437, 440, 447
  miscommunication during client handoff,
    437
  practice simulations for improving, 441–442
  as priority, 441
  reluctance to report errors, 440
  standardization benefits for, 438
  team training, 446, 448
  technology used for, 448
Safety communication
  changes for improving, 439
  checklists for, 443
  competencies, 442f
  goals for, 438–439

health provider collaborations for, 444–445, 446

poor, 437, 444

profession-specific differences in, 440

standardized tools for, 443

strategies for, 440*b*

teaching strategies for nurses to improve, 441–444

SBAR format, 37–38, 38*t*, 443–444, 444*b*, 445*t*, 446*b*, 476, 477, 477*b*, 478*b*

Schemata, 13

Schizophrenia, 71, 340, 345–346, 346*b*

School-age children

communication with, 356, 358–360

teaching strategies for, 318*t*

Scope of practice, 26

Searchable databases, 512

Secondary appraisal, 395, 396*f*

Secondary group, 222

Secondary prevention, 291, 299

Secure messaging, 513, 516

Self, therapeutic use of, 88–89

Self-actualization, 11, 11*b*, 372–373

Self-awareness

about death, 149*b*

culture, 203*b*

description of, 64, 88–89, 89*b*, 130, 177–178

health promotion through, 309

unintentional bias, 203

Self-concept

aspects of, 63, 81

characteristics of, 62, 63*f*

cultural identity, 69

definition of, 62–63, 81

environment and, relationship between, 63–64

features of, 63–64

functions of, 63–64

in infancy, 65

life experiences effect on, 70*b*

as nursing diagnosis, 68–76

possible selves, 63

self-assessments, 64*b*

spiritual, 77, 78

theoretical models of, 64–65

Self-differentiation, 249

Self-disclosure, 96–97, 97*b*

Self-efficacy, 77–81

definition of, 77, 298

description of, 300

development of, 77, 300–301

Self-esteem, 74–76

assessment of, 74–76

communication effects on, 76

definition of, 74

evaluation of, 76

therapeutic strategies for, 76

Self-fulfilling prophecy, 63, 370

Self-help groups, 77, 238–239

Self-management skills, 329–332

Self-roles, 228, 229*t*

Self-talk, 73–74

Selye, Hans, 393

Sender, 14

Sensorimotor stage, 350*t*

Sentinel events, 437–438

Separation anxiety, 355

Shaping, 316–317

Shared decision making, 472, 473*f*

Sibling position, 249, 250, 268

Sick role, 137

Silence, 166, 187–188, 188*b*

Single-parent family, 247

Situational crisis, 416

Situational leadership, 241

Situational self-esteem, 74

Skinner, B.F., 316

Slang, 172

"Smart Rooms," 512–513

Smartphones, 511, 516

SNOMED-CT. *See* Systematized nomenclature of medical-clinical terms

Social cognitive competency, 171

Social isolation, 378

Social justice, 48, 126*t*

Social learning theory, 298–299

Social networking, 485–486

Social policy statement, 25

Social relationships, 84*t*

Social support

assessment of, 401–402

crisis intervention uses of, 422

description of, 74, 75*b*

for older adults, 378–379

stress management with, 398–399, 401–402

Social worth, 48

Societal emotional process, 250

Sorrow, chronic, 146–147

Speech deficits, 339, 344–345, 345*b*

Speech-generating devices, 343

Spiritual distress, 78, 80*b*, 155

Spiritual growth, 155

Spiritual needs, 78–79

Spiritual rituals, 79

Spiritual self-concept, 77

Spiritual well-being, 79, 155

Spirituality

assessment of, 78–80

description of, 77

end-of-life care, 154–155

evaluation of, 81

existential view of, 155

meditation, 81

in older adults, 378–379

prayer, 81

religion vs, 77

strategies for, 80–81

stress effects on, 402

Staff conflict, 457–458

Stages of dying, 142–143

State Board of Nursing, 25

Statutory laws, 26

Stereotypes/stereotyping, 110–111, 111*b*, 200*b*

Stimulus stress model, 394

Storytelling, 358, 359*b*

Stranger anxiety, 357

Stranger role, 89

Stress

allostasis model of, 394, 395*f*

anger associated with, 401

anticipatory guidance for, 405–406

anxiety associated with, 400

assessment of, 399–404

behavioral observations associated with, 400

biological models of, 393–395

burnout caused by, 409–412, 411*f*, 411*t*, 412*b*

characteristics of, 393

children, 404

community resources for management of, 402, 403*b*

coping with. *See* Coping, stress

cultural differences, 399

definition of, 392

expression of feelings during, 405

factors that affect, 399*b*

family affected by, 403, 407

gender differences in response to, 393

general adaptation syndrome, 394

health care sources of, 399–401

high levels of, 393

hostility caused by, 401

levels of, 393

mild, 393

moderate, 393

nurses in palliative care setting, 159–160

occupational, 409–412

older adults, 404

parents of physically ill child, 366

physiologic response models, 393–394

primary appraisal of, 395, 396*f*

priority setting for, 406

psychosocial models of, 393–395

reduction strategies for, 404–407

secondary appraisal, 395, 396*f*

social support for, 398–399, 401–402

sources of, 393*b*, 399–401

spirituality affected by, 402

stimulus model of, 394

tolerance levels for, 392–393

transactional model of, 394–395

Stress management

biofeedback, 408

client efforts for, 406–407

community resources for, 402, 403*b*

guided imagery for, 409

healthy lifestyle for, 407

meditation, 408, 408*b*

mind/body therapies, 407–409, 408*b*, 409*b*

older adults, 404

progressive relaxation, 408, 409*b*

social support for, 398–399, 401–402

tai chi for, 408–409

therapies for, 407–409

yoga for, 408–409

Stressor, 392
Subculture, 198
Sublimation, 397t
Subsystems, 248–249, 250
Suicidal ideation, 428
Suicide, 427–429
  adolescent, 360
  demographics of, 428
  precaution protocols for, 428
  reporting of, 428
  risk assessment, 427
  statements about, 427
  survivors of, 146
Sullivan, Harry Stack, 9, 65
Summarization, 186–187, 187b
Sundowning, 388
Supervision of unlicensed personnel, 459
Support groups
  description of, 238–239, 238t, 239b
  Internet, 518
  parents of physically ill child, 367
Support system, 463–464
Suprasystems, 248–249
Surrogate role, 89
Symbolic interactionism, 64
System oriented continuity of care, 19
Systematized nomenclature of medical-clinical
    terms, 501

T
Tai chi, 408–409
Taxonomies, 495–499, 496t, 497b
Teach-back method, 331
Teaching role, 89, 122t
Team culture, 439
Team meetings, 464, 474–475
Team training, 446, 448
TeamSTEPPS, 446, 465, 474, 475b, 509t
Technology. See also Health information
      technology
  communication uses of, 195
  health care delivery use of, 19–20
  medication error prevention using,
      447–448
  safety improvements using, 448
Teenagers. See Adolescents
Telecare, 512–513
Telehealth, 19, 380, 492, 513–514
Telemicroscopes, 344
Tellatouch, 344
Temper tantrums, 387, 388
Tertiary prevention, 292
Text instant messaging, 513, 516
Theory, 2–5
  critiquing of articles, 5b
  definition of, 2
  development of, 2–3
  evidence-based practice and, 17
  frameworks of
    clinical practice application of, 7–8
    description of, 5, 7–8

family. See Family, theoretical frameworks
      of
  health promotion. See Health promotion,
      theoretical frameworks for
  health teaching. See Health teaching,
      theoretical frameworks of
  grand, 5
  as guide to practice, 5–7
  historical development of, 2–3
  holistic, 7
  levels of, 4–5
  mid-range, 5
  practice, 5
  types of, 2
Therapeutic communication, 175–176.
      See also Communication
  characteristics of, 176f
  components of, 176–177
  conflict resolution uses of, 280
  definition of, 175
  description of, 15
  environmental effects on, 178–179
  factors that affect, 177
    environmental, 178–179
    personal, 177
  humor, 193–194
  metaphors, 193
  personal factors that affect, 177
  professional self-awareness effects,
      177–178
  purpose of, 176–179
  reframing, 194
  specialized strategies for, 193–194
  technology used in, 195
  themes, 183, 184b
  timing of, 179
Therapeutic conversation
  description of, 175–176
  personal space in, 178–179
Therapeutic groups, 223, 225t, 231.
      See also Group
  activity groups, 236–238
    in long-term settings, 237
    in psychiatric settings, 236
  communication characteristics of, 231
  co-leadership, 230
  format of, 231
  self-help groups, 238–239
  size of, 231–232
  structure of, 231
  support groups, 238–239, 238t, 239b
  therapy groups, 236–237
  types of, 235–240
Therapeutic relationships
  barriers to, 108–113
    anxiety, 108–110, 109b, 109t, 110b
    bias, 110–111
    cultural, 112
    gender differences, 113
    overinvolvement, 87, 111
    personal space violation, 111–112, 112b

  reduction of, 115
  stereotyping, 110–111, 111b
  summary of, 117
  tips to reduce, 115b
boundary crossings, 86
boundary violations, 86
characteristics of, 84–86
clarifying the purpose of, 91–92
clients
  client-centered nature, 85
  description of, 83–84, 85
  needs of, 92–93
concepts in, 83–89
defining the problem, 93–94
definition of, 83
goals of, 94
improvement in, concepts for, 103, 104
  caring, 104–105
  empathy, 106–107
  empowerment, 105–106
  mutuality, 107
  respect, 104
  trust, 106, 106b, 107b
  veracity, 107–108
levels of involvement in, 87–88, 87f
nurse's role in, 83
participant observation, 93
phases of, 89–100
  orientation, 91–94
  preinteraction, 90–91
  termination, 97–98
  working, 94–97
professional boundaries, 85–86, 101
self, 88–89
short-term, 98–100
trust, 92
Therapy groups, 236–237
Thinking
  critical. See Critical thinking
  types of, 44–45
Three-generational family, 247
Throughput, 248
Time lines, 258–259, 260f
Time orientation, 208, 217
Toddlers, 357
Token gifts, 98
Torts, 26–27
Touch, 167, 192–193, 344, 387
Transactional model of stress, 394–395
Transcendent wisdom, 372
Transference, 8
Transforming Care At the Bedside, 448
Transition(s)
  handoffs for, 477–481
  planning of, 479t
  sending and receiving teams for, 480b
Transitional cues, 332
Transitional objects, 357
Transparent decision making, 148–150
Transtheoretical model of change, 296–297,
    298b

Trauma. *See also* Disaster management
children and, 433–434
citizen responders to, 433
coping with, 433–434
mass, 429, 430*t*
older adults and, 433–434
Triage assessment system, 425
Triangles, 249
Trust, 92, 106, 106*b*, 107*b*, 171–172, 212,
354
Trust vs. mistrust stage, 66*t*
Trustfulness, 48

U

Unclear communication, 466*t*
Unconditional acceptance, 110–111
Uncooperative clients, 419*t*
Undoing, 397*t*
Uniform Emergency Volunteer Health
Practitioners Act, 432
Universal client identifier numbers, 494
Universal norms, 225
Universal nursing languages and codes,
505–506
Universality, 224*b*
Unknown self, 64
Unlicensed personnel, 459, 460*b*, 504–505
U.S. Preventive Services Task Force, 287, 304,
304*b*
Utilitarian/goal-based model, 45–46

V

Validation therapy, 387
Value judgments, 203

Values
clarification of, 51–52, 57
identifying of, 57
personal, 50–51
professional, 50–51, 54–55, 55*b*
Veracity, 48, 107–108
Verbal communication, 164–166, 165*t*,
281
Verbal medical orders, 504
Verbal responses, 176–177, 188–192
Violence, 426–427, 426*b*, 427*t*,
464–465
Violent clients, 287–288
Vision loss, 338–339, 343–344, 375
Visiting Nurse Association, 519
Visual aids
communication with school-age child using,
359–360
health teaching uses of, 327, 328*f*
Voice pitch and tone, 284
Voice synthesizers, 344

W

Watson, Jean, 8, 8*b*
Web portals for client education, 514
Well-being, 292, 292*f*
Western cultures, 69
Win–win situation, 274
Wireless devices, 509–511, 509*f*, 510*b*, 510*f*,
516
Wireless text communication, 342
Wisdom, 372, 372*b*
Wong-Baker FACES Pain Rating Scale, 148*f*,
376

Work environment, 131–132
bullying in, 452
code of behavior in, 453
collegiality culture in, 452–453
conflict resolution in, 454–459
barriers to, 455–456, 456*b*
conflict sources, 455, 455*b*
goal setting, 455
nurse-nurse, 457–458
physician-nurse, 456–457
culture of regard in, 454
definitions, 453
disruptive behaviors in, 452, 453
group process, 464–465
healthy, standards for, 452–453
incivility in, 453
respect in, 454, 465
support system, 463–464
Work groups
description of, 240
group concepts applied to, 240–242
leadership styles, 240–242
organizational, 464–465
stage development leader tasks applied to,
242–244
World Health Organization, 337, 438, 468
Worldview
African American, 212
definition of, 197
Written handbooks, 327–328
Written medical orders, 503–504

Y

Yoga, 408–409

ONLINE RESOURCES

Chapter 3

American Association of Colleges of Nursing (AACN): www.aacn.org/

American Nurses Association, Center for Ethics and Human Rights (ANA): www.nursingworld.org/

American Academy on Communication in Healthcare (AACH): www.aachonline.org/

National Bioethics Advisory Commission: bioethics.georgetown.edu/nbac/human/overvol1.html/

Chapter 6

Discrimination: www.employeeissues.com

Chapter 7

Commission on Collegiate Nursing Education, *Standards for accreditation of baccalaureate and graduate degree nursing programs*, 2008: www.aacn.nche.edu/Accreditation/pdf/standards.pdf

Chapter 8

Agency for Healthcare Research and Quality, *End-of-life care and outcomes:* www.ahrq.gov/downloads/pub/evidence/pdf/eolcare/eolcare.pdf.

American Association of Suicidology: www.suicidology.org (Click on "Suicide loss survivors.")

American Foundation for Suicide Prevention: www.afsp.org (Click on "Surviving Suicide Loss.")

Institute for Clinical Systems Improvement, *Consensus project for quality palliative care:* www.icsi.org/guidelines_and_more/palliative_care_11918.html.

Chapter 12

American Group Psychotherapy Association: www.groupsinc.org/

American Society of Group Psychotherapy and Psychodrama (ASGPP): www.asgpp.org/

Association for Specialists in Group Work
- Professional Training Standards: www.asgw.org/PDF/training_standards.pdf
- Best Practices Guidelines: www.asgw.org/PDF/best_Practices.pdf
- Principles for Diversity Competent Group Workers: www.asgw.org/PDF/Principles_for_Diversity.pdf

Chapter 15

American Academy of Family Physicians Foundation Health Education Program: www.aafpfoundation.org/cgi-bin/hepp.pl

Centers for Disease Control and Prevention: www.cdc.gov/

Healthy People: www.healthypeople.gov/

Healthy People 2010 Health Communication Focus Area: www.healthypeople.gov/documentHTML/Volume1/11HealthCom.htm

Motivational Interviewing: www.motivationalinterviewing.org.

Office of Disease Prevention and Health Promotion: odphp.osophs.dhhs.gov/

Partnership for Clear Health Communication: www.askme3.org

Pfizer Clear Health Communication Initiative: www.pfizerhealthliteracy.com

World Health Organization: www.who.int/topics/health_promotion/en/

Chapter 17

American Foundation for the Blind: www.afb.org/

National Institute on Deafness and Other Common Disorders: www.nidc.nih.gov/

United States Preventive Health Services Task Force] Agency for Healthcare Research and Quality (USPSTF), *The Guide to Clinical Preventive Services: Recommendations of the US Preventive Services Task Force*, 2008: www.ahrq.gov/ or epss.ahrq.gov/ePSS/

US Department of Health & Human Services, Office of Civil Rights: www.hhs.gov/ocr/

Chapter 18

Healthy People 2010: hp2010.nhlbihin.net/

Healthy People 2020: www.healthypeople.gov/hp2020/

University California Library Systems: *Communicating with your Child:* www.mdconsult.com/das/patient/body/115729442-4/788918080/10068/18752.html

US Department of Health & Human Services, Maternal and Child Health Bureau: www.hhs.gov/mch

Chapter 19

Alzheimer's Foundation: www.alzprevention.org

American Geriatrics Society, *An online edition of the book Geriatrics at your fingertips:* www.geriatricsatyourfingertips.org/

American Geriatrics Society Practice Guidelines: www.americangeriatrics.org/staging/products/positionpapers/aan_dementia.shtml

Claude D. Pepper Older Americans Independence Center at Yale University: pepper.med.yale.edu/pages/pubs_list.htm

Committee on Aging, *Aging and the right of older persons: Statement for the Human Rights Commission:* ngo.fawco.org

Elder maltreatment: www.cdc.gov/ncipc

Harford Institute for Nurses, *Evidence based assessments, Interventions, Care plans:* www.consultgerirn.org

National Center on Elder Abuse: www.ncea.aoa.gov

National Institute on Aging: www.nia.nih.gov

National Institute of Justice: www.ojp.usdoj.gov/nij/topics/crime/elder-abuse/welcome.htm

Chapter 20

American Institute of Stress: www.stress.org

National Center for Complementary and Alternative Medicine at the National Institutes of Health (NCCAM): www.nccam.nih.gov

National Institute for Occupational Safety and Health (NIOSH): www.cdc.gov/niosh

Chapter 21

American Academy of Pediatrics: www.aap.org/disasters

American Association of Suicidology: www.suicidology.org

American Foundation for Suicide Prevention: www.afsp.org

Emergency Mental Health and Traumatic Stress: mentalhealth.samhsa.gov/cmhs/EmergencyServices/after.asp

Federal Emergency Management Agency: www.fema.gov/kids/teacher.htm

International Society for Traumatic Stress Studies: www.istss.org/resources/index.cfm

National Alliance for the Mentally Ill: www.nami.org